Personal Health Reporter

ISSN 1061-4125

Personal Health Reporter

Excerpts from current articles on 148 medical conditions and treatments and other health issues

Alan M. Rees and Charlene Willey, Editors

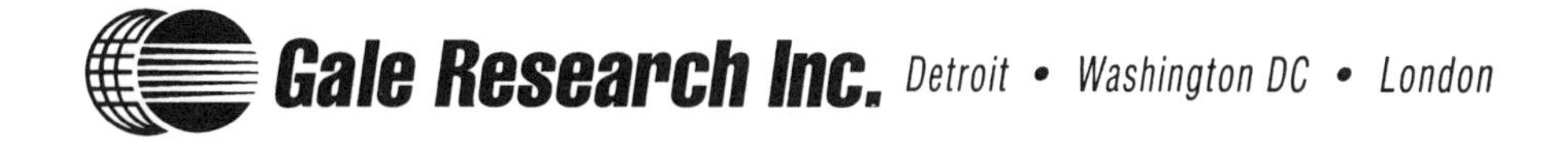

Alan M. Rees, *Editor*
Charlene D. Willey, *Editor*
Connie Fawcett, *Data Entry Associate*

Gale Research Inc. Staff

Lawrence W. Baker, Christine B. Hammes, *Senior Developmental Editors*

Sandra C. Davis, *Text Permissions Supervisor*
Maria L. Franklin, Josephine M. Keene, Michele M. Lonoconus,
Denise M. Singleton, Kimberly F. Smilay, *Permissions Associates*
Brandy C. Johnson, Shelly A. Rakoczy, Shalice Shah, *Permissions Assistants*

Benita L. Spight, *Data Entry Supervisor*
Gwendolyn Tucker, *Data Entry Group Leader*
Beverly Jendrowski, *Data Entry Associate*

Mary Beth Trimper, *Production Director*
Evi Seoud, *Assistant Production Manager*
Shanna Heilveil, *Production Assistant*

Cynthia Baldwin, *Art Director*
Bernadette M. Gornie, *Cover Designer*
Kathleen A. Hourdakis, *Page Designer*

∞™ This book is printed on acid-free paper that meets the minimum requirements of American National Standard for Information Sciences—Permanence Paper for Printed Library Materials, ANSI Z39.48-1984.

ISBN 0-8103-8392-6
ISSN 1061-4125
Printed in the United States of America by Gale Research Inc.
Published simultaneously in the United Kingdom
by Gale Research International Limited
(An affiliated company of Gale Research Inc.)

Table of Contents

Preface

Health ranks high on the American agenda. The pursuit of health is a powerful force in contemporary American society with health care accounting for some fourteen percent of the U.S. gross national product. The Commerce Department anticipates that health care spending will increase an average of twelve to thirteen percent annually over the next five years. Health care has also become an increasingly important political issue. Concerned citizens, physicians, corporations, public officials, economists, and the 37 million Americans without health insurance are calling for sweeping changes in the organization, financing, and delivery of American health care. In many other countries, medical consumers exercise very limited choice with respect to when, where, and how often they receive health care. However, Americans are forced to make intelligent and informed decisions in regard to access, quality, and cost of their personal health care. Unfortunately, in our highly competitive health care marketplace, consumers typically lack the requisite information for such informed decision making. Medical information is often poorly presented and simplified almost to the point of distortion. The weekly announcements in the media of "breakthroughs" result in confusion and false expectations. The American public is forced to seek out and filter reliable and useful information from the conflicting information supplied by journalists, television doctors, hospital marketing specialists, promoters, and public relations advocates.

The essential problem confronting consumers is not the lack of information but rather the confusion produced by the necessity to seek out and reconcile fragmentary information, contradictory claims, and conflicting opinions. Individual decision-making is further complicated by the complexity of the issues and the lack of consensus among the experts. What is the "truth" in relation to such topics as breast implants, the safety of drugs such as Prozac and Halcion, the best means of reducing cholesterol levels, and the use of aspirin in preventing heart attacks? What is the meaning of "reduced fat," "low sodium," and "light" in the nutritional Tower of Babel? Not surprisingly, individuals turn to dial-up experts in the form of Doctors by Phone, Ask A Nurse, and Pharmacy Question—Ask the Pharmacist.

Broad Range of Topics

To provide integrated and orderly access to the vast outpouring of medical information, *Personal Health Reporter (PHR)* assembles extracts of essential, useful, and authoritative information on a variety of topics of concern to consumers, culled from the most current and reliable sources. *PHR* goes beyond the compiling of lists of information sources and avoids overwhelming readers with large amounts of full text. The extracts are carefully selected to provide informative explanation and definition of each topic, the nature and dimensions of the problem, alternative approaches in terms of current treatment, methods of coping, and probable outcome. The extracts selected are derived from professional and popular medical journals, dictionaries, manuals, newsletters, general interest magazines, government reports, pamphlets, medical textbooks, popular medical guides and encyclopedias, and national newspapers. We have attempted to portray the present consensus with regard to treatment modalities. Where no such consensus exists, the selected extracts reveal such differences of opinion.

The subjects in this first edition are arranged alphabetically. *PHR* covers 148 topics in a variety of medical interests, including:

- **Diseases and disorders**
  - Arthritis
  - Diabetes
  - Eating disorders
  - Lyme disease
- **Syndromes**
  - Carpal tunnel syndrome
  - Chronic fatigue syndrome
  - Premenstrual syndrome
  - Sudden infant death syndrome
- **Common medical problems**
  - Constipation
  - Diarrhea
  - Food poisoning
  - Jet lag
- **Health concerns of women**
  - Endometriosis
  - Estrogen replacement therapy
  - Hysterectomy
  - Yeast infections
- **Health problems of children**
  - Attention deficit disorder
  - Colic
  - Measles
- **Mental health**
  - Depression
  - Obsessive compulsive disorder
  - Phobias and panic disorders
  - Schizophrenia
- **Substance abuse**
  - Alcoholism
  - Crack/cocaine
  - Drug abuse
  - Smoking
- **Medical tests and diagnostic methods**
  - CAT scans
  - Magnetic resonance imaging (MRI)
  - Prenatal testing
- **Medical and surgical procedures**
  - Chemotherapy
  - Dilation and curettage (D&C)
  - Liposuction
  - Vasectomy
- **Nutritional topics**
  - Cholesterol
  - Dietary fat
  - Dietary fiber
  - Pesticide residues in foods

- **Alternative medicine**
  - Chiropractic
  - Homeopathy
- **New technology**
  - In vitro fertilization
  - Laser surgery
  - Organ transplants
- **Consumer advocacy**
  - Choosing a physician
  - Hospital mortality rates
  - Medical malpractice
  - Medical records
  - Quackery
- **Cost concerns**
  - Health insurance
  - Health maintenance organizations (HMOs)
  - Medicare
  - Nursing homes

Sources

A number of databases were searched to identify significant content. These include *Medline, Cumulative Index to Nursing and Allied Health Literature, Health Reference Center,* and the *Consumer Health and Nutrition Index.* Extensive searching yielded a large amount of relevant information sources. Extracts offering readable and reliable information were identified and selected from:

- **Professional medical journals**
  - *American Family Physician*
  - *Journal of the American Medical Association (JAMA)*
  - *Lancet*
  - *New England Journal of Medicine*
  - *Patient Care*
- **Specialty journals**
  - *American Journal of Obstetrics and Gynecology*
  - *Journal of Urology*
- **Nursing journals**
  - *Nursing91*
  - *RN*
- **Popular health magazines**
  - *American Health*
  - *FDA Consumer*
  - *In-Health*
  - *Prevention*
- **Health newsletters**
  - *Environmental Nutrition*
  - *Harvard Health Letter*
  - *Health Facts*
  - *Health Letter*
  - *Johns Hopkins Medical Letter*
  - *Mayo Clinic Health Letter*
  - *Tufts University Diet & Nutrition Letter*
  - *University of California Berkeley Wellness Letter*
  - *University of Texas Lifetime Health Letter*

- **Reference and textbooks**
  Mosby's Medical, Nursing and Allied Health Dictionary

- **Encyclopedias and home medical guides**
  AMA Family Medical Guide
  American Medical Association Encyclopedia of Medicine
  Columbia University College of Physicians and Surgeons Home Medical Guide
  Mayo Clinic Family Health Book

- **Pamphlet publications from . . .**
  Government agencies such as the National Cancer Institute
  Pharmaceutical companies
  Professional societies
  Voluntary health associations

- **General interest magazines**
  Insight
  Newsweek
  Time
  U.S. News and World Report

- **National newspapers**
  The New York Times
  Wall Street Journal

- **Government publications**
  National Institutes of Health Consensus Conference reports

Extracts Provide General Overview

Extracts were selected in order to present a balanced view of each topic. Typical headings used to arrange and label extracts are:

- Overview
- Definition of Terms
- Signs and Symptoms
- Detection and Diagnosis
- Staging
- Treatment Methods
- Effectiveness
- Safety
- Risk Factors
- . . . in Children
- . . . in Women
- Outcome Management
- Rehabilitation
- Recovery
- Coping
- Prevention

More detailed and complex topics contain additional headings. Close attention has been paid to identifying information in relation to conflicting points of view and alternative treatment methods for controversial topics such as breast cancer and heart bypass surgery.

Also included under each topic are lists of relevant organizations, support and advocacy groups, books, pamphlets, and related articles.

The 148 topics in this first edition of *Personal Health Reporter* cannot cover all topics of interest to medical consumers. Subsequent editions will contain additional topics and will update previously covered topics with new information as needed.

We believe that *Personal Health Report* brings together diverse sources of authoritative information on a multitude of topics. The information extracted will supply a composite and balanced view that will significantly reduce the need to seek out, obtain, and digest the full text of multiple published sources. Very few libraries can hope to acquire the full range of health informational materials of interest to consumers. Public libraries by definition and mission do not acquire expensive professional medical publication. Conversely, medical libraries in academic medical centers and hospitals do not stock popular health journals, books, magazines, and consumer pamphlets. *Personal Health Reporter* should save considerable library staff time in identifying and reproducing information, while broadening the range of relevant and useful material available to the public in both public library and clinical settings.

Many thanks to Larry Baker, Christine Hammes, Barbara Beach, and John Schmittroth for editorial assistance and encouragement.

Comments and suggestions regarding future editions are welcome and should be addressed to the Editor, Gale Research Inc., 835 Penobscot Bldg., Detroit, MI 48226.

Alan M. Rees and Charlene D. Willey
Cleveland, Ohio
October 1992

Permissions Acknowledgments

The editor wishes to thank the copyright holders of the excerpted articles included in *Personal Health Reporter (PHR),* as well as the permissions managers of many book and magazine publishing companies who assisted in securing reprint rights. The following is a list of the copyright holders who have granted permission to reprint material in this volume of *PHR.* Every effort has been made to trace copyright, but if omissions have been made, please contact the editor.

Copyrighted excerpts in *PHR* were reprinted from the following periodicals:

About Hysterectomy (Surgical Removal of the Uterus), n.d. Reprinted by permission of the American College of Surgeons.—***About Kidney Stones,*** 1988. Reprinted by permission of the National Kidney Foundation.—***Addiction & Recovery,*** June 1990; August 1990. Both reprinted by permission of International Publishing Group.—***Adverse Reactions to Foods: A Patient Guide,*** November 1985. Reprinted by permission of the American Academy of Allergy and Immunology.—***Alpha-Fetoprotein Screening, Public Health Information Sheet,*** January 1991. Reprinted by permission of the March of Dimes Birth Defects Foundation.—***American Baby,*** May 1990. © 1991 by Cahners Publishing Company. Reprinted by permission of the publisher.—***American Family Physician,*** May 1988; December 1988; January 1989; February 1989; March 1989; May 1989; June 1989; November 1989; December 1989; January 1990; February 1990; March 1990; April 1990; May 1990; June 1990; October 1990; November 1990; January 1991; February 1991. All reprinted by permission of *American Family Physician.*—***American Health,*** July-August 1989 for "When Prenatal Tests Bring Bad News: Few Support Services Help Couples Cope" by Magda Krance; April 1990 for "Can You Trust Generic Drugs? In the Wake of Scandal, Here's What You Need To Know" by Caryl S. Avery. *American Health Magazine,* © 1989, 1990. Both reprinted by permission of the respective author. November 1989; March 1990; July/August 1990; September 1990; November 1990; May 1991. *American Health Magazine* © 1989, 1990, 1991 by the respective authors. All reprinted by permission of the publisher.—***The American Journal of Medicine,*** 85(supp 2A): August 29, 1988; 88(supp 6A): June 20, 1990. Both reprinted by permission of the publisher.—***American Journal of Nursing,*** August 1988; December 1990. Both reprinted by permission of the publisher.—***American Medical News,*** April 20, 1990; June 8, 1990; January 21, 1991; May 13, 1991. Copyright 1990, 1991 American Medical Association. All reprinted by permission of *American Medical News.*—***American Review of Respiratory Diseases,*** no. 2, August, 1990. Reprinted by permission of the American Lung Association.—***Anaphylaxia,*** November 1988. Reprinted by permission of the American Academy of Allergy and Immunology.—***Annals of Internal Medicine,*** 108 (3): March 1988. Reprinted by permission of the publisher.—***Answers about AIDS,*** April 1988. Reprinted by permission of the American Council on Science and Health.—***Arthritis: Basic Facts, Answers to Your Questions,*** 1989. Used by permission of the Arthritis Foundation.—***Arthritis Information: Osteoarthritis,*** 1990. Copyright © 1990. Used by permission of the Arthritis Foundation.—***Bestways,*** 17,

December 1989. Reprinted by permission of Bestways, Inc.—***British Medical Journal,*** no. 6710, November 18, 1989; no. 6731, April 21, 1990. Both reprinted by permission of the publisher.—***The Brown University Child Behavior and Development Letter,*** February 1989. Reprinted by permission of Manisses Communications Group, Inc.—***Changing Times Magazine,*** February 1989; April 1991. Copyright © 1989, 1991 by The Kiplinger Washington Editors, Inc. Both reprinted by permission of the publisher.—***Chlamydia Is Not a Flower. It's a Sexually Transmitted Disease with Devastating Effects,*** Abbott Laboratories, 1989.—***Chronic Myelogenous Leukemia,*** 1988. Reprinted by permission of the Leukemia Society of America.—***Circulation,*** 81, no. 5, for "The Cholesterol Facts: A Summary of the Evidence Relating Dietary Fats, Serum Cholesterol, and Coronary Heart Disease. A Joint Statement by the American Heart Association and the National Heart, Lung, and Blood Institute." by the Task Force on Cholesterol Issues. © Copyright 1990 by the American Heart Association. Reproduced with permission of the publisher.—***Clozapine,*** 1990. Reprinted by permission of the National Alliance for the Mentally Ill.—***Cocaine: Facts and Dangers,*** April 1990. Reprinted by permission of the American Council on Science and Health.—***Consultant,*** 31 January, 1991. Reprinted by permission of the publisher.—***Consumer Reports,*** January 1989; August 1990; February 1991. Copyright 1989, 1990, 1991 by Consumers Union of United States, Inc., Yorkers, NY 10703. All excerpted by permission from *Consumer Reports.*—***Consumer Reports Health Letter,*** September 1989; February 1990; June 1990; July 1990; September 1990; October 1990; December 1990; January 1991. Copyright 1989, 1990, 1991 by Consumers Union of United States, Inc., Yonkers, NY 10703. All excerpted by permission from *Consumer Reports Health Letter.*—***Coronary Artery Bypass Graft Surgery,*** no. 50-1027, 1989. © Copyright 1989 by American Heart Association. Reproduced with permission of the publisher.—***Critical Care Medicine,*** 17(12), December 1989. © by Williams & Wilkins, 1989. Reprinted by permission of the publisher.—***CUTIS,*** July 1990. Reprinted by permission of the publisher.—***Diabetes Forecast,*** November 1989; March 1990. Copyright © 1989, 1990 by American Diabetes Association, Inc. Reproduced with permission from *Diabetes Forecast.*—***Diabetes in the News,*** January-February 1991. Reprinted by permission of the publisher.—***Diagnostic Criteria from DSM-III-R,*** 1987. Both reprinted by permission of the publisher.—***Diet and Health: Implications for Reducing Chronic Disease Risk,*** May 1989. © 1989 by the National Academy of Sciences. Reprinted with permission of the National Academy Press, Washington, DC.—***Diabetic Retinopathy,*** November 1990. Reprinted by permission of the National Eye Institute.—***Dialysis,*** 1989. Reprinted by permission of the National Kidney Foundation, Inc.—***Dilation and Curettage (D & C),*** ACOG Patient Education Pamphlet APO62. Washington, DC, 1989. Reprinted by permission of the American College of Obstetricians and Gynecologists.—***DM: Disease-a-month,*** March 1989; April 1990. Both reprinted by permission of Mosby-Yearbook, Inc.—***The Doctor's People Newsletter,*** 2, February 1989.—***Down Syndrome,*** 1988. Reprinted by permission of the National Down Syndrome Congress.—***"E" Is for Exercise,*** no. 51-1023, 1989. © 1989 by American Heart Association. Reproduced with permission of the publisher.—***East West,*** 20, November 1990 for "A Woman's Guide to Birth Control," by Gene Bruce. Reprinted by permission of the author.—***East West Journal,*** November 1989 for "Chiropractic's New Wave: Controversial New Ideas, Tools, and Techniques Are Transforming This Spine-Oriented Therapy" by Nathaniel Mead. Reprinted by permission of the author.—***Employee Health & Fitness,*** 12, no. 6, June 1990. Reprinted by permission of the publisher.—***Environmental Nutrition,*** May 1989; August 1989; August 1990. All reprinted by permission of the publisher.—***Executive Edge,*** 21, no. 7, July 1990.—***Executive Health Report,*** June 1989; February 1990; May 1990, June 1990; October 1990; March 1991. All reprinted with permission of *Executive Health's Good Health Report,* P. O. Box 8880, Chapel Hill, NC 27515.—***Executive Health's Good Health Report,*** 28, no. 5, February 1992. Reprinted by permission of *Executive Health's Good Health Report,* P. O. Box 8880, Chapel Hill, NC 27515.—***Fact Sheet on Heart Attack, Stroke and Risk Factors,*** no. 51-1027, 1987. © Copyright 1987 by American Heart Association. Reproduced by permission of the publisher.—***Facts about Coronary Artery Bypass Surgery,*** NIH Publication No. 87-2891, 1987. Reprinted by permission of the National Heart, Lung, and Blood Institute.—***Facts About Herpes Simplex,*** American Academy of Dermatology, 1987.—***Facts About Muscular Dystrophy,*** May 1990.—***Facts about SIDS,*** July 1989. Reprinted by permission of SIDS Alliance.—***Facts About Stroke,*** 1989. Reprinted by permission of the American Heart Association.—***Family Circle,*** July 24, 1990. Copyright © 1990 The Family Circle, Inc. All rights reserved. Reprinted by permission of *Family Circle Magazine.*—***Fast Food and the American Diet,*** 1985. Reprinted by permission of the American Council on Science and Health.—***Fibrocystic Breast Disease: What Should I Know about It?*** 1987.—***Fluoridation,*** September 1990. Reprinted by permission of the American Council on Science and Health.—***Food Additives and Hyperactivity,*** 1982. Reprinted by permission of the American Council on Science and Health.—***Food and Life: A Nutrition Primer,*** July 1990. Reprinted by permission of the American Council on Science and Health.—***Genetic Counseling,*** December 1987. Reprinted by permission of the March of Dimes Birth Defects Foundation.—***Geriatrics,*** November 1988; August 1989; April 1990. All reprinted by permission of the publisher.—***The Genetics of Cystic Fibrosis,*** Reprinted by permission of the Cystic Fibrosis Foundation.—***Glamour,*** April 1991 for "Endometriosis Update" by Nancy Monson. Reprinted by permission of the author. March, 1991. Copyright © 1991 by The Conde Nast Publications. Reprinted by permission of the publisher.—***Gum Disease:***

Be Tested to See If You Have It, September 1989. Reprinted by permission of the American Academy of Periodontology.—***Harvard Health Letter,*** June 1991. © 1991, President and Fellows of Harvard College. Reprinted by permission of the publisher.—***Harvard Medical School Health Letter,*** January 1989; August 1989; January 1990; May 1990. © 1989, 1990 President and Fellows of Harvard College. Reprinted by permission of the publisher.—***Hay Fever,*** 1986. Reprinted by permission of the American Council on Science and Health.—***Health,*** March 1990; May 1990; October 1990; February 1991; March 1991.—***Health Care and Finances: A Guide for Adult Children and Their Parents,*** December 1987. Reprinted by permission of the American Council of Life Insurance, Health Insurance Association of America.—***Health News,*** October 1988; April 1989; June 1990; October 1990; December 1990; February 1991. All reprinted by permission of *Health News.*—***Health Tips,*** December 1987-January 1988; March 1988; December 1988-January 1989; May 1989; no. 362, June 1989; no. 435, July-August 1989; no. 524, July-August 1989; no. 130, September 1989; no. 72, October 1989; no. WH-53, December 1989-January 1990; no. 345, December 1989-January 1990; no. WH-54, February 1990; March 1990; no. 123, March 1990; no. 445, April 1990; no. 453, April 1990; no. 461, May 1990; no. 108, August 1990; no. 305, November 1990; no. WH-31, March 1991; no. 426, March 1991; no. 490, March 1991; no. 491, March 1991. © 1987, 1988, 1989, 1990, 1991 CMA. All reprinted by permission of the California Medical Association. (HEALTH TIPS is a publication of the California Medical Education and Research Foundation, prepared and edited by physician members of the California Medical Association. HEALTH TIPS are intended to provide general medical information. Differences in individual cases may suggest alternative treatments or services. HEALTH TIPS should not be treated as a substitute for the advice of a physician. Specific questions should be directed to your physician.)—***Health News (University of Toronto),*** April 1988; December 1988; December 1989; August 1990; February 1991; April 1991; June 1991. All reprinted by permission of *Health News.*—***HealthFacts,*** (published by the center for Medical Consumers, 237 Thompson St., New York, NY 10012), April 1988; September 1989; July 1990; August 1990; September 1990; March 1991; April 1991; May 1991. All reprinted by permission of the publisher.—***Healthline,*** July 1990.—***Heartcorps,*** March/April 1989; July/August 1989. July-August 1989 for "All About Balloon Angioplasty" by Albert E. Raizner, M.D. Reprinted by permission of the author.—***Herpes: The Good News Is that It Can Now Be Controlled,*** 1985. Reproduced with permission of the Burroughs Wellcome Co.—***Herpes Zoster (Shingles),*** American Academy of Dermatology, 1988.—***HMOs: Are They Right for You?*** 1991. Reprinted by permission of the American Council on Science and Health.—***Hospital Practice,*** March 30, 1990. Reprinted with permission of the publisher.—***How to Buy a Hearing Aid,*** July 1, 1991. Reprinted with permission by the American Speech Language Hearing Association.—***How to Prevent Sexually Transmitted Diseases,*** ACOG Patient Education Pamphlet APO09, Washington, DC, 1991. Reprinted by permission of The American College of Obstetricians and Gynecologists.—***Important Facts About Endometriosis,*** ACOG Patient Education Pamphlet APO13. Washington, DC, 1983. Reprinted by permission of the American College of Obstetricians and Gynecologists.—***In Health,*** July/August 1990. Copyright © 1990. Excerpted from *In Health.*—***Independent Living,*** 5. Aug./Sept. 1990. Reprinted by permission of the publisher.—***Information about Insulin,*** December 1990. Reprinted by permission of Juvenile Diabetes Foundation International/The Diabetes Research Foundation.—***IVF & GIFT: A Patient's Guide to Assisted Reproductive Technology,*** Reprinted by permission of the American Fertility Society.—***JAMA,*** Feb. 13, 1987; March 20, 1987; April 8, 1988; May 13, 1988; January 27, 1989; March 3, 1989; April 14, 1989; June 9, 1989; July 28, 1989; March 23/30, 1990; June 20, 1990; December 12, 1990. Copyright © 1987, 1988, 1989, 1990 American Medical Association. All reprinted by permission of the publisher.—***The Johns Hopkins Medical Letter: Health After 50,*** September 1989; October 1990; November 1990; December 1990; February 1991; March 1991; April 1991. © Medletter Associates, 1989, 1990, 1991. Excerpted from the *Johns Hopkins Medical Letter: Health After 50.*—***The Journal of Family Practice,*** 30, no. 2, 1990 for "The Risks and Benefits of Exercise During Pregnancy" by Robert W. Jarski and Diane L. Trippett. Copyright © 1990. Reprinted by permission of Appleton & Lange, Inc. and Robert W. Jarski.—***Journal of the American Geriatrics Society,*** August 1989. Reprinted by permission of the American Geriatric Society.—***Ladies' Home Journal,*** February 1991. © Copyright 1991, Meredith Corporation. All rights reserved. Reprinted from *Ladies' Home Journal* Magazine.—***Lancet,*** August 30, 1986; September 30, 1989; May 5, 1990. Reprinted by permission of the publisher.—***Life With Diabetes: Diabetes Defined,*** 1987. Reprinted by permission of the Michigan Diabetes Research and Training Center.—***Living with Your Pacemaker,*** no. 50-1003, 1986. © Copyright 1986 by American Heart Association. Reproduced with permission of the publisher.—***Longevity,*** December 1989/January 1990 for "Beams of Life" by Morton Hunt. Reprinted by permission of Georges Borchardt, Inc. on behalf of the author. October 1990 for "Don't Let Stress Number Your Days" by Gurney Williams III. © 1990, Longevity International, Ltd. Reprinted by permission of the publisher. February 1990.—***Macular Degeneration: Major Cause of Central Vision Loss,*** Reviewed 1990. Reprinted by permission of the American Academy of Ophthalmology.—***Manage,*** March 1990. Reprinted by permission of the National Management Association.—***Mayo Clinic Health Letter,*** March 1990; September 1990; November 1990; December 1990; February 1991; May 1991. All reprinted by permission of the publisher.—***Mayo Clinic Proceedings,*** 65, no. 2, February 1990; 65, no.

6, June 1990. Both reprinted by permission of the publisher.—***McCall's,*** October 1990. Copyright © 1990 by *McCall's Magazine.* Reprinted by permission of the publisher.—***Medical Aspects of Human Sexuality,*** February 1991; February 1991. Both reprinted by permission of the publisher.—***Medical Clinics of North America,*** January 1989. Reprinted by permission of W. B. Saunders Co.—***Medical Selfcare,*** March/April 1989; November/December 1989. Both reprinted by permission of Island Publishing Company, Inc.—***Medical Update,*** May 1989; December 1990; February 1991; March 1991. Copyright © 1989, 1990, 1991 Medical Education and Research Foundation. All rights reserved. All reprinted by permission of Medical Education and Research Foundation, P. O. Box 567, Indianapolis, IN 46206.—***Medical World News,*** February 27, 1989; March 27, 1989; February 12, 1990; July, 1990. All reprinted by permission of the publisher.—***Melanoma/Skin Cancer: You Can Recognize the Signs,*** American Academy of Dermatology, 1989.—***Men's Health,*** 5 October, 1990. Copyright 1990 Rodale Press, Inc. All rights reserved. Reprinted by permission of *Men's Health Magazine.*—***The Menopause Time of Life,*** NIH Pub. No. 86-2461, July 1986, National Institute on Aging.—***Mood Disorders: Depression and Manic Depression,*** n.d. Reprinted by permission of the National Alliance for the Mentally Ill.—***Mothering,*** v. 56, Summer 1990 for "Drugs and Breastmilk" by L.S. Moses II. Excerpted with permission from *Mothering* and the author.—***NCAHF Newsletter,*** July/August 1989; September/October 1990. Both reprinted by permission of the publisher.—***NCI Cancer Weekly,*** (Currently entitled *Cancer Weekly*), December 24, 1990. Reprinted by permission of *Cancer Weekly.*—***Network News,*** January-February 1990.—***The New England Journal of Medicine,*** January 21, 1988; March 31, 1988; June 2, 1988; January 5, 1989; March 2, 1989; March 9, 1989; November 30, 1989; January 18, 1990; January 25, 1990; June 7, 1990; April 25, 1991. Copyright © 1988, 1989, 1990, 1991 by the Massachusetts Medical Society. All reprinted by permission of the publisher.—***New Techniques for Treating Kidney Stones: Extracorporeal Shock Wave Lithotripsy,*** 1987. Reprinted by permission of the National Kidney Foundation.—***The New York Times,*** February 14, 1989; March 2, 1989; August 3, 1989; December 12, 1989; December 28, 1989; March 6, 1990; September 5, 1990; October 11, 1990; October 13, 1990; October 25, 1990; November 9, 1990; November 13, 1990; December 4, 1990; December 10, 1990; February 7, 1991; February 8, 1991; February 20, 1991; March 7, 1991; April 11, 1991; April 23, 1991; April 25, 1991; April 28, 1991; June 30, 1991; July 10, 1991; August 9, 1991. Copyright © 1989, 1990, 1991 by The New York Times Company. All reprinted by permission.—***New York Times National,*** September 5, 1990. Copyright © 1990 by The New York Times Company. Reprinted by permission.—***The Newsletter For People With Lactose Intolerance And Milk Allergy,*** n.d. Reprinted by permission of the publisher.—***Newsweek,*** December 18, 1989; November 12, 1990; December 3, 1990; July 15, 1991. © 1989, 1990, 1991, Newsweek, Inc. All rights reserved. All reprinted by permission of the publisher.—***Nonsteroidal Anti-Inflammatory Drugs (NSAID) and Ulcers,*** 1989. Copyright © 1989. Used by permission of the Arthritis Foundation.—***Nonsteroidal Anti-Inflammatory Drugs (NSAIDs): Questions and Answers,*** 1990. Copyright © 1990. Used by permission of the Arthritis Foundation.—***Nursing 89,*** June 1989. Reprinted by permission of the publisher.—***Nutrition Forum,*** 6 January/February, 1989. Reprinted by permission of the publisher.—***Nutrition Reviews,*** 47, no. 5, May 1989 for "National Academy of Sciences Report on Diet and Health" by the Interdisciplinary Committee on Diet and Health. Reprinted by permission of Springer-Verlag Publishers.—***Nutrition Today,*** June 1989 for "An Overview of the Eating Disorders Anorexia Nervosa and Bulimia Nervosa" by D. B. Woodside and P. E. Garfinkel; September-October 1989 for "Morbid Obesity: Weighing the Treatment Options" by Armour Forse, Peter N. Benotti and George Blackburn. © by Williams & Wilkins, 1989. Both reprinted by permission of the publisher and the respective authors. February 1989. © by Williams & Wilkins, 1989. Reprinted by permission of the publisher.—***Obstetrics and Gynecology,*** 72, no. 1, July 1988. Reprinted with permission from The American College of Obstetricians and Gynecologists.—***Panic Disorder,*** n.d. Reprinted by permission of the National Alliance for the Mentally Ill.—***Parents,*** March 1989 for "What Are Uterine Fibroids?" by Paula Adams Hillard. Reprinted by permission of the author.—***Parents' Magazine,*** 64, July 1989 for "The Earliest Prenatal Test" by Paula Adams Hillard; 66, March 1991 for "All about Allergies" by Stephen Perrine. Both reprinted by permission of the respective author.—***Parents Pediatric Report,*** 7(4), April 1990.—***The Parkinson Handbook: A Guide for Parkinson Patients and Their Families,*** n.d. National Parkinson Foundation.—***Patient Care,*** September 30, 1987; April 15, 1988; May 15, 1988; August 15, 1988; February 28, 1989; August 15, 1989; November 30, 1989; August 15, 1990; June 15, 1991. 1987, 1988, 1989, 1990, 1991. Copyright, © Medical Economics Publishing, a division of Medical Economics Co., Inc., Montvale, N.J., 07645. All rights reserved. All reproduced with permission.—***Pediatric Clinics of North America,*** June 1990. Reprinted by permission of W. B. Saunders Co.—***Pediatrics,*** June 1987; August 1989; September 1989; January 1990. Copyright © 1987, 1989, 1990. All reproduced by permission of *Pediatrics.*—***Pediatrics for Parents,*** January 1988; May 1988; May 1989; August 1989; September 1989. All reprinted by permission of the publisher.—***People's Medical Society Health Letter,*** July 1991.—***Peoples's Medical Society Newsletter,*** December 1989; June 1990. Both reprinted by permission of the People's Medical Society.—***Pesticides and Food Safety,*** June 1989. Reprinted by permission of the American Council on Science and Health.—***Plain Talk About Depression,*** DHHS Pub. No. (ADM) 89-1639, 1989. Reprinted by permission of the National Institute of Mental Health, Office of Scientific Information.—

Plain Talk about Handling Stress, DHHS Pub. No. (ADM) 85-502, 1985. Reprinted by permission of the National Institute of Mental Health.—***Poison Ivy,*** American Academy of Dermatology, 1990.—***Position Paper on Chiropractic,*** 1985. Reprinted by permission of the National Council Against Health Fraud, Inc.—***Premenstrual Syndrome,*** ACOG Patient Education Pamphlet APO57, Washington, DC, 1985. Reprinted by permission of the American College of Obstetricians and Gynecologists.—***Preventing Epilepsy,*** 1983. Reprinted by permission of the Epilepsy Foundation of America.—***Prevention,*** May 1988; February, 1991. Copyright 1991, Rodale Press, Inc. All rights reserved. Reprinted by permission of *Prevention.*—***Priorities,*** Summer 1989; Winter 1990; Spring 1990.—***Progress Report on Alzheimer's Disease,*** National Institute on Aging, 1990. ***Psoriasis,*** American Academy of Dermatology, 1987.—***The Public Citizen Health Research Group Letter,*** December 1990; February 1991; March 1991; May 1991; August 1991.—***Public Health Reports,*** October 30, 1987 for "Proceedings of the National Conference on Women's Health. Series: Special Topic Conference on Women's Health" by the National Conference on Women's Health; September/October 1989 for "Supplement 2-4" by the National Conference on Women's Health. Both reprinted by permission of the publisher.—***Public Health Reports Supplement,*** September/October 1988. Reprinted by permission of the publisher.—***Questions and Answers about Epilepsy,*** 1985. Reprinted by permission of the Epilepsy Foundation of America.—***Reader's Digest,*** April 1990. Excerpted with permission from *Reader's Digest,* 1989 for "Heart Failure" by Thomas J. Moore. Copyright © 1989 *Reader's Digest.* Reprinted by permission of *Reader's Digest* and Random House, Inc. 1989 for "Balanced Nutrition: Beyond the Cholesterol Scare" by Frederick Stare, Robert Olson and Elizabeth Whelan. © 1989. Reprinted by permission of *Reader's Digest* and Bob Adams, Inc.—***Redbook,*** September 1990; February 1991. Copyright © 1990, 1991 by The Hearst Corporation. All rights reserved. Both reprinted by permission of Redbook Magazine.—***The Responsible Use of Alcohol: Defining the Parameters of Moderation,*** January 1991. Reprinted by permission of the American Council on Science and Health.—***RN,*** October 1989; December 1989; December 1990. All excerpted by permission of Medical Economics Publishing/RN.—***Schizophrenia: Questions and Answers,*** DHHS Pub. No. (ADM) 86-1457, 1986. Reprinted by permission of the National Institute of Mental Health.—***Science News,*** June 3, 1989; July 22, 1989; November 11, 1989; March 2, 1991. Copyright 1989, 1991 by Science Services, Inc. All reprinted by permission from *Science News.*—***Searching for a Way Out: Smoking Cessation Techniques,*** March 1985. Reprinted by permission of the American Council on Science and Health.—***Self,*** September 1990 for "Herpes Update: Safe Sex Hasn't Slowed the Spread of This Virus, But Treatments Are on the Horizon" by Annette Spence. Reprinted by permission of the author.—***Sickle Cell Anemia, Public Health Education Information Sheet,*** Genetic Series, February 1989. Reprinted by permission of the March of Dimes Birth Defects Foundation.—***Sleep Apnea,*** July 1989. Reprinted by permission of the American Lung Association.—***So You Have High Blood Cholesterol,*** June 1989. Reprinted by permission of the National Heart, Lung, and Blood Institute.—***Survey of Ophthalmology,*** 32, no. 6, May-June 1988 for "Age-Related Macular Degeneration" by Neil M. Bressler, Susan B. Bressler and Stuart L. Fine. Reprinted by permission of the authors.—***Time,*** October 1, 1990; November 5, 1990; December 24, 1990; July 8, 1991; July 15, 1991. Copyright 1990, 1991 The Time Inc. Magazine Company. All reprinted by permission of the publisher.—***Total Health,*** February 1990 for "Sports Injuries Are Preventable" by Rick McGuire. Copyright © 1990 Trio Publications. Reprinted by permission of the publisher.—***Tufts University Diet and Nutrition Letter,*** February 1988; August 1988; December 1988; October 1989; April 1990; August 1990. All reprinted by permission of the publisher.—***U.S. News & World Report,*** July 25, 1988; April 3, 1989; July 24, 1989; April 2, 1990; April 30, 1990. Copyright, 1988, 1989, 1990, *U.S. News & World Report.* Reprinted by permission of the publisher.—*Understanding Allergy,* 1986. Reprinted by permission of the National Jewish Center for Immunology and Respiratory Medicine.—***Understanding and Living with Glaucoma: A Reference Guide for Patients and Their Families,*** 1990. Reprinted by permission of the Foundation for Glaucoma Research.—***Understanding Angina,*** no. 50-1031, 1991. © Copyright 1991 by American Heart Association. Reproduced with permission of the publisher.—***Understanding Asthma,*** 1985. Reprinted by permission of the National Jewish Center for Immunology and Respiratory Medicine.—***Understanding Immunology,*** 1985. Reprinted by permission of the National Jewish Center for Immunology and Respiratory Medicine.—***The University of California, Berkeley Wellness Letter,*** January 1989; December 1989; March 1990; May 1990; November 1990; March 1991; May 1991. © Health Letter Associates, 1989, 1990, 1991. Reprinted by permission of the publisher.—***University of Texas Lifetime Health Letter,*** September 1989; May 1990; June 1990; September 1990; October 1990; November 1990; January 1991; February 1991; July 1991. All reprinted with permission from the *University of Texas Lifetime Health Letter,* Houston.—***University of Toronto Faculty of Medicine Health News,*** April 1990; October 1990; April 1991; June 1991. All reprinted by permission of *Health News.*—***University of Toronto Health News,*** April 1990. Reprinted by permission of *Health News.*—***Urinary Tract Infections,*** ACOG Patient Education Pamphlet APO50, Washington, DC, 1984. Reprinted by permission of the American College of Obstetricians and Gynecologists.—***Urologic Clinics of North America,*** August 1987 for "Vasovasostomy" by E. S. Yarbro and S. S. Howards; November 1989 for "Early Detection of Prostrate Cancer" by P. T. Scardino. Both reprinted by permission of W. B. Saunders Company.—***Urticaria-Hives,*** American

Academy of Dermatology, 1987.—***Useful Information on Alzheimer's Disease,*** DHHS Pub. No. (ADM) 90-1696, 1990. Reprinted by permission of the National Institute of Mental Health.—***Useful Information on Anorexia Nervosa & Bulimia,*** DHHS Pub. No. (ADM) 87-1514, 1987. Reprinted by permission of the National Institute of Mental Health.—***Useful Information On . . . Sleep Disorders,*** DHHS Pub. No. (ADM) 87-1541, 1987. Reprinted by permission of the National Institute of Mental Health.—***Useful Information on Paranoia,*** 1989. Reprinted by permission of the National Institute of Mental Health.—***Useful Information on Phobias and Panic,*** DHHS Pub. No. (ADM) 89-1472, 1989. Reprinted by permission of the National Institute of Mental Health.—***Vaginitis: Causes and Treatments,*** ACOG Patient Education Pamphlet APO28, Washington, DC, 1984. Reprinted by permission of the American College of Obstetricians and Gynecologists.—***Vibrant Life,*** March-April 1990 for "Your Menstrual Period: As Unique As You Are" by Janet E. Shepherd. Reprinted by permission of the publisher and the author.—***Viral Hepatitis: Everybody's Problem?*** Reprinted by permission of the American Liver Foundation.—***Weight Watchers Women's Health and Fitness News,*** October 1990; December 1990. Copyright © 1990 *Weight Watchers Magazine.* Reprinted by permission of the publisher.—***What is Multiple Sclerosis?*** 1988. Reprinted by permission of the National Multiple Sclerosis Society.—***What You Should Know about P.T.C.A.,*** no. 70,-064A, 1985. © 1985 by American Heart Association. Reproduced by permission of the publisher.—***When You Need an Operation: About Cataract Surgery in Adults,*** n.d. Reprinted by permission of the American College of Surgeons.—***Working Woman,*** 15, January, 1990. Copyright © 1990 by WWT Partnership. Reprinted with permission from *Working Woman* magazine.

Copyrighted excerpts in *PHR* were excerpted from the following books:

American Medical Association. From ***The American Medical Association Encyclopedia of Medicine.*** American Medical Association, 1989. Copyright © 1989 by Dorling Kindersley Ltd. and the American Medical Association. Reprinted by permission of Random House, Inc.—American Psychiatric Association. From ***Let's Talk Facts About Depression.*** American Psychiatric Association, 1988. Reprinted by permission of the publisher.—Annas, George J. From "Informed Consent," in ***The Rights of Patients.*** Second edition. Southern Illinois University Press, 1990. Reprinted by permission of the publisher.—Bausell, R. Barker, Michael A. Rooney, and Charles B. Inlander. From ***How to Evaluate and Select a Nursing Home.*** Addison-Wesley, 1988. © 1988, with People's Medical Society. Reprinted with permission of Addison-Wesley Publishing Company.—Bender, Stephanie DeGraff, and Kathleen Kelleher. From ***PMS: A Positive Program to Gain Control.*** The Body Press, 1986.—Bennett, William I., and others. From ***Your Good Health: How to Stay Well, and What to do When You're Not.*** Edited by William I. Bennett, and others. Copyright © 1987 by the President and Fellows of Harvard College. Reprinted by permission of the publisher.—Bigger, J. Thomas, Jr. From "Angina," in ***The Columbia University College of Physicians & Surgeons Complete Home Medical Guide.*** 2nd edition. Crown Publishers, 1989. Reprinted by permission of the publisher.—Clayman, Charles B. From ***The American Medical Association Family Medical Guide.*** Edited by Charles B. Clayman. Copyright © 1982 by The American Medical Association. Reprinted by permission of Random House, Inc.—Glanze, Walter D., Kenneth N. Anderson, and Lois E. Anderson. From ***Mosby's Medical, Nursing, & Allied Health Dictionary.*** 3rd edition. Mosby, 1990.—Horowitz, Lawrence C. From ***Taking Charge of Your Medical Fate.*** Ballantine, 1990. Reprinted by permission of Random House, Inc.—Landers, Daniel V. From "The Treatment of Vaginitis: Trichomonas, Yeast, and Bacterial Vaginosis," in ***Clinical Obstetrics and Gynecology.*** J. B. Lippincott Company, 1988.—Larson, David, M.D. (ed.) From ***The Mayo Clinic Family Health Book.*** Copyright © 1990 by the Mayo Foundation for Medical Education and Research. Reprinted by permission of the Mayo Foundation for Medical Education and Research, and William Morrow & Company, Inc., Publishers, New York.—Love, Susan. From ***Dr. Susan Love's Breast Book.*** Addison-Wesley, 1990. © 1990, 1991 by Susan M. Love, M.D. Reprinted with permission of Addison-Wesley Publishing Company.—Richardson, Sarah. From ***Homeopathy: The Illustrated Guide.*** Harmony Books, 1988. Reprinted by permission of the publisher.—Rothman, David J., and Donald F. Tapley. From "Evidence of Patients' Wishes," in ***The Columbia University College of Physicians and Surgeons Complete Home Medical Guide.*** Second edition. Crown Publishers, 1989. Reprinted by permission of the publisher.—Schroeder, Steven A., and others. From ***Current Medical Diagnosis & Treatment 1991.*** Appleton & Lange, 1991. Reprinted by permission of the publisher.—Sobel, David M., and Tom Ferguson. From "CT Scan—Body," in ***The People's Book of Medical Tests.*** Simon & Schuster, 1985. Copyright © 1985 by David M. Sobel, M.D. and Tom Ferguson, M.D. Reprinted by permission of Summit Books, a division of Simon & Schuster, Inc.—Stern, Jeffrey L. From ***Everyone's Guide to Cancer Therapy.*** Andrews and McMeel, 1991. Reprinted by permission of Andrews and McMeel. In Canada by Somerville House Books Ltd.—Stewart, Felicia, M.D. From ***Understanding Your Body.*** Bantam Books, 1987. Copyright © 1987 by Felicia Stewart, M.D., Felicia Guest, Gary Stewart, M.D., and Robert Hatcher, M.D. Used by permission of Bantam Books, a division of Bantam Doubleday Dell Publishing Group, Inc.—Utian, Wulf H., and Ruth S. Jacobowitz. From ***Managing Your***

Personal Health Reporter

ACNE

OVERVIEW

Technically called acne vulgaris, this skin disease affects millions of Americans annually. It can vary from quite mild to extremely severe. About 80 percent of all teenagers develop acne, but the disease may also start as late as age 25 or 30, particularly in women.

No one knows for sure exactly what causes acne, or why it usually begins in adolescence. But a number of factors, most importantly heredity, play a role. If one of your parents had acne, there's a good chance you will, too. If both had it, "the gun is pointed directly at you," says FDA dermatologist Carnot Evans, M.D.

Acne develops when the sebaceous glands and the lining of the skin duct begin to work overtime, as they do in adolescence. The glands produce more sebum, making the skin more oily. Normally the lining of the duct sheds cells that are carried to the surface of the skin by the sebum.

When the duct is blocked, cells and sebum accumulate, forming a plug (comedo). If the plug stays below the surface of the skin, it is called a "closed" comedo or whitehead. If the plug enlarges and pops out of the duct, it is called an "open" comedo or blackhead because the top is dark. This is not dirt and will not wash away. The discoloration is due to a buildup of melanin, the dark pigment in the skin.

Pilosebaceous [related to a hair follicle and its oil gland] units are found all over the body, but there are more on the face, upper chest, and back, which explains why acne usually occurs in these places.

There are two main types of acne: non-inflammatory and inflammatory. In non-inflammatory acne, there are usually just a few whiteheads and blackheads on the face. A relatively mild type of acne, it can be treated effectively with nonprescription medicines, or, in the case of blackheads, with the prescription drug Retin-A. The majority of people with acne have this type.

With inflammatory acne, the whiteheads become inflamed, and pimples and pustules develop. In its most severe form, inflammatory acne can cause disfiguring cysts and deep, pitting scars of the face, neck, back, chest, and groin. Prescription drugs and sometimes surgery are needed to treat inflammatory acne.

SOURCE:
Snider, Sharon. "Acne: Taming That Age-Old Adolescent Affliction." *FDA Consumer* (October 1990): 17.

COMEDONES (BLACKHEADS)

Mild acne is marked by a predominance of comedones. In addition to comedones, moderate acne is characterized by a limited number of papules and pustules with some erythema. Severe acne consists predominantly of nodules (cysts), although comedones, papules, and pustules are also present. The goals of treatment are to decrease sebum output, reduce and prevent comedones, and control bacterial proliferation.

SOURCE:
Pochi, Peter E., Alan R. Shalita, and David A. Whiting. "An Update on Acne Management." *Patient Care* 23 (February 28, 1989): 85.

MILD ACNE

What can you do to clear up mild acne?

[FDA dermatologist Carnot] Evans suggests the following:

- Get a nonprescription acne medicine and apply regularly. Over-the-counter drugs containing sulfur, resorcinol, salicylic acid, and benzoyl peroxide are all effective for treating mild acne.
- Use ordinary hygiene on affected areas, washing your face once or twice daily with your usual soap or cleanser. Deodorant soaps may be used, but they are of no particular value for acne.
- Avoid any food or drink you know is a trigger.

If these measures don't work, Evans advises, see a dermatologist.

While it might be tempting to pick at pimples and squeeze blackheads, this can injure the skin and underlying tissues. Doctors advise patients not to pick pimples. Medical instruments called comedo extractors are used to remove blackheads. Some doctors may suggest that their patients use such an instrument themselves. Other doctors would rather remove the blackheads in their office or clinic because of a risk of scarring.

SOURCE:
Snider, Sharon. "Acne: Taming That Age-Old Adolescent Affliction." *FDA Consumer* (October 1990): 18–19.

USE OF TRETINOIN (RETIN-A)

Topical tretinoin is a highly effective comedolytic agent that limits abnormal follicular keratinization and reduces the number of comedones. General guidelines for choosing a topical formulation call for a

- Gel for oily or combination skin (patches of oily and dry skin)
- Cream for dry, sensitive skin
- Liquid for patients who fail to respond to a gel or cream

Some experts recommend using the cream in winter and the gel in summer. Many patients cannot tolerate the liquid, which is the most irritating form of this drug.

Start tretinoin therapy cautiously; redness, peeling, and itching often occur before the patient's skin adjusts to the medication. Initiate therapy with 0.01% of the gel or 0.025% of the cream. Instruct the patient to rub the medication into the affected areas of the face every second or third night about one-half hour after washing and thoroughly drying the skin. Tell him or her to apply the medication about one-half hour before retiring. This therapy "window" renders the skin less sensitive to irritation from the medication and allows time for it to be absorbed, preventing its rubbing off on the pillow during sleep. Caution the patient to avoid applying any medication on hypersensitive areas, such as around the eyes, near the nostrils, or in the corners of the mouth.

The patient should be told that in about a third of cases, acne worsens during the first 3-4 weeks of therapy, with transient outbreaks of pustules, but that treatment should continue. The outbreak is self-limited in most patients, and therapeutic benefits become visible in approximately 2 months.

If the patient does not respond to the medication after a six-week trial, gradually increase the concentration to 0.025% of the gel or 0.05–0.1% of the cream, applied nightly. Consider a trial of 0.05% tretinoin liquid in patients who fail to respond to maximum concentrations of the gel or cream. Prior therapy with other forms of tretinoin may contribute to tolerance of tretinoin liquid.

Because tretinoin causes photosensitivity, advise the patient to avoid direct sun exposure during the middle of the day, if possible. As a precaution, recommend a noncomedogenic sun block of SPF 15 or higher, as well as wearing a hat during unavoidable exposure to the sun.

If the clinical response is unsatisfactory or the patient has papules or pustules in addition to comedones, prescribe benzoyl peroxide as a supplement to tretinoin. Benzoyl peroxide is a potent antibacterial agent: daily application produces significant reduction in the follicular population of Propionibacterium acnes. Some patients may be unable to tolerate this combined regimen, however, if the drugs are started concomitantly. As a precaution, begin therapy with one drug for 1-2 weeks and then add the second, or instruct the patient to use the drugs on alternate days.

SOURCE:
Pochi, Peter E., Alan R. Shalita, and David A. Whiting. "An Update on Acne Management." *Patient Care* 23 (February 28, 1989): 86.

USE OF ISOTRETINOIN (ACCUTANE)

For very severe, disfiguring acne unresponsive to the treatments mentioned, the doctor may prescribe isotretinoin, commonly known as Accutane. Also a vitamin A derivative, Accutane is taken orally in capsule form. It is highly effective for treating severe cystic acne and preventing the deep pits and scars that result.

Scientists do not know exactly how Accutane works, but evidence suggests that it reduces the size of the sebaceous gland and the amount of sebum secreted. In any case, it completely clears up the disease in many people.

Women should use Accutane with extreme caution, however, because it can cause miscarriage and birth defects. If a woman becomes pregnant while taking the drug, there is a great possibility that the baby will be born deformed. Therefore, Accutane's use is tightly regulated by the FDA. Doctors may only prescribe it for a woman who has had a negative pregnancy test and does not intend to become pregnant while taking it, and who has signed a consent form that she has been duly informed of its side effects.

In addition to the danger of fetal malformation and miscarriage, there are a number of minor side effects associated with Accutane. Ninety percent of those who take the drug experience inflammation of the lips (and less frequently of the eyes), and 80 percent experience drying of the skin, nose or mouth.

SOURCE:

Snider, Sharon. "Acne: Taming That Age-Old Adolescent Affliction." *FDA Consumer* (October 1990): 19.

DANGERS OF ISOTRETINOIN (ACCUTANE)

As of now, there are a total of 79 serious Accutane birth defects reported in the U.S. (through 1989 but not all 1989 data is in yet). Because there is well-documented underreporting of adverse drug reactions, it is likely that at least three times more have actually occurred than have been reported. Thus, we estimate about 237 serious Accutane syndrome birth defects have occurred in the United States alone. This is clearly the worst epidemic of preventable serious birth defects we have ever seen in the United States. Equally tragic are the several thousand women who have had induced abortions because they found they were pregnant when they started Accutane or became pregnant while taking the drug and were understandably frightened of the 25 percent risk of a seriously deformed child if they carried the pregnancy to term. In these women, the fear of having a baby with an Accutane-caused birth defect in effect coerced them into deciding to have an abortion.

Gross overprescribing continues because of the inadequacy of various "voluntary" industry measures (such as doctor education) taken, short of severely restricting the distribution of the drug.

SOURCE:

"Accutane." *People's Medical Society Health Letter* (July 1990): 9–10.

USE OF ANTIBIOTICS

Consider adding oral antibiotics to the regimen in patients with:

- Acne that does not respond well to topical therapy
- No tolerance for topical medication
- Extrafacial acne—the back, shoulders, and chest, for example, where topical medications are less effective.

Whenever feasible, the patient taking an oral antibiotic should use topical therapy concomitantly. This may reduce the amount of oral antibiotic required and, possibly, all need for it. In addition, some experts recommend that patients with extrafacial acne scrub affected areas of the body with povidone/iodine (Betadine) each evening in the shower, using a long-handled brush. Applying benzoyl peroxide to trouble spots expedites healing of lesions. A spouse or parent can help apply the medication on the patient's back.

Tetracycline is the antibiotic of choice because of its safety, efficacy, and low cost. Start therapy with 500 mg bid, either one hour before or two hours after meals, to maximize absorption. Continue this dosage for 1-2 months. If treatment is effective, gradually reduce the daily dosage by 250 mg every 6 weeks, with the expectation that the patient might be managed with topical therapy alone. Caution the patient to avoid excessive exposure to sunlight while on tetracycline or to use a sunblock of SPF 15 or higher when outdoors. Ask female patients to inform you if symptoms of vaginal candidiasis occur while taking tetracycline or another antibiotic, so that you can prescribe concomitant treatment for the infection. Keep in mind, however, that oral contraceptives are diminished in efficacy while a woman is taking tetracycline and that another form of birth control is indicated. This antibiotic is also not advisable during pregnancy. Animal studies show that tetracycline crosses the placenta and can have toxic effects on the developing fetus. The drug also can cause permanent discoloration of the teeth if it is taken during the second half of pregnancy.

If the patient does not respond to tetracycline therapy after an eight-week trial or cannot tolerate the drug, or when tetracycline is contraindicated, prescribe oral erythromycin, 250–300 mg bid or tid. An advantage of erythromycin is that it can be taken with meals, which most patients find more convenient.

Minocycline (Minocin) is an excellent alternative for patients who fail to respond satisfactorily to either tetracycline or erythromycin. This antibiotic achieves a high intrafollicular concentration and has a more prolonged effect than does tetracycline. A 200 mg dose of minocycline given daily is equivalent to about 1,500 mg of tetracycline. The drawbacks to minocycline are its higher cost than generic tetracycline or erythromycin and the higher incidence of vestibular toxicity.

SOURCE:

Pochi, Peter E., Alan R. Shalita, and David A. Whiting. "An Update on Acne Management." *Patient Care* 23 (February 28, 1989): 85-95.

RESOURCES

ORGANIZATIONS

American Academy of Dermatology. P.O. Box 1601, Evanston, IL 60204-1601.

American Dermatological Association. 1900 Randolph Road, Suite 174, Charlotte, NC 28207.

RELATED ARTICLES

"Acne Drug Causes Birth Defects." *Brown University Child Behavior and Development Letter* (September 1990): 5.

"Acne Pointers." *Parents' Pediatric Report* (December 1989): 78–79.

Feuerstein, Phyllis. "Acne: Yes, There's Help." *Current Health* (February 2, 1989): 10–11.

Husten, Larry. "A New Look at Acne: Clearing Up Myths." *Weight Watchers Women's Health and Fitness News* (September 1989): 5–6.

Marwick, Charles. "Additional Steps Proposed to Ensure Antiacne Drug Used Only in Appropriate Patient Population." *JAMA* 263, no. 23 (June 20, 1990): 3125–3126.

ACQUIRED IMMUNE DEFICIENCY SYNDROME (AIDS)

(*See also:* IMMUNE SYSTEM AND AUTOIMMUNE DISEASES)

OVERVIEW

The letters A-I-D-S stand for Acquired Immune Deficiency Syndrome. When a person is sick with AIDS, he/she is in the final stages of a series of health problems caused by a virus (germ) that can be passed from one person to another chiefly during sexual contact or through the sharing of intravenous drug needles and syringes used for "shooting" drugs. Scientists have named the AIDS virus "HIV or HTLV-III or LAV." These abbreviations stand for information denoting a virus that attacks white blood cells (T-Lymphocytes) in the human blood. Throughout this [article], we will call the virus the "AIDS virus." The AIDS virus attacks a person's immune system and damages his/her ability to fight other disease. Without a functioning immune system to ward off other germs, he/she now becomes vulnerable to becoming infected by bacteria, protozoa, fungi, and other viruses and malignancies, which may cause life-threatening illness, such as pneumonia, meningitis, and cancer.

These are different names given to AIDS virus by the scientific community: HIV-Human Immunodeficiency Virus; HTLV-III-Human T-Lymphotropic Virus Type III; LAV Lymphadenopathy Associated Virus.

There is presently no cure for AIDS. There is presently no vaccine to prevent AIDS.

When the AIDS virus enters the blood stream, it begins to attack certain white blood cells (T-Lymphocytes). Substances called antibodies are produced by the body. These antibodies can be detected in the blood by a simple test, usually two weeks to three months after infection. Even before the antibody test is positive, the victim can pass the virus to others by methods that will be explained.

Once an individual is infected, there are several possibilities. Some people may remain well but even so they are able to infect others. Others may develop a disease that is less serious than AIDS, referred to as AIDS Related Complex (ARC). In some people, the protective immune system may be destroyed by the virus and then other germs (bacteria, protozoa, fungi and other viruses) and cancers that ordinarily would never get a foothold cause "opportunistic diseases"—using the opportunity of lowered resistance to infect and destroy. Some of the most common are Pneumocystis carinii pneumonia and tuberculosis. Individuals infected with the AIDS virus may also develop certain types of cancers such as Kaposi's sarcoma. These infected people have classic AIDS. Evidence shows that the AIDS virus may also attack the nervous system, causing damage to the brain.

Some people remain apparently well after infection with the AIDS virus. They may have no physically apparent symptoms of illness. However, if proper precautions are not used with sexual contacts and/or intravenous drug use, these infected individuals can spread the virus to others. Anyone who thinks he or she is infected or involved in high risk behaviors should not donate his/her blood, organs, tissues, or sperm because they may now contain the AIDS virus.

AIDS-Related Complex (ARC) is a condition caused by the AIDS virus in which the patient tests positive for AIDS infection and has a specific set of clinical symptoms. However, ARC patients' symptoms are often less severe than those with the disease we call classic AIDS. Signs and symptoms of ARC may include loss of appetite, weight loss, fever, night sweats, skin rashes, diarrhea, tiredness, lack of resistance to infection, or swollen lymph nodes. These are also signs and symptoms of many other diseases and a physician should be consulted.

Only a qualified health professional can diagnose AIDS, which is the result of a natural progress of infection by the AIDS virus. AIDS destroys the body's immune (defense) system and allows otherwise controllable infections to invade the body and cause additional diseases. These opportunistic diseases would not otherwise gain a foothold in the body. These opportunistic diseases may eventually cause death.

Some symptoms and signs of AIDS and the "opportunistic infections" may include a persistent cough and fever associated with shortness of breath or difficult breathing and may be the symptoms of Pneumocystis carinii pneumonia. Multiple purplish blotches and bumps on the skin may be a sign of Kaposi's sarcoma. The AIDS virus in all infected people is essentially the same; the reactions of individuals may differ.

The AIDS virus may also attack the nervous system and cause delayed damage to the brain. This damage may take years to develop and the symptoms may show up as memory loss, indifference, loss of coordination, partial paralysis, or mental disorder. These symptoms may occur alone, or with other symptoms mentioned earlier.

The number of people estimated to be infected with the AIDS virus in the United States is about 1.5 million. All of these individuals are assumed to be capable of spreading the virus sexually (heterosexually or homosexually) or by sharing needles and syringes or other implements for intravenous drug use. Of these, an estimated 100,000 to 200,000 will come down with AIDS Related Complex (ARC). It is difficult to predict the number who will develop ARC or AIDS because symptoms sometimes take as long as nine years to show up. With our present knowledge, scientists predict that 20 to 30 percent of those infected with the AIDS virus will develop an illness that fits an accepted definition of AIDS within five years. The number of persons known to have AIDS in the United States to date is over 25,000; of these, about half have died of the disease. Since there is no cure, the others are expected to also eventually die from their disease.

The majority of infected antibody positive individuals who carry the AIDS virus show no disease symptoms and may not come down with the disease for many years, if ever.

There is no known risk of non-sexual infection in most of the situations we encounter in our daily lives. We know that family members living with individuals who have the AIDS virus do not become infected except through sexual contact. There is no evidence of transmission (spread) of AIDS virus by everyday contact even though these family members shared food, towels, cups, razors, even toothbrushes, and kissed each other.

SOURCE:

U.S. Department of Health and Human Services. *Surgeon General's Report on Acquired Immune Deficiency Syndrome.* 1990. pp. 9-13.

WOMEN AND AIDS

Over 15,000 women in the United States have developed AIDS; proportionately, women are the fastest growing group of AIDS patients. In New York City, AIDS is the leading cause of death for women aged 25 to 34.

In the United States, about ten percent of people with AIDS are women. A woman is most at risk for AIDS if she has shared I.V. needles, or if she has had sex without a condom with someone who was infected with the AIDS virus. Women who have used I.V. drugs or had sex with I.V. drug users, gay or bisexual men, or hemophiliacs since 1977 are at higher risk of having been exposed to the AIDS virus. A woman may also be at risk if her sex partner has had sex without a condom with anyone at high risk. The more sex partners a woman has had, the greater the risk.

A woman who has sex only with other women and does not use I.V. drugs is at extremely low risk unless her partners have high risk contacts or use I.V. drugs. A woman who has sex with both men and women is far more at risk through sex with men.

You can't tell by looking at someone whether or not he or she is infected with the AIDS virus. Many people who are infected don't even know it themselves; therefore, you should always take the precautions listed below.

You can take steps to prevent transmission of the AIDS virus. Unless you KNOW that a sex partner is not infected:

- Don't allow blood (including menstrual blood), semen, urine, vaginal secretions, or feces to enter your vagina, anus or mouth.
- Use latex condoms with nonoxynol-9 (but not "natural" or "lambskin") for vaginal, oral, and anal sex. The AIDS virus cannot get through a condom if the condom is properly used and does not break. Use only water-based lubricants. Oil-based lubricants (like Vaseline or baby oil) increase the risk of the condom breaking.
- Spermicide containing nonoxynol-9, in foams, jellies or creams, should be used in addition to latex condoms for extra protection.

If you suspect you might have been exposed to the AIDS virus, you can get a blood test to see if you have antibodies to the AIDS virus. If you test positive, it does NOT mean that you have or will get AIDS. Antibody-positive people should assume they are contagious, but everyone—whether they test positive or negative—should be careful.

If you think you might be infected, talk with your doctor or other health care worker who is knowledgeable about AIDS before getting pregnant. If you are carrying the AIDS virus, your baby could be born infected and become ill with AIDS. Most babies born with AIDS don't live for more than a few years. The AIDS virus can also be passed to a baby through breast milk.

SOURCE:
California Medical Association. "Women and AIDS." *HealthTips* index WH-31 (March 1991): 1-2.

CHILDREN AND AIDS

In the United States, over 2500 children under the age of 13 have developed AIDS symptoms as of this date.

In most of the children with AIDS, the only known risk factor was having a mother or father who engaged in high-risk behavior, primarily intravenous drug use. Newborns receive the virus through the transmission of contaminated blood or blood products, but this risk has been virtually eliminated by universal blood screening procedures.

Most children infected with the AIDS virus perinatally become ill very early in life, usually under one year of age. The immunodeficiency often does not become medically evident until three to six months of age. Symptoms include failure to grow normally, chronic diarrhea, repeated severe colds and pneumonias, and extensive yeast infections. Failure to achieve neurologic milestones or a loss of previously achieved milestones is also indicative of AIDS in children. These conditions almost always result in death. Full-blown AIDS is likely to develop more rapidly in an infected infant than in an infected adult. This may occur because an infant's immune system is underdeveloped at the time the infection takes place.

Because AIDS is a fairly new and often misunderstood disease, some people are afraid of allowing children with AIDS in schools or other public places. Complete, authoritative studies have shown that there is no medical reason for excluding children with AIDS from the classroom. Exceptions to this rule might be children with behavioral problems such as habitual biting, inability to control their bladder or bowel, or open sores or rashes that cannot be covered.

Parents and others caring for children with AIDS should be aware of the special needs of the child. Children with AIDS do not fight off infections from common illnesses as well as a healthy child. The signs of minor infections should be noted immediately and carefully monitored. The usual immunization schedule should be altered and children with AIDS should be given inactivated polio virus vaccine instead of live polio virus vaccine. Infants are recommended to receive the usual mumps, measles, and rubella vaccine and other vaccinations as usual. Just as with every other child, care givers should wear gloves when changing diapers, cleaning up body excretions, and when there is a risk of contact with blood. Every effort should be made to keep the child's life as normal as possible to avoid victimizing children who already carry a heavy physical and emotional burden.

SOURCE:
California Medical Association. "Children and AIDS." *HealthTips* index 491 (March 1991): 1.

TRANSMISSION

Research and experience has proven that the AIDS virus is not transmitted through casual everyday contact. The AIDS virus, known as HIV, is quite fragile and cannot reproduce outside the human body. The virus is easily destroyed by household bleach. The virus does not linger on clothing or objects handled by persons with AIDS and is not transmitted through the air or by mosquitoes. Family members caring for people with AIDS over extended periods of time have never become infected as a result without direct blood contact. Of the tens of thousands of health care workers who care for those infected with the virus, those with AIDS-related conditions and AIDS itself, only a few have become infected with the virus—usually as a result of contaminated blood which has been injected from a needlestick. There have been no reports of development of AIDS in school children or co-workers who have had casual contact with people with AIDS or those infected with HIV. There is absolutely no risk of contracting the AIDS virus by donating blood. Transmission by any means other than sexual contact, mother to child, or contact with infected blood or tissue has never been demonstrated.

Research shows that infected blood and sexual discharges must enter the body to spread the disease. Tears and saliva have not been associated with transmission of the virus although they may contain small amounts of HIV. The body's first defense to any infection is intact skin, which provides a barrier to any invading organism. The AIDS virus cannot be transmitted by a hug, a water fountain, swimming pools, door knobs, shared pens, or surfaces in restrooms.

The incubation period for AIDS—the period of time from the virus entering the body to the onset of disease symptoms—is not absolutely known. Studies have shown it is usually more than seven years. However, if someone has been infected with the AIDS virus, it will show up in an AIDS antibody test four weeks to six months after infection in most cases. Of individuals infected for five years, about 25 percent will have developed AIDS. Another 30 to 35 percent of infected individuals will develop less severe symptoms of AIDS infection, a condition called AIDS-related complex (ARC). Half of the people infected ten years ago remain well today.

AIDS is transmitted through three main routes. The most common mode of transmission is the transfer of sexual secretions through sexual contact. This is accomplished through exposure of mucous membranes of the rectum, vagina, or mouth to blood, semen, or vaginal secretions containing HIV. Blood or blood products can transmit the virus, most often through the sharing of contaminated syringes and needles. Finally, HIV can be spread during pregnancy from mother to fetus. Research shows that there is a 30–50 percent chance that an infected woman will spread the virus to her fetus.

SOURCE:
California Medical Association. "AIDS Transmission: The Risk of Acquiring AIDS." *HealthTips* index 490 (March 1991): 1–2.

* * *

Transmission of human immunodeficiency virus (HIV) is known to occur perinatally, through sexual contact, and after exposure to infected blood or blood products. The possibility that breast milk may transmit HIV continues to be evaluated. There is no epidemiologic evidence that contact with saliva, tears, or urine has resulted in HIV infection. However, because HIV has (in some cases rarely) been isolated from these body fluids, guidelines have been developed to reduce more extensive exposures to such secretions. Laboratory and epidemiologic data strongly indicate that HIV is not transmitted through immune globulin preparations, the hepatitis B vaccine, or contact with insects. Increasing evidence from many studies also indicates that HIV is not transmitted through casual contact. All individuals need to be aware of how HIV is and is not transmitted, to reduce high-risk behaviors and to avoid unnecessary fears and actions.

SOURCE:
Lifson, Alan R. "Do Alternate Modes for Transmission of Human Immunodeficiency Virus Exist?" *JAMA* 259, no. 9 (March 4, 1988): 1353-1356.

SYMPTOMS

Although the initial symptoms of the disease vary widely and most of the symptoms can be indicators of many other non-AIDS related medical problems, medical attention should be sought immediately if any of the following symptoms develop:

- rapid weight loss of unknown cause (more than 10 lbs. in 2 months for no reason);
- the appearance of swollen or tender glands (lymph nodes) for no apparent reason, lasting for more than four weeks;
- unexplained shortness of breath, frequently accompanied by a dry cough, and not due to allergies or smoking;
- persistent diarrhea;
- intermittent high fever or soaking night sweats of unknown origin;
- a marked change in illness pattern—either frequency, severity, or length of sickness;
- the appearance of one or more purple spots on the surface of the skin or inside the mouth;

If you develop any of these symptoms, see your physician. There is a blood test for antibodies to the virus which causes AIDS. Although this test cannot tell you if you have or will develop the disease, it can tell you if you are infected with the virus and can pass it on to others. A thorough medical history and physical examination, some routine lab tests, and biopsy of any suspicious lesions will help in the diagnosis of this complex disease. Although there is no known cure for AIDS as yet, medical advances towards controlling the disease are being made each day. There are also several preventive medications that may be used to prevent the development of some AIDS-related infections.

SOURCE:
California Medical Association. "Acquired Immunodeficiency Syndrome (AIDS): An Overview." *HealthTips* index 426 (March 1991): 1–2.

TREATMENT WITH AZT

Therapy with zidovudine [AZT] is recommended for both symptomatic and asymptomatic HIV-infected individuals whose CD4 [helper lymphocyte] cell counts are below 500, at a total daily dose of 500 mg.

For persons with initial CD4 cell counts close to 500 (+100), the count should be repeated before initiation of zidovudine therapy. Optimally, two consecutive CD4 cell counts below 500 should be obtained at least 1 week apart before initiation of therapy.

There is no laboratory marker other than CD4 cell count that is necessary in deciding when to initiate zidovudine therapy.

SOURCE:
"Recommendations for Zidovudine: Early Infection." *JAMA* 263, no. 12 (March 23–30, 1990): 1606, 1609. Copyright 1990, American Medical Association.

TREATMENT—AZT DOSAGES AND SIDE EFFECTS

The initial dosage of zidovudine is 200 mg every four hours. The medication originally was given around the clock, but many physicians now omit the middle-of-the-night dose so that the patient can have an uninterrupted night's sleep. Studies have shown that using lower-dose zidovudine therapy (500 mg per day) in patients whose CD4 cell counts are below 200 per mm^3 and 500 per mm^3 is less toxic than the standard 1,200 mg per day regimen and is equally effective. For asymptomatic seropositive patients with CD4 counts below 500 per mm^3, the dosage is 500 mg per day in divided doses (100 mg every four hours while awake).

Side effects often occur with zidovudine therapy. They are usually transient and frequently include gastrointestinal complaints, headache and fatigue. Impaired hematopoiesis appears to be the most serious toxic effect associated with zidovudine therapy. It is manifested by granulocytopenia and anemia, which generally appear about six to eight weeks after initiation of high-dose treatment. Impaired hematopoiesis indicates myelosuppression. Toxicity is exacerbated by concomitant use of acetaminophen, indomethacin (Indameth,

Indocin), aspirin or probenecid (Benemid, Probalan); these drugs increase the serum half-life of zidovudine. Concomitant use of ganciclovir (Cytovene) has been shown to cause severe myelosuppression. The patient should always be warned of these drug interactions.

SOURCE:
Brooke, Grace Lee, and others. "HIV Disease: A Review for the Family Physician. Part I. Evaluation and Conventional Therapy." *American Family Physician* 42, no. 4 (October 1990): 978.

KAPOSI'S SARCOMA AND AIDS

Kaposi's sarcoma is the most common malignancy in AIDS patients. The incidence varies widely among risk groups, occurring in approximately one-third of homosexual men with AIDS but in only 4 percent of heterosexual intravenous drug users. For unknown reasons, the rate of Kaposi's sarcoma is falling in the homosexual AIDS population . . . .

Kaposi's sarcoma most commonly begins as asymptomatic, widespread, violaceous patches or plaques on the trunk and extremities. The lesions usually range from 1 to 2 cm in size. Typically, the number of lesions increases with time. However, the lesions may remain stable for many years and may even resolve spontaneously. The course of Kaposi's sarcoma generally appears to parallel the course of HIV disease. . . .

The management of cutaneous Kaposi's sarcoma may be divided into local and systemic therapies. Radiation therapy is excellent for treating cosmetically disturbing lesions of the face, ulcerative lesions of the oral mucosa, and lower extremity lesions that are producing edema. Other local measures such as cryotherapy and intralesional vinblastine injections may be used for cosmetic improvement of limited cutaneous disease.

SOURCE:
Berger, Timothy G., Marian L. Obuch, and Ronald H. Goldschmidt. "Dermatologic Manifestations of HIV Infection." *American Family Physician* 41, no. 6 (June 1990): 1737, 1738.

PREVENTION

The only sure way to protect yourself from contracting AIDS sexually is to abstain from sex outside a mutually faithful relationship with a partner whom you know is not infected with the AIDS virus. Otherwise, risks can be minimized if you:

- Don't have sexual contact with anyone who has symptoms of AIDS or who is a member of a high risk group for AIDS.
- Avoid sexual contact with anyone who has had sex with people at risk of getting AIDS.
- Don't have sex with prostitutes.
- Avoid having sex with anyone who has multiple and/or anonymous sexual partners.
- Avoid oral, genital and anal contact with your partner's blood, semen, vaginal secretions, feces or urine. Unless you know with absolute certainty that your partner is not infected, a latex condom should be used during each sexual act, from start to finish. Use of a spermicidal agent may provide additional protection.
- Avoid anal intercourse altogether.
- Don't share toothbrushes, razors or other implements that could become contaminated with blood with anyone who is, or who might be infected with the AIDS virus.
- Exercise caution regarding procedures, such as acupuncture, tattooing, ear piercing, etc., in which needles or other unsterile instruments may be used repeatedly to pierce the skin and/or mucous membranes. Such procedures are safe if proper sterilization methods are employed or disposable needles are used. Ask what precautions are being taken before undergoing such procedures.
- If you know that you will be having surgery in the near future, and you are able, consider donating blood for your own use. This will eliminate completely the already small risk of contracting AIDS through a blood transfusion. It will also eliminate the more substantial risk of contracting other bloodborne diseases, such as hepatitis, from a transfusion.

If you are a homosexual or bisexual man who does not use IV drugs:

The only sure way to protect yourself from contracting AIDS sexually is to abstain from sex outside a mutually faithful relationship with a partner whom you know is not infected with the AIDS virus. Otherwise, risks can be minimized if you:

- Don't have sexual contact with anyone who is or who might be infected with the AIDS virus.
- Avoid having multiple and/or anonymous sexual partners.
- Avoid having sex with anyone who has multiple and/or anonymous sexual partners. Don't have sexual contact with a sexual partner of someone who has AIDS.
- Avoid oral, genital and anal contact with your partner's blood, semen, vaginal secretions, feces or urine. Unless you know with absolute certainty that your partner is not infected, a latex condom should be used during each sexual act, from start to finish. It's best to avoid anal intercourse altogether, however.
- Don't share toothbrushes, razors or other implements that could become contaminated with blood with anyone who has, or might have, AIDS.
- Don't have sexual contact with individuals who use IV drugs.

If you are an IV drug user:

- Get professional help in terminating your drug habit.
- If you are unable to get off drugs, do not share needles and syringes. You should be aware that some street sellers are resealing previously used needles and selling them as new.
- If, knowing the risks, you decide to use a needle or syringe that may not be sterile, clean it with bleach before use.
- Avoid sexual contact (homosexual or heterosexual) with others who use IV drugs or who are otherwise at risk for AIDS.
- Don't share toothbrushes, razors or other implements that could become contaminated with blood with anyone who has, or might have, AIDS.

SOURCE:
American Council on Science and Health. *Answers about AIDS.* 6th ed. April 1988. pp. 38–40.

RESOURCES

AIDS HOTLINES
Centers for Disease Control. (800) 321-AIDS.

LyphoMed. (800) PCP-7003.

National AIDS Hotline. U.S. Public Health Service. (800) 342-AIDS.

National Gay and Lesbian Crisis Line. (800) 221-7044, (212) 529-1604 (NY State).

National Institute of Allergy and Infectious Diseases. (800) TRIALS-A.

National Institutes of Health. (800) AIDS-NIH.

Project Inform. (800) 822-7422.

ORGANIZATIONS
AIDS Action Council. 729 Eighth St. SE, Suite 200, Washington, DC 20003.

National AIDS Information Clearinghouse. P.O. Box 6003, Rockville, MD 20850.

National AIDS Network. 1012 14th St. NW, Suite 601, Washington, DC 20005.

National Association of People with AIDS. 2025 I St. NW, Suite 415, Washington, DC 20006.

PAMPHLETS
American Academy of Dermatology:

Skin Conditions Related to AIDS. 1988.

American National Red Cross:

Caring for the AIDS Patient at Home. #329507. 1986. 6 pp.

Children, Parents, and AIDS. #329540. 1988. 11 pp.

Drugs, Sex, and AIDS. #329539. 1988. 12 pp.

HIV Infection and AIDS. #329560. 1989. 12 pp.

Living with HIV Infection. #329548. 1990. 9 pp.

Teenagers and AIDS. #329536. 1988. 12 pp.

Women, Sex, and AIDS. #329537. 1988. 14 pp.

California Medical Association:

"AIDS and HIV Antibody Testing." *HealthTips* index 489 (October 1987): 2 pp.

National Institute of Allergy and Infectious Diseases:

AIDS Clinical Trials: Talking It Over. NIH Pub. No. 89-3025. 1989. 32 pp.

Understanding the Immune System. NIH Pub. No. 89-529. 1989. 40 pp.

National Institute of Mental Health:

When Someone Close Has AIDS. DHHS Pub. No. (ADM) 89-1515. 1989. 15 pp.

National PTA:

How to Talk to Your Children about AIDS. 1988.

U.S. Public Health Service:

America Responds to AIDS.

How You Can and Cannot Become Infected with AIDS. n.d.

What Is HIV Infection? And What Is AIDS? n.d.

BOOKS
AIDS Project Los Angeles. *AIDS: A Self-Care Manual.* Betty Clare Moffatt, Judith Spiegal, and others (eds.) Santa Monica, CA: IBS Press, 1987. 306 pp.

Fettner, Ann Giudici and William A. Click. *The Truth about AIDS: Evolution of an Epidemic.* New York: Holt, 1985.

Gong, Victor, and Norman Rudnick (eds.). *AIDS: Facts and Issues.* New Brunswick, NJ: Rutgers University Press, 1986. 388 pp.

Kubler-Ross, Elisabeth. *AIDS—The Ultimate Challenge.* New York: Macmillan, 1987. 330 pp.

Shilts, Randy. *And the Band Played On: People, and the AIDS Epidemic.* New York: St. Martin's Press, 1987. 630 pp.

Sontag, Susan. *AIDS and Its Metaphors.* New York: Farrar, Straus and Giroux, 1988. 95 pp.

RELATED ARTICLES
Brooke, Grace Lee, and George F. Safran. "HIV Disease: A Review for the Family Physician. Part II. Secondary Infections, Malignancy and Experimental Therapy." *American Family Physician* 42, no. 5 (November 1990): 1299–1308.

Health and Public Policy Committee, American College of Physicians. "The Acquired Immunodeficiency Syndrome (AIDS) and Infection with the Human Immunodeficiency Virus (HIV)." *Annals of Internal Medicine* 108, no. 3 (March 1988): 460–469.

Henry, Keith, Joseph Thurn, and Daniel Anderson. "Testing for Human Immunodeficiency Virus: What to Do If the Result Is Positive?" *Postgraduate Medicine* 85, no. 1 (January 1989): 293–309.

U.S. Preventive Services Task Force. "Counseling to Prevent HIV Infection and Other Sexually Transmitted Diseases." *American Family Physician* 41, no. 4 (April 1990): 1179–1187.

ALCOHOLISM

(*See also:* DRUG ABUSE)

OVERVIEW

Alcoholism is a primary, progressive, chronic disease characterized by a growing compulsion to drink. Scientists do not know precisely what causes this disease, but research suggests that physiological factors, such as heredity and metabolism, play an important role in determining who becomes alcoholic. Children of alcoholics are three to four times more likely than others to develop this disease, but people with no known history of family alcoholism may also be at risk. Since researchers have not yet identified the factors that predispose 10 percent of all drinkers to become alcoholic, anyone who drinks takes that chance. Alcoholism has no known cure and, if left unchecked, ends in death. Only abstinence can stop the disease's progress.

According to the National Council on Alcoholism (NCA), more than 22 million alcoholics live in the United States today. Following conventional wisdom, which holds that every alcoholic directly affects four others, 88 million people in this country are adversely affected by alcoholism in a family member, friend, or other associate. A recent Gallup poll closely supports this estimate: Approximately 81 million people—nearly half the adults in the United States—have been hurt by someone else's drinking.

In recent years Americans have become more knowledgeable about alcoholism and more willing to seek help. Nevertheless, the stigma with which society has branded this disease remains deeply impressed. Many people wonder how alcoholism can be called a disease when the individual, by choosing to drink, perpetuates the cycle of drunkenness. They reason that alcoholics must be responsible for bringing on the condition and conclude that they are either weak people who can't control themselves or bad people who ought to know better. They fail to understand that alcoholism is a physiological condition, like diabetes and other illnesses, to which some people are genetically predisposed.

No one sets out to become addicted to alcohol. Many recovering alcoholics say that their first drink filled them with profound enjoyment, as if they had found a magical elixir. In retrospect they can see that from the very beginning their bodies processed alcohol abnormally. Other alcoholics remember no early clues. But for all alcoholics, whether subtle signs appear with the first drink or only after many years of drinking, the disease progresses surreptitiously, long before they exhibit obvious symptoms that would cause them or their families to suspect a problem. It begins to work on them in secret, altering not only their body chemistry, but also their judgments, feelings, and perceptions. At first, alcoholics seem to respond to alcohol no differently than the majority of drinkers. Such early warning signs as preoccupation with alcohol and frequent drinking are socially acceptable and may fail to cause alarm.

A high tolerance for alcohol—the ability to drink it in great quantities without appearing to be drunk—is a notable early warning sign. As the disease progresses, tolerance changes. In middle-stage alcoholics, tolerance increases: They require more alcohol to achieve the desired effect. They drink more than they intend to, experience tensions in their family relationships, deny having a problem with alcohol, and become resentful and depressed. They may also hide their bottles and make attempts to drink less. In late-stage alcoholics, tolerance decreases: They cannot achieve the desired effect no matter how much they drink. Rather than get high from alcohol, they just get sick. Late-stage alcoholics drink in spite of adverse consequences. They experience deep cravings for alcohol, severe withdrawal symptoms, and malnutrition.

Also known as alcoholic amnesia, blackouts can occur in any stage of the disease. An alcoholic in a blackout may appear to behave normally, so that a casual observer might not guess he or she is drunk. Later on, however, the alcoholic will have no recollection of what was said or done. Blackouts can last from several minutes during a night of drinking up to several days during a prolonged period of binge drinking. They are one of the more frightening symptoms that alcoholics experience.

The symptoms of this disease generally don't become clear until the middle or late stage. By then alcoholics have lost the ability to evaluate themselves realistically and to recognize their illness, much to their family's bewilderment and chagrin.

Alcoholism is called a family disease. Family members unwittingly enable the alcoholic to drink, and they invariably suffer the consequences of erratic alcoholic behavior. Although they may not be alcoholic themselves, they nevertheless begin to take on the symptoms of the disease—becoming compulsive, irrational, and unable to assess their behavior. (Hence they are called "co-alcoholics" or "codependents.") As co-alcoholics get caught up in the cycle of addiction, they tend to become so concerned with the alcoholic in their lives that they lose sight of themselves. They may nag, scold, threaten, count the alcoholic's drinks, make excuses for the alcoholic's behavior. By focusing exclusively on the alcoholic, they deny their own needs and ultimately make themselves sick with worry, hostility, and shame.

Children of alcoholics grow up in an environment that is at best unpredictable and at worst abusive. They learn not to count on their parents, not to talk about the alcohol problem with other family members, and not to share the secret with outsiders. In an atmosphere of denial and shame, they learn three basic rules, as therapist Claudia Black has noted: Don't talk. Don't trust. Don't feel. They grow into adulthood with no sense of normal behavior, bear feelings of low self-esteem, and may be intensely loyal to people who do not deserve their loyalty. Many adult children of alcoholics marry alcoholics, work for alcoholics, or become alcoholics themselves.

This disease deludes its victims, alcoholics and co-alcoholics alike. It often takes years before family members recognize an alcohol problem in their home. Alcoholics are usually the last to see it. To break the barriers of denial takes time. To make the first step toward recovery—recognizing and admitting the loss of control—takes courage. All family members need help and education to recover from physical and psychological damage and to learn to care for themselves again.

SOURCE:

Yoder, Barbara. *The Recovery Resource Book.* New York: Simon & Schuster, 1990. pp. 32–34.

STATISTICS

An estimated 10.5 million U.S. adults exhibit some symptoms of alcoholism or alcohol dependence and an additional 7.2 million abuse alcohol, but do not yet show symptoms of dependence.

Alcohol use is associated with a wide variety of diseases and disorders, including liver disease, cancer and cardiovascular problems.

Cirrhosis of the liver caused almost 27,000 deaths and was the ninth leading cause of death in the United States in 1984.

Fetal exposure to alcohol is one of the leading known causes of mental retardation in the Western world and can be totally prevented.

Accidental death, suicide, and homicide are significant causes of death, particularly for young men under age 34; nearly half of these violent deaths are alcohol-related.

More than 20,000 alcohol-related motor vehicle fatalities annually are attributed to alcohol abuse and these deaths are relatively more frequent among younger Americans.

In 1986, alcohol abuse in the U.S. was estimated to cost $128.3 billion. Lost employment and reduced productivity accounted for more than half this amount.

Health care for accidents and illnesses related to alcohol abuse, including alcoholism, liver cirrhosis, cancer, and diseases of the pancreas, was estimated to cost $16.5 billion.

It is estimated that 20 to 40 percent of all U.S. hospital beds are occupied by persons whose health conditions are complications of alcohol abuse and alcoholism.

Blacks, especially males, are at extremely high risk for acute and chronic alcohol-related diseases such as cirrhosis, alcoholic fatty liver, hepatitis, heart disease, and cancers of the mouth, larynx, tongue, esophagus and lung.

Chronic alcohol abusers can develop clinical signs of cardiac dysfunction, and up to 50 percent of excess mortality in alcoholics and heavy drinkers can be attributed to cardiovascular disorders.

Chronic alcohol consumption is associated with a significant increase in hypertension.

Heavy alcohol consumption is a well-documented cause of neurological problems, including dementia, blackouts, seizures, hallucinations, and peripheral neuropathy.

SOURCE:

"Alcohol's Toll." *Addiction & Recovery* (June 1990): 52.

ALCOHOLISM IN ADOLESCENTS

Alcohol is the substance most commonly misused by teenagers; other than tobacco, it is the drug used at the earliest age. Substance abuse among adolescents has increased so markedly during the past three decades that 40 of 50 states have again set 21 as the minimum drinking age. Today, alcohol is a major cause of morbidity and mortality among young people.

Adolescent alcohol abuse has social, psychologic, economic and medical consequences. Alcohol-related motor vehicle accidents are responsible for a large number of highway crashes and fatalities (8,000 deaths per year in the 15 to 24 age group). In many cases, suicide and violent crimes, the second and third leading causes of death among young people, are alcohol-related. Alcohol use is frequently involved when adolescents have early sexual intercourse, resulting in unplanned and unwanted pregnancies and contributing to alcohol-related birth defects. Alcohol abuse often contributes to family violence. Finally, youths who abuse alcohol are much less likely to complete high school and to find and maintain steady employment, with resulting long-term economic consequences and adverse effects on family stability.

Alcohol abuse, as well as other substance abuse, causes developmental delays in adolescents, because it interferes with the normal steps of maturation. Heavy use of alcohol can be used to mask other problems; it can also serve as a "rite of passage" to adulthood when healthier avenues seem inaccessible or as a way to appear comfortable in unfamiliar social situations. . . .

When questioned about the behavioral consequences of alcoholism, teenagers often blame parents or other authority figures for their difficulties or fail to see drinking-related problems as serious. They may believe that adults are overreacting. Denial or unwillingness to consider alcohol abuse a problem then becomes another piece of supporting diagnostic information for the physician.

Considerable research describes a behavioral constellation that makes alcohol abuse more likely. Adolescents who abuse alcohol are more likely also to be regular smokers, to be sexually active without using birth control, to be experiencing problems both at home and at school, to have friends who drink regularly and to avoid participation in religious activities. Screening for these factors can often be a way of obtaining historical information that supports or relieves adult suspicions about alcohol abuse in teenagers.

In considering the diagnosis of alcohol abuse in adolescents, information from parents, other family members and, sometimes, peers is also important. Siblings may be more attuned to what is happening with an alcohol-dependent brother or sister than are the parents. Parents of teenagers who abuse alcohol are often slow to become aware of the abuse; when they do become aware of it, they tend to misjudge and underestimate the extent of the problem.

SOURCE:
Alexander, Beth. "Alcohol Abuse in Adolescents." *American Family Physician* 43 (February 1991): 527, 531.

FETAL ALCOHOL SYNDROME (FAS)

The issue of alcoholic beverage consumption during pregnancy and the potential risk of injury to the fetus is no longer a subject of debate. It is widely accepted that a fully developed fetal alcohol effect (FAE) can occur in offspring of women who consume excessive alcohol. The debate revolves around the question of how much alcohol will produce these effects. It is accepted that one need not be an alcoholic to injure the fetus, but in such an individual other contributing factors such as poor nutrition, smoking, drug abuse, etc., in addition to alcohol abuse, must also be considered.

One of the largest studies on the effects of alcohol on the fetus has been carried out at Boston University.

This study showed no clinically significant effects on the fetus if the mother consumed less than one ounce of alcohol per day. Nevertheless, it is frequently advised that would-be mothers abstain from alcohol intake during pregnancy or restrict their intake to a maximum of one or two drinks on rare occasions. These restrictions are examples of prudent rules that are given because sufficient human scientific information is not yet available to specify a "safe level," and because it is well known that individuals respond differently to the same amount of alcohol.

A summary on FAS, excerpted from [*Food for Health: A Nutrition Encyclopedia*. Pegus Press, 1986. p. 16.] is given below:

"Fetal addiction and fetal alcohol syndrome (FAS). When the mother is an addictive alcoholic, her child may be born addicted and experience withdrawal symptoms within the first week of life.

"Heavy drinking during pregnancy can also cause the fetal alcohol syndrome. Most common in the FAS are prenatal growth deficiencies, usually more severe with respect to birth length than weight, and postnatal growth deficiencies persisting through early childhood. Failure to thrive is reported despite adequate calorie intake and excellent foster care in the first year of life. Often, the infant has an abnormally small head. Mental deficiency or developmental delay are almost always present. Fine motor dysfunction including tremulousness, weak grasp, and poor eye-hand coordination are present in most children with FAS. . . .

"There are still a number of unanswered questions about fetal alcohol syndrome, such as the risk of moderate drinking, whether the risk to the fetus is greater at particular times during pregnancy, and the influence of other factors such as smoking and nutrition. While research continues on these and other issues, caution is advised. . . ."

SOURCE:
American Council on Science and Health. *The Responsible Use of Alcohol: Defining the Parameters of Moderation.* January 1991. pp. 14–15.

DRUNK DRIVING

It's true: Drinking and driving don't mix, and statistics prove it. In the United States, traffic accidents are the leading cause of death for people between the ages of 5 and 34; and, in more than half of all fatal crashes, alcohol is involved. Nearly one-third of all alcohol-related traffic fatalities are caused by problem drinkers or alcoholics, who are more likely than other drivers to have blood alcohol concentration (BAC) levels well above 0.10, the level at which most states consider a driver to be legally drunk. Drivers 16 to 24 years old account for 42 percent of all fatal alcohol-related crashes, although they represent only 20 percent of licensed drivers. In most states it is illegal for youth under 18 years of age to drive with a BAC of 0.05 or higher.

Tough laws adopted over the past decade have undoubtedly deterred some people from driving after drinking or from repeating that offense after a first arrest. Between 1970 and 1986 arrests for driving under the influence (DUI) increased nearly 223 percent, while the number of licensed drivers increased by just 42 percent. Yet apprehending drunk drivers presents a formidable task. Of every 2,000 drunk drivers, only one is likely to be arrested. And of those in jail for DUI, nearly half have been previously sentenced to probation, jail, or prison for DUI. Most repeat offenders—95 percent—are men, 80 percent unmarried men, with a median age of 32.

Raising the drinking age to 21 has reduced per capita arrests for DUI among 18- to 20-year-olds by more than 14 percent since 1983, when most states passed new drinking-age laws. As of 1988 all states had raised the drinking age to 21. Another effective measure has been to increase excise taxes on beer. States with relatively high excise taxes have lower death rates from motor vehicle accidents among 15- to 24-year-olds.

Despite all these measures drunk driving continues to be the most frequently committed crime in the United States, surpassing by three times the total for all other violent crimes. Estimates of the economic costs of drunk driving range from $11 billion to $24 billion each year. And the death toll continues to soar. In 1987 an estimated 23,632 people died in alcohol-related crashes—51 percent of the total traffic fatalities for that year. Two out of five Americans will be involved in an alcohol-related crash at some point in their lives.

Individuals can positively affect this problem. We can be responsible hosts, making sure that our guests don't get drunk or, if they do get drunk, that they don't drive. We can be alert to drunk drivers on the road, keep clear of their path, and stop to report them to police. And we can get involved in lobbying organizations and support educational efforts to prevent drunk driving. Finally, we must remember this: If we drink, even one can be too many for the road.

SOURCE:

Yoder, Barbara. *The Recovery Resource Book.* New York: Simon & Schuster, 1990. pp. 121.

TREATMENT

A. Psychologic: The most important consideration for the physician is to suspect the problem early and take a nonjudgmental attitude, though this does not mean a passive one. The problem of denial must be met, preferably with significant family members at the first meeting. This means dealing from the beginning with any enabling behavior of the spouse or other significant people. This is particularly true when the problem has become a "chronic rescue operation." There must be an emphasis on the things that can be done. This approach emphasizes the fact that the physician cares and strikes a positive and hopeful note early in the treatment. Valuable time should not be wasted trying to find out why the patient drinks; come to grips early with the immediate problems of how to stop the drinking. Total abstinence (not "controlled drinking") should be the primary goal.

B. Social: Get the patient into Alcoholics Anonymous (AA) and the spouse into Al-Anon. Success is usually proportionate to the utilization of AA, religious counseling, and other resources. The patient should be seen frequently for short periods and charged an appropriate fee.

Do not underestimate the importance of religion, particularly since the alcoholic is often a dependent person who needs a great deal of support. Early enlistment of the help of a concerned religious adviser can often provide the turning point for a personal conversion to sobriety.

One of the most important considerations is the job; it is usually lost or in jeopardy. The business community has become painfully aware of the problem, with the result that about 70% of the Fortune 500 companies offer programs to their employees to help with the problem of alcoholism. In the latter case, some specific recommendations to employers can be offered: (1) Avoid placement in jobs where the alcoholic must be alone, e.g., traveling buyer or sales executive. (2) Use supervision but not surveillance. (3) Keep competition with others to a minimum. (4) Avoid positions that require quick decision making on important matters (high stress situations).

C. Medical: Hospitalization is not usually necessary or even desirable at this stage, which is not an acute one. It is sometimes used to dramatize a situation and force the patient to face the problem of alcoholism, but generally it should be used on medical indications. . . .

Disulfiram [Antabuse] blocks the metabolism of alcohol with acetaldehyde buildup, with the result that unpleasant symptoms of headaches, flushing, and nausea occur within 30 minutes after exposure and may progress to more serious signs and symptoms, including hypertension, shock, and coma. Disulfiram is helpful in deterrence, particularly binge drinking. There should be no surreptitious use of the drug. The patient should have full knowledge of the consequences of using alcohol with the drug (including elixirs and sunscreens with alcohol). Cardiac disease and psychoses are contraindications to the use of disulfiram. Side effects without concomitant alcohol use include impotence, liver damage (obtain hepatic baseline studies), drowsiness, and fetal anomalies in pregnant women. The initial dose is 500 mg orally daily (after abstention from alcohol for 12 hours), reduced to 250 mg daily after a week. Disulfiram impairs elimination of caffeine and interacts with phenytoin, sedatives, and narcotics. A disulfiram regimen need not interfere with other treatment approaches such as AA.

D. Behavioral: Conditioning approaches have been used in many settings in the treatment of alcoholism, most commonly as a type of aversion therapy. For example, the patient is given a drink of whiskey and then a shot of apomorphine, and proceeds to vomit. In this way a strong association is built up between the vomiting and the drinking. Although this kind of treatment has been successful in some cases, many people do not retain the learned aversive response.

SOURCE:

Schroeder, Steven A., and others. *Current Medical Diagnosis & Treatment 1992.* Norwalk, CT: Appleton & Lange, 1992. pp. 819-820.

RESOURCES

ORGANIZATIONS

Al-Anon. 1372 Broadway, New York, NY 10018.

Alcoholics Anonymous. P.O. Box 459, Grand Central Station, New York, NY 10163.

American Council on Alcoholism. 8501 LaSalle Rd., Suite 301, Towson, MD 21204.

Hazelden Foundation. Box 11, Center City, MN 55012.

Johnson Institute of Rehabilitation. 509 South Euclid Avenue, St. Louis, MO 63110.

National Clearinghouse for Alcohol and Drug Information. P.O. Box 2345, Rockville, MD 20852.

National Council on Alcoholism. 12 W. 21st St., New York, NY 10010.

PAMPHLETS

Al-Anon:

Al-Anon Is for Adult Children of Alcoholics. 1987.

Al-Anon, You and the Alcoholic. 1988.

American Council on Alcoholism:

The Most Frequently Asked Questions About. . . Drinking and Pregnancy. 1988.

Johnson Institute:

Alcoholism: A Treatable Disease. 20 pp.

Blackouts and Alcoholism. 9 pp.

National Clearinghouse for Alcohol and Drug Information:

Alcohol and the Body. MS 251. 1988.

Facts about Alcohol. RP 0106. 1988.

BOOKS

Alcoholics Anonymous. *Twelve Steps and Twelve Traditions.* New York, 1953.

Gold, Mark S. *The Facts about Drugs and Alcohol.* New York: Bantam, 1987. 120 pp.

Goodwin, Donald W. *Is Alcoholism Hereditary?* 2nd edition. New York: Ballantine, 1988. 259 pp.

Kinney, Jean, and Gwen Leaton. *Loosening the Grip: A Handbook of Alcohol Information.* St. Louis: Times Mirror/Mosby, 1987. 369 pp.

Mueller, L. Ann, and Katherine Ketcham. *Recovery: How to Get and Stay Sober.* New York: Bantam, 1987. 220 pp.

Mumey, Jack. *The Joy of Being Sober.* Chicago: Contemporary Books, 1984. 214 pp.

RELATED ARTICLES

"Acamprosate, Citalopram, and Alcoholism." *The Lancet* 337 (March 30, 1991): 770.

Barringer, Felicity. "Youthful Drinking Persists: With Teens and Alcohol, It's Just Say When." *The New York Times* (June 23, 1991): Section 4.

Gordis, Enoch, and others. "Finding the Gene(s) for Alcoholism." *JAMA* 263 (April 18, 1990): 2094-2095.

ALLERGY

OVERVIEW

Researchers have found that, ironically, allergy results from malfunctioning of the immune system, a collection of cells and molecules which exists to protect us from harm.

Simply stated, allergy happens because of an educational error.

Normally, the body learns to defend itself through experience—by encountering, battling and remembering one enemy after another. For decades, medical science has taken advantage of this ability by using vaccination to create immunity, the immunologic "memory" of a disease.

Allergic reactions occur after the immune system mistakenly learns to recognize innocent foreign substances as potentially harmful. Such substances are called allergens. Among those that most frequently cause problems are pollens, mold spores, house dust mites, animal danders and foods. They can come into contact with the body in different ways—for example, through inhalation, ingestion, or just by touching the skin. Allergic responses also can be triggered by environmental conditions such as cold temperatures.

An element of the immune system that plays a central role in allergy is the antibody, a "scout" molecule whose job is to identify foreign invaders so the body's powerful weapons of defense can be deployed with precision and speed. Antibodies are produced by a class of white blood cells known as B lymphocytes, which in turn are regulated by another key group of blood cells, the T lymphocytes. It is not yet known where in this system the "mistake" that leads to allergy occurs.

In 1965, scientists at the National Jewish Center for Immunology and Respiratory Medicine discovered a particular class of antibody called immunoglobulin (IgE). This molecule plays a significant role in a common type of allergy.

The following story illustrates how this kind of allergy can develop: Over a field of ragweed plants floats an invisible cloud of pollen grains, which are soon carried by the wind into a nearby town. The pollen is inhaled by a child whose body has never been exposed to this substance before.

Because of some defect or genetic predisposing factor, this person's immune system overreacts. It produces large numbers of IgE antibodies, all specially designed to respond to ragweed pollen. Several of the antibodies attach themselves to cells in the child's nasal passages and upper respiratory tract. These cells, known as mast cells, contain strong chemicals called mediators, the best-known of which is histamine.

On a later occasion, when the child inhales the same kind of pollen again, proteins from the pollen bind in lock-and-key fashion to the specially designed antibodies on the surface of the mast cells. This sets off an explosion of sorts as the mediators burst from inside the mast cells, destroying the pollen but also damaging surrounding tissues.

The end result is symptoms—the sneezing, sniffling, stuffed-up head and red, watery eyes that are well-known hallmarks of the condition commonly known as "hay fever." (This is actually a misnomer, since neither hay nor fever is involved in the reaction. The official medical term is allergic rhinitis.)

The child in this example began with an "ignorant" immune system which unfortunately learned something untrue: "This foreign substance that has come into the body is extremely dangerous. The next time this 'enemy' is encountered, chemical defenses must be at hand to get rid of it fast, even if the body itself must suffer in the process."

Any organ system can be affected by allergy. Those most often involved are the skin, the respiratory tract, the digestive system, and the blood vessels. In addition to allergic rhinitis, some common allergic conditions are eczema (a scaly skin rash) and urticaria (hives). A rare type of allergy caused by cold temperatures is cold urticaria. Asthma is often, although not always, triggered by allergy.

Sometimes, an allergic reaction will occur far from the area of the body where initial contact with the allergen is made. For example, a substance that is swallowed may cause eczema.

Allergic responses vary widely in their severity. The most serious type of reaction is anaphylaxis, an immediate, dramatic attack often characterized by itching and flushing of the skin followed by more serious symptoms such as severe vomiting and diarrhea, spasm of the larynx, constriction of respiratory passages, and swelling of blood vessels. Some allergens are more commonly associated with anaphylaxis than others—for example, certain insect venoms and drugs such as penicillin and, among foods, fish, peanuts, nuts, eggs and seeds.

If not treated promptly and properly, anaphylaxis can result in death. Fortunately, the tendency to have such serious reactions is rare.

The fundamental cause of allergy still is not known. The problem clearly has a tendency to run in families—an allergic individual is much more likely to have relatives who are allergic than would be expected on the basis of chance. But non-hereditary factors apparently play a part as well. Evidence of this is the fact that infants who are breast-fed are less likely to develop allergies than bottle-fed babies.

Why an individual becomes sensitive to some substances and not to others also remains a mystery.

Another crucial question involves the timing of allergic responses. Some allergy attacks occur immediately after exposure to an offending substance, while others take minutes or hours.

Not all allergic reactions happen in the same way as the pollen allergy in the illustration. For example, scientists theorize that the biological mechanisms leading up to delayed reactions are different from those that result in short-term allergic responses.

SOURCE:
National Jewish Center for Immunology and Respiratory Medicine. *Understanding Allergy*. 1986. pp. 1–3.

HAY FEVER

Hay fever is the most common allergic disease in this country. It has been estimated that 18–20 million Americans suffer from hay fever, which is about half of all persons in the country believed to have some type of allergic disease. About one-third of hay fever sufferers also have asthma. Figures for hay fever probably somewhat underestimate the number of cases because many people do not seek professional treatment for their symptoms and not every hay fever sufferer has symptoms throughout his or her life. . . .

Hay fever is an allergic reaction to pollen produced by trees, grasses, or weeds. It may also be caused by spores from molds (a type of fungus). Often an individual is sensitive to more than one of these irritants (allergens).

The term "hay fever" is extremely misleading because the allergic reaction one suffers is rarely associated with hay, and fever is not a symptom of the reaction. Scientific descriptions of the symptoms of the disease go back to the 1500s, but the name was coined in England in the early 1800s when numerous individuals suffered from runny noses, itchy eyes, and congestion (symptoms generally associated with colds and fevers) during the fall hay harvest. In 1866, the first theory of the association between hay fever and pollen was published, but the theory remained largely ignored until the early 1900s. . . .

Due to the seasonal nature of the presence of pollen and mold spores, hay fever is also called "seasonal allergic rhinitis." Rhinitis is defined as an inflammation of the mucous membranes of the nose. This term is used to distinguish hay fever from "perennial allergic rhinitis" in which the individual suffers throughout the year and is generally allergic to a variety of substances including house dust, the house mite, animal danders, and often pollens and mold spores. Occupational allergens (dusts and odors) may also be important.

SOURCE:
American Council on Science and Health. *Hay Fever*. 1986. pp. 2–3.

FOOD ALLERGIES

Since no uniform definitions exist for the various terms, the Committee on Adverse Reactions to Foods of the American Academy of Allergy and Immunology suggests the following be used:

Adverse reaction to a food: A general term that is used to describe any abnormal reaction to a food or food additive that is eaten, whether caused by allergic or non-allergic mechanisms.

Food allergy, hypersensitivity or sensitivity to a food: An abnormal immunologic reaction in which the body's immune system overreacts to ordinary harmless things. Irritating and uncomfortable symptoms also may result after eating a food or food additive. The word "allergy" is frequently over-used and misused. The reaction actually only occurs in some people, usually as the result of a genetic factor, and may be noticeable after just a small amount of the food or food additive is eaten. (Wheezing after consuming milk or dairy products is an example.)

Food intolerance: An abnormal physical response to a food or food additive that is eaten and is not proved to be immunologic, i.e., milk sugar (lactose) intolerance, where the individual lacks the enzymes to break down the milk sugar for proper digestion.

Food poisoning: A severe allergic reaction caused by a food or food additive without immune system mechanisms being involved. Toxins (poisons or bacteria) may be either contained within the food or released by microorganisms or parasites contaminating food products.

Pharmacologic food reaction: An adverse reaction in which a chemical found in a food or food additive produces a drug-like (pharmacologic) effect, i.e., caffeine in coffee causing "the jitters."

Food allergens, those parts of foods that cause allergic reactions, are usually proteins. Most of these allergens can still cause reactions even after they are cooked or have undergone digestion in the intestines. Numerous food proteins have been studied to establish allergen content. The most thoroughly studied allergens include cow's milk, egg white, shrimp, and peanut. Allergens also have been found in codfish, soybeans, and crab. Recent studies conducted in the United States indicate that the proteins in cow's milk, egg, peanut, wheat, and soy are the most common food allergens.

All foods come from either a plant or an animal source. Foods are grouped into families according to their origin. For example, black-eyed peas, kidney beans, lima beans, peas, soybeans, and peanuts are some of the members of the pea (legume) family, whereas asparagus, chives, garlic, onion and shallot are members of the lily family. In some food groups, especially legumes and seafoods, an allergy to one member of a family may result in the persons being allergic to other members of the same group (known as cross-reactivity). Persons allergic to peanuts are more likely to be allergic to soybeans, peas, and other legumes than to walnuts or pecans. However, some persons may be allergic to both peanuts and walnuts. These allergies are called coincidental allergies.

Soybeans are being used more frequently as protein extenders and food supplements. Thus, the potential for developing an allergy to soybeans also is increasing.

Within animal groups of foods, cross-reactivity within food families is not seen as often. For example, people allergic to cow's milk can usually eat beef, and patients allergic to eggs can usually eat chicken.

Cooking some proteins usually reduces their ability to cause a reaction, but not always, and in fact the heating process may actually make some proteins more allergenic. The protein of cow's milk is composed of two types: casein (80%) and whey (20%). Most of these proteins are not affected by heating. Persons allergic to eggs usually react only to the egg white, which contains several proteins, and again, cooking or heating does not make these proteins non-allergenic. Natural processes such as ripening also may affect the allergenic properties of a food. For example, tomatoes become more allergenic as they ripen.

SOURCE:
American Academy of Allergy and Immunology. *Adverse Reactions to Foods: A Patient Guide.* November 1985. pp. 2–3.

HIVES

Hives are localized swellings (wheals) of the skin or mucous membranes that usually occur in groups on any part of the skin. They usually last 1 to 6 hours before fading away, leaving no trace. No single hive lasts more than 36 hours. Swellings lasting longer are not hives. Hives vary in size, from as small as a pencil eraser to as large as a dinner plate. Hives may join together to form larger hives. When hives are forming, the swellings itch, burn, or sting.

What produces a hive is blood plasma leaking into the skin through tiny gaps between the cells lining small blood vessels in the skin. A natural chemical called "histamine" causes these gaps to appear. Histamine is released from cells called "mast cells" which lie abundantly along the blood vessels in the skin. Histamine is released by an allergic reaction or by pharmacological mechanisms. The term "pharmacological mechanisms" refers to certain natural chemicals in some foods (i.e. strawberries, lobsters, clams) or in certain drugs (i.e., morphine, codeine) which cause the mast cells to empty their "packets" of histamine thus producing the reddening and swelling in the skin. An allergic reaction is produced when a person makes a protein called an antibody against some foreign substance, usually a natural or synthetic protein called antigen. When the antibody reacts to the antigen, histamine is released by the mast cells. So whether an allergic or pharmacological reaction occurs, the mast cell is the site of action. . . .

Urticaria [pruritic skin eruption] is classified according to how long the attacks last and how frequently they occur. Acute urticaria is a single attack of hives occurring once or twice during a person's lifetime. The bouts of hives can last hours or perhaps as long as a week before the attack stops. The most common known cause is an infection or a drug. Acute urticaria can occur with such infections as chicken pox, certain upper respiratory viral infections, mononucleosis, serum hepatitis, and rheumatic fever. Patients who develop hives and swelling of the joints after receiving penicillin or other drugs fit into this category. They should not take the same or related drug again.

SOURCE:
American Academy of Dermatology. *Urticaria-Hives.* 1987. pp. 1, 2.

ANAPHYLACTIC SHOCK

Anaphylaxis is a medical emergency which is an acute systemic (affecting the whole body) allergic reaction. It occurs after exposure to an antigen (allergen) to which a person was previously sensitized.

Anaphylaxis is caused by an immunologic mechanism which involves an IgE (immunoglobulin) antibody that attaches to a mast cell or basophil and reacts with a certain allergen. This causes the release of many chemicals or mediators. Mediators are chemical substances that attract or activate other parts of the immune system; the best known mediator is histamine.

Anaphylactoid reactions have symptoms similar to those of anaphylaxis, but are triggered instead by non-IgE mechanisms which directly cause the release of these mediators. These include reactions to non-steroidal, anti-inflammatory drugs (i.e., aspirin, ibuprofen). . . .

The signs and symptoms of anaphylaxis include: anxiety, itching of the skin, headache, nausea and vomiting, sneezing and coughing, abdominal cramps, hives and swelling of tissues such as lips or joints, diarrhea, shortness of breath and wheezing, low blood pressure, convulsions, and loss of consciousness. The eyes may itch, water and swell. Additional symptoms include: itching of the mouth and throat, hoarseness, change of voice, nasal congestion, chest pain and tightness, a feeling of warmth and flushing, redness of the skin, cramping of the uterus and the feeling of having to urinate.

Thus, anaphylaxis can affect various organ systems including the skin, upper and lower respiratory tracts, cardiovascular system, eyes, uterus and the bladder. . . .

Anaphylaxis is a medical emergency. The best therapy is prevention. Physicians should take a careful history from the patient before prescribing certain medications or administering general anesthesia. Patients with known drug or insect allergy, severe food reactions, or anaphylaxis should wear a Medic-Alert bracelet or necklace at all times. Such persons also should know how to self-administer epinephrine (adrenalin). The sooner the reaction is treated, the less severe it will be.

SOURCE:
American Academy of Allergy and Immunology. *Anaphylaxis.* November 1988. pp. 1-2, 3.

TREATMENT

The best treatment for allergies is to avoid the offending substance; indeed, for food allergies, that's the only treatment, [Kathy] Lampl [co-director of the Allergy Center, Silver Springs, MD] says. But there are effective methods of dealing with inhalant allergies. If you suffer from occasional, seasonal rhinitis (hay fever), over-the-counter antihistamines may relieve your symptoms quite effectively by counteracting the release of histamines. Many over-the-counter antihistamines have a sedating effect, but nonsedating varieties are available by prescription from your family physician. Either may be taken in tandem with decongestants, which help dry up the nasal membranes and lessen congestion (some over-the-counter remedies already contain decongestants).

Over-the-counter nasal decongestants may help relieve the stuffy nose and breathing difficulties associated with allergies, but they can have serious drawbacks. "I'm often very leery of introducing people to topical decongestants," says [Donald] Kennerly [assistant professor of internal medicine at the Division of Allergy and Immunology, University of Texas Southwestern Medical Center, in Dallas]. Many patients, after a week of use, find they don't work as well, so instead of following the package directions, they begin using them more frequently, five or six times a day. They become physically addicted." Patients find themselves unable to breathe without the medication, and withdrawal from the drug is uncomfortable.

Another option in allergy treatment is immunotherapy, or allergy shots. Small amounts of the specific allergen are injected, in ever increasing doses, once or twice a week until a "maintenance level" is reached—the highest dose tolerable without causing a serious reaction. Once it has been reached, shots can be given every two to four weeks.

"There is a controversy as to how long to continue immunotherapy once the maintenance level has been reached," he continues. He says he usually stops the therapy after two and a half to three years. "Half to two thirds of the patients will stay better for life," he estimates. "For the rest, symptoms will return slowly over the next four to ten years." He adds that although immunotherapy can be restarted, the second treatment must start from the beginning.

SOURCE:
Perrine, Stephen. "All about Allergies." *Parents' Magazine* 66 (March 1991): 204–205.

MEDICATIONS

When environmental controls are not enough to suppress the symptoms of pollen allergies, medication can usually bring relief. Antihistamines have long been the hallmark of allergy therapy. But to be fully effective, they must be taken before symptoms and used around the clock during the pollen season. They work by blocking the action of histamine and thus must be in place before histamine acts.

Traditional antihistamines cause drowsiness, which can be a problem for people who have to remain alert at work and disastrous for people who have to drive or to operate hazardous equipment. Furthermore, after a while, individual antihistamines lose effectiveness, but switching to a drug from another one of the classes of antihistamines can get around this limitation.

Two antihistamines, Seldane and Hismanal, that are nonsedating and do not lose effectiveness with regular use, are available by prescription. Decongestants, which are stimulants, are also sometimes used to reduce swelling of nasal passages, but these can be unduly drying and can cause rebound congestion if used for more than several days at a time. Another remedy that many doctors prefer to decongestants is cromolyn, an ingredient in some prescription nasal sprays that prevents the release of histamine. If all else fails, steroids may be administered orally, by injection or by nasal spray.

SOURCE:
Brody, Jane E. "Old Advice As Well As New Hope for Millions Who Are Allergic to the Pollens of Springtime." *The New York Times* (April 11, 1991): Health.

RESOURCES

ORGANIZATIONS

American Academy of Allergy and Immunology. 611 East Wells Street, Milwaukee, WI 53202.

Asthma & Allergy Foundation of America. 1717 Massachusetts Ave. NW, Suite 305, Washington, DC 20036.

National Institute of Allergy and Infectious Diseases. Office of Communications, 9000 Rockville Pike, Bethesda, MD 20892.

National Jewish Center for Immunology and Respiratory Medicine. 1400 Jackson Street, Denver, CO 80206.

PAMPHLETS

American Academy of Allergy and Immunology:

Helpful Hints for the Allergic Patient. 1990.

What Is an Allergic Reaction? 1990.

American Council on Science and Health:

Food Allergies. 1989.

Asthma and Allergy Foundation of America:

Allergy in Children. n.d.

Drug Allergy. n.d.

Exercise and Allergy. n.d.

Food Allergy. n.d.

Hay Fever. n.d.

The Immune System. n.d.

Insect Stings. n.d.

Mold Allergy. n.d.

Poison Ivy Allergy. n.d.

Pollen Allergy. n.d.

Questions and Answers about Asthma and Allergic Diseases. n.d.

Sinusitis. n.d.

Skin Allergy. n.d.

California Medical Association:

"Hay Fever Misery." *HealthTips* 31 (March 1986).

National Institute of Allergy and Infections Diseases:

Pollen Allergy. NIH Pub. No. 87-493. 1987. 20 pp.

National Jewish Center for Immunology and Respiratory Medicine:

Education: Your Child and Asthma. 1986. 20 pp.

Understanding Allergy. 1986. 5 pp.

Understanding Asthma. 1985. 10 pp.

Understanding Immunology. 1985.

BOOKS

Carper, Steve. *No Milk Today: How to Live with Lactose Intolerance.* New York: Simon & Schuster, 1986. 286 pp.

Golos, Natalie, and Frances Golos Golbitz. *Coping with Your Allergies.* New York: Simon & Schuster, 1986. 396 pp.

Orenstein, Neil S., and Sarah L. Biggham. *Food Allergies: How to Tell If You Have Them; What to Do about Them If You Do.* New York: Perigee/Putnam's, 1987. 161 pp.

Weinstein, Allan M. *Asthma: The Complete Guide to Self Management of Asthma and Allergies for Patients and Their Families.* New York: McGraw-Hill, 1987. 350 pp.

RELATED ARTICLES

"Allergy Warfare." *U.S. News and World Report* (February 20, 1989): 68-79.

Bernstein, I. Leonard. "Proceedings of the Task Force on Guidelines for Standardizing Old and New Technologies Used for the Diagnosis and Treatment of Allergic Diseases." *The Journal of Allergy and Clinical Immunology* 82, no. 3, part 2 (September 1988): 487-490, 523-526.

Klein, Gerald L. "Treatment of Hay Fever: Allergen Avoidance and Medication to Control Symptoms." *Postgraduate Medicine* 85, no. 6 (May 1, 1989): 193-200.

"Legitimate Allergy Tests: Three Reliable Ways to Find Out If You Have an Allergy." *Mayo Clinic Health Letter* 8 (April 1990): 5-6.

Tamasky, Paul R., and Van Arsdel, Paul P. Jr. "Antihistamine Therapy in Allergic Rhinitis." *The Journal of Family Practice* 30, no. 1 (1990): 71-80.

ALZHEIMER'S DISEASE

OVERVIEW

When elderly people suffer memory lapses or become confused periodically, friends and family are inclined to blame this behavior on "old age." Oftentimes, the behavior is due to a disorder known as Alzheimer's disease—the most common form of dementia among the elderly. It is estimated that 500,000 to 1.5 million older Americans are affected by it, although some estimates are as high as 2.5 million.

Alzheimer's disease was first described in 1906 by German neurologist Alois Alzheimer. The disease causes irreversible changes in nerve cells in certain vulnerable areas of the brain. It is characterized by nerve cell loss, abnormal tangles within nerve cells and deficiencies of several chemicals which are essential for the transmission of nerve messages. The disorder leads to behavioral and personality changes, forgetfulness, confusion, inability to learn new material, paranoia and motor activity problems. Language difficulties are also common in Alzheimer's disease. The disease typically progresses to the stage where it is difficult for the patient to be understood by others or understand others, and in the final stages the patient is bedridden.

The cause of Alzheimer's disease is not known. For many years, it was incorrectly believed that the hardening of the arteries (atherosclerosis), which can cause the blood vessels of the brain to narrow, led to Alzheimer's. Today a number of other factors, both genetic and environmental, are suspected of contributing to its development. Although the cause of the disease is unknown, genetics may play a role; the risk of Alzheimer's is higher among those who have relatives afflicted by it. Other possible causes include viral infections, inadequate diet and a deficiency of certain brain chemicals. There may be a link between aluminum and Alzheimer's disease, but scientific evidence on this is still inconclusive and the instances are rare.

It is important to diagnose Alzheimer's disease accurately in order to ensure that the mental impairment is not reversible. An estimated 5–10% of all mental deterioration in persons over 65 is due to reversible conditions such as depression, underlying physical disease (metabolic disorders, cardiovascular disease or pernicious anemia), excessive and inappropriate drug use, loss of social support or change in social environment. In order to diagnose Alzheimer's disease a physician must take a detailed medical history and a complete inventory of any prescription and over-the-counter drugs the patient is taking. Diagnosis also requires a set of laboratory examinations, such as blood and urine tests, and in most cases a CAT scan or magnetic resonance imaging (MRI) to detect structural abnormalities of the head and brain.

Although there is currently no cure for Alzheimer's disease, a great deal can be done to manage it. Treatment may include prescription medications and other therapies which help decrease depression. Proper diet, daily exercise and continued intellectual stimulation and social contact are extremely important for someone with Alzheimer's. Memory aids such as a prominent calendar, lists of daily tasks and labels on frequently used items can help compensate for memory loss and confusion. Family and friends should provide a comfortable and stimulating environment, and always try to give simple, easy to understand instructions. Day care programs may provide needed rest for care givers and support groups are often found to be helpful. The Alzheimer's Association sponsors support groups in many communities throughout the country. Current research into new drug treatments and dietary supplements is encouraging and provides hope for the future treatment of the disease.

SOURCE:
California Medical Association. "Alzheimer's Disease." *HealthTips* index 453 (April 1990): 1-2.

PREVALENCE

Studies done in the mid-1970's estimated that 2.5 million older Americans suffer from Alzheimer's disease. Now, NIA-supported scientists have given us reason to believe that the current number may be closer to 4 million, and that this figure may double or triple in the next century if more is not done to cure or prevent the disease.

Beginning in 1982, Dr. Denis Evans and his colleagues at Harvard Medical School in Boston, Massachusetts conducted a census of 32,000 people living in East Boston, a well-defined, stable, working-class community. More than 80 percent of the 4,485 residents over age 65 then participated in the first stage of examination by responding to a questionnaire concerning medical and social problems, and by taking a brief memory test.

Of these, 467 were selected for more extensive evaluation to rule out the presence of conditions other than Alzheimer's disease. The evaluation included a neurological examination, a brief psychiatric evaluation, laboratory tests, a brief review of medical history, and a review of current medications.

What Dr. Evans and his colleagues found was that more than 10 percent of the people over age 65 had probable Alzheimer's disease, and the prevalence of the disease rose more rapidly with age than previously suspected. Of those people between the ages of 65 and 74 years, 3 percent had probable Alzheimer's disease, as compared to 18.7 percent in the age 75 to 84 year group and a striking 47.2 percent over age 85. This translates to about 4 million Americans who might currently suffer from Alzheimer's disease.

Based on Census Bureau projections for the numbers of people 85 and older, Dr. Evans estimates that there could be a seven-fold increase in the numbers of oldest victims of Alzheimer's disease, contributing to a total of between 10 and 14 million people over 65 with Alzheimer's disease by the middle of the next century.

SOURCE:
National Institute on Aging. *Progress Report on Alzheimer's Disease*. 1990. pp. 1-2.

ETIOLOGY

Whether Alzheimer's is triggered by a virus, a toxin or anything else, there is no question that genes can help determine one's susceptibility. For one thing, people with Down syndrome, a genetic disorder involving an extra copy of the 21st chromosome, almost always develop Alzheimer's if they survive into their 40s. Moreover, Alzheimer's clearly runs in some families, following the classic pattern of dominant inheritance. (In these families, each child or sibling of an Alzheimer's victim stands a 50 percent chance of developing the disease himself.) Familial Alzheimer's disease, or FAD, may account for 10 to 30 percent of all cases. But its very existence suggests that a single gene can cause the illness. If the identity and function of that gene could be pinned down, notes Dr. David Drachman, head of neurology at the University of Massachusetts Medical Center, in Worcester, it would reveal much about the nature of Alzheimer's.

SOURCE:
Cowley, Geoffrey. "Medical Mystery Tour: What Causes Alzheimer's Disease, and How Does It Ruin the Brain." *Newsweek* (December 18, 1989): 60, 63.

ALZHEIMER'S DISEASE—AND ALUMINUM

An increased aluminum content in brain tissue of patients with AD had been reported, but analyses of bulk brain and the cores of neuritic plaques have shown no quantitative differences in aluminum content in samples from patients with AD and mentally normal elderly individuals.

SOURCE:
Mozar, H. N., and others. "Perspectives on the Etiology of Alzheimer's Disease." *JAMA* 257, no. 11 (March 20, 1987): 1503-1507. Copyright 1987, American Medical Association.

IMPACT ON FAMILY MEMBERS

The patient's immediate environment can similarly interfere with coping, adding to the level of impairment. Modifying the surroundings can reduce stresses imposed by environmental factors. There is the matter of safety, as in the need to protect the person from wandering toward a stairway and subsequently falling. There is the matter of lowering the individual's frustration level, such as by placing different cues in the immediate environment to combat memory loss and to reduce resulting stress and disorganization. There is the matter of finding the most protective but least restrictive setting for care which at some point may involve a move away from home to a nursing home or other care facility well equipped to deal with those who have Alzheimer's disease.

Stress on the family can take a toll on patient and caregiver alike. Caregivers are usually family members—either spouses or children—and are preponderantly wives and daughters. As time passes and the burden mounts, it not only places the mental health of family caregivers at risk, it also diminishes their ability to provide care to the Alzheimer's disease patient. Hence, assistance to the family as a whole must be considered.

As the disease progresses, families experience increasing anxiety and pain at seeing unsettling changes in a loved one, and they commonly feel guilt over not being able to do enough. The prevalence of reactive depression among family members in this situation is disturbingly high—caregivers are chronically stressed and are much more likely to suffer from depression than the average person. If caregivers have been forced to retire from positions outside the home, they feel progressively more isolated and no longer productive members of society.

The likelihood, intensity, and duration of depression among caregivers can all be lowered through available interventions. For example, to the extent that family members can offer emotional support to each other and perhaps seek professional consultation, they will be better prepared to help their loved one manage the illness and to recognize the limits of what they themselves can reasonably do.

SOURCE:
National Institute of Mental Health. *Useful Information on Alzheimer's Disease.* DHHS Pub. No. (ADM) 90-1696. 1990. pp. 14–15.

ALZHEIMER'S DISEASE—AND SPOUSES

Spouses are the main source of care for elderly people needing help. They provide the most extensive and comprehensive care, and are typically responsible for the most disabled older people. Furthermore, spouses maintain the role of caregiver longer, tolerate greater levels of disability than other caregivers, and are more likely to be care providers than care managers. Yet, their own advanced old age and concomitant chronic health problems yield caregiving spouses, a group at risk for serious physical and mental health problems. . . .

Across all indicators of mental health, spouse caregivers are more depressed, express higher levels of negative affect, are more likely to use psychotropic drugs, and have more symptoms of psychological distress than the population matched for age and gender.

In terms of physical health, the inclusion of several measures of both objective and subjective health reveal that the health of spouse caregivers is substantially poorer than the physical health of older people in the general population. Although caregivers use medical services (doctor visits, hospital stays), either at similar or lower rates than the population, and report spending less time in bed than the general population, these findings may be attributed more to the inability to allocate time to their own needs than to their actual health status. In addition, problems related to finding alternative care for the impaired spouse may prohibit caregivers from tending to their own health problems.

Caregiving spouses do, however, report higher rates of diabetes, arthritis, ulcers, and anemia than the population. Female caregivers also report more hypertension and heart trouble.

SOURCE:
Pruchno, R. A., and Potashnik, S. L. "Caregiving Spouses: Physical and Mental Health in Perspective." *Journal of the American Geriatrics Society* 37 (August 1989): 697, 702–703.

RESOURCES

ORGANIZATIONS

Alzheimer's Association. 70 E. Lake Street, IL 60601. (800) 621-0379.

Alzheimer's Disease Education and Referral Center. P.O. Box 8250, Silver Spring, MD 20907-8250.

National Council on the Aging, Family Caregivers Program. 600 Maryland Avenue SW, Washington, DC 20024.

National Institute on Aging. Information Center, 2209 Distribution Circle, Silver Springs, MD 20910. (301) 495-3455.

BOOKS

Aronson, M. K. (ed.). *Understanding Alzheimer's Disease.* New York: Scribners, 1988.

Guthrie, Donna. *Grandpa Doesn't Know It's Me.* New York: Human Sciences Press, 1986.

Mace, Nancy L., and Peter V. Rabins. *The 36-Hour Day: A Family Guide to Caring for Persons with Alzheimer's Disease.* Revised edition. Baltimore: Johns Hopkins University Press, 1991.

Reisberg, B. *Guide to Alzheimer's Disease.* New York: Free Press, 1983.

U.S. Congress, Office of Technology Assessment. *Summary. Confused Minds, Burdened Families: Finding Help for People with Alzheimer's and Other Dementias.* Washington, DC: U.S. Government Printing Office, 1990.

RELATED ARTICLES

Black, K. S., and P. L. Hughes. "Alzheimer's Disease: Making the Diagnosis." *American Family Physician* 36, no. 5 (November 1987): 196–202.

Dreary, I. J., and L. J. Whaley. "Recent Research on the Causes of Alzheimer's Disease." *British Medical Journal* 297, no. 6652 (October 1, 1988): 807–810.

Evans, D. A., and others. "Prevalence of Alzheimer's Disease in a Community Population of Older Persons: Higher than Previously Reported." *JAMA* 262, no. 18 (November 10, 1989): 2551–2556.

Kukull, W. A., and E. B. Larson. "Distinguishing Alzheimer's Disease from Other Dementias." *Journal of the American Geriatrics* 37 (June 1989): 521–527.

Levy, R. "Are Drugs Targeted at Alzheimer's Disease Useful?" *British Medical Journal* 300 (April 28, 1990): 1131–1132.

Mozar, H. N., and others. "Perspectives on the Etiology of Alzheimer's Disease." *JAMA* 257, no. 11 (March 20, 1987): 1503–1507.

Pfeiffer, E. "What's New in Alzheimer's Disease?" *Postgraduate Medicine* 83, no. 5 (April 1988): 107–109, 112–115.

"Practical Considerations in Managing Alzheimer's Disease I: A Geriatrics Panel Discussion." *Geriatrics* 42, no. 9 (September 1987): 78–94.

"Practical Considerations in Managing Alzheimer's Disease II: A Geriatrics Panel Discussion." *Geriatrics* 42, no. 10 (October 1987): 55–65.

Warshaw, Gregg A. "New Perspectives in the Management of Alzheimer's Disease." *American Family Physician* 42, no. 5, supplement (November 1990): 41S–47S.

ANABOLIC STEROIDS

OVERVIEW

The sports world was stunned in 1988 when Canadian sprinter Ben Johnson was stripped of his Olympic gold medal for using anabolic steroids, a day after apparently setting a world record in the 100-meter dash. But Johnson wasn't alone: Steroid use has exploded among top-level athletes, and it's spreading fast to health clubs and gyms across America, where millions of men, women and teenagers are buying huge quantities of the drugs from illegal vendors.

Their main goal is muscle. Anabolic steroids, also known as "'roids" or "juice," are synthetic versions of the hormone testosterone, which in its natural form is responsible for males' sexual differentiation in the womb and sexual development at puberty. When injected or taken orally, steroids can help make muscles bigger and stronger in just a few months. Unfortunately, the Charles Atlas look comes with some not-so-pretty side effects, including personality changes, high blood pressure, increased risk of heart disease and stroke, and possible long-term liver damage.

This hasn't kept an estimated 2 million to 3 million Americans, most of them men, from gobbling up the drugs like candy. A 1987 national survey of 3,400 12th-grade boys found that 6.6% had taken steroids, which translates into a national figure of 250,000 to 500,000 adolescents who have used or are currently using steroids. Two-thirds said they started using steroids by age 16, most to improve sports performance, but one out of four users took them simply to improve appearance. Growing numbers of female athletes are also taking steroids, despite their inevitable masculinizing effects.

One sign of steroids' allure is that so many of these so-called healthy users are willing to put up with disturbing physical changes from the drugs. Because steroids mimic the actions of testosterone, they shut down men's natural testosterone production; the testicles can begin to shrink—a change that may be irreversible—and after an initial burst of erotic energy, sexual interest drops off sharply. Other common side effects include breast growth (in men), male pattern baldness, acne and increased facial and body hair. Users may also develop inflamed hair follicles.

But as bad as these side effects sound, there's increasing evidence that far more serious changes can be traced to steroid use, some of which may go unnoticed for many years:

- Doctors have found that within just a few weeks steroids, especially the oral kinds, reduce levels of high-density lipoproteins (HDL's), increasing the risk of heart disease. In one 10-week study of bodybuilders on steroids, their HDL levels dropped an average of 63%. Some investigators think steroid use can thus significantly raise the lifetime risk of heart attack.
- There is evidence in animal studies that high doses of steroids cause blood platelets to clump together, which can trigger strokes and heart attacks. While the numbers are still very low, there are several reports of young bodybuilders dying suddenly in this way.
- Steroid use has been associated with increased risk of liver disorders (with oral steroids only), kidney disease, immune system disturbances and reproductive system disruptions. Again, the incidence of serious illness is low, and some of these conditions may clear up after steroid use has stopped, but long-term liver damage has also been reported.
- Sperm counts of 15 male athletes on steroids fell by an average of 73% during a two-month period.

- Steroids' negative side effects among female users include male pattern baldness, facial hair growth, thickened vocal cords and a deepened voice, and an enlarged clitoris. These changes appear to be permanent and may occur after just a few months of steroid use.
- Teenage steroid users face special risks, since the hormones can cause permanent changes where development is still under way, such as in the reproductive and skeletal systems. By causing the long bones to stop growing prematurely, the drugs may prevent teens from reaching full height.

The longer a person uses steroids and the more he takes, the greater the risks.

SOURCE:
Fultz, Oliver. "'Roid Rage: Anabolic Steroid Use Is Exploding—With Shattering Consequences." *American Health* 10 (May 1991): 60, 62.

ANABOLIC (TISSUE BUILDING) EFFECTS

Anabolic steroids are more precisely characterized as anabolic-androgenic steroids. They include testosterone, the primary male sex hormone, and all chemically altered derivatives of testosterone that have anabolic (tissue-building) and androgenic (masculinizing) properties. Synthetic anabolic steroids have greater anabolic activity than androgenic activity when compared with testosterone; in large quantities, however, the synthetic steroids also have strong androgenic effects. Anabolic steroids have medical indications in the treatment of refractory anemias, hereditary angioedema, certain breast cancers, hypogonadism and starvation states.

Athletes use anabolic steroids in the belief that these drugs increase body mass, muscle tissue, strength and aggressiveness. Testosterone and the synthetic anabolic steroids combine with an androgen receptor in skeletal muscles and other organs. This steroid/receptor complex stimulates production of RNA/DNA, which in turn leads to increased protein synthesis. In muscle, increased amounts of actin and myosin are produced under the influence of anabolic steroids. These force-producing contractile proteins result in increased strength.

SOURCE:
Hough, David O. "Anabolic Steroids and Ergogenic Aids." *American Family Physician* 41 (April 1990): 1157–1158.

FEDERAL REGULATION

Anabolic Steroids as Controlled Substances: New federal legislation adds certain anabolic steroid substances to Schedule III of the Controlled Substances Act (CSA), which is enforced by the Drug Enforcement Administration (DEA).

The new law applies the Schedule III registration, reporting, record keeping, prescribing, investigating, penalty, and other provisions of the CSA to anabolic steroids. Under Schedule III, only properly registered practitioners can issue prescriptions for anabolic steroids. Prescriptions are refillable a maximum of five times within 6 months from the date of issuance for substances that are controlled through Schedule III.

The new legislation also establishes criminal penalties under the Federal Food, Drug, and Cosmetic Act for distributing human growth hormone for nonmedical uses. The DEA, as well as the FDA, is authorized to investigate offenses concerning the distribution of human growth hormone.

This new legislation, part of the Omnibus Crime Control Act of 1990, was targeted at the growing trends in use, abuse, and diversion of anabolic steroids for nonmedical purposes. A recent American Medical Association Council on Scientific Affairs report (*JAMA*. 1990: 264; 2923–2927) described the legislative, legal, and professional education activities that have been applied by federal and state agencies and other organizations to address the anabolic steroid abuse problem.

SOURCE:
Nightingale, Stuart L. "Anabolic Steroids As Controlled Substances." *JAMA* 265, no. 10 (March 13, 1991): 1229.

EFFECTIVENESS OF STEROIDS

Many athletes believe that steroids can improve their performance. Reports are abundant in the scientific and popular literature that numerous athletes, both male and female, regularly treat themselves with high doses of anabolic-androgenic steroid compounds in hopes of achieving a competitive edge.

The results of various tests have failed to show any consistent improvement in aerobic performance, as measured by maximal oxygen uptake, or running or swimming times. Experienced weight-trainers have found increases in strength, however, when anabolic-androgenic steroids were supplemented with a high-protein diet.

SOURCE:
Minelli, Mark J. "Athletes at Risk: Steroids." *Addiction & Recovery* 10 (August 1990): 30.

RESOURCES

ORGANIZATION
American College of Sports Medicine. P.O. Box 1440, Indianapolis, IN 46204.

PAMPHLET
Food and Drug Administration:

Anabolic Steroids: Losing at Winning. DHHS Pub. No. (FDA) 90-3171. 1990. 5 pp.

RELATED ARTICLES

Buckley, William, and others. "Anabolic Steroid Use In Teens on the Rise." *Parents' Pediatric Report* (February 1989): 6.

Cowart, Virginia S. "Blunting 'Steroid Epidemic' Requires Alternatives, Innovative Education." *JAMA* 264 (October 3, 1990): 1641.

Paterson, Ellen R. "Steroids and Sports." *RQ* 29 (Fall 1989): 20-22.

Ramotar, Juliet E. "Getting Tougher on Steroid Abuse." *The Physician and Sportsmedicine* 19 (February 1991): 46.

Woolley, Bruce H. "The Latest Fads to Increase Muscle Mass and Energy: A Look at What Some Athletes Are Using." *Postgraduate Medicine* 89, no. 2 (February 1, 1991): 195-205.

ANEMIA

OVERVIEW

If you are feeling fatigued, and believe the ads about "tired blood," you might think that taking an iron supplement will cure iron deficiency anemia and pep you right up. In truth, however, most fatigue is not related to tired blood; most anemia comes on without any noticeable symptoms at all; and most anemia in older adults is not due to low iron intake, but rather to slow intestinal bleeding.

Anemia is one of the most common disorders among older adults. It is usually discovered not by a person reporting symptoms to a doctor—but rather by the complete blood count your doctor periodically orders. Indeed, screening for anemia is one of the important reasons for doing a complete blood count.

Anemia is not a normal consequence of aging, as had been thought until recently. Nor is anemia itself a disease, it is, rather, a manifestation of any one of a number of different disorders or diseases that affect your red blood cells—ranging from iron deficiency anemia to the less common types, such as hemolytic and aplastic anemia. All the anemias have different origins, and different treatments. We focus here on the three most common, which have their origin in vitamin or mineral deficiencies.

Iron deficiency anemia arises from too little iron in your body to make sufficient hemoglobin. Most of the blood cells of your body, including the red blood cells that perform the crucial task of picking up oxygen in your lungs and taking it throughout your system, are produced in the marrow that lies within certain bones.

The principle component of these red blood cells, the substance that enables them to transport oxygen, is a special protein, hemoglobin—and a necessary component of hemoglobin is iron. A decrease in the quality or quantity of hemoglobin, or in the number of red blood cells themselves, results in a reduced oxygen-carrying capacity in your blood—which is to say, in anemia (from the Greek, meaning "a lack of blood").

By far the most frequent cause of iron deficiency among older adults is excessive blood loss, which takes iron from the body faster than it can be replaced. This is usually the result of slow, persistent bleeding from any number of intestinal lesions—for example, an ulcer, polyps, or cancer. The frequent use of aspirin, ibuprofen, or other non-steroidal anti-inflammatory drugs can also result in chronic blood loss from irritation of the stomach lining. Bleeding from the intestines, when severe, generally shows up as black tarry stools, or even frankly bloody stools; or most commonly, however, the bleeding is very slow and not readily apparent (so called "occult blood").

It is possible, too, that iron deficiency anemia can be caused by too little iron in your diet—though this is very unusual, except among menstruating women whose diets have a limited iron content. Most iron in red blood cells is recycled to make new red blood cells—and the amount of iron lost in the recycling process is so miniscule (just 1 mg a day for men, 2 mg for menstruating women) that most diets easily compensate for the loss, except those on severe weight-loss plans and impoverished people who have little variety of food sources. (Because your body only absorbs 10% of the iron you consume, you need to have 10 mg of iron per day—an amount easily provided by a balanced diet of about 1,700 calories.)

Another possible cause of this type of anemia is an inability of the digestive system to absorb iron—most often because part of the stomach or intestine has been removed surgically. But this, too, is uncommon. Again, the most common cause of iron deficiency anemia is slow bleeding.

As you might imagine, the symptoms of iron deficiency anemia—when and if they do appear—are paleness (because it is the pigmented red cells flowing near the skin that produce the pinkness of your complexion), a feeling of weakness (because oxygen is required to use energy), fatigue, and, in more severe cases, shortness of breath, heart palpitations and an increased heart rate, especially during exertion (as the heart tries to compensate for the lack of oxygen in the system by pumping out more blood), and even chest pains (not totally because the blood flow is impeded, as in coronary artery disease, but because the blood can't carry sufficient oxygen to the heart). Certain nutritional anemias may manifest as a sore tongue or tiny cracks at the corners of your mouth.

But you should not, under any circumstances, attempt to treat yourself if you feel "anemic." Adding iron-rich foods or multivitamins with iron to your diet, or taking Geritol, is almost certainly just a way of ignoring the problem. Taking iron supplements may not address the underlying condition (such as an ulcer or a cancer) that is causing the anemia.

Vitamin B-12 deficiency, or pernicious anemia, most often occurs among older adults. Except among strict vegetarians, or those who have had certain forms of digestive-tract surgery, B-12 deficiency is the result of an impaired ability of the digestive tract to absorb the B-12 that is a normal part of your diet. For some reason, the condition occurs more often in fair-haired older people of northern European descent.

Vitamin B-12 is essential for the production of red blood cells; if it is deficient in your system, the production of red blood cells declines. B-12 is vital also to the maintenance of the nervous system, so a B-12 deficiency produces not only the usual symptoms of anemia, but leads to damage of the brain and spinal cord—which can show up in numbness and tingling in the hands and feet, a disturbed sense of balance with a change in walking gait, and mental disturbances such as confusion, personality changes, and depression. Because so much B-12 is stored in the liver, it can take a long time for a deficiency to develop. If you have a close relative who has had pernicious anemia, your risk of having it yourself is increased. You ought to inform your physician and be certain to have the appropriate blood tests. The disorder is commonly called pernicious anemia because it used to be untreatable, though today it can almost always be effectively treated.

Current treatment usually consists of a life-long regimen of monthly B-12 injections. Neither diet nor any oral supplement can help, since the underlying problem is non-absorption of B-12 from the gastrointestinal tract. If the deficiency is caught and treated promptly, you should recover completely.

Folic acid deficiency is usually caused by an inadequate intake of folic acid, a vitamin mainly supplied by the fresh green leafy vegetables, mushrooms, lima beans, and kidney beans in your diet. Since the body cannot store folic acid, a dietary deficiency will ordinarily show up in only a few weeks as anemia, because folic acid, like B-12, is essential in the production of red blood cells. Folic acid deficiency may occur among older people who have, for whatever reason, a poor diet. It is particularly common among heavy alcohol drinkers. This form of anemia is simple to treat with folic acid tablets for a short period of time—followed by an attentiveness to including a range of green vegetables in your diet. Treatment may be less simple if the deficiency results from an inability to absorb folic acid in the digestive tract—though this is less common.

The bottom line: Anemia is common among older adults, and the most common form of it is iron deficiency anemia. But do not treat yourself with iron supplements; rather, see your physician if you have any "anemic" symptoms. Above all, be sure to have a periodic blood test.

SOURCE:

"Anemia: Different Causes, Different Cures." *The Johns Hopkins Medical Letter, Health After 50* (February 1991): 4–5.

TAKING IRON SUPPLEMENTS

If your doctor prescribes iron supplements, ask your druggist for the cheapest generic available. Coated, time-release, or combination pills cost much more and may actually impede the iron's absorption into your system.

- Take your pill with at least eight ounces of fluid.
- Take it between meals to maximize iron absorption, but, if it causes stomach upset, take the pill with food or right after a meal.
- If you take iron in liquid form, mix it with water or fruit juice and drink it through a straw so that it doesn't stain your teeth. (If you do get stains, brush your teeth with baking soda or 3% hydrogen peroxide.)
- If you miss a dose, skip it; don't double up on doses.
- Keep your medicine out of reach of children. As few as three or four adult iron tablets can cause serious poisoning in young children.
- Do not store iron tablets in your bathroom medicine cabinet, since heat or moisture may cause the medicine to break down. Keep them in a cool, dry place.
- While you are taking iron, consume the following foods in only very small amounts, and then only an hour before or two hours after your iron tablet: tea, coffee, cheese, eggs, ice cream, and milk, because they decrease absorption; and whole-grain breads and cereals, because they are already iron-fortified.
- Check with your doctor if you have any of the more common side effects of iron supplements (constipa-

tion, diarrhea, heartburn), particularly if you experience nausea or vomiting.

- If you are taking a long-acting or enteric-coated iron tablet, such as Enseals or Fero-Gradumet, and your stools do not turn black, check with your doctor, since the tablets may not be breaking down properly. If your stools are black and tarry, and are accompanied by cramps, soreness, or sharp pains in the stomach, or red streaks in the stool, check with your doctor at once, since this may indicate gastrointestinal bleeding.
- Do not take an iron supplement for more than six months without checking back with your doctor.

SOURCE:
"Anemia: Different Causes, Different Cures (Taking Iron Supplements)." *The Johns Hopkins Medical Letter, Health After 50* (February 1991): 5.

SICKLE CELL ANEMIA

[Sickle cell anemia] is an inherited blood disease which can cause bouts of pain, damage to vital organs, and for some, death in childhood or early adulthood. Its effects vary greatly from one person to another, and from one time to another in the same person. Most people with sickle cell anemia enjoy reasonably good health much of the time.

Oxygen-carrying red blood cells are normally round and flexible. But under certain conditions, the red blood cells of a person with sickle cell anemia may change into a crescent or sickle shape within the blood vessels. Sickled cells tend to become trapped in the spleen and elsewhere and are destroyed. This results in a shortage of red blood cells which, when severe, can cause the patient to be pale, short of breath, and easily tired. Patients may be prone to certain infections which can worsen their condition, and their physical growth and development are often slower than normal.

Sometimes certain conditions may worsen a patient's anemia. This can happen when red blood cells are either destroyed, not produced in sufficient amounts, or are removed from circulation. For example, infections and other problems can speed up destruction of red blood cells. A tell-tale sign of this is the yellowing of the whites of patients' eyes. Reduced red blood cell production can be caused by a viral infection or a vitamin deficiency, especially during in pregnant women with the disease. Large numbers of red blood cells may be trapped by the spleen. This occurs primarily in young children.

Infants and young children with sickle cell anemia also are vulnerable to potentially life-threatening infections that spread quickly through the blood. Recently it has been shown that regular doses of penicillin taken by mouth can prevent development of these serious infections, when the disease is diagnosed early and treatment is started immediately. Penicillin may need to be continued over a period of several years, until the child's own immune system is capable of fighting off infection.

What Is a Sickle Cell Crisis?

At times, sickled cells become stuck in tiny blood vessels. When other red blood cells pile up behind this jam, they lose oxygen and this causes them to sickle, so that vessels may become totally blocked.

These sickling crises usually occur in bones and in organs of the abdomen or chest. They deprive the tissues of oxygen. They are often very painful and, if long-lasting, can destroy areas of tissue. Crises that damage vital organs such as the brain, lungs and kidneys may lead to disability or even death. . . .

In the United States, most cases of sickle cell anemia occur among blacks, and Hispanics of Caribbean ancestry. About one in every 400 to 600 blacks and one in every 1,000 to 1,500 Hispanics inherit sickle cell disease. The disease also affects some people of Arabian, Greek, Maltese, Sicilian, Sardinian, Turkish and southern Asian ancestry.

SOURCE:
March of Dimes Birth Defects Foundation. *Sickle Cell Anemia.* (Public Health Education Information Sheet, Genetic Series.) February 1989. pp. 1, 2.

RESOURCES

RELATED ARTICLES

Farley, Patrick C., and Jaime Foland. "Iron Deficiency Anemia: How to Diagnose and Correct." *Postgraduate Medicine* 87, no. 2 (February 1, 1990): 89–93, 96, 101.

Goldberg, Mark A., and others. "Treatment of Sickle Cell Anemia with Hydroxyurea and Erythropoietin." *The New England Journal of Medicine* 323 (August 9, 1990): 366–372.

Rodgers, Griffin P. "Recent Approaches to the Treatment of Sickle Cell Anemia." *JAMA* 265, no. 16 (April 24, 1991): 2097–2101.

Segal, Marian. "New Hope for Children with Sickle Cell Disease." *FDA Consumer* 23 (March 1989): 14–19.

Welborn, Jeanna L., and Meyers, Frederick J. "A Three-Point Approach to Anemia." *Postgraduate Medicine* 89, no. 2 (February 1, 1991): 179–183, 186.

ANGINA PECTORIS

OVERVIEW

Angina pectoris, the medical term for pain behind the sternum (breastbone), is a common manifestation of coronary artery disease. The pain is caused by reduced blood flow to a segment of heart muscle [myocardial ischemia]. It usually lasts for only a few minutes, and an attack is usually quickly relieved by rest or drugs, such as nitroglycerin. Also, it is possible to have myocardial ischemia without experiencing angina.

Typically, angina is a pressing or squeezing pain that starts in the center of the chest and may spread to the shoulders or arms (most often on the left side, although either or both sides may be involved), the neck, jaw, or back. It is usually triggered by extra demand on the heart: exercise, an emotional upset, exposure to cold, digesting a heavy meal are common examples. There are, however, some people in whom an attack may occur while sleeping or at rest. This type of angina may be caused by a spasm in a coronary artery, which most commonly occurs at the site of atherosclerotic plaque in a diseased vessel.

Most people with angina learn to adjust their lives to minimize attacks. There are cases, however, when the attacks come frequently and without provocation—a condition known as unstable angina. This is often a prelude to a heart attack, and requires special treatment, primarily with drugs.

In most instances, drugs are recommended for the treatment of angina before surgery is considered. The major classes of drugs used to treat angina include the following.

Nitrates. These come in several forms: as nitroglycerin tablets to be slipped under the tongue during or in anticipation of an attack; as ointment to be absorbed through the skin; as long-acting medicated skin discs; or as long-acting tablets. The latter three forms are used mostly to prevent rather than relieve attacks. The nitrates work by reducing the oxygen requirements of the heart muscle.

Beta-blocking Drugs. These agents act by blocking the effect of the sympathetic nervous system on the heart, slowing heart rate, decreasing blood pressure, and thereby reducing the oxygen demand of the heart. Recent studies have found that these drugs also can reduce the chances of dying or suffering a recurrent heart attack if they are started shortly after suffering a heart attack and continued for 2 years.

Calcium-channel Blocking Drugs. These drugs are prescribed to treat angina that is thought to be caused by coronary artery spasm. They can also be effective for stable angina associated with exercise. All muscles need varying amounts of calcium in order to contract. By reducing the amount of calcium that enters the muscle cells in the coronary artery walls, the spasms can be prevented. Some calcium-channel blocking drugs also decrease the workload of the heart and some lower the heart rate as well.

SOURCE:

Bigger, J. Thomas, Jr. "Angina." In *The Columbia University College of Physicians & Surgeons Complete Home Medical Guide.* 2nd ed. Crown Publishers, 1989. p. 391.

SIGNS AND SYMPTOMS

Taken from Latin, angina means "strangling," and pectoris means "chest." A strangling sensation in the chest is an apt description of the condition, observes Houston heart specialist H.V. "Skip" Anderson, M.D. Coronary chest pain arises from atherosclerosis, a disease process in which fatty deposits (plaque) form inside the arteries of the heart, causing them to narrow.

Among people with angina, the inside diameter of the arteries remains adequate for ordinary blood flow but inadequate to meet the demands of exercise or sudden and strong emotional reactions. Inadequate blood flow means an inadequate oxygen supply for the heart—leading to the painful "strangling" sensation in the chest.

Classic or typical angina occurs predictably with physical exertion or strong emotional reactions and goes away just as predictably with rest. Occasionally, the pain may radiate to the left arm and shoulder or up to the jaw. Most people describe the pain as a kind of squeezing pressure, tightness or heaviness.

In some instances, chest pain results from other types of heart problems, including diseases that affect the heart muscle itself or the valves that control blood flow through the heart.

Occasionally, ulcers, gallstones, abnormal contractions of the esophagus or severe anxiety and panic attacks can cause chest pain.

"Unfortunately, however, typical chest pain in a man over age 40 or a woman over age 50 has a strong association with coronary artery disease," says Dr. Anderson, an assistant professor of medicine at The University of Texas Medical School at Houston. "It's not 100%, but it's 90% or greater."

SOURCE:
"Angina: A Warning Sign of Heart Disease." *The University of Texas Lifetime Health Letter* 3 (February 1991): 3.

USE OF NITROGLYCERIN

Nitroglycerin is usually effective in relieving anginal chest discomfort. It also can be used to prevent anginal pain. It is usually taken in tiny tablets placed under the tongue to dissolve but may also be prescribed as an oral spray. The nitroglycerin tablets are inexpensive and quick-acting. Keep a fresh, sealed supply of the tablets on hand at all times. As a general rule, avoid transferring your nitroglycerin tablets out of the original, dark glass bottle since the tablets are sensitive to heat, light and air. Do not keep cotton in the bottle because it will absorb the nitroglycerin. Always use the medicine as directed by your doctor.

Be sure to carry the nitroglycerin with you at all times. Take a tablet just before starting an activity you know is likely to cause anginal discomfort. Also, take a tablet when the discomfort does not subside within a minute or two after you have stopped the activity, or if it occurs when you are not physically active. Let your doctor know what usually causes your angina so that he can advise you about preventing attacks.

It may take several tablets a day to control your symptoms. Nitroglycerin is safe and not habit forming, so don't be afraid to take it. Ask your doctor what to do if nitroglycerin is not effective in relieving your angina completely or if the pain begins to increase in frequency or severity.

In some people, nitroglycerin causes a short headache or a feeling of fullness in the head. Often these symptoms will disappear after you have taken nitroglycerin several times. If not, your doctor may want to reduce the dosage in each tablet.

Some Tips on Nitroglycerin

- If your angina is not relieved after taking 3 tablets within a 10-minute period, seek medical attention promptly. If your doctor is not immediately available, go to your local hospital emergency room.
- Ask your doctor about refilling your nitroglycerin prescription at six-month intervals since old tablets can lose their strength; tablets that are effective should cause stinging or burning under the tongue.
- Your doctor may also prescribe longer-acting nitroglycerin compounds which are taken by mouth or applied to the skin as an ointment or a skin patch.

SOURCE:
American Heart Association. *Understanding Angina*. pp. 6–7.

STABLE ANGINA—TREATMENT

The therapeutic goals for the patient with angina pectoris are to minimize the frequency and severity of angina and to improve functional capacity at a reasonable cost and with as few side effects as possible. An integrated approach necessitates attention to conditions that might be aggravating angina, such as anemia or hypertension. Alterations in life-style and personal habits, such as cessation of cigarette smoking, are often necessary and should be continually reinforced by the physician. Certain concomitant diseases, such as chronic obstructive pulmonary disease, may influence the selection of drug therapy. Nitrates, β-adrenergic blockers, and calcium entry blockers are the major classes of drugs that can be used alone or in combination in a program that is designed for the individual patient. . . .

Aspirin and other antiplatelet agents, such as sulfinpyrazone, have shown no consistent antianginal effect, and, except for patients with unstable angina or acute myocardial infarction, their effect on reducing cardiovascular mortality in patients with stable angina remains unclear. Nevertheless, many physicians still recommend low-dose aspirin therapy (325 mg once daily or even every other day) because this approach is usually safe, inexpensive, and well tolerated.

SOURCE:
Shub, Clarence. "Stable Angina Pectoris: 3. Medical Treatment." *Mayo Clinic Proceedings* 65, no. 2 (February 1990): 256, 270.

RESOURCES

ORGANIZATION

American Heart Association. 7320 Greenville Ave., Dallas, TX 75231.

RELATED ARTICLES

Beyerle, Andrea, Gunther Reiniger, and Werner Rudolph. "Long-Acting, Marked Antiischemic Effect Maintained Unattenuated During Long-Term Interval Treatment with Once-Daily Isosorbide-5-Mononitrate in Sustained-Release Form." *The American Journal of Cardiology* 65 (June 15, 1990): 1434–1437.

California Medical Association. "Living with Angina." *HealthTips* index 271 (September 1982): 1–2.

Gleeson, Barbara. "Loosening the Grip of Anginal Pain." *Nursing 91* 21, no. 1 (January 1991): 33–39.

Munger, Thomas M., and Jae K. Oh. "Unstable Angina." *Mayo Clinic Proceedings* 65 (March 1990): 384–406.

"Painless Angina." *Harvard Medical School Health Letter* (February 1989): 3–4.

Wilcox, Ian, and others. "Risk of Adverse Outcome in Patients Admitted to the Coronary Care Unit with Suspected Unstable Angina Pectoris." *The American Journal of Cardiology* 64 (October 15, 1989): 845–848.

ANGIOPLASTY

(*See also:* HEART ATTACK; HEART BYPASS SURGERY)

OVERVIEW

Percutaneous transluminal coronary angioplasty (PTCA) is a nonsurgical procedure designed to dilate (widen or expand) narrowed coronary arteries. It works like this:

First, a doctor inserts a thin plastic tube (a catheter) into an artery in your arm or leg. He or she then guides this catheter to the aorta (the large artery that conducts blood from the heart to the rest of the body). From there it passes into the coronary arteries.

As the doctor guides the catheter to the coronary arteries, the procedure is monitored by a special x-ray camera called a fluoroscope. Once the catheter is passed into the narrowed coronary artery, a second, smaller catheter with a balloon on its tip is passed through the first catheter. You can think of this as one "pipe" passed through another.

As this second catheter is passed through the first, the balloon remains deflated; however, once the balloon tip reaches the narrowed part of the coronary artery, it's inflated. When the balloon is inflated, it compresses the plaque and enlarges the diameter of the opening within the blood vessel. After that, the balloon is deflated and the catheters are withdrawn.

The result of this procedure is that the blood vessel is dilated, and blood can flow more easily through the (formerly narrowed) part of the coronary artery.

Before your doctor considers PTCA, you'll undergo a variety of tests, including a cardiac catheterization. During this catheterization, a special dye will be injected into your coronary arteries and x-ray pictures will be taken to see where coronary artery disease is present. This procedure is called "coronary arteriography."

SOURCE:
American Heart Association. *What You Should Know about P.T.C.A.* 1985. pp. 2–5.

RISKS

Anyone facing angioplasty meanwhile can get a few key answers by asking his or her doctor these questions:

- How many angioplasties have you done?

The SCA [Society for Cardiac Angiography and Interventions] will probably recommend a minimum of 125 procedures during training and at least 50 a year thereafter. Many experts, however, believe a practitioner should do at least two a week to keep skills in the tricky procedure well honed.

- What percentage of your patients have a heart attack, die or suffer a complication during the procedure requiring surgery?

In the most experienced hospitals, about 1 percent of angioplasty patients die, 4.3 percent suffer a heart attack and 3.4 percent require emergency surgery. Numbers considerably higher than these may be cause for having the procedure elsewhere.

- Will there be surgical backup in case of emergency?

It's mandatory in case a vessel is punctured or a heart attack occurs during angioplasty.

Be sure to get a second opinion if the doctor doing the diagnosis would also perform the angioplasty. It's common practice for bypass surgery, and critics say angioplasty should meet the same standard.

You can always look into the possibility of a bypass; the chance that a vessel will reclose is much smaller. But neither angioplasty nor bypass surgery cures heart disease. Only a regime that incorporates diet, exercise and healthy habits can reduce risk.

SOURCE:
Carey, Joseph. "New Caution on the Heart Balloon: Critics of Angioplasty Worry about Inflated Success Claims." *U.S. News & World Report* 105 (July 25, 1988): 65.

STENOSIS (CONSTRICTION OR NARROWING)

The tendency of the dilated plaque to renarrow after angioplasty is called restenosis. An inevitable consequence of dilating the plaque and artery with the balloon is injury to the artery wall at the site of inflation. This injury is usually minor. A healing process begins immediately and takes several months to be completed. There are two major components of this healing process. First, there is a deposition of a group of blood cells called platelets, which form a coating on the inner wall of the artery. Second, the muscle cells of the artery wall are stimulated to regenerate and bolster the wall of the artery. When these two processes respond appropriately, the artery heals with the inner channel enlarged and there is little concern about this lesion renarrowing in the future. Occasionally, however, either of these two processes may respond in an exaggerated manner. Platelets can initiate clot formation on the inner wall of the artery. Excessive proliferation of artery muscle cells can thicken the wall of the artery. In either case, the net result is a renarrowing of the inner channel, or restenosis.

Restenosis occurs in approximately one out of four patients. To date, no drug or therapeutic action has been found to effectively prevent restenosis. A major research effort, however, is underway to study ways to lessen the occurrence of this frustrating problem.

If restenosis occurs, most patients can undergo another angioplasty. Occasionally, a third or even fourth angioplasty may be necessary before the artery remains open or patent.

SOURCE:
Raizner, Albert E. "All About Balloon Angioplasty." *HeartCorps* 2 (July-August 1989): 43.

LASER ANGIOPLASTY

Laser angioplasty, when reduced to Star Wars-like simplicity, has been alluring to both physicians and the general public since its introduction some 10 years ago. One popular interpretation of the technique: a little poof of light, and the plaque is gone.

But in practical terms, the technology has been plagued by logistical problems, including devising effective delivery and guidance systems and a lack of precise understanding of how lasers actually ablate plaque and interact with the cardiovascular system.

Laser systems have been turning over very rapidly during the past decade, with each new generation addressing a problem of the previous one. But now the pace seems to have slowed, with the technology entering a period of reevaluation and assessment of laser angioplasty's role.

"As sometimes happens in medicine, the glamour and excitement came ahead of practical applications," said Klemens Barth, MD, director of interventional vascular radiology at Georgetown University Hospital in Washington, D.C. Laser angioplasty "has been referred to as a technique looking for an application. Now we are cooling off and trying to find the best application."

The excitement began with the realization that laser energy could recanalize occluded vessels. At the same time, the limitations of balloon angioplasty were becoming apparent: for example, balloon angioplasty cannot cross totally occluded vessels and is associated with a high restenosis rate.

At the very least, it was hoped laser angioplasty could function as an adjunct to balloon angioplasty. At the most, it was hoped it could function as a stand-alone system producing better patency rates than balloon angioplasty. Above all, it was hoped that a laser system could be designed to work in the coronary arteries. . . .

One of the early researchers in thermal angioplasty was Timothy Sanborn, MD, director of laser angioplasty research at Mt. Sinai Hospital in New York City. While maintaining that hot-tipped lasers do have a narrow role in treating peripheral vascular disease, he acknowledges that wider applications have not developed. Reported negative results with the hot tipped lasers stem from physicians applying the technique to unsuitable candidates, he said. . . .

Ironically, thermal angioplasty does not even take advantage of the unique properties of laser energy. The hot tipped simply converts laser energy into thermal energy. Other cheaper energy sources, such as radio frequencies, have been used to create a hot tipped. Furthermore, when thermal angioplasty is used as an adjunct to balloon angioplasty, the total system still suffers from the limitations of the balloon procedure.

SOURCE:
Brown, Elizabeth. "Laser Advancements Spur Debate on Role in Angioplasty." *American Medical News* 33 (April 20 1990): 18.

ANGIOPLASTY OR CORONARY ARTERY BYPASS SURGERY?

People whose angina has not been relieved by medications are candidates for this procedure [angioplasty]. The ideal candidate has only one narrowed artery, although many persons with several areas of narrowing can undergo PTCA [percutaneous transluminal coronary angioplasty]. The decision to recommend PTCA rather than bypass surgery is based on the location, number, and severity of blockages as well as the overall function of the heart.

However, the procedure does not cure the underlying disease. In fact, the procedure may have to be repeated to reopen the same or another artery that becomes blocked.

In future years, physicians may be able to remove plaque by using laser light or mechanical devices. . . .

If you have mild angina or have recovered from a heart attack with no continuing symptoms, you are probably best treated by medication or other means rather than by a bypass or other operation.

Although there have been controversial aspects of coronary artery bypass surgery, especially in the early days of its use, the consensus now favors this treatment in appropriate situations: for those with a blocked left main coronary artery; for those with disease in multiple vessels and poor function of the left ventricle (the main pump of the heart); and for those with debilitating angina. For these persons, a bypass procedure is of clear value in most cases and life is clearly prolonged.

SOURCE:
Larson, David E. *Mayo Clinic Family Health Book*. New York: William Morrow and Company. pp. 813, 814.

RESOURCES

RELATED ARTICLES

Faxon, F. P., N. Ruocco, and A. K. Jacobs. "Long-Term Outcome of Patients After Percutaneous Transluminal Coronary Angioplasty." *Circulation* 81, no. 3, supplement (March 1990): 9–13.

Holmes, David R., Jr., and Ronald E. Vlietstra. "Balloon Angioplasty in Acute and Chronic Coronary Artery Disease." *JAMA* 261, no. 14 (April 14, 1989): 2109–2115.

Naunheim, Keith S., and others. "The Changing Mortality of Myocardial Revascularization: Coronary Artery Bypass and Angioplasty." *Annals of Thoracic Surgery* 46, no. 6 (December 1988): 666–674.

Popma, Jeffrey J., and Gregory J. Dehmer. "Management of Patients after Coronary Angioplasty." *American Family Physician* 41, no. 1 (January 1990): 121–129.

ANTI-INFLAMMATORY DRUGS

OVERVIEW

When the FDA approved over-the-counter sales of ibuprofen in 1984, the drug became one of the most widely used pain relievers in the United States. Sold under brand names such as Motrin, Advil, and Midol, ibuprofen is one of a family of drugs known as nonsteroidal anti-inflammatory drugs, or NSAIDs, most of which are still available only by prescription. Stronger than aspirin, these drugs have a remarkable ability not only to relieve pain but also reduce inflammation in a host of conditions, including arthritis, painful menstrual periods, muscle aches, and headaches.

The drugs are especially useful in treating arthritis. They act specifically against the body's production of prostaglandins (PGs), those mysterious molecules that are somehow involved in all kinds of bodily processes—some good, some bad. In the kidney, for example, PGs are instrumental in maintaining adequate blood flow; in the stomach, they protect its lining against stomach acids. On the other hand, PGs are somehow involved in the pathological process that leads to inflammation of joints (arthritis), tendons (tendonitis), and muscles (myositis). By inhibiting the production of PGs, ibuprofen drugs relieve pain and promote healing in these inflammatory diseases—but in the process, they may produce undesirable and sometimes severe side effects by inhibiting the good PGs in the kidney and stomach.

NSAIDs are related to aspirin, and persons with a particular sensitivity to aspirin (the so-called aspirin syndrome, which produces asthma and nasal polyps) may not tolerate NSAIDs either. Similarly, some patients are susceptible to kidney or stomach damage as the result of the action of NSAIDs on the prostaglandins in those organs. Although they pose no great risk to young, healthy persons who use them intermittently, elderly patients may have more of a problem because they are more apt to have chronic arthritis and similar conditions requiring heavy and continuous use of the drugs.

Although estimates place only 1 in 6,000 elderly patients on NSAIDs with gastrointestinal bleeding, the risk of this or other complications increases when more of these drugs are taken, especially for longer periods. Some relief seems now to be available in a new drug, misoprostol (Cytotec), which has recently received FDA approval. Related to the prostaglandin that keeps stomach acid in check, the drug has been shown to heal ulcers and related stomach lining damage caused by NSAIDs. It does, however, have some undesirable side effects of its own—and it is very expensive. For those who must take NSAIDs but who also suffer from their side effects, it may be a useful adjunct to therapy.

The common NSAIDs still requiring a prescription are naproxen (Naprosyn), piroxicam (Feldene), indomethacin (Indocin), tolmetin sodium (Tolectin), mefenamic acid (Ponstel), diflunisal (Dolobid), and diclofenac sodium (Voltaren). The risk of adverse reactions seems to rise with the daily doses of these drugs, and the elderly, as well as those having kidney disease, heart failure, excessively high blood pressure, or chronic heart disease, should be particularly careful about using over-the-counter ibuprofen. Also, ibuprofen should not be given to patients with ulcerative colitis, active peptic ulcer disease, or gastritis; the drug should be used with caution if there is a history of these disorders. With proper medical supervision, however, these drugs can safely be used by persons who may not have previously obtained significant and lasting pain relief.

SOURCE:

"Are We Having an NSAIDs Epidemic?" *Medical Update* 14, no. 8 (February 1991): 1–2.

BASIC TYPES—GENERIC AND BRAND NAMES

EXAMPLES OF PRESCRIPTIONS AND OVER-THE-COUNTER (NSAIDs)

Generic Name	Some Brand Names
Aspirin compounds	Anacin, Bayer, BC Powder, Bufferin, Discalcid, Ecotrin, Trilisate, Zorprin
Diclofenac sodium	Voltaren
Diflunisal	Dolobid
Fenoprofen calcium	Nalfon
Flurbiprofen	Ansaid
Ibuprofen	Advil, Medipren, Motrin, Nuprin, Rufen
Indomethacin	Indocin
Ketoprofen	Orudis
Meclofenamate sodium	Meclomen
Mefenamic acid	Ponstel
Naproxen	Naprosyn
Naproxen sodium	Anaprox
Phenylbutazone	Butazolidin
Piroxicam	Feldene
Sulindac	Clinoril
Tolmetin sodium	Tolectin

SOURCE:
Arthritis Foundation. *Nonsteroidal Anti-Inflammatory Drugs (NSAIDs): Questions and Answers*. 1990. p. 2.

THERAPEUTIC USE

How you take a drug can be very important to both its effectiveness and safety. Sometimes it can be almost as important as what you take. Timing, what you eat and when you eat, proper dose, and many other factors can mean the difference between feeling better, staying the same, or even feeling worse.

Indomethacin and phenylbutazone should always be taken with food. Meclofenamate may be taken with meals. For other NSAIDs, however, your doctor may tell you to take the first several doses 30 minutes before or two hours after eating. This will help the medicine relieve the symptoms more quickly.

Like food, antacids may prevent an upset stomach when taking NSAIDs. However, both food and some over-the-counter antacids may interfere with an NSAID's effectiveness. Ask your doctor for the best approach for a particular NSAID.

Tablets and capsules should be washed down with eight ounces of water to help prevent the drugs from irritating the delicate lining of the esophagus and stomach. In addition, to let gravity help move the pills along—don't lie down for at least 15 to 30 minutes after each dose.

Be sure to take the right number of tablets or capsules for each dose. Liquid doses are best measured in special spoons available from your pharmacist. Teaspoons or tablespoons from the kitchen drawer are rarely the right dosage size.

In general, only take a missed dose within two to four hours of its originally scheduled time. However, because the duration of action of NSAIDs varies, contact your doctor for specific advice. DO NOT DOUBLE DOSES. Be sure to refill your prescriptions soon enough to avoid missing any doses.

Most NSAIDs start to relieve pain symptoms in about an hour. However, for long-term inflammation and for severe or continuing arthritis, relief may not come for a week to several weeks.

How long you will need to take the medicine depends on the condition being treated. Make sure you understand your doctor's instructions.

Common side effects include nausea, cramps, indigestion, and diarrhea or constipation. Other side effects can include increased sensitivity to sunlight, nervousness, confusion, headache, drowsiness, or dizziness. If you have any of these side effects, notify your doctor.

Occasionally, NSAIDs can cause ulcers or bleeding in the stomach or small intestine. Warning signs include severe cramps, pain, or burning in the stomach or abdomen; diarrhea or black tarry stools; severe, continuing nausea, heartburn, or indigestion; or vomiting of blood or material that looks like coffee grounds. If any of these side effects occurs, stop taking the medicine and call your doctor immediately.

Other serious but rare reactions are:

- Anaphylaxis—Signs of this severe allergic reaction are very fast or difficult breathing, difficulty in swallowing, swollen tongue, gasping for breath, wheezing, dizziness, or fainting. A hive-like rash, puffy eyelids, change in face color, or very fast but irregular heartbeat or pulse may also occur. If any of these occurs, get emergency help at once.
- With phenylbutazone, sore throat or fever can be early signs that the drug has impaired the bone marrow's ability to produce blood cells. Call your doctor immediately. Because of the seriousness of this side effect, phenylbutazone is usually prescribed as a last resort and then for short periods only.
- Unusual swelling of the fingers, hands or feet, weight gain, or decreased or painful urination can indicate worsening of an underlying heart or kidney condition. If any of these symptoms occurs, call your doctor.
- During pregnancy or while breast-feeding, these drugs should not usually be taken.
- People 65 and older are more likely to experience the side effects of NSAIDs and get sicker with those effects than younger adults.
- Alcoholic beverages should be avoided, as they increase the potential for stomach problems while taking NSAIDs.

- Don't take acetaminophen or aspirin or other salicylates with NSAIDs unless directed by your doctor. Taking these drugs along with NSAIDs may increase the risk of side effects.
- Tell your physician if you are taking any other medication—prescription or nonprescription.
- Before any surgery or dental work, tell the physician or dentist that you are taking NSAIDs.
- Don't drive or operate machines if the medicine makes you confused, drowsy, dizzy, or lightheaded. Learn how the medicine affects you.
- Increased sensitivity to sunlight can occur in some people. To avoid the risk of a serious burn, stay out of direct sunlight, especially between 10 A.M. and 3 P.M.; wear protective clothing; and apply a sunblock with a skin protection factor of at least 15.

SOURCE:
Stehlin, Dori. "Nonsteroidal Anti-Inflammatory Drugs." *FDA Consumer* (June 1990): 33–34.

RISK OF ULCERS

Most people can take NSAIDs without serious stomach problems. Scientists do not yet know how to predict who will get ulcers. Research to date suggests that you may be at risk for getting an ulcer from NSAIDs if you have one or more risk factors.

- over age 60
- severe disability from other chronic diseases
- smoking
- prior history of ulcers
- use of cortisone-type drugs and NSAIDs

If you can check one or more of the possible risk factors for ulcers from NSAIDs, talk with your doctor about ways to reduce your risk for getting an ulcer.

If you are on NSAIDs, there are several steps you can take now that may help reduce your risk for ulcers. These steps include the following:

- stop smoking
- drink limited amounts of alcohol
- take exactly the amount of NSAIDs your doctor prescribes, no more
- let your doctor know if you are taking aspirin or other over-the-counter NSAIDs
- watch for and report signs of an ulcer to your doctor

In addition to the changes you can make, your doctor may suggest several ways to reduce your chances for getting an ulcer from NSAIDs. If you are at high risk, your doctor may recommend the following:

- stop using NSAIDs
- use the lowest possible dose of NSAIDs
- take a drug that may prevent stomach ulcers: generic name—misoprostol; brand name—Cytotec

SOURCE:
Arthritis Foundation. *Nonsteroidal Anti-Inflammatory Drugs (NSAID) and Ulcers*. 1989. pp. 6–7.

* * *

Nonsteroidal anti-inflammatory drugs (NSAIDs) are a significant cause of gastric mucosal injury and bleeding, particularly in elderly patients. The mechanism of this injury appears to be, at least in part, a disruption of normal cytoprotective mechanisms by the inhibition of prostaglandin production. Acute injury results from the local effect of some drugs and may resolve with time. Chronic injury may occur with any NSAID and may often be asymptomatic until a complication occurs. Treatment of either lesion centers around NSAID withdrawal and standard ulcer therapy. Although routine prophylaxis of all patients is not indicated, those patients with a history of NSAID injury or other risk factors may need preventive measures if they are treated with NSAIDs. Oral prostaglandins, such as misoprostol, are effective in the prevention of NSAID-induced injury. The efficacy of sucralfate and H2-blockers in this setting appears promising but requires further study.

SOURCE:
Moore, John G., and David J. Bjorkman. "NSAID-Induced Gastropathy in the Elderly: Understanding and Avoidance." *Geriatrics* 44, no. 8 (August 1989): 51.

RESOURCES

ORGANIZATION
Arthritis Foundation. P.O. Box 19000, Atlanta, GA 30326. Or local affiliate.

RELATED ARTICLES

Bakris, George L., and Sidney R. Kern. "Renal Dysfunction Resulting from NSAIDs." *American Family Physician* 40, no. 4 (October 1989): 155–204.

"Gastrointestinal Side Effects Associated with NSAID Use." *American Family Physician* 40, no. 6 (December 1989): 167.

Gay, George R. "On Other Side Effects of NSAIDs." *JAMA* 264 (November 28, 1990): 2677-2678.

Hochberg, Marc C. "NSAIDs: Patterns of Usage and Side Effects." *Hospital Practice* 11, no. 3 (May 15, 1989): 167–174.

Rashad, Shawk, and others. "Effect of Non-Steroidal Anti-Inflammatory Drugs on the Care of Arthritis." *The Lancet* 2 (April 2, 1989): 519–522.

Williams, James H, and Daniel O. Clegg. "Basic Therapy of Rheumatoid Arthritis: Nonsteroidal Anti-Inflammatory Drugs." *Comprehensive Therapy* 16, no. 5 (May 1990): 58–64.

ARTHRITIS

OVERVIEW

Arthritis is a serious disease that causes pain and loss of movement. It affects the movements you rely on for everyday activities. Arthritis is usually chronic. This means that it can last on and off for as long as a lifetime. There are over 100 kinds of arthritis, which can affect many different parts of the body. Joints are most often affected. People of all ages, including children and young adults, can develop arthritis. . . .

The word arthritis literally means joint inflammation ("arth" = joint; "itis" = inflammation) and refers to more than 100 different diseases. . . .

Inflammation is a reaction of the body that causes swelling, redness, pain, and loss of motion in an affected area. It is the major physical problem in the most serious forms of arthritis. Normally, inflammation is the way the body responds to an injury or to the presence of disease agents such as viruses or bacteria. During this reaction, many cells of the body's defense system, called the immune system, rush to the injured area to wipe out the cause of the problem, clean up damaged cells, and repair tissues that have been hurt. Once the "battle" is won, the inflammation normally goes away and the area become healthy again.

But in many forms of arthritis, the inflammation does not go away as it should. Instead, it becomes part of the problem, damaging healthy tissues of the body. This may result in more inflammation, more damage, and so on in a continuing cycle. The damage that occurs can change the bones and other tissues of the joints, sometimes affecting their shape, and making movement hard and painful. Diseases in which the immune system malfunctions and attacks healthy parts of the body are called autoimmune diseases.

SOURCE:
Arthritis Foundation. *Arthritis: Basic Facts, Answers to Your Questions*. 1990. pp. 1-2, 3.

RHEUMATOID ARTHRITIS

Arthritis—pain and inflammation of joints—has many forms. Rheumatoid arthritis can be one of the most disabling types of arthritis. Its course is variable—from just a few symptoms to severe, painful deformities. Three times as many women as men are affected, usually at a fairly young age (between 25 and 50). The disease may come on slowly or appear suddenly.

Rheumatoid arthritis typically affects the small finger joints, wrists, knees and toes. All joints of the body, however, are potential targets. Along with swelling and pain of joints, some of the early symptoms of the disease may include fatigue, loss of appetite, weight loss and fever. Stiffness in the joints and surrounding muscles that lasts for several hours after getting up in the morning is a regular symptom. Sometimes the disease involves other organs, causing damage to the heart, lungs, eyes, skin and nerves.

Many individuals with rheumatoid arthritis feel that their arthritis is influenced by the weather, stress, temperature and exercise. A few have periods of remission when the disease seems to have gone away. Unfortunately, in almost all the cases the symptoms eventually return.

The cause of rheumatoid arthritis is unknown. Some scientists feel that it may result from an infection, but there is no evidence that it is contagious. For whatever reason, the joint lining becomes very inflamed and thickened, slowly destroying cartilage and bone. The goal of treatment is to halt the inflammation and prevent the destruction of joints.

Medical supervision is a must. This form of arthritis can be crippling, other organs may be affected and all treatments may, on occasion, cause side effects. Doctors now have many ways of treating rheumatoid arthritis. Large doses of aspirin or aspirin-like drugs are effective in reducing pain and inflammation. If the arthritis is aggressive, other drugs, including anti-malarials, cortisone (steroids) or gold therapy may be used. A recently approved medication, methotrexate, is often effective if these other drugs are not satisfactory. All these drugs require close supervision since they may have hazardous side effects.

Rest, heat and physical therapy are important adjuncts to drug therapy. Proper diet and exercise will also help patients retain mobility and strength. Joint deformity or pain is sometimes so severe that surgery is the best alternative. A patient can have added years of mobility due to the hip, elbow, shoulder and knee replacements that can be performed today. The use of a splint or brace can also help straighten some joints. Although surgery cannot cure all deformities, advances in the field have given rheumatoid patients, who previously would have been wheelchair-bound, the ability to continue relatively normal lives.

One form of chronic arthritis which is less widely known is one that attacks children—juvenile rheumatoid arthritis. It may start with symptoms as general as fever and rash, and it may take a long time for a definite diagnosis to be reached. Other children complain of swelling and stiffness in a few scattered joints. When the disease threatens the function of the joints, skilled professional treatment is called for to prevent permanent deformity. The disease in its juvenile form often stops progressing within ten years, but the damage may be permanent and cause further deterioration of the joints. The major concern for the child, parent and doctor is to provide treatment that will spare the child deformity which persists long after the disease itself has disappeared.

SOURCE:
California Medical Association. "Rheumatoid Arthritis." *HealthTips* index 123 (March 1990): 1–2.

OSTEOARTHRITIS

Osteoarthritis is a disease that causes the breakdown of joint tissue, leading to joint pain and stiffness. It can affect any joint, but commonly occurs in the hips, knees, feet, and spine. It may also affect some finger joints, the joint at the base of the thumb, and the joint at the base of the big toe. It rarely affects the wrists, elbows, shoulders, ankles, or jaw, except as a result of injury or unusual stress.

Osteoarthritis is one of the oldest and most common diseases of man. It probably affects almost every person over age 60 to some degree, but only some have it badly enough to notice any symptoms. Osteoarthritis is also known by many other names, such as degenerative joint disease, arthrosis, osteoarthrosis, or hypertrophic arthritis.

Although there is no cure for osteoarthritis, proper treatment can help relieve the symptoms and prevent or correct serious joint problems.

SOURCE:
Arthritis Foundation. *Arthritis Information: Osteoarthritis.* 1990. pp. 1–2.

DRUG THERAPY

Today, the first pharmaceutical line of defense against arthritis is the NSAIDs (nonsteroidal anti-inflammatory drugs), which include the salicylates, such as aspirin, prescribed at higher than usual doses. Coated and timed-release preparations can lessen the risk of gastrointestinal bleeding, the major side effect of these drugs.

The NSAIDs block release of prostaglandins, which trigger inflammation. Some more commonly used NSAIDs include ibuprofen, flurbiprofen, indomethacin, and naproxen. Currently, 15 NSAIDs are available.

Drugs called disease modifiers are used in rheumatoid arthritis patients who have had symptoms for at least six months and for whom NSAIDs no longer control swelling of joints. One such treatment is gold injected into a joint, which helps about 50 percent of patients, but unfortunately remains effective in only 5 to 15 percent of them after five years of use.

"No one knows how it works, but it is not an anti-inflammatory," says [Dottie] Pease, [Consumer Safety Officer at FDA's pilot drug evaluation department]. The physical presence of gold in the joint may reduce swelling, or the metal may chemically react with a biochemical in some as yet unknown way.

Another disease modifier is methotrexate, an anti-cancer drug that tempers the runaway cell division in the synovial joint. If these disease modifiers do not work, agents that suppress the immune response, such as cyclophosphamide, may be tried.

Biologics Block Cytokines

Unraveling the immune imbalances that underlie some forms of arthritis, and investigating how drugs alter immune function to quell inflammation are opening up an entirely new avenue to treating arthritis—the use of "biologics," or body chemicals. A prime target for new arthritis drugs is blocking cytokine production, a different approach to halting prostaglandin synthesis, which is the mechanism of most existing arthritis drugs.

Innovative approaches under way include work at Nova Pharmaceuticals in Baltimore with unusual amino acids that, in test animals, block the release of inflammation-provoking cytokines from activated T cells (a specialized type of white blood cell). Laboratory research at Immunex Corporation in Seattle, Synergen Corporation in Boulder, Colo., and Hoffmann-La Roche in Nutley, N.J., focuses on using interleukin-1 to prevent inflammation. Interleukin-1 is an immune system chemical that must bind to the lining inside joints to start the inflammatory process.

SOURCE:
Lewis, Ricki. "Arthritis: Modern Treatment for That Old Pain in the Joints." *FDA Consumer* 25, no. 6 (July-August, 1991): 21.

DRUG THERAPY—GASTROINTESTINAL DAMAGE

A campaign is underway by the Arthritis Foundation to alert the public to the potential risks of gastric ulcers from the continued use of nonsteroidal anti-inflammatory drugs. These drugs, used regularly by arthritis patients, relieve pain and inflammation. Unfortunately, they can also produce "silent" ulcers that cause no pain or symptoms until bleeding occurs and/or the stomach wall perforates. The foundation says the incidence of gastric ulcers in chronic users of nonsteroidal anti-inflammatory drugs (NSAIDs) is estimated at somewhere between 10 and 20 percent, based on several published reports.

The drugs are the mainstay of arthritis therapy throughout the world," says Dr. Arthur Grayzel, the Foundation's senior vice president for medical affairs. "It is important for people taking these drugs to understand the possible risks and be aware of the potential for ulcers and what can be done to prevent and treat them."

In February, the Food and Drug Administration issued a revision in the working of prescription drug inserts. The inserts now must state that "gastrointestinal damage can occur without causing symptoms in persons taking nonsteroidal anti-inflammatory drugs." The only drug currently approved by the FDA to prevent ulcers stemming from NSAID use is misoprostol (brand name Cytotec), a medication available only by prescription. The foundation urges regular users of NSAIDs to discuss concerns about possible ulcers with their physicians. It the meantime, it will be making radio-and-TV public service announcements, as well as providing a toll-free telephone number for consumers to use in getting physician referrals and notification of local Arthritis Foundation services.

SOURCE:
"Arthritis Drug Alert." *Medical Update* 12 (May 1989): 2.

GENETIC LINK

Scientists said today that they had identified a genetic defect that appeared to cause at least some cases of arthritis.

The discovery is the first to suggest that some cases of osteoarthritis might have roots in the genes. But it was not immediately clear how many cases might be the result of this or other genetic defects. Osteoarthritis is the most common form of arthritis, afflicting 16 million Americans, including most of those over 70 years old.

The researchers, from Case Western Reserve University in Cleveland and Thomas Jefferson University in Philadelphia, studied members of an Ohio family prone to severe arthritis that develops early in life. The researchers found that those affected had a genetic defect that resulted in an abnormal collagen, the principal building block of cartilage, the tough material that covers and protects the bony surfaces in joints. In osteoarthritis, the normally smooth cartilage is torn and frayed.

The research, published in the *Proceedings of the National Academy of Sciences,* raises the possibility of devising specific new treatment for what is now an inexorably progressive condition, either by manipulating collagen or the defective genes themselves. Currently doctors treat the pain rather than the underlying disease. The research also offers the strongest evidence to date that collagen plays a major role in joint destruction.

"It's a landmark discovery, one that will probably lead to more research which will help sufferers," said Dr. Henry J. Mankin, chief of orthopedics at the Massachusetts General Hospital in Boston.

SOURCE:
Rosenthal, Elisabeth. "Genetic Link Suggested in One Form of Arthritis." *New York Times National* (September 5, 1990): A1.

RESOURCES

ORGANIZATION
Arthritis Foundation. P.O. Box 19000, Atlanta, GA 30326. Or local affiliate.

PAMPHLETS
Arthritis Foundation:

Coping with Pain: The Battle Half Won. 1987.

Guide to Medications: How to Use Them Wisely. 1989.

Rheumatoid Arthritis. 1987.

BOOKS

Brown, Thomas McPherson, and Henry Scammel. *The Road Back: Rheumatoid Arthritis—Its Cause and Its Treatment.* New York: Evans, 1988. 212 pp.

Kantrowitz, Fred G. *Taking Control of Arthritis.* Fairfield, OH: Consumer Reports Books, 1990.

Lorig, Kate, and James F. Fries. *The Arthritis Helpbook: A Tested Self-Management Program for Coping with Your Arthritis.* Revised ed. Reading, MA: Addison-Wesley, 1986. 266 pp.

Sayce, Valerie, and Ian Fraser. *Exercise for Arthritis.* Fairfield, OH: Consumer Reports Books, 1989. 96 pp.

Sheon, Robert P., and others. *Coping with Arthritis: More Mobility, Less Pain.* New York: McGraw-Hill, 1987. 375 pp.

Sobel, Dana, and Arthur C. Klein. *Arthritis: What Works.* New York: St. Martin's Press, 1989.

RELATED ARTICLES

Altman, Roy D. "Osteoarthritis: Differentiation from Rheumatoid Arthritis, Causes of Pain, Treatment." *Postgraduate Medicine* 87, no. 3 (February 15, 1990): 66–72.

"Arthritis: Heat Works." *Good Housekeeping* 209 (October 1989): 138–143.

Birnbaum, Neal S., Lynn H. Gerber, and Richard S. Panush. "Self-Help for Arthritis Patients." *Patient Care* (August 15, 1989): 69–72, 77, 80–82, 84, 91.

Corman, Lourdes C. "Rheumatoid Arthritis: New Developments in Treatment." *Postgraduate Medicine* 89, no. 2 (February 1, 1991): 75–88.

Gall, Eric. "Coping with Arthritis." *Executive Health Report* (August 1989): 1–3.

Roth, Sanford H. "New Directions in Treating Rheumatoid Arthritis." *Consultant* 29, no. 4 (April 1988): 67–80.

Stehlin, Dori. "Nonsteroidal Anti-Inflammatory Drugs." *FDA Consumer* (June 1990): 33, 35.

"Voltaren: The Mickey Mantle Drug is Associated with Severe Liver Damage." *Harvard Health Letter* (May 1991): 10.

Wilder, Ronald L. "Treatment of the Patient with Rheumatoid Arthritis Refractory to Standard Therapy." *JAMA* 259, no. 16 (April 22/29, 1988): 2446–2449.

Ziff, Morris. "Rheumatoid Arthritis—Its Present and Future." *The Journal of Rheumatology* 17, no. 2 (1990): 127–133.

ASTHMA

OVERVIEW

Fifteen million people—seven percent of those who live in the United States—have asthma. It is the number one cause for school absenteeism among all chronic diseases. It is the number six cause for hospitalization of all diseases and the number one cause for hospitalization of children.

It is estimated that $4.5 billion is spent every year on medically related charges for the treatment of asthma. That includes hospital and doctor visits. This is an extremely important disease that kills as many as 4,000 Americans a year.

Asthma is a disease of the airways, the tubes through which people breathe. The causes of airflow obstruction in asthma are swelling of the airways, excessive mucus production, inflammation of the airways with eosinophils and neutrophils, and airway smooth muscle contraction. Asthmatic airways are full of secretions, mucus containing eosinophils and neutrophils—white blood cells—that reflect the underlying inflammation. The epithelial cells that line the airways have been lifted off and the airways are denuded. The muscles contract, closing the airways, and the glands are very reactive and produce large quantities of mucus.

Asthma is an inability to breathe out. Normally when people breathe in, they lower their diaphragms, raise their ribs, and breathe in. It is an active process. To breathe out, they stop breathing in. Breathing out is passive. They breathe out because the lungs are made of elastic tissue, like a rubber band. When a person stops breathing in, the lungs try to assume their relaxed size and do so by letting the air out—if there is no obstruction.

Asthmatic airways have excess mucus, are swollen and inflamed, and have their muscles contracted. As people with asthmatic airways breathe in, they open up their chests and their lungs get bigger. As a result, the airways get bigger and they can move air around these obstructions. They have opened up the airways. When they stop breathing in to breathe out, these obstructions close, thereby trapping the air in the lungs.

Take a deep breath to the maximum and do not let it out for the next minute. Breathe at the top of your lungs and do not let out any air. That is what it feels like to have asthma. Asthmatics trap 2 liters of air in their chests, which is the amount of air in a basketball. They have to breathe at the top of their lungs. It is exhausting and feels terrible.

SOURCE:
National Institute of Allergy and Infectious Diseases. *Allergic Diseases.* NIH Pub. No. 91-3221. April 1991. pp. 13-15.

CAUSES AND EFFECTS

The most common signs of asthma are a feeling of tightness in the chest, coughing, difficulty inhaling and exhaling and noisy breathing ("wheezing"). Not all of these symptoms occur in every case.

The parts of the lung most directly affected by asthma are the bronchi and smaller bronchioles, the tubes through which oxygen passes into the body and carbon dioxide is expelled. During an attack, these airways narrow when the muscles around them tightly contract ("bronchospasm"). The membranes lining the inner walls of the air passages become swollen and inflamed, and the glands within these walls produce excess mucus or phlegm.

An asthma attack can be brief or it can last for several days. A very severe, prolonged attack can threaten a person's life. This condition, which requires specialized treatment in a hospital, is known as "status asthmaticus."

The negative effects of asthma on the body generally last only as long as the attack itself. Asthma does not cause serious, permanent damage to the lungs or heart. Persistent severe asthma can lead to secondary health problems such as chronic fatigue if it is not properly controlled.

A popular notion is that children can outgrow asthma. In some cases symptoms may decrease or disappear, perhaps because the airways get larger with normal growth, but the tendency toward asthma will always remain.

Asthma can begin at any age, in adults as well as children. The "triggers" of attacks, and the combinations in which they occur, vary from person to person.

Allergy can trigger asthma, although not all asthmatics are allergic and not all people with allergies have asthma. In allergic individuals, the immune system become sensitized to one or more substances known as allergens. Among the most common are pollens, house dust, mold spores, foods and animal danders. On later contact with the allergen, the allergic asthmatic's body produces chemicals that irritate his "twitchy" airways and bring on an attack. In the majority of adults with asthma, no specific allergic trigger can be identified.

Exercise frequently leads to wheezing and coughing in people who have asthma. This may be due to cooling or drying of the airways and is related to the amount on has to breathe during the exertion. Preventive treatment with certain medications (cromolyn and inhaled bronchodilators) usually helps. Physical activity is possible for all asthmatics and is crucial to their good health. Each must simply learn his level of tolerance.

Some people have idiosyncratic (unexpected) asthmatic reactions to normally harmless medicines and other chemicals. The allergic immune response is not involved. One example of such a substance is aspirin, which asthmatics should avoid unless it is prescribed by a doctor after careful testing. A small percentage of asthmatics are sensitive to tartrazine, a widely used yellow food coloring. Others react negatively to metabisulfite, a preservative sometimes added to fresh fruits and vegetables in grocery stores and restaurants and also found in wine and other foods.

Exposure to job-related triggering factors can cause asthma, and is often suspected when an adult with no history of the disease suddenly develops symptoms. Occupational asthma can be allergic or nonallergic, can affect workers of all kinds, and can be traced to a number of sources, from bacteria to wood dust to the chemicals in synthetic fibers.

Respiratory infection is a major asthma trigger. Irritation of the airways by tobacco smoke, perfume, air pollution and fumes from paint or household cleaners also can lead to attacks, as can exposure to cold air, sudden changes in temperature or humidity, and even laughing. Sinus inflammation and polyps (growths) in the sinuses or nose can also make asthma worse.

Strong emotions can bring on asthma symptoms, but this does not mean that the disease is of psychological origin. No amount of stress will bring on an attack unless a person already has hyperreactive airways. Asthma begins in the lungs, not in the head.

SOURCE:
National Jewish Center for Immunology and Respiratory Medicine. *Understanding Asthma.* 1985. pp. 2-3.

MANAGEMENT

The primary goal of asthma management is to eliminate all of the symptoms and maintain normal pulmonary function with the safest medical program. Important management issues, which are often overlooked, include identification and management of respiratory allergy to dust mites, pets and occupational exposures; appropriate (sparing) use of antibiotics; proper dosing and instruction in the use of aerosol corticosteroids; recognition and management of nocturnal asthma, and continuing assessment of the severity of asthma by measuring and monitoring pulmonary function. Adherence to these and other principles of management will help achieve the goal of symptom-free asthma.

SOURCE:
Li, James T. C. "Five Steps Toward Better Asthma Management." *American Family Physician* 40, no. 5 (November 1989): 201.

MEDICATIONS

Most of the medications useful in controlling asthma fall into three major groups:

1. **Bronchodilators** work by increasing the diameter of the air passages, easing the flow of gases to and from the lungs.

THEOPHYLLINE, one of the most effective asthma drugs, relaxes the muscles around the bronchi and makes these muscles less irritable, preventing airway constriction.

Theophylline is usually taken orally. Its level in the blood is crucial to its effectiveness, but the optimal blood level varies in different patients and can be changed by medications, diet and other factors. Theophylline does not become less effective with long use, cause dependency or have serious lasting side-effects.

Acute (short-term) problems that can result from taking theophylline are nausea and vomiting, loss of appetite, diarrhea, rapid heart beat, headaches, dizziness, insomnia, nervousness and personality changes. The physician usually can eliminate these effects by reducing the dosage.

The generic drug theophylline is sold under a variety of names. Some of them are Aerolate, Bronkodyl, Elixophyllin, Quibron, Slo-phyllin, Theo-dur, Theolair, Theospan and Uniphyl. Other drugs related to theophylline include aminophylline (Somophyllin) and oxtriphylline (Choledyl). Theophylline is also used in "combination drugs," for example Asbron, Marax, Quadrinol, Tedral and Verequad.

EPINEPHRINE (adrenalin) also works by dilating the bronchi. It is a short-acting medication, excellent for temporary relief of severe symptoms but not for everyday use.

Epinephrine is usually injected. (It is available in a metered-dose inhaler, but its use in this form is rarely recommended.) The side effects of epinephrine include increased heart rate, headache, jitteriness, blanching of the skin and sometimes nausea and vomiting.

Much more commonly used are inhaled beta-2 agents, medications related to epinephrine and similar in their effects. They are longer-lasting and have fewer cardiovascular side-effects. Examples are albuterol (Proventil, Ventolin), ephedrine, isoetherine (Bronkosol), Isoproterenol (Isuprel), metaproterenol (Alupent, Metaprel), and terbutaline (Brethine, Bricanyl). Some of these can also be taken orally but are much less effective in acute attacks.

ATROPINE SULFATE opens the airways by blocking reflexes through nerves that control the bronchial muscles. It is highly effective for some asthma patients.

Atropine sulfate is taken by inhalation. Since it affects bodily secretions, it can cause dry mouth, thirst and urinary retention. Other side effects are rapid heart beat and blurred vision.

A derivative of this drug which has fewer side effects is ipratropium (Atrovent). It is taken by metered-dose inhaler.

2. Cromolyn (Intal) appears to act by making the airways less sensitive to factors that trigger attacks. It can be useful to reduce reactions known but unavoidable allergens, and is also helpful when taken before exercise or exposure to some irritants. It is used only for prevention and has no value once symptoms have begun.

Cromolyn is inhaled. It has just a few known side effects. These include throat irritation and coughing, both of which can be controlled by bronchodilator drugs. Skin rashes occur rarely and resolve when the medication is discontinued.

3. Steroids reduce inflammation and swelling in the airways and allow other medicines to work better. They are effective anti-asthma drugs, but their potential for serious side effects limits their use.

Most steroids are taken orally. They can increase appetite, leading to weight gain. They can also cause puffiness of the face, extra growth of soft hair, acne, mood changes, high blood pressure, thinning of the bones, gastric ulcer, blood coagulation disorders, cataracts, and slowing of growth in children. Taking them increases the likelihood that hidden diabetes will become active.

It is extremely rare for one individual to experience all of these side effects. Most come only with long-term use, and can be minimized by careful scheduling of medication by the doctor.

The steroid most commonly prescribed for asthma is prednisone (Deltasone, Meticorten, Paracort). Methylprednisolone (Medrol) and prednisolone (Delta Cortef, Sterane) are also frequently used. Steroids that most doctors consider less desirable because of their severe side effects are dexamethasone (Decadron) and triamcinolone (Aristocort, Kenacort).

Beclomethasone (Beclovent, Vanceril) is taken by inhalation. It does not have as many side effects as other steroids. It can cause soreness in the mouth or throat, so the patient must gargle with mouthwash after each use. Inhaled steroids are not effective for acute severe attacks of asthma. Patients taking this form of medication should consult their physician immediately if their asthma begins to worsen, since dosage may need to be adjusted.

SOURCE:
National Jewish Center for Immunology and Respiratory Medicine. *Understanding Asthma.* 1985. pp. 6-7.

TREATMENT

There is evidence that the prevalence and severity of asthma are rising. The number of deaths from asthma may also be rising, contrary to the trend for other common treatable conditions. These alarming increases are occurring despite a marked increase in prescribed asthma therapy, which suggests that currently available therapy is inadequate or is not being used optimally. In the past, attention has been concentrated on bronchoconstrictor mechanisms and possible abnormalities of airway smooth muscle in asthma, with consequent emphasis on bronchodilator therapy. Recently, it has been recognized that chronic asthma involves a characteristic inflammatory response in the airways. This has important therapeutic implications and provides some insight into the action of antiasthma therapy.

Although it has long been recognized that fatal asthma is associated with marked inflammatory changes in the submucosa of the airways, it is now apparent that inflammation is present even in patients with very mild asthma. Biopsies of bronchial tissue from patients with asthma have demonstrated that infiltration by inflammatory cells, particularly eosinophils and lymphocytes, and epithelial shedding are prominent features. Bronchoalveolar lavage has also revealed an increased proportion of inflammatory cells, particularly eosinophils, in patients with asthma, and the number of cells increases after allergen challenge. . . .

In the light of recent research emphasizing the inflammatory component of asthma, it seems important to stress the advantage of long-term antiinflammatory therapy. . . .

Earlier introduction of antiinflammatory agents, such as corticosteroids or cromolyn sodium, is strongly recommended. Effective suppression of airway inflammation reduces the need for bronchodilator therapy and may reduce the morbidity and, perhaps, mortality of asthma.

SOURCE:
Barnes, Peter J. "A New Approach to the Treatment of Asthma." *The New England Journal of Medicine* 321, no. 22: (November 30, 1989): 1517-1518, 1523, 1525.

USE OF INHALED STEROIDS

The most important finding in the last five years concerns the role played by inflammation. Asthma, even in its mildest form, is now recognized as an inflammatory disease, not solely one of bronchial constriction. This has radically altered the way drugs are prescribed. . . .

The drug treatment of asthma has always been aimed at relieving the constriction of the bronchial tubes, or air passages to the lungs. For children and adults, the most commonly prescribed antiasthma drugs come from two chemical families: theophylline and the beta-adrenergics. They are called bronchodilator drugs because they open the air passages by relaxing the muscles of the walls. Doctors often prescribe one from each "family" for an additive effect. Another commonly prescribed drug is cromolyn, which reduces the lungs' response to allergens. . . .

In the U.S., inhaled steroids are not commonly used as an initial treatment, and oral steroids are reserved for severe asthma that is resistant to all other treatments. Much of the credit for attempting to change the American approach to drug therapy goes to British physician Peter J. Barnes of the National Heart and Lung Institute and Brompton Hospital in London. This panelist's reputation had preceded him with the publication of "A New Approach to the Treatment of Asthma" in *The New England Journal of Medicine* (30 November 1989). The alarming increase in asthma prevalence, severity and possibly the number of deaths in industrialized countries, wrote Dr. Barnes, are occurring despite a marked rise in the prescription of antiasthma drugs, which suggests that currently available therapy is either inadequate or not being used optimally.

"[In England] we are rapidly increasing the use of inhaled steroids early in the course of treatment because now we understand that asthma is a chronic disease," Dr. Barnes told *HealthFacts* in an interview after his presentation. "For any other condition in which inflammation was the normal part of the problem, it would be inconceivable not to treat with anti-inflammatory drugs.

Doctors are only treating the symptoms, he explained, when they prescribe bronchodilators without an antiinflammatory drug. The practice was described as dangerous because it masks the inflammation, which is thought to be a factor in the bronchodilator-related deaths from asthma. As the air passages to the lungs become inflamed, they get narrower and narrower. The asthmatic who uses an inhaled bronchodilator gets immediate relief, but it can be a false sense of security since the inflammation left untreated continues to close off the airways.

SOURCE:
"Asthma: Deaths Continue to Rise. New Treatment Approach Offered." *HealthFacts* 15, no. 134 (July 1990): 1, 3-4.

RESOURCES

ORGANIZATIONS

American Academy of Allergy and Immunology. 611 East Wells Street, Milwaukee, WI 53202.

American College of Allergy and Immunology. 800 E NW Highway, Suite 1080, Palatine, IL 60067.

American Lung Association. 1740 Broadway, New York, NY 10019.

Asthma and Allergy Foundation of America. 1717 Massachusetts Ave. NW, Suite 305, Washington, DC 20026.

National Jewish Center for Immunology and Respiratory Medicine. 1400 Jackson Street, Denver, CO 80206.

BOOK

Hannaway, P. J. *The Asthma Self-Help Book.* Lighthouse Press, 1989.

PAMPHLET

National Jewish Center for Immunology and Respiratory Medicine:

Your Child and Asthma. 1986. 20 pp.

RELATED ARTICLES

American Academy of Pediatrics. "AAP (American Academy of Pediatrics) Issues Statement on Exercise-Induced Asthma in Children." *American Family Physician* (October 1989): 314.

"Asthma: Deaths Continue to Rise: New Treatment Approach Offered." *HealthFacts* 15, no. 134 (July 1990): 1-6.

Franklin, P. "Review of Acute Severe Asthma (Status Asthmaticus)." *Western Journal of Medicine* (May 1989): 552.

Hannaway, P. J. "Rid Your Home of Asthma 'Bugs.'" *Prevention* (April 1990): 57-63.

Hargreave, Frederick E., Jerry Dolovich, and Michael T. Newhouse (eds.). "The Assessment and Treatment of Asthma: A Conference Report." *Journal of Allergy and Clinical Immunology* 85, no. 6 (June 1990): 1098-1111.

Hoffman, Stephen. "Turning Around." *Harvard Health Letter* 16, no. 7 (May 1991): 5-7.

Hoffman, Stephen. "Rethinking Therapy." *Harvard Health Letter* 16, no. 8 (June 1991): 1-4.

Thomas, P. "Mild Asthma, Too, Needs Steroids." *Medical World News* 31 (June 25, 1990): 11.

Warner, J. O., and others. "Management of Asthma: A Consensus Statement." *Archives of Disease in Childhood* 64 (July 1989): 1065-1079.

Weinberger, Miles. "Antiasthmatic Therapy in Children." *Pediatric Clinics of North America* 36, no. 5 (October 1989): 1251-1284.

ATTENTION DEFICIT DISORDER

OVERVIEW

A syndrome affecting children, adolescents, and, rarely, adults characterized by learning and behavior disabilities. The symptoms may be mild or severe and are associated with functional deviations of the central nervous system without signs of major neurologic or psychiatric disturbance. The people affected are usually of normal or above average intelligence. Symptoms include impairment in perception, conceptualization, language, memory, and motor skills, decreased attention span, increased impulsivity and emotional lability, and usually, but not always, hyperactivity. The condition is 10 times more prevalent in boys than in girls and may result from genetic factors, biochemical irregularities, or perinatal or postnatal injury or disease. There is no known cure, and symptoms often subside or disappear with time. Medication with methylphenidate, pemoline, or the dextroamphetamines is frequently prescribed for children with hyperactive symptoms, and some form of psychotherapeutic counseling is often recommended. Some treatments include abstinence from certain foods and food additives. Also called hyperactivity, hyperkinesis, minimal brain dysfunction.

SOURCE:
Glanze, Walter D., Kenneth N. Anderson, and Lois E. Anderson, (eds.). "Attention Deficit Disorder." In *Mosby's Medical, Nursing, and Allied Health Dictionary*. St. Louis: C. V. Mosby, 1990. p. 109.

AMERICAN PSYCHIATRIC ASSOCIATION—DIAGNOSTIC CRITERIA

314.01 Attention-deficit Hyperactivity Disorder

Note: Consider a criterion met only if the behavior is considerably more frequent than that of most people of the same mental age.

A. A disturbance of at least six months during which at least eight of the following are present:

(1) often fidgets with hands or feet or squirms in seat (in adolescents, may be limited to subjective feelings of restlessness)

(2) has difficulty remaining seated when required to do so

(3) is easily distracted by extraneous stimuli

(4) has difficulty awaiting turn in games or group situations

(5) often blurts out answers to questions before they have been completed

(6) has difficulty following through on instructions from others (not due to oppositional behavior or failure of comprehension), e.g., fails to finish chores

(7) has difficulty sustaining attention in tasks or play activities

(8) often shifts from one uncompleted activity to another

(9) has difficulty playing quietly

(10) often talks excessively

(11) often interrupts or intrudes on others, e.g., butts into other children's games

(12) often does not seem to listen to what is being said to him or her

(13) often loses things necessary for tasks or activities at school or at home (e.g., toys, pencils, books, assignments)

(14) often engages in physically dangerous activities without considering possible consequences (not for the purpose of thrill-seeking), e.g., runs into street without looking

Note: The above items are listed in descending order of discriminating power based on data from a national field trial of the DSM-III-R criteria for Disruptive Behavior Disorders.

B. Onset before the age of seven.

C. Does not meet the criteria for a Pervasive Developmental Disorder.

Criteria for Severity of Attention-Deficit Hyperactivity Disorder:

Mild: Few, if any, symptoms in excess of those required to make the diagnosis and only minimal or no impairment in school and social functioning.

Moderate: Symptoms of functional impairment intermediate between "mild" and "severe."

Severe: Many symptoms in excess of those required to make the diagnosis and significant and pervasive impairment in functioning at home and school and with peers.

SOURCE:
"314.01 Attention-deficit Hyperactivity Disorder." In *Diagnostic Criteria from DSM-III-R*. Washington, DC: American Psychiatric Association, 1987. pp. 56–57.

THE FEINGOLD DIET

In 1973, Dr. Benjamin Feingold, a California pediatric allergist, proposed that salicylates (naturally occurring substances present in many fruits, some vegetables, and a number of other foods), artificial food colors, and artificial flavors were causes of hyperactivity. He suggested a diet free of these substances for treatment and prevention of the condition.

Dr. Feingold presented his recommendations in two popular books, and his ideas have received widespread media coverage. Many parents of children with behavior problems adopted the suggested diet, and some of them have reported a noticeable improvement in their children's behavior.

Since behavioral problems are complex, variable disorders that can be affected by many factors (including the power of suggestion), these parental observations must be interpreted cautiously. They are valuable because they suggest that a relation might exist between hyperactivity and certain food ingredients, and because they indicate that further investigation of this possible link would be worthwhile. But these informal observations alone cannot prove that this link exists.

To determine conclusively whether a substance affects behavior, carefully controlled scientific experiments must be performed. In the past six years, researchers have conducted several well-designed, controlled experimental tests of Dr. Feingold's theory and diet, involving hundreds of hyperactive children. In this report, the American Council on Science and Health briefly reviews these experiments and evaluates their results.

On the basis of its review of the scientific evidence, the American Council on Science and Health (ACSH) concludes that artificial food colors, artificial flavors, and the salicylate-containing foods specified by Dr. Feingold are not significant causes of hyperactivity in children. ACSH therefore does not recommend that these substances be eliminated or restricted in the diets of hyperactive children in an attempt to improve their conditions. Changes in food processing, food labeling, or food-related public policies in an effort to prevent or control hyperactivity in children are unwarranted.

The available evidence does not completely eliminate the possibility that a limited relationship might exist between certain food colors and hyperactivity. If this is so, however, it would affect only a very small number of hyperactive children.

ACSH also concludes that no physical harm is done by removing artificial flavors and colors from the diet. The placebo effect of these diet modifications and the changes in family dynamics associated with this dietary regimen may lead to behavioral improvement in some children. This potential benefit should be weighed against the potentially harmful long-term educational impact of communicating to a child that consumption of artificial colors and flavors controls behavior, when it does not.

SOURCE:
American Council on Science and Health. *Food Additives and Hyperactivity*. 1982. pp. 2–3.

METABOLIC DYSFUNCTION EXPLANATION OF ATTENTION DEFICIT DISORDER

Almost any teacher can identify the hyperactive kids in the class. They're the ones who simply can't sit still. Because they tend to be disorganized and have trouble focusing their attention and controlling their impulses, they frequently do poorly in school, get in trouble with their parents and teachers and are unpopular with other children. Scientists have long been unable to pinpoint the cause of the problem. While kids fidgeted, the experts argued over whether the disorder had psychological or biological roots.

Now, for the first time, research recently published in *The New England Journal of Medicine* suggests that attention deficit hyperactivity disorder (ADHD) is related to a metabolic dysfunction in the brain. In a study of adults who have been hyperactive since childhood (and who are parents of hyperactive children), researchers at the National Institute of Mental Health in Bethesda, Md., found reduced activity in those areas of the brain that control attention and movement. Dr. Alan J. Zametikin, the principal author of the study, says the findings are good news for the parents of hyperactive kids.

"This shows this is not the result of bad parenting," says Zametikin. "This is a medical problem." He adds that parents might now feel less concerned about using medication to control the disorder, which affects about 4 percent of school-age children.

It has long been known that many hyperactive children benefit from low doses of amphetamines (such as Ritalin). While the drugs don't provide a cure, they often seem to help the kids focus their attention and sit still. In the past, experts who believed in a psychological explanation for hyperactivity have criticized the use of drugs to control it. Instead, they urged parents to employ behavior-modification techniques, training in social skills, remedial education and family therapy. In an editorial accompanying the new study results in *The New England Journal of Medicine*, Dr. Gabrielle Weiss points out that even when medication is used, augmenting it with such therapy is a good idea.

Finding an effective treatment is crucial since many children don't outgrow the problem. In fact, up to 60 percent of hyperactive children become hyperactive adults. There is also evidence that the disability is often inherited. Now there's hope that the new finding will lead to earlier diagnosis and even better medication.

SOURCE:
"A New View on Hyperactivity." *Newsweek* (December 3, 1990): 61.

USE OF METHYLPHENIDATE (RITALIN) AND OTHER STIMULANT MEDICATIONS

The Food and Drug Administration has approved three stimulant drugs as safe and effective for ADHD: methylphenidate (Ritalin), dextroamphetamine (Dexedrine), and pemoline (Cylert). Methylphenidate is the treatment of choice, though one of the other drugs may produce a better response in some children. When properly administered, stimulants help nearly all patients, often dramatically. As blinders filter out distracting stimuli for a racehorse, so does a stimulant given to a child. The result is increased concentration for the task at hand: running a horse race or learning a math problem.

At least 750,000 U.S. children received stimulants for hyperactivity and inattentiveness in 1987, and this figure may grow to more than a million by the early 1990s, according to an article in the Oct. 21, 1988, *Journal of the American Medical Association*. Authors Daniel Safer, M.D., and John Krager, M.D., reporting on a study of Baltimore County schools, described as "understandable" the finding that an increased number of teenagers and girls are being given drug therapy. "There is now substantial evidence that stimulants are as useful for teenagers as for their elementary school counterparts," they wrote, and "the gender ratio for medication treatment is now approaching the hyperactivity-inattentiveness gender ratio found in the classrooms." But, citing other studies, they expressed concern that "a growing number of inattentive, nonhyperactive, primarily learning-impaired students are being treated with stimulants."

In an accompanying editorial, Sally Shaywitz, M.D., and Bennett Shaywitz, M.D., both of the Yale University School of Medicine, agreed with Safer and Krager that it's improper to treat learning disorders with stimulants. Of factors contributing to school failure, they wrote, "only attention-deficit disorder . . . can be ameliorated by a treatment program incorporating stimulant therapy." They agreed that part of the increased stimulant use was due to increased awareness and diagnosis of children who primarily have inattention. "Many experienced clinicians and investigators would argue that stimulants treat not hyperactivity, but rather attentional difficulties that interfere with school function, a belief supported by studies from many investigative groups. . . ."

Stimulants are not appropriate for every child with attention disorder. For instance, they are not intended for anyone with a primary psychiatric illness (such as schizophrenia, in which the person loses touch with reality) because they can worsen the disturbances. They can aggravate emotional problems, such as anxiety. They can bring out tics (involuntary movements) in a patient with a family history of tics; stimulants don't cause tics, however. And, even a correctly administered stimulant can cause adverse effects, for no drug is completely without risk. The side effects most frequently reported are decreased appetite and insomnia. Less common are drowsiness, hypersensitivity, weight loss, headache, nausea, and blood pressure changes. Whether a child should be given stimulants is a case-by-case decision in which the benefits are weighed against the risks.

In the past, most stimulant treatments for ADHD were prescribed only for two to three years and only for children. But today, treatment may extend over longer periods and may be given to adolescents and adults. . . .

Stimulants clearly are not intended to be the sole treatment. FDA requires that labeling on the drugs state that they be used "as an integral part of a total treatment program which typically includes other remedial measures (psychological, educational, social)."

SOURCE:
Farley, Dixie. "Helping Children with Attention Disorder." *FDA Consumer* 23 (February 1989): 12, 14.

RESOURCES

ORGANIZATIONS

ADDA: Attention Deficit Disorder Association, c/o Ms. Linda Phillips. Child Development Center, University of California at Irvine, Irvine, CA 92715.

CHADD: Children with Attention Deficit Disorder. 499 Northwest 70th Avenue #308, Plantation, FL 33117.

BOOKS

Greenhill, Laurence L., and Betty B. Osman. *Ritalin: Theory and Patient Management.* New York: Mary Ann Liebert, Inc, 1991. 320 pp.

Ingersoll, Barbara. *Your Hyperactive Child: A Parent's Guide to Coping with Attention Deficit Disorder.* New York: Doubleday, 1988.

RELATED ARTICLES

Cowart, Virginia S. "The Ritalin Controversy: What's Made This Drug's Opponents Hyperactive? *JAMA* 259, no. 17 (May 6, 1988): 2521-2523.

Garber, Stephen W., Marianne Daniels Garber, and Robyn Freedman Spizman. "Is Your Child Hyperactive? Inattentive? Impulsive? Distractible?" *Redbook* 175 (October 1990): 32–35.

Safer, Daniel J., and John M. Krager. "A Survey of Medication Treatment for Hyperactive-Inattentive Students." *JAMA* 260 (October 21, 1988): 2256–2258.

Shaywitz, Sally E., and Bennett A. Shaywitz. "Increased Medication Use in Attention-Deficit Hyperactivity Disorder: Regressive or Appropriate? (editorial)" *JAMA* 260 (October 21, 1988): 2270–2272.

Stevenson, Richard D., and Mark L. Wolraich. "Stimulant Medication Therapy in the Treatment of Children with Attention Deficit Hyperactivity Disorder." *Pediatric Clinics of North America* 36, no. 5 (October 1989): 1183–1197.

Weiss, Gabrielle. "Hyperactivity in Childhood." *The New England Journal of Medicine* 323 (November 15, 1990): 1413–1415.

AUTISM

OVERVIEW

Autism is a condition in which children are unable to develop normal relationships with others. It is a disease of the central nervous system, which is diagnosed by the presence of characteristic disturbances in development. About 4 to 5 of every 10,000 children are autistic, and 10 to 14 per 10,000 have some form of pervasive developmental disorder (PDD). PDD means that some, but not all, symptoms of autism are present. Autism is a lifelong disease and ranges in severity—there are mild cases in which the individuals may live independently, and severe forms in which the patients require social support and medical supervision throughout their lives.

There are physical bases for autism's development, including genetic, infectious and traumatic factors. The most common cause is probably viral infection during the first trimester of pregnancy; rubella is one of the best studied culprits. Autism affects males four times more often than females, and there is a genetic basis for the disease. A couple who already has an autistic child has an eight percent chance of having a second autistic.

Two types of onset are reported. In one, the patient appears to have symptoms from the first months of life. In the second, an apparently normal course of development occurs until age 18–24 months, when the symptoms become manifested.

The symptoms vary greatly but also follow a general pattern. Not all symptoms are present in all autistic children. Autistic infants may act relatively normal during their first few months of life before they become less responsive to their parents and other stimuli. They may have difficulty with feeding or toilet training; may not smile in recognition of their parents' faces; and may put up resistance to being cuddled. As they enter toddlerhood, it becomes increasingly apparent that these children have a world of their own. They do not play with other children or toys in the normal manner; autistic children remain aloof and prefer to play alone.

Skills for verbal and nonverbal communication, such as speech and facial expressions, develop peculiarly. Symptoms range from mutism to prolonged use of echoing or stilted language. When language is present it is often concrete, unimaginative and immature.

Another symptom of autism is an extreme resistance to change of any kind. Autistic children tend to want to maintain the established pattern in their behavior and their environment. They develop rituals in play, oppose change (such as moving certain furniture) or may become obsessed with one particular topic.

Other behavioral abnormalities may also exist, or may be present in a transitory manner: staring at hands or flapping arms and hands, walking on tiptoe, rocking, tantrums, strange postures, unpredictable behavior and hyperactivity. There is always a risk of danger since an autistic child has poor judgment about the safety of many situations. For instance, an autistic child may run into a busy street without any sign of fear.

Ninety percent of autistic children also have some degree of mental retardation. It is very important, however, to properly diagnose autism since confusion may result in inappropriate and ineffective treatment. Deafness is often the first suspected diagnosis since they do not respond normally to the sounds they hear. Their appearance and muscle coordination are normal. Occasionally, an autistic child has an outstanding skill, such as an incredible rote memory or musical ability; such children may be referred to as "autistic savants."

Appropriate early intervention is important for autistic children. Psychiatrists or psychologists can determine if the child is autistic, and this is usually done after the age of 30 months. The diagnosis may be made earlier at a special diagnostic center for autism. Once the diagnosis has been made, everyone involved, including the parents, physicians and specialists, needs to discuss what is best for the child. In most cases, parents are encouraged to take care of the child at home. Special education classes are available for autistic children. Treatment requires structured behaviorally-based programs geared to the patient's developmental level. Parents are encouraged to participate in all aspects of the patient's care and treatment, and should be educated in behavioral techniques. The more specialized instruction and behavior therapy the child receives, the more likely it is that the condition will improve. Medication is only administered to treat specific symptoms such as seizures, hyperactivity, extreme mood changes or self-injurious behaviors.

It is important to recognize the effect that an autistic child can have on the rest of the family. Other children may be affected since the autistic child requires so much of their parents' attention. It can be devastating for parents to learn that their child is autistic, so counseling and support may be helpful.

The outlook for each child depends on his or her intelligence and language ability, and it frequently cannot be determined until adolescence since developmental spurts occur up to that age. The number and proportion of mild cases that have come to clinical attention has not been estimated. Very few autistic people are independent as adults. A majority can be taught to live in community-based homes, although they may require supervision throughout adulthood.

SOURCE:

California Medical Association. "Autism." *HealthTips* Index 508 (December-January 1989): 1–2.

DIAGNOSTIC CRITERIA—AMERICAN PSYCHIATRIC ASSOCIATION

Autistic Disorder

At least eight of the following sixteen items are present, these to include at least two items from A, one from B, and one from C.

Note: Consider a criterion to be met only if the behavior is abnormal for the person's developmental level.

A. Qualitative impairment in reciprocal social interaction as manifested by the following:

(The examples within parentheses are arranged so that those first mentioned are more likely to apply to younger or more handicapped, and the later ones, to older or less handicapped, persons with this disorder.)

(1) marked lack of awareness of the existence or feelings of others (e.g., treats a person as if he or she were a piece of furniture; does not notice another person's distress; apparently has no concept of the need of others for privacy)

(2) no or abnormal seeking of comfort at times of distress (e.g., does not come for comfort even when ill, hurt, or tired; seeks comfort in a stereotyped way, e.g., says "cheese, cheese, cheese" whenever hurt)

(3) no or impaired imitation (e.g., does not wave bye-bye; does not copy mother's domestic activities; mechanical imitation of others' actions out of context)

(4) no or abnormal social play (e.g., does not actively participate in simple games; prefers solitary play activities; involves other children in play only as "mechanical aids")

(5) gross impairment in ability to make peer friendships (e.g., no interest in making peer friendships; despite interest in making friends, demonstrates lack of understanding of conventions of social interaction, for example, reads phone book to uninterested peer)

B. Qualitative impairment in verbal and nonverbal communication, and in imaginative activity, as manifested by the following:

(The numbered items are arranged so that those first listed are more likely to apply to younger or more handicapped, and the later ones, to older or less handicapped, persons with this disorder.)

(1) no mode of communication, such as communicative babbling, facial expression, gesture, mime, or spoken language

(2) markedly abnormal nonverbal communication, as in the use of eye-to-eye gaze, facial expression, body posture, or gestures to initiate or modulate social interaction (e.g., does not anticipate being held, stiffens when held, does not look at the person or smile when making a social approach, does not greet parents or visitors, has a fixed stare in social situations)

(3) absence of imaginative activity, such as playacting of adult roles, fantasy characters, or animals; lack of interest in stories about imaginary events

(4) marked abnormalities in the production of speech, including volume, pitch, stress, rate, rhythm, and intonation (e.g., monotonous tone, questionlike melody, or high pitch)

(5) marked abnormalities in the form or content of speech, including stereotyped and repetitive use of speech (e.g., immediate echolalia or mechanical repetition of television commercial); use of "you" when "I" is meant (e.g., using "You want cookie?" to mean "I want a cookie")'; idiosyncratic use of words or phrases (e.g., "Go on green riding" to mean "I want to go on the swing"); or frequent irrelevant remarks (e.g., starts talking about train schedules during a conversation about sports)

(6) marked impairment in the ability to initiate or sustain a conversation with others, despite adequate speech (e.g., indulging in lengthy monologues on one subject regardless of interjections from others)

C. Markedly restricted repertoire of activities and interests, as manifested by the following:

(1) stereotyped body movements, e.g., hand-flinching or -twisting, spinning, head-banging, complex whole-body movements

(2) persistent preoccupation with parts of objects (e.g., sniffing or smelling objects, repetitive feeling of texture of materials, spinning wheels of toy cars) or attachment to unusual objects (e.g., insists on carrying around a piece of string)

(3) marked distress over changes in trivial aspects of environment, e.g., when a vase is moved from usual position

(4) unreasonable insistence on following routines in precise detail, e.g., insisting that exactly the same route always be followed when shopping

(5) markedly restricted range of interests and a preoccupation with one narrow interest, e.g., interested only in lining up objects, in amassing facts about meteorology, or in pretending to be a fantasy character

D. Onset during infancy or childhood

Specify if childhood onset (after 36 months of age).

SOURCE:
"299.00 Autistic Disorder." In *Diagnostic Criteria from DSM-III-R.* Washington, DC: American Psychiatric Association, 1987. pp. 49–51.

GENETIC ORIGINS

A surprisingly large percentage of parents and siblings of autistic individuals display language and personality features reminiscent of autism, suggesting a genetic component for this early-onset developmental disorder, reports Susan E. Folstein, a psychiatrist at Johns Hopkins.

In 2 ½-hour interviews, Folstein and her colleagues tested the general mental ability, social skills and language skills of normal parents and siblings of 40 autistic patients and a control group of 20 matched families of children with Down's syndrome. They concluded that about 30 percent of the family members of autistic subjects suffered pronounced reading and spelling difficulties as children and/or displayed language deficits as adults, particularly in social communication. They tended to be disorganized and overly detailed when speaking, Folstein says. In contrast, none of the controls showed pronounced deficits in these areas, she reports.

Autism, which appears in four out of every 10,000 children worldwide, is characterized by late speech development, repetitive or stereotyped behavior and an inability to develop social relationships, Folstein notes. She says her findings and previous studies indicate the behavior of parents or siblings is not the cause of autism. Instead, she suggests the disease might arise from a recessive genetic defect. If two parents carry the relevant genes—leading to slight abnormalities in those individuals—then their child could inherit a more deleterious genetic combination resulting in autism, Folstein hypothesizes.

The ongoing study, which includes a research team in London, will eventually involve 240 "autistic" and 80 control families, she told *Science News*.

SOURCE:
Wickelgren, Ingrid. "Genetic Evidence for Autism." *Science News* 135 (June 3, 1989): 349.

TREATMENT

The best-known behavioral treatment program for autistics began in the early 1960s at the University of California, Los Angeles, under the direction of O. Ivar Lovaas. In 1970, Lovaas and his co-workers admitted 38 autistics, all around 3 years of age, to a long-term study. They randomly assigned each child to one of two groups: 19 received intensive behavioral treatment, and 19 received minimal treatment. In addition, they tracked another 21 autistic youngsters who were not part of the program and who received no behavioral treatment.

For two or more years, intensive-treatment autistics underwent 40 hours a week of one-to-one treatment at home, administered by students trained in Lovaas' program. The children also entered public preschools. Parents received instruction in behavioral techniques to extend the treatment to all a child's waking hours.

Most behavioral treatment programs today employ the same training elements used by the staff, parents and, when possible, preschool teachers in the Los Angeles study. These include clear instructions to the child, prompting to perform specific behaviors, immediate praise and rewards for performing those behaviors, a gradual increase in the complexity of reinforced behaviors, and definite distinctions of when and when not to perform the learned behaviors.

Over three years, Lovaas, his co-workers and the parent-therapists aimed to reduce the children's aggressive behavior (in extreme cases, they used a loud "no" or a slap on the thigh), teach them to imitate adults' actions, establish appropriate play with toys and with other children, develop speech and language skills, teach basic reading, writing and arithmetic, and promote the verbal expression of feelings.

Children in the minimal-treatment group received fewer than 10 hours a week of one-to-one training from the staff. They were often enrolled in special education classes rather than public preschools. Their parents received no training as home therapists.

If any child in the project proved capable of starting first grade around age 6, contact with the Lovaas program was largely stopped, although occasional family consultations continued.

By age 7, minimal-treatment children in the study fared poorly. Their IQ scores, averaging around 55 at the study's outset, remained largely unchanged, and only one achieved normal social and academic functioning in a public school. The rest were in classes for autistic and retarded children.

In marked contrast, nine intensive-treatment children passed first grade in public school. Their IQ scores ranged from 94 to 120, in the normal to above-average range. Only two children in the intensive-treatment group had an IQ of 30 or less and were placed in classes for the autistic and retarded; the remainder had "mildly retarded" IQs and passed first grade in classes for the language-impaired.

SOURCE:

Bower, Bruce. "Remodeling the Autistic Child: Parents Join Clinicians to Transform the Tragedy of Autism." *Science News* 136 (November 11, 1989): 312–313.

RESOURCES

ORGANIZATION

Autism Research Institute. 4182 Adams Ave., San Diego, CA 92116.

RELATED ARTICLES

Merz, Beverly. "Evidence of New Physical, Genetic Links in Autism." *JAMA* 261, no. 21 (June 2, 1989): 3067.

Pascoe, Elizabeth Jean. "Can Autism Be Cured?" *Woman's Day* (March 5, 1991): 50–53.

BACK PAIN

(*See also:* CHIROPRACTIC)

OVERVIEW

At least once in their lives, about 80 percent of Americans will experience a bout of low back pain that can range from a dull, annoying ache to absolute agony. According to *American Family Physician*, on any given day 6.5 million Americans are under some sort of treatment for low back pain.

After headaches, low back pain is the most common ailment in the United States and is topped only by colds and flu in time lost from work. Low back pain has been described as a 20th century epidemic, the nemesis of medicine, and an albatross of industry. When all the costs connected with it are added up—job absenteeism, medical and legal fees, social security disability payments, workmen's compensation, long-term disability insurance—the bill to business, industry and the government has been estimated to total at least $16 billion each year. Those most often affected are young adults in their most productive years, from ages 17 to 45.

It is believed that many cases of low back pain are due to stresses on the muscles and ligaments that support the spine. Our sedentary jobs and lifestyle make us vulnerable to this type of damage. Too much time in front of the TV, not enough exercise, poor posture, and poor sleeping habits (including sleeping on the stomach) weaken muscles. Weak muscles, especially abdominal muscles, cannot support the spine properly. Obesity, which afflicts 34 million Americans, is another factor—it increases both the weight on the spine and the pressure on the discs.

When the body is in poor shape, it doesn't take much to overstretch (strain) a muscle or put a small tear in (sprain) a ligament. The medical word for backaches arising from either of these conditions is lumbosacral strain (or sprain). Sometimes, a sudden twist or fall can bring on muscle spasm—sudden, involuntary contractions that can be excruciatingly painful. A spasm immobilizes the muscles over the injured area, possibly acting as a kind of splint to protect muscles or joints from further damage.

Jobs that involve bending and twisting, or lifting heavy objects repeatedly—especially when the loads are beyond a worker's strength—are no better for the back than are sedentary jobs. Certain occupations, such as truck driving or nursing, are particularly hard on the back. The truck driver must contend with sitting for long periods (actually worse for the back than standing), the vibration of the vehicle, and lifting and straining at the end of the day when muscles are fatigued and more susceptible to damage. (Truck driving ranks first in workmen's compensation cases for low back pain.) Football, gymnastics, and other strenuous sports can also damage the lower back.

Because many people are familiar with the term "slipped" disc, this problem is mistakenly believed to be the chief cause of most low back pain. But in fact, slipped discs are responsible for only 5 percent to 10 percent of the cases. Actually, the term itself is inaccurate because the disc doesn't slip at all; it bulges out between two vertebrae. In some cases, the tough tissues that contain the disc are weakened by injuries that allow the soft gel-like center to protrude. If the protrusion presses on a nerve root, pinching it against the bone, the result is pain in the area of the body served by that nerve. Doctors can tell which disc in the lower back is causing the problem by the part of the body affected, usually the legs.

The protruded part of the disc does not slip back into place. Scar tissue forms around the protrusion and walls it in. If the outer tissues continue to be stressed, they will weaken further and, in time, the slightest activity—a sneeze or cough—may cause the disc to burst through its capsule, or rupture.

As might be expected, pain from disc disease can rank pretty high on the pain index. To make matters worse, if a nerve root is irritated in any one place, it tends to become irritable along its whole length. A ruptured disc that presses on nerve roots in the low back (lower lumbar or high sacral areas) causes sciatica, a condition in which sharp, shooting pains begin in the buttock and run down the back of the thigh and the inside of the leg to the foot. Tingling, numbness and weakness may follow. If the pressure on the nerve root is not relieved, the leg muscles will eventually waste away, or atrophy.

SOURCE:

Zamula, Evelyn, II. "Back Talk: Advice for Suffering Spines." *FDA Consumer* 23 (April 1989): 28–35.

CONSERVATIVE TREATMENTS

Trite as it sounds, the best advice is usually: "Go to bed, take aspirin, and if it's not better in a couple of days, call your doctor." When back pain is not the only symptom, however, immediate medical help must be sought.

Loss of bladder or bowel control—either incontinence or difficulty voiding—indicates that the nerve roots at the tail end of the spinal cord (the *cauda equina*) are being injured, and immediate surgery may be required. A major back injury, say in an automobile accident, requires prompt attention. Evidence of systemic illness—particularly fever or weight loss—also needs to be pursued. Finally, if the legs are weak, tingling, or numb, progressive nerve damage may be occurring, and a doctor should be called.

In the majority of cases by far, localized back pain comes from "strain" of muscles and ligaments. Relatively limited protrusion of a disk that impinges on nerve roots is a much less frequent cause, though not a rare one. In either case, the first things to do are:

- Lie down on any bed or couch and in any comfortable position or positions.
- Use anti-inflammatory medication (aspirin, ibuprofen, or prescription drugs).
- Apply heat or cold, whichever feels better.

This is called "conservative" therapy—medical jargon meaning that no surgical procedure is performed. Conservative therapy is not merely symptomatic; these measures have specific benefits. First, lying on one's side or back with the hips and knees somewhat flexed relieves all kinds of forces that a vertical position, or even sitting, imposes on the disks, ligaments, and muscles of the spine. Second, aspirin and its relatives are anti-inflammatory drugs. Not only do they relieve pain (and thus reduce one of the triggers of reflex muscle spasm), they also reduce inflammation in injured tissues. To get the anti-inflammatory effect requires more than the usual painkilling dose; at least 2 tablets every 4 hours (but not during the hours of sleep) are typically required. Finally, cold applied immediately after an injury helps to prevent swelling and pain; later on, heat appears to reduce swelling and promote recovery.

Muscle relaxants, particularly cyclobenzaprine (Flexeril), may be prescribed for patients with low-back pain. I personally do not feel that they have much to contribute, and I worry that relaxing spasm may actually be counterproductive, undoing what amounts to the protective effect of contracted spinal muscles.

On a conservative regimen, pain due to strain is usually relieved within 2 to 3 days; a minimally protruding disk may also resume its shape sufficiently to decompress the affected nerve root. Even if pain persists longer than this, however, there is not necessarily any reason to take more drastic measures. Conservative therapy can require as long as 6 weeks to take hold. If there has been little progress at 6 weeks, the likelihood is quite small that greater improvement will follow. If there has been improvement, but no total recovery, the prudent course may still be to "wait it out," provided the patient is willing to do so and there is no evidence of nerve damage.

We're not talking about absolute bed rest at any stage of conservative management. Realistically, few people will manage to stay in bed constantly for more than a couple of days, and even at the beginning, when pain is most severe, getting up to go to the bathroom or to eat a meal may be better for both morale and the back than trying to achieve the contortions necessary to do these things in bed. One well-designed study has shown that people with an attack of low-back pain responded to only a couple of days of true bed rest followed by the judicious resumption of activity; 7 days in bed just increased absentee rates without otherwise affecting recovery.

Conservative therapy is a balancing act. The specific benefit of a horizontal position is that it relieves pressure on the lumbar spine. The disadvantages of strict bed rest are:

- loss of muscle conditioning—setting the stage for further episodes of strain
- loss of bone
- vulnerability to blood clotting
- depression
- a sense of weakness or malaise

Current practice is to think more in terms of "controlled activity" than strict bed rest.

SOURCE:

White, Augustus A. "Back Pain: Treatment." *Harvard Medical School Health Letter* 15 (January 1990): 4–5.

CHYMOPAPAIN INJECTIONS

Over a decade ago, chymopapain injections received a considerable amount of media attention as a non-surgical treatment for herniated disks, a common cause of chronic back pain. Unfortunately, the ongoing controversy over its value has not been settled by a panel of experts convened with that goal in mind (*JAMA*, 18 August 1989). The 36 physician members, selected for their expertise in this area, were asked to review all published reports on the injection of chymopapain (an enzyme derived from the papaya plant) as a treatment for herniated, or ruptured, spinal disks. The condition is the result of a break in the cartilage surrounding each disk, which in turn releases the gelatinous substance that separates and cushions the bones of the spine. Pressure on the spinal nerve roots causes severe and often disabling pain.

The chymopapain is injected directly into the bulging disk in an effort to accelerate its reduction and thus alleviate symptoms. The procedure received Food and Drug Administration approval in 1982 for certain people with herniated disks of the lower, or lumbar, spine. It is recommended only after conservative measures, such as bed rest, analgesics, and exercise, have failed. Evaluating the efficacy of back treatment has always presented problems because back pain often recedes with time and conservative measures. Researchers who followed people with untreated back pain found that 60 percent of people return to work in one week and 90 percent are working by six weeks.

The risks include anaphylaxis, a severe and sometimes fatal response, and damage to the spinal cord. The former accounts for the most frequent major complication with studies showing the rate of adverse allergic reactions varying from 0.4 percent to 4.2 percent. One unexplained finding concerned gender differences: women are six to ten times more likely than men to be sensitive to chymopapain. The procedure's death rate from all causes is about one in 4,000; whereas, the rate of disastrous neurologic complications is one in 2,000.

SOURCE:
"Expert Group Assesses Non-Surgical Treatment." *HealthFacts* 14 (September 1989): 4.

CHIROPRACTIC TREATMENT

Cherkin and MacCornack compared the satisfaction with providers among enrollees in a Washington state HMO who experienced treatment for low back pain from either family physicians or chiropractors. Patients of DCs [doctors of chiropractic] were three times as likely as patients of family physicians to report that they were very satisfied with the care they received (66% vs. 22%). DC-patients were much more likely to have been satisfied with the amount of information they were given, to have perceived that their provider was concerned about them, and to have felt that their provider was comfortable and confident in dealing with their problem. The researchers state: "Although the more positive evaluations of chiropractors may be related to differences in the patient populations. . . it is suggested that a potentially more potent force—the therapeutic effect of the patient and provider interaction itself—may explain the observed differences."

Comment: These results are not surprising, and the researchers' conclusions seem appropriate; however, it is important to bear in mind that the DCs are highly specialized in not only treating low back pain, but many also specialize in the psychology of patient satisfaction. Family physicians are not low back pain specialists. I recall the book *Backache Relief* by back-pain sufferer Arthur Klein and science writer David Sobel. They consulted 492 back-pain sufferers located through ads placed in 24 newspapers and magazines. This self-selected population rated physiatrists (MDs who specialize in physical medicine and rehabilitation) as 300% more effective than chiropractors and orthopedists. Painkillers, muscle relaxants, and anti-inflammatory drugs were rated no better than placebos by this group. The problem with physiatrists is finding one!

SOURCE:
"Chiropractors Rated Better than Family Physicians by Back Pain Patients." *NCAHF Newsletter* 12 (July-August 1989): 3.

* * *

Consider back manipulation by a physician or chiropractor. Manipulation of the spinal vertebrae (with the familiar "crack," as gas escapes from the synovial fluid in the joint) succeeds in relieving backache for some cases, depending on the underlying cause. It often brings speedier improvement than standard medical approaches alone. Manipulation works best for certain types of low back pain such as facet joint problems and sacroiliac irritation rather than those due to herniated discs, spinal instability or spinal stenosis (narrowed spinal canal). Although techniques vary greatly from one manipulator to another, many patients use chiropractic manipulation in addition to physician care. One Canadian study found that 97 per cent of chiropractors refer patients to physicians for further care and 84 per cent had been referred to a chiropractor by a physician, noting that 10 to 15 sessions at most are usually needed—additional sessions rarely bring extra benefit. Many back patients benefit from about two weeks of daily chiropractic manipulation. Although manipulation often brings psychological as well as practical support, in the long run there's no evidence that manipulated backs fare better than those treated by heat, painkillers and muscle relaxants. Manipulation is unlikely to cure the underlying back problem, although it may temporarily relieve the pain, increase flexibility and is something practical to do.

SOURCE:
"Back Pain Update." *University of Toronto Faculty of Medicine Health News* 8 (2) (April 1990): 2.

USE OF TENS UNITS

A number of treatments are widely prescribed for chronic back pain, but few have been rigorously evaluated. We examined the effectiveness of transcutaneous electrical nerve stimulation (TENS), a program of stretching exercises, or a combination of both for low back pain.

Patients with chronic low back pain (median duration, 4.1 years) were randomly assigned to receive daily treatment with TENS (n=36), sham TENS (n=36), TENS plus a program of exercises (n=37), or sham TENS plus exercise (n=36).

After one month, no clinically or statistically significant treatment effect of TENS was found on any of 11 indicators of outcome measuring pain, function, and back flexion; there was no interactive effect of TENS with exercise. Overall improvement in pain indicators was 47 percent with TENS and 42 percent with sham TENS (P not significant). The 95 percent confidence intervals for group differences excluded a major clinical benefit of TENS for most outcomes. By contrast, after one month patients in the exercise group had significant improvement in self-rated pain scores, reduction in the frequency of pain, and greater levels of activity as compared with patients in the groups that did not exercise. The mean reported improvement in pain scores was 52 percent in the exercise groups and 37 percent in the nonexercise groups (P=0.02). Two months after the active intervention, however, most patients had discontinued the exercises, and the initial improvements were gone.

We conclude that for patients with chronic low back pain, treatment with TENS is no more effective than treatment with a placebo, and TENS adds no apparent benefit to that of exercise alone.

SOURCE:
Deyo, Richard A., Nicolas E. Walsh, and others. "A Controlled Trial of Transcutaneous Electrical Nerve Stimulation (TENS) and Exercise for Chronic Low Back Pain." *The New England Journal of Medicine* 322 (23) (June 7, 1990): 1627–1634.

SURGERY

The vast majority of people with low-back pain—even those with some disk disease, will not need surgery. In general, surgery is only useful for problems in 4 broad categories: (1) disk displacement (a protruded or "slipped" disk), (2) painful (and abnormal) motion of one vertebra in relation to another, (3) narrowing of the spinal canal itself from overgrowth of bone (spinal stenosis), or (4) some cases in which misalignment of one vertebra on another (spondyloisthesis) leads to pain.

If there is clear evidence in the physical examination that function of a nerve root is impaired, and if one of the diagnostic imaging techniques confirms an anatomical abnormality accounting for pressure on that root, surgery is worth considering. If there are signs of rapidly progressive nerve damage—increasing weakness in a leg, loss of bladder or bowel function—surgery moves high on the list of options. It must also be considered when pain is unremitting or getting worse.

Both criteria for surgery should be met: neurological abnormalities and pressure on the implicated nerve root, as shown by an appropriate imaging technique. Bear in mind that diagnostic images often show evidence of spinal abnormalities in people without symptoms. Unless there are signs of nerve compression, it is quite possible that the pain comes from another source.

Even evidence of nerve compression is not an automatic reason to operate. Signs of compression often subside after a period of controlled activity. As a rule, all nonsurgical approaches should be exhausted first, provided that delaying surgery does not jeopardize the patient's health. There's a flip side to this, though. The longer a painful situation persists, the less likely surgery is to help. Decisions about surgery must take into account the individual patient's situation—and preferences.

SOURCE:
White, Augustus A. "Back Pain: Treatment." *Harvard Medical School Health Letter* (January 1990): 5–6.

RESOURCES

BOOK

White, Augustus M. III. *Your Aching Back: A Doctor's Guide to Pain Relief.* Fairfield, OH: Consumer Reports Books, 1990. 336 pp.

ADDITIONAL ARTICLES

"Back Injury Patients' Recovery Time Varies with Insurance Type." *Medical World News* 29 (February 8, 1988): 125.

"Back Pain: Don't Take the Problem Lying Down." *Mayo Clinic Nutrition Letter* 3 (May 1990): 6–7.

Bassam, Bassam A. "Low Back Pain: The Challenge of Accurate Diagnosis and Management." *Postgraduate Medicine* 87, no. 4, (March 1990): 204–215, 218.

Bennett, Dana L. and others. "Comparison of Integrated Electromyographic Activity and Lumbar Curvature during Standing and during Sitting in Three Chairs." *Physical Therapy* 69 (November 1989): 902.

Boachie-Adjei, Oheneba. "Conservative Management of Low Back Pain: An Evaluation of Current Methods." *Postgraduate Medicine* 84, no. 3 (September 1, 1988): 127–133.

"Chiropractors and Low Back Pain." *The Lancet* 336 (July 28, 1990): 220.

"Doctors' Home Remedies: 50 Self-Care Tips to Beat Aches, Pains, Injuries and More." *Prevention* 42 (August 1990): 33–45.

"Functional Rehab: Helping the '5 Percent' Back to Work." *The Back Letter* 4 (June 1990): 6.

"Investigation of Failed Low Back Surgery." *The Lancet* 1 (April 29, 1989): 939–940.

"Manipulation Study Shows Mixed Results." *The Back Letter* 4 (July 1990): 6.

Mills, Simon and Finando, Steven J. "Comparing the Backache Cures: Would You Turn to Acupuncture, Chiropractic, Homeopathy, Herbalism, Osteopathy, or Conventional Western Medicine?" *East West Journal* 19 (September 1989): 58–63.

"Patient Evaluation of Low Back Pain Care." *American Family Physician* 40 (October 1989): 283–284.

"Percutaneous Lumbar Diskectomy for Herniated Disks." *JAMA* 261 (January 6, 1989): 105–109.

Reilly, K. and others. "Differences between a Supervised and Independent Strength and Conditioning Program with Chronic Low Back Syndromes." *Journal of Occupational Medicine* 31 (June 1989): 547–550.

Setterberg, Fred. "How I Got My Back Up." In *Health* 4, no. 2 (March-April 1990): 40–49.

Spoelhof, Gerard and Michael Bristow. "Back Pain Pitfalls." *American Family Physician* 40, no. 4 (October 1989): 133–138.

"Study Debunks TENS: No Better Than Placebo?" *Back Letter* 4 (July 1990): 4.

"TENS Proves Ineffective for Low Back Pain." *Executive Health Report* 26 (September 1990): 8.

Webster, Barbara S. and Stover H. Snook. "The Cost of Compensable Low Back Pain." *Journal of Occupational Medicine* 32 (January 1990): 13–15.

BREAST CANCER

OVERVIEW

[Breast cancer is] a malignant neoplastic disease of breast tissue, the most common malignancy in women in the United States. The incidence increases exponentially with age from the third to the fifth decade and reaches a second peak at age 65, suggesting that breast cancer in premenopausal women may be related to ovarian hormonal function and in postmenopausal patients to adrenal function. Based on the great prevalence of breast cancer in affluent countries, especially in high socioeconomic groups, it is thought that a high fat diet may be a causative factor, but the relationship is unproven and the origin is unknown. Risk factors include a family history of breast cancer, nulliparity, exposure to ionizing radiation, early menarche, late menopause, obesity, diabetes, hypertension, chronic cystic disease of the breast, and, possibly, postmenopausal estrogen therapy. Women who are over 40 years of age when they bear their first child and patients with malignancies in other body sites also have an increased risk of developing breast cancer. Initial symptoms, detected in most cases by self-examination, include a small painless lump, thick or dimpled skin, or nipple retraction. As the lesion progresses, there may be nipple discharge, pain, ulceration, and enlarged axillary glands. The diagnosis may be established by a careful physical examination, mammography, and cytologic examination of tumor cells obtained by biopsy. Infiltrating ductal carcinomas are found in about 75% of cases, and infiltrating lobular, infiltrating medullary, colloid, comedo, or papillary carcinomas in the others. Tumors are more common in the left than in the right breast and in the upper and outer quadrant than in other quadrants. Metastasis through the lymphatic system to axillary lymph nodes and to bone, lung, brain, and liver is common, but there is evidence that primary carcinomas of the breast may exist in multiple sites and that tumor cells may enter the bloodstream directly without passing through lymph nodes.

SOURCE:
"Breast Cancer." In *Mosby's Medical & Nursing Dictionary*. 3d ed. St. Louis: C.V. Mosby, 1990. p. 158.

SYMPTOMS

Women's breasts vary in size, shape, and texture. And each woman's breasts change throughout her lifetime. Changes can be related to age, the menstrual cycle, pregnancy, birth control pills or other hormones, menopause, or injury.

It is normal for the breasts to feel lumpy and uneven. Sometimes the breasts feel tender, especially right before the menstrual period. That's why it is important for all women to learn to examine their breasts. By practicing monthly breast self-examination (BSE), women learn what's normal for their own breasts, and they are more likely to notice anything unusual that might be a warning sign of cancer. All women should also have their breasts checked regularly by a doctor.

Breast cancer can cause a number of symptoms. Listed below are some of the warning signs to watch for:

- A lump or thickening in the breast or armpit;
- A change in the size or shape of the breast;
- Discharge from the nipple;
- A change in the color or texture of the skin of the breast or areola (such as dimpling, puckering, or scaliness).

Pain is generally not an early warning sign of breast cancer. However, any changes in the breast should be reported to a doctor without delay. Symptoms can be caused by cancer or by a number of less serious conditions. Early diagnosis is especially important for breast cancer because the disease responds best to treatment before it has spread. The earlier breast cancer is found and treated, the better a woman's chances for complete recovery.

SOURCE:
National Cancer Institute. *What You Need To Know about Breast Cancer.* NIH Pub. No. 88-1556. January 1988. pp. 4-5.

STAGING

In breast cancer, the following staging system is used:

- Carcinoma in situ is very early breast cancer. Cancer is present only in the immediate area in which it developed.
- Stage I means the tumor is no larger than 2 centimeters (cm)—about 1 inch—and has not spread outside the breast.
- Stage II means the tumor is from 2 to 5 cm—roughly 2 inches—and/or has spread to the lymph nodes under the arm.
- Stage III means the cancer is larger than 5 cm—about 2 inches—involves the underarm lymph nodes to a greater extent, and/or has spread to other lymph nodes or other tissues near the breast.
- Stage IV means the cancer has spread to other organs of the body, most often the lungs, bones, liver, or brain.

SOURCE:
National Cancer Institute. *What You Need To Know about Breast Cancer.* NIH Pub. No. 88-1556. January 1988. pp. 7-8.

TREATMENT METHODS

There are four standard ways to treat breast cancer: surgery, radiation therapy, chemotherapy, and hormone therapy. The doctor may decide to use just one method or a combination, depending on the woman's individual treatment needs. In some cases, the patient may be referred to other doctors who specialize in the different kinds of cancer treatment.

Surgery is the most common treatment for breast cancer. The purpose of surgery is to remove the tumor in the breast and, usually, to remove the underarm lymph nodes. The nodes are removed because they filter the lymph fluid that circulates through the breast and other parts of the body, and they are one of the first places to which breast cancer spreads. Cancer cells in the lymph nodes indicate that there may be cancer elsewhere in the body.

Radiation therapy (also called x-ray therapy, radiotherapy, cobalt treatment, or irradiation) uses high-energy rays to damage cancer cells and stop them from growing. Like surgery, radiation therapy is a local treatment; it affects only the cells in the treated area. Radiation may come from an outside source or from radioactive materials placed directly in the breast. Sometimes both are used. The patient receives external radiation treatments as an outpatient, usually 5 days a week for 5 or 6 weeks. At the end of that time, an extra "boost" of radiation is usually given to the treatment site. The boost may be either external (using electron beam therapy) or internal (using an implant). A short hospital stay is required for implant radiation.

Chemotherapy uses drugs to stop the growth of cancer cells. Chemotherapy may be given in different ways—by mouth or by injection into a muscle or vein. Because the drugs enter the bloodstream and travel through the body, chemotherapy is a systemic treatment. It can act on cancer cells outside the breast area. Some of these drugs are given in cycles so that treatment periods alternate with rest periods. Depending on the specific drugs, most patients take their chemotherapy as an outpatient at the hospital, at the doctor's office, or at home. Sometimes it may be necessary to stay in the hospital for a period of time so the effects of the treatment can be watched.

Hormone therapy is used to prevent cancer cells from getting the hormones they need to grow. This treatment may include the use of drugs that interfere with hormone activity or surgery that removes hormone-producing organs. Like chemotherapy, hormone therapy can act on cells all over the body.

Patients with early stage breast cancer (stage I and stage II) are most often treated with surgery or a combination of surgery and radiation therapy. The type of operation depends on the size and location of the tumor, the type of cancer, the age and general health of the woman, and the size of her breast. The possibility of plastic surgery to reconstruct the breast following treatment is another consideration. Decisions about treatment must also take into account the experience of the doctor and the desires of the patient.

A number of different operations are used to treat breast cancer:

- Modified radical mastectomy removes the breast, the underarm lymph nodes, and the lining over the chest muscles (but leaves the muscles). Today this is the most common operation for breast cancer.
- Lumpectomy removes just the breast lump and is followed by radiation therapy. Most surgeons also remove the underarm lymph nodes.
- Total or simple mastectomy removes just the breast. Sometimes a few of the underarm lymph nodes closest to the breast are also removed.
- Partial or segmental mastectomy removes the tumor, some of the normal breast tissue surrounding it, and the lining of the chest muscle below the tumor. Usually some of the underarm lymph nodes are removed. In most cases, radiation therapy follows the surgery.
- Radical mastectomy (also called the Halsted radical mastectomy) removes the breast, chest muscles, all of

the underarm lymph nodes, and some additional fat and skin. This procedure was the standard operation for many years. It is still used occasionally; but for most patients, less extensive surgery is just as effective.

Patients with carcinoma in situ may have a mastectomy or less extensive surgery. As with other types of breast cancer, the type of operation depends on many factors. Also, depending on the specific type of breast cancer involved, the lymph nodes may be removed, and radiation therapy may be advised.

For some patients with early stage breast cancer, chemotherapy or hormone therapy may be suggested along with the primary treatment (surgery or radiation therapy). Doctors may recommend this additional treatment, called adjuvant therapy, when cancer is found in the underarm lymph nodes or when lab tests show that the cancer cells are likely to spread. The purpose of adjuvant therapy for early stage patients is to prevent a recurrence by killing any undetected cells that may remain in the body.

Adjuvant therapy is usually recommended for patients who have cancer cells in the lymph nodes, which means that some cells may have reached other parts of the body. Whether to use chemotherapy or hormone therapy depends mainly on the woman's menopausal status and whether or not the cancer is hormone dependent.

Patients with stage III breast cancer usually have both local and systemic treatment. The local treatment may be mastectomy and/or radiation therapy. The systemic treatment may include chemotherapy and/or hormone therapy.

Chemotherapy and/or hormone therapy are used to treat stage IV breast cancer. In addition, patients may have limited surgery or radiation therapy to control the tumor in the breast. Also, radiation may be useful to treat breast cancer that has spread to other parts of the body.

SOURCE:
National Cancer Institute. *What You Need To Know about Breast Cancer.* NIH Pub. No. 88-1556. January 1988. pp. 9-13.

LUMPECTOMY VERSUS MASTECTOMY

Some 150,000 American women will be diagnosed with breast cancer this year. As many as 80 percent of them will be in the early stages of disease. According to a panel for the National Institutes of Health, early breast cancer is usually best treated by a limited operation that preserves the breast.

In the limited procedure, commonly called lumpectomy, only the tumor itself is removed. In mastectomy, the more common operation, the entire breast is removed. A lumpectomy, however, is always followed by daily radiation therapy for about five weeks. A mastectomy for early breast cancer does not usually require follow-up radiation therapy.

If the cancer hasn't spread beyond the breast, the panel concluded, lumpectomy followed by radiation generally gives the same excellent chance of survival as mastectomy. When the cancer has spread, neither procedure alone is adequate; drug treatment (chemotherapy and hormone therapy) would be necessary.

But not all cases of early breast cancer are best treated by lumpectomy. Sometimes there's more than one area of cancer in the breast. Sometimes the size or location of a tumor requires surgery that would seriously disfigure the breast. In those cases, a mastectomy is the preferred procedure. And some women choose mastectomy rather than go through radiation treatments.

When women undergo mastectomy, the panel recommended that they consider breast reconstruction to "improve the cosmetic result." However, some women may prefer a prosthetic device (artificial breast) or nothing at all.

SOURCE:
"Lumpectomy vs. Mastectomy." *Consumer Reports Health Letter* (October 1990): 79.

ADJUVANT THERAPY

Recent studies have shown that women with early stage breast cancer may benefit from adjuvant (additional) therapy following primary treatment (mastectomy or lumpectomy with radiation therapy). These studies indicate that many breast cancer patients whose underarm lymph nodes show no sign of cancer (known as node negative) may benefit from chemotherapy or hormonal therapy after primary treatment. (These findings do not apply to women with preinvasive or in situ breast cancer.)

Until now, women whose underarm lymph nodes were free of cancer usually received no additional therapy because they have a relatively good chance of surviving the disease after primary treatment. But scientists know that cancer may return in about 30 percent of these women. Adjuvant therapy may prevent or delay the return of cancer.

Based on these findings, the National Cancer Institute has alerted doctors to consider using adjuvant therapy for their node negative breast cancer patients. Although there is strong evidence of the benefits of adjuvant therapy, there also are certain risks and expenses. Therefore, each woman should discuss her treatment options with her doctor.

SOURCE:
National Cancer Institute. *Breast Cancer Treatment Update: Adjuvant Therapy May Benefit Patients with Early Stage Disea'* (flyer). GPO: O-238-647. 1989.

BREAST RECONSTRUCTION

Breast reconstruction is a surgical procedure in which a plastic surgeon rebuilds the breast contour after a mastectomy. If the patient wishes, the surgeon can recreate the nipple and/or areola (the circle of pigmented skin around the nipple).

Many women choose reconstruction so that they won't need to wear an artificial breast form (prosthesis), as well as to restore their whole-body image.

Susan Love, M.D., a surgical oncologist at the Dana Farber Cancer Institute's Breast Evaluation Center in Boston, recalls the words of one of her patients:

"When I was wearing my prosthesis every day, when I looked at my body and it was concave where there had been a breast, I felt that I was a cancer patient, that I was living with that every single day. With the reconstruction, I feel that I'm healthy again—that I can go on with my life."

According to the National Cancer Institute, virtually every woman who undergoes a mastectomy can have her breast artificially restored. Neither age nor type of cancer surgery is an obstacle. Reconstruction is still possible even if a woman's skin has been damaged by radiotherapy or her chest muscles have been removed during cancer surgery.

It's important to remember, however, that breast reconstruction is a cosmetic procedure. The surgery will restore breast appearance but not breast function or sensation.

SOURCE:
"Breast Reconstruction: Helping Restore Self-Esteem." *The University of Texas Lifetime Health Letter* 2, no. 10 (October 1990): 4.

LONG TERM SURVIVAL

The critical factor for long term survival in breast cancer is whether the underarm lymph nodes are also cancerous. If the lymph nodes test negative and show no signs of malignancy the chances are good for disease-free survival. Most studies suggest excellent survival in node-negative women after removal of tumours less than one cm across. Over the long haul, those with invasive breast cancer but negative nodes do better than those with positive nodes. Based on present statistics, about 85 per cent of node-negative patients are alive and well five years after removal of a cancerous breast lump, and 70 per cent are doing well 10 years later. On the other hand, if some of the lymph nodes show signs of cancer the odds for survival drop. Women with breast cancer who have malignant nodes have a higher risk of recurrence, depending on the number of cancer-ridden nodes and the type of malignancy. Women with breast cancer aren't really free of recurrence risks for 15, 20 or more years. Nonetheless, some women with ominous nodes at biopsy survive for many decades!

SOURCE:
"Breast Cancer Update: Part One." *University of Toronto Faculty of Medicine Health News* 9, no. 3 (June 1991): 5.

RESOURCES

ORGANIZATIONS

American Cancer Society. 1599 Clifton Road NE, Atlanta, GA 30329.

Office of Cancer Communications. National Cancer Institute, Building 31, Bethesda, MD 20892. (800) 4-CANCER.

BOOK

Love, Susan M. *Dr. Susan Love's Breast Book.* Addison-Wesley, 1990. 455 pp.

PAMPHLETS

National Cancer Institute, Office of Cancer Communications:

Adjuvant Therapy: Facts for Women with Breast Cancer. NIH Pub. No. 87-2877. July 1987. 10 pp.

Breast Cancer: Understanding Treatment Options. NIH Pub. No. 87-2675. September 1987. 19 pp.

Mastectomy: A Treatment for Breast Cancer. NIH Pub. No. 87-658. August 1987. 24 pp.

Radiation Therapy: A Treatment for Early Stage Breast Cancer. NIH Pub. No. 87-659. September 1987. 21 pp.

ADDITIONAL ARTICLES

"Adjuvant Chemotherapy of Early Breast Cancer." *The Medical Letter on Drugs and Therapeutics* 32, no. 818 (May 18, 1990): 49-52.

Angier, Natalie. "Some Genetic Pieces Are Falling Into Place in Breast Cancer Puzzle." *New York Times.* Tuesday, December 25, 1990.

Baker, Nancy C. "Relative Risk: How Families Face Up to Breast Cancer." *Good Housekeeping* (April 1991): 96, 98, 100, 104.

"Breast Cancer: Early Decisions." *Harvard Medical School Health Letter* 13, no. 5 (March 1988): 1-4.

"Breast Cancer Part Two: Treatment." *University of Toronto Faculty of Medicine News* 9, no. 4 (August 1991): 1-4.

"In Pursuit of a Terrible Killer." *Newsweek* (December 10, 1990): 66-68.

Komaki, Ritsuko, James D. Cox, and others. "Stage I and II Breast Carcinoma: Treatment with Limited Surgery and Radiation Therapy Versus Mastectomy." *Radiology* 174, no. 1 (January 1990): 255-257.

"New Options for Breast Cancer." *Health After 50* (June 1990): 2-3.

Schwade, James G., David S. Robinson, and Neil Love. "Primary Localized Breast Cancer: Treatment Options and Informed Choices." *Postgraduate Medicine.* 86, no. 5 (October 1989): 181-192.

"Treatment of Early-Stage Breast Cancer: NIH Consensus Conference." *JAMA* 265, no. 3 (January 16, 1991): 391-397.

Wallis, Claudia. "A Puzzling Plague." *Time* (January 14, 1991): 48-52.

BREAST FEEDING

OVERVIEW

When deciding whether or not to breastfeed their baby, new parents need guidance, reassurance, accurate information and emotional support to wend their way through the wealth of conflicting data from the media, caregivers and well-meaning friends. Breastmilk, specifically tailored to human development by the long process of evolution, supplies all the nutrients necessary for optimal infant development. Besides its specific nutrients, breastmilk also contains anti-infective agents—antibodies and living cells (such as white blood cells) that ward off infection and protect newborns against many bacteria, viruses, fungi and parasites during the first few postnatal months. Formula manufacturers have not yet managed to duplicate precisely the many properties of that complex, living fluid, human milk.

While breastfeeding is the optimal nutrition for babies in the first few post-birth months, this doesn't mean that babies fed modern, scientifically researched, meticulously produced, and carefully selected formula will be nutritionally deprived, but simply that mothers should get enough information beforehand so that they can make an informed choice about how to feed their infants. They should know about the benefits of breastmilk and how it compares to formula. But if, for whatever reason, a woman cannot or doesn't want to nurse her baby—perhaps because of job commitments, an illness (such as hepatitis) or because she must take certain drugs—she needn't feel less competent as a mother. Better to bottle feed than to feel uncomfortable and insecure about nursing.

SOURCE:
"Breast is Still Best." *Health News* 7, no. 5 (April 1989): 8.

MOTHER-INFANT RELATIONSHIP

The unique feature of breastfeeding relevant to infant development is that mother and baby are involved in a system based on mutuality. Their need for each other goes beyond the feeding of a hungry baby signaling his need for food, as in bottle feeding. In the breastfeeding couple, the system remains in balance because the mother offers the breast both in response to the baby's signal and in response to the signals of her own body. The mother's breasts fill with milk and she needs to relieve the pressure by nursing. As she nurses, the hormone prolactin, called the "mothering hormone," is released, adding a feeling of relaxation and well-being. Such an effect can be a positive reinforcement of breastfeeding.

The infant's hunger produces physical demands for feeding. His crying stimulates the hormones of the mother to release the milk from her breast, known as the "milk ejection reflex," even before she is holding her baby and before he begins sucking. Left to their own scheduling, without the imposition of routines, mother and baby adjust their behavior and sleep patterns to meet these mutual needs. A sufficient supply of milk is created to maintain the infant during periods of rapid growth.

Because both derive physical comfort from nursing, their interdependence keeps them in close, frequent contact. The proper positioning of the baby at the breast allows for skin-to-skin contact, eye contact, and reinforcement of maternal feelings through the effect of the released hormones. The baby passively receives immunizations all during the breastfeeding period offering protection from illness. For the first six months, this system needs no additional supplements to be adequate.

The amount of milk produced does not depend on the size of a woman's breasts or the adequacy of her diet, but on the frequency and length of the feeding per day. A fully breastfeeding mother may produce a quart of milk per day. Even malnourished women produce sufficient milk of generally high quality for their babies.

SOURCE:
Popper, B. K., and C. K. Culley. "Breast Feeding Makes a Comeback—for Good Reason." *The Brown University Child Behavior and Development Letter* 5, no. 4 (February 1989): 1.

BREAST DISORDERS DURING LACTATION

The number of mothers who breast-feed their infants is on the rise because of patient education and support from perinatal nurses and physicians. In addition to greater social acceptance of breast feeding, mothers recognize cost effectiveness, availability of the food source to the infant and enhanced mother-infant bonding as reasons to try breast feeding. Improved infant nutrition and health through passive immunity are other reasons that physicians may mention to encourage women to consider nursing. The family physician should not only be prepared to support the mother who decides to nurse, but should also be familiar with the common breast disorders that may occur during lactation.

Such disorders range from relatively minor problems, such as sore nipples, milk stasis and mastitis, to more serious conditions, such as abcesses and neoplasms. Inflammatory changes are easily treated with frequent breast emptying; infectious processes require antibiotics. Surgical intervention may be needed for some conditions. Pregnancy or lactation should not delay or alter the diagnosis and treatment of suspected breast carcinoma.

SOURCE:
Olsen, C. G., and R. E. Gordon, Jr. "Breast Disorders in Nursing Mothers." *American Family Physician* 41, no. 5: (May 1990): 1509.

MILK STORAGE

More and more new mothers are opting to breast-feed their infants, a practice wholeheartedly endorsed by the American Academy of Pediatrics because of its nutritional as well as psychological benefits. But the fact that so many breast-feeding mothers are also working mothers presents a problem. To be sure, a nursing mother can use a breast pump to extract milk during the work day, but several hours may pass before her milk is fed to the baby. And that raises the question of how it can be stored safely.

Obviously, refrigeration is the preferred method of storage, says Laurence Finberg, MD, chairman of the American Academy of Pediatrics' committee on nutrition. But mothers who do not have access to refrigerators need not worry. Researchers reporting in the *Journal of Pediatrics* have discovered that breast milk can be left at room temperature for up to six hours with very little risk. In other words, unlike cow's milk, nonrefrigerated mother's milk is a poor breeding ground for organisms that can cause illness. The reason is that human milk contains appreciable amounts of protective substances, such as lactoferrin, that inhibit bacterial proliferation.

To be on the safe side, working mothers who want to store their milk at room temperature should keep it out of sunlight and in a cool place to insure the least possible growth of bacteria.

SOURCE:
"Storing the Mother's Milk." *Tufts University Diet and Nutrition Letter* 5, no. 1 (February 1988): 7.

USE OF BREAST PUMPS

If you plan to go back to work within a few month of giving birth but want your baby to continue to drink your breast milk while you are at the office, you can pump (express) it and store it in the refrigerator to be given to the baby during the day. Some women prefer pumping by hand, a matter of placing the thumb and index finger on the areola about an inch away from the nipple, pressing gently inward toward the chest, squeezing the two fingers together, and pushing back and squeezing on the breast while catching the milk in a clean container. Others prefer breast pumps.

Full-service electric pumps are the most efficient, but they are also prohibitively expensive for most women and fairly expensive to rent (although no more expensive to rent than to purchase formula). Other options, all generally costing less than $50, include a number of good hand pumps that are either operated manually or powered by batteries or wall-socket electricity.

It doesn't really matter which you use, according to LaLeche League International, an organization that offers information and support to breast-feeding mothers, as long as you're comfortable with it. Most important, points out Laleche League medical information liaison Julie Stock, is pumping the milk in a relaxed environment—while watching the baby asleep, for instance, or while looking at a picture of the baby if you're at the office—so that the "letdown" mechanism, which allows the milk to reach the nipple from farther up in the breast, will work smoothly. The only pump Ms. Stock advises against is the hand-operated kind that is shaped like a bicycle horn. Because it's cheap, you may be tempted to buy it, but it's both ineffective and difficult to sterilize, and it can cause serious damage to breast tissue.

SOURCE:
"When Deciding Between Feeding by Breast or by Bottle." *Tufts University Diet and Nutrition Letter* 8, no. 10 (December 1990): 4.

BREAST FEEDING—AND BIRTH CONTROL

Women who breast feed can resume sexual relations soon after giving birth, just as can women who do not breast feed. Nursing is not a form of birth control. It is true that the risk of pregnancy is decreased compared to someone who is not nursing, but you can become pregnant before you begin to menstruate again after pregnancy.

There are many methods of birth control available, but you should not take birth control pills while you are breast feeding. Talk with your doctor about the different types, and together you can select the method that is best for you.

SOURCE:
Breast Feeding Your Baby. *HealthTips* 2 (March 1988): 7.

EFFECT OF SOCIAL DRUGS

Studies reveal that tobacco, black tea, alcohol, coffee and other caffeine-based substances, as well as marijuana and other street drugs, can negatively affect the quantity or quality of breastmilk. Although some of these substances may produce only minimal alterations, it is difficult, if not impossible, to determine a "safe" limit.

Cigarette smoking, even in small amounts, is contraindicated. To begin with, the smoke inhaled by a baby can cause as many problems as the nicotine ingested in the milk. Babies of mothers who smoke more than 20 cigarettes a day have more vomiting and nausea that those whose mothers do not smoke. In addition, mothers who smoke have decreased levels of milk production, as well as both higher levels of DDT (from the tobacco leaves) and lower levels of vitamin C in their milk; and their children have a greater susceptibility to upper respiratory infections.

Caffeine, one of the most frequently ingested drugs in society, is present not only in coffee, black tea, chocolate, and cola drinks, but also in such over-the-counter medications as stimulants, pain relievers, diuretics, cold remedies, and weight-control aids. Whereas only about 1 percent of the caffeine ingested by a nursing mother appears in her milk, the amount passed on can accumulate in baby's system. Nursing mothers who consume small amounts of caffeine will therefore want to watch for side effects in their babies. The most common responses are wakefulness and hyperactivity—behaviors that are sometimes misdiagnosed as colic. Such side effects can disappear within one week of eliminating caffeine from the diet.

Although alcohol is known to negatively affect the growth and development of a fetus, most studies exploring its impact on the breastfed infant are inconclusive. Small amounts of alcohol may be safe and may even stimulate the let-down reflex. Large amounts, however, can reduce or block the transport of hormones needed to activate this reflex. Alternatives to alcohol are visualization, deep breathing, and other relaxation techniques.

SOURCE:
Moses, L. S., II. "Drugs and Breastmilk." *Mothering* 6 (Summer 1990): 68.

RESOURCES

ORGANIZATION
LaLeche League International. P.O. Box 1209, Franklin Park, IL 60131.

BOOKS

Eiger, Marvin S., and Sally Wendkos Olds. *The Complete Book of Breastfeeding.* Revised ed. New York: Bantam, 1987. 224 pp.

Kamen, Betty, and Si Kamen. *Total Nutrition for Breast-feeding Mothers.* Boston: Little, Brown, 1986. 266 pp.

La Leche League International. *The Womanly Art of Breastfeeding.* 4th revised edition. New York: New American Library. 1987. 422 pp.

Mason, Diane, and Diane Ingersoll. *Breastfeeding and the Working Mother: The Complete Guide for Today's Nursing Mother.* New York: St. Martin's Press, 1986. 212 pp.

Reukauf, Diane M., Mary A. Trause. *Commonsense Breastfeeding: A Practical Guide to the Pleasures, Problems, and Solutions.* New York: Athenaeum, 1987. 194 pp.

RELATED ARTICLES

"Breast Feeding and the Working Mother." *American Family Physician* (November 1989): 205.

"Breast Not Necessarily Best." *The Lancet* (March 19, 1988): 624–626.

Cherry, Sheldon H. "Deciding Whether to Breast-Feed." *Parents* 66, no. 9 (September 1991): 175–178.

Gray R. H. and others. "Risk of Ovulation during Lactation." *The Lancet* 335 (January 6, 1990): 25–29.

Howie, P. W. and others. "Protective Effect of Breast Feeding against Infection." *British Medical Journal* 300 (January 5, 1990): 11–16.

Seltzer, Vickie S., and Fred Benjamin. "Breast-Feeding and the Potential for Human Immunodeficiency Virus Transmission." *Obstetrics & Gynecology* 75, no. 4 (April 1990): 713–715.

CARPAL TUNNEL SYNDROME

OVERVIEW

It starts with a tingling sensation in the fingers. Over the next few months, the tingling may progress to numbness and a burning or aching pain. At first, the discomfort strikes only at night. Then it lingers in the morning. The pain may radiate up the arm. By then, even a simple task like buttoning a shirt may be difficult.

That's the way carpal tunnel syndrome typically progresses. The carpal tunnel is a narrow channel formed by the bones and ligaments of the wrist. Tendons that flex the fingers thread through the carpal tunnel alongside the median nerve, which provides sensation to the thumb and the index, middle, and ring fingers. Sometimes, the sheaths around those tendons become swollen and compress the median nerve, triggering the symptoms of carpal tunnel syndrome. If left untreated, the nerve can eventually suffer permanent damage, leaving you without the full use of your hand.

Carpal tunnel syndrome is one of several increasingly common "repetitive-motion ailments" brought on by such tasks as long hours at a typewriter, computer keyboard, or assembly line. Other contributing factors include pregnancy; underlying conditions such as arthritis, diabetes, and hypothyroidism; and fractures, infections, or cysts in the wrist. The syndrome is most common among women in their 40's through 60's.

Preventing problems

If your activities or some other factor makes you susceptible to carpal tunnel syndrome, certain steps can reduce the risk.

Since bending the wrist up and down compresses the tunnel, try to adjust your posture to minimize such bending. Adjusting the height of your seat, for example, may allow you to type with your wrists in a neutral rather than a flexed or extended position. When possible, use hand tools with fat, easy-to-grip, specially curved handles that you can use without bending your wrist. Stopping to rest your hands periodically also helps.

Treating the syndrome

When simple self-help measures don't help, professional treatment of the wrist probably will. Therapies range from splinting to surgery, depending on how advanced the condition is.

Wrist splinting. Immobilizing the wrist temporarily with a lightweight plastic splint usually helps. The splint prevents movement and supports the wrist in a neutral position, relieving pressure on the irritated median nerve. The splint may be worn round the clock or only at night. Symptoms subside permanently in some people after wearing the splint for a few weeks.

Oral antiinflammatory drugs. Nonprescription antiinflammatory drugs—aspirin or ibuprofen—may help reduce the inflammation and pain of carpal tunnel syndrome. If those don't work, your doctor may prescribe stronger antiinflammatory pills. For maximum benefit, medications can be used in addition to splinting.

Cortisone injection. If that combination doesn't provide relief, a cortisone injection directly into the carpal tunnel may do the trick. At first, the injection can actually increase discomfort. But after a day or two, the inflammation subsides and symptoms ease. If they recur, you could try a second injection or consider surgery.

Surgery

Severe or chronic symptoms can signal nerve damage. To prevent further deterioration, surgery is often required. Surgery may also be necessary to relieve acute carpal tunnel syndrome, when severe symptoms appear suddenly.

The procedure, carpal tunnel release, is relatively fast and simple. It's usually performed on an outpatient basis, often under local anesthesia. The surgeon cuts the ligament that forms the carpal tunnel. That relaxes the rigid tunnel and frees the compressed nerve. Two or three weeks later, you can begin to use your hand, though you may not regain complete function for up to three months.

The procedure usually relieves pain immediately and permanently without reducing strength in the hand. Numbness, however, often lingers for a year or more. If the hand has gone untreated for several years, it may never recover completely.

Some surgeons report that most people who have had the operation can safely return to their old activities without triggering symptoms all over again. Others believe that those activities should be avoided or modified to prevent relapse.

SOURCE:
"When Overworked Hands Hurt: A Common Disorder Called Carpal Tunnel Syndrome Can Result from Overdoing Simple Tasks Like Typing." *Consumer Reports Health Letter* 3 (January 1991): 5-6.

DIAGNOSIS

The gold standard for diagnosing carpal tunnel syndrome, nerve conduction testing, is costly. Although the sensitivity of nerve conduction testing is approximately 90 percent, the specificity has not been established. Clinical history and physical examination, including provocative maneuvers, are appropriate screening tools, but their diagnostic accuracy is not well established. Katz and colleagues assessed the value of the history and physical examination findings in the diagnosis of carpal tunnel syndrome.

The study included 110 patients referred to a neurophysiology laboratory for electrophysiologic evaluation of upper extremity complaints of diverse causes. The majority of patients had experienced numbness, pain and tingling. Seventy-two percent indicated that their symptoms were worse at night and awakened them from sleep. Medical history, demographic and physical examination data, and a hand pain diagram were obtained from each patient before nerve conduction testing was performed. The hand pain diagram depicted both hands in dorsal and palmar views. Each patient marked the areas on the diagram that corresponded to the location of symptoms. The diagrams were categorized as either indicating classic, probable or possible carpal tunnel syndrome, or as unlikely to indicate the diagnosis. Associations between clinical data and nerve conduction results were examined in univariate and multivariate analyses.

Forty-four (40.0 percent) of the patients were diagnosed as having carpal tunnel syndrome. The best predictors were the hand pain diagram rating and Tinel's sign. The combination of Tinel's sign [indication of irritability of a nerve] and a probable or classic diagram rating had a positive predictive value of 0.71. Other findings from the physical examination (two-point discrimination, thenar [ball of the thumb] atrophy, thumb strength and Phalen's sign) and the history were less useful. Only 9 percent of the patients under 40 years of age with possible or unlikely diagram ratings had carpal tunnel syndrome. The authors believe that this finding may suggest that subsets of patients presenting with symptoms of carpal tunnel syndrome may be managed without performing nerve conduction studies. (*Annals of Internal Medicine*, March 1, 1990, vol. 112, p. 321.)

SOURCE:
"Carpal Tunnel Syndrome." *American Family Physician* 42 (October 1990): 1096-1097.

SPORTS AS A RISK FACTOR

Besides work involving repetitive hand movements, other risk factors include being female (women are twice as likely as men to get CTS); being pregnant (because of fluid retention); or having arthritis, diabetes or thyroid problems. For office workers and others already at risk for developing CTS, some advice from Susan Toth Cohen, an occupational therapist and assistant clinical professor at Thomas Jefferson University in Philadelphia on protecting themselves while at play:

Weight lifting: If you wrap your wrists too tightly, the straps can cause swelling and make your hands stiff. "But as a reminder to keep your wrists straight, the straps are great."

Running: Avoid clenching or squeezing your hands while running. Hand weights may also aggravate the condition.

Aerobics: Heavy hand weights cause the wrist to bend down, stressing it. Lighter weights won't cause this problem.

Exercise machines: On stair-climbers, avoid leaning on the handrails during increased speeds, which places the wrist in an unnatural position. The continuous flexing and extending of the wrist on stationary bicycles and rowers can aggravate CTS symptoms.

Racket sports: Gripping the racket correctly and keeping aware of wrist position is the best defense against CTS. Racquetball players should avoid crashing into walls to retrieve balls; that stresses hands trying to offset the crash. If you do develop symptoms of CTS while playing racquetball, squash or tennis, you may be wise to find another sport. "But don't assume if you have pain or tingling in your hand or wrist, you have CTS," she says. "See your doctor."

SOURCE:
"Carpal Tunnel Syndrome: Worsened by Some Sports." *Executive Edge* 21, no. 7 (July 1990): 6.

PREVENTION

Roger Stephens, Ph.D., a government ergonomist, [notes], "In my experience, about only one in four patients with true, work-induced CTS can return to the job successfully. We're seeking many job changes."

Obviously, it's a much better idea to prevent CTS in the first place. The key is body mechanics. "Sometimes changing the height of your chair or the way you hold a tool can cure the problem," Stephens says. Things you can do:

- Type with your arms parallel to the floor and wrists in neutral, "floating" above the keyboard. Adjust the height of your keyboard, desktop or chair to eliminate any cocking of the hands. Don't rest your wrists on the edge of the desk. That compresses the carpal area.
- If you have a detachable keyboard with a long cord, change your position occasionally. For instance, rest the keyboard on your lap.
- Consider a wrist rest, a soft pad that extends toward you from under the keyboard. Ergonomic Design, Inc., (303) 452-8006, sells one for about $50. Sit-Rite, (800) 235-4204, markets an adjustable rest for about $350.
- Switch from a conventional computer mouse to a track ball, which looks like a pool ball resting in a cup. "We see more and more engineers and designers getting CTS," says David Rempel, M.D., a University of California-San Francisco ergonomist and expert in occupational medicine. One reason is that clicking and dragging a mouse is tough on tendons. A track ball is easier to lock and release.
- Use larger tool handles. "Too small and they can press directly on the tendons and median nerve in the palm," explains Dr. Rempel. Buy soft covers that enlarge tool handles, or make your own with duct tape and foam rubber.
- Avoid working in the cold, when tendons are less flexible, more likely to become irritated and swollen.
- Avoid repetition. "Take a break lasting 5 to 10 minutes every hour and shorter pauses every 5 to 10 minutes," advises Dr. [David] Thompson, [a Stanford University ergonomist]. "Shake out your hands, roll your head on your shoulders, get up and walk around, anything to relax and get the blood flowing."

SOURCE:
Olsen, Eric. "Wrist Stop." *Men's Health* 5 (October 1990): 32–33.

RESOURCES

RELATED ARTICLES

"Carpal Tunnel Syndrome: If You Have This Annoying Hand Condition, There's Light at the End of the Tunnel." *Mayo Clinic Health Letter* 8 (April 1990): 1–2.

Cotton, Paul. "Symptoms May Return after Carpal Tunnel Surgery." *JAMA* 265 (April 17, 1991): 1922–1923.

Haase, Gunter R., Alexander C. Johnson, and Oscar M. Reinmuth. "Coping with Carpal Tunnel Syndrome." *Patient Care* 24 (July 15, 1990): 127–130.

"Preventing CTS." *The University of California, Berkeley Wellness Letter* 7 (April 1991): 7.

Shellenbarger, Teresa. "When You're Asked about Carpal Tunnel Syndrome." *RN* (July 1991): 40–42.

CAT SCANS (COMPUTED TOMOGRAPHY)

(*See also:* MAGNETIC RESONANCE IMAGING [MRI])

DEFINITION

An x-ray technique that produces a film representing a detailed cross section of tissue structure. The procedure is painless, noninvasive, and requires no special preparation. Computed tomography employs a narrowly collimated beam of x-rays that rotates in a continuous 360-degree motion around the patient to image the body in cross-sectional slices. An array of detectors, positioned at several angles, records those x-rays that pass through the body. The image is created by computer using multiple attenuation readings taken around the periphery of the body part. The computer calculates tissue absorption, displays a printout of the numeric values, and produces a visualization of the tissues that demonstrates the densities of the various structures. Tumor masses, infractions, bone displacement, and accumulations of fluid may be detected. Formerly called computerized axial tomography.

SOURCE:
Glanze, Walter D., Kenneth N. Anderson, and Lois E. Anderson (eds.). "Computed Tomography (CT)." In *Mosby's Medical, Nursing, and Allied Health Dictionary*. 3d ed. St. Louis: C.V. Mosby, 1990. p. 289.

OVERVIEW

In this test a computerized axial tomography (CAT or CT) scanner is used to produce a series of cross-sectional x-ray images of a selected part of the body. A computer operates the scanner, and the resulting picture represents a slice of the body. Areas above and below the chosen slice do not appear on the image. The computer can then combine the information in several slices to create other images of the structures inside the body. These images can detect many conditions that cannot be seen in regular x-rays.

The scanner produces images by passing a pencil-thin beam of x-rays through a particular area of the body. The x-ray tube moves rapidly around the chosen slice, creating a 360-degree picture. It takes the machine only a few seconds to photograph each slice, and 10–30 slices are usually taken.

The x-ray beam is picked up by an electronic device that records the information and sends it to a computer for processing. The computer then displays the chosen slice on a TV screen. Information from several slices can be combined to create a view across the body from any angle.

Information from the scans is stored in the computer's memory and can be converted into images on a video screen at any time. Photographs of the video screen are taken to record significant findings. The information is then kept in storage on a disk or tape so that it can be examined again if necessary.

It is no overstatement to say that CT scanning has revolutionized the practice of making images of the human body. The CT scanner is the greatest advance in diagnostic imaging since the discovery of x-rays. It produces pictures with 10–20 times the detail of regular x-rays, and it can be used to make images of parts of the body that were previously difficult or impossible to obtain.

However, CT scans are more expensive than regular x-rays, and scanners are not available in all areas. And because the technique is relatively new, some doctors may be unfamiliar with all its uses.

CT scans of the body are used to diagnose a wide variety of conditions, including the following:

- **Chest (Thorax)**—To locate suspected tumors, including Hodgkin's disease, in the space between the lungs (mediastinum); to help decide whether small lumps in the lung are cancer; to distinguish bulges (aneurysms) of the aorta (a large artery which passes down the back of the chest cavity) from tumors of the chest; and to investigate the spread of tumors into the chest from elsewhere in the body.
- **Kidney**—To confirm the presence of stones, obstructions, tumors, congenital abnormalities, infections, and other diseases of the kidneys.
- **Liver**—To diagnose tumors, abscesses, and bleeding.
- **Biliary Tract**—To evaluate jaundice (yellowing of the skin).
- **Pancreas**—To determine if there is a tumor or inflammation of the pancreas. The CT scan is replacing the use of ultrasound as the test of choice for examination of the pancreas. Although it costs more and involves radiation exposure, it can be much more accurate in many conditions. CT scans do a much better job than ultrasound in distinguishing between benign and malignant tumors of the pancreas.
- **Adrenals**—To look for tumors.
- **Spleen**—To evaluate suspected injury and other abnormalities.
- **Spine**—To investigate suspected tumors, injuries, deformities, and other problems of the backbone, discs, and spinal canal. . . .

This test is performed in a hospital radiology department or office by a radiologist and an x-ray technician. You will be asked to lie on a table which is connected to the large CT scanner. You will be positioned so that the body part to be examined lies in the middle of the large scanner ring. The ring contains the x-ray tube and detector.

After the procedure begins, the table on which you are lying will move a small distance every few seconds—this is to position you for each new slice. The mechanism inside the scanner will move around your body and may make clicking or buzzing sounds. It is especially important that you hold completely still while the scan is being taken. Otherwise, repeat scans may be needed.

During the test you will be alone in the room. A technician will be keeping a close watch through an observation window, and you will be able to talk to him or her by a two-way intercom.

An x-ray contrast material may be used to highlight internal structures. This material may be given by mouth, by an injection, or in some cases via an enema. If contrast enhancement is to be used, a preliminary set of CT scans will be done, the contrast medium will be administered, and the CT scans will be repeated.

Afterward you will be asked to wait while the radiologist reviews the scans to be sure that they contain all the required information. Occasionally repeat or additional scans are required.

This test usually takes from 30 minutes to 1½ hours, but because delays and repeats are common, you should allow 2 hours or more.

SOURCE:
Sobel, David S., and Tom Ferguson. "CT Scan—Body." In *The People's Book of Medical Tests*. New York: Simon & Schuster, 1985. pp. 253–254.

COMMON APPLICATIONS

Most trauma, emergency, and critical care imaging requirements are best met by CT. It is difficult or impossible with current technology to ensure continuous monitoring of vital functions during MRI scanning.

CT is generally preferred for postoperative follow-up and is still preferred, often because of availability and lower cost, as an initial method for imaging most abnormalities of the maxillary sinuses, nasal turbinates, lungs, mediastinum, pancreas, spleen, liver, and pelvis. It is also preferred for middle ear diseases involving the ossicles, osteomeatal stenosis, routine examination of hydrocephalic patients, examination of post-stroke patients and patients with encephalomalacia, and progress studies of patients with cerebral atrophy.

Because bone does not emit any appreciable MRI signal and therefore cannot be seen on MRI scans, CT is preferred whenever fine bone detail is required. CT is also the most informative study for the evaluation of some tumors, particularly meningiomas, although the newly approved paramagnetic contrast agent, gadolinium diethylenetriamine pentaacetic acid (Gd-DTPA), is improving MRI's ability to image such lesions.

SOURCE:
Cushmore, Frederick N., Walter Kucharczyk, and David L. Rodibaugh. "MRI: When You Can't Afford Not To." *Patient Care* 23 (February 28, 1989): 33.

RESOURCES

RELATED ARTICLES

Anderson, Robert E. "Magnetic Resonance Imaging Versus Computed Tomography—Which One?" *Postgraduate Medicine* 85, no. 3 (February 15, 1989): 79–83, 86–87.

Weck, Egon. "A Primer on Medical Imaging. Part One." *FDA Consumer* 23 (April 1989): 24–27.

CATARACTS

OVERVIEW

A cataract is a clouding of the normally clear and transparent lens of the eye. It is not a tumor or a new growth of skin or tissue over the eye, but a fogging of the lens itself. Normally the lens of the eye is clear. When a cataract develops, the lens becomes as cloudy as a frosted window.

Located near the front of the eye, the lens focuses light on the retina at the back of the eye. Light passes through it to produce a sharp image on the retina. When a cataract forms, the lens can become so opaque and unclear that light cannot easily be transmitted to the retina. Often, however, a cataract covers only a small part of the lens and, if sight is not greatly impaired, there is no need to remove the cataract. If a large portion of the lens becomes cloudy, sight can be partially or completely lost until the cataract is removed.

There are many misconceptions about cataracts. For instance, cataracts do not spread from eye to eye, though they may develop in both eyes at the same time. A cataract is not a film visible on the outside of the eye, is not caused from overuse of the eyes, and using the eye does not make it worse. Cataracts usually develop gradually over many years; rarely they develop over a few months. Finally, cataracts are not related to cancer and having a cataract does not mean a patient will be permanently blind.

There are many types of cataracts. Most are caused by a change in the chemical composition of the lens resulting in a loss of transparency. These changes can be caused by aging, injuries to the eye, certain diseases and conditions of the eye and body, and heredity or birth defects.

The normal process of aging may cause the lens to harden and turn cloudy. These are called senile cataracts and are the most common type. They can occur as early as age 40.

Children as well as adults of any age can develop cataracts. When cataracts appear in children, they are sometimes hereditary or can be caused by infection or inflammation which affect the pregnant mother and the unborn baby. These are called congenital cataracts and are present at birth.

Eye injuries can cause cataracts in patients of any age. A hard blow, puncture, cut, intense heat or chemical burn can damage the lens, resulting in a traumatic cataract. Certain infections or diseases of the eye such as diabetes, can also cause the lens to cloud and form a secondary cataract.

Depending on the size and location of the cloudy areas in a lens, a person may or may not be aware that a cataract is developing. If the cataract is located on the outer edge of the lens, no change may be noticed in vision, but if the cloudiness is located near the center of the lens, it usually interferes with clear sight. As cataracts develop there may be hazy, fuzzy, and blurred vision. Double vision may also occur when a cataract is beginning to form. The eyes may be more sensitive to light and glare, making night driving difficult. There may be a need to change eyeglass prescriptions frequently.

As the cataract worsens, stronger glasses no longer improve sight. It may help to hold objects closer to the eye to read and do close-up work.

The pupil, which is normally black, may undergo noticeable color changes and appear to be yellowish or white.

SOURCE:

American Academy of Ophthalmology. *Cataract: Clouding the Lens of Sight*. April 1987. pp. 1-4.

* * *

A cataract is a cloudy area inside the eye that interferes with vision. The only way a cataract can be eliminated is through a surgical procedure. Some people who have cataracts can see well enough to go about their day-to-day activities, however, and an operation is not always necessary for them. . . .

Cataracts cause a gradual loss of transparency in a part of the focusing mechanism of the eye, which is called the lens. The lens has a soft central nucleus and a soft outer part (cortex) within a clear capsule. The lens sits behind the iris (the colored part of the eye) and in the center of the pupil (the dark opening of the iris that changes size with the amount of light that strikes the eye).

As cataracts become progressively larger and more cloudy, they produce a steadily increasing but painless loss of vision. The degree of visual loss varies with the location and the extent of the cataract. If the cataract is small and in the center of the lens, a person often can see around it. If it is large, the cataract will prevent light from passing through the lens and will blur vision more.

Some cataracts have no obvious cause, but they are associated with certain diseases or other circumstances. Cataracts are often found in older people, and they are particularly common in older diabetics. They may occur in people who have metabolic disorders, and they sometimes affect individuals who have chronic inflammations of the eye. Cataracts occasionally may follow a severe injury to the eye or the ingestion of toxic chemicals or drugs.

SOURCE:
American College of Surgeons. *When You Need an Operation: About Cataract Surgery in Adults.* n.d. pp. 1-2.

SYMPTOMS

Symptoms of developing cataracts include double or blurred vision, sensitivity to light and glare (which may make driving difficult), less vivid perception of color, and frequent changes in eyeglass prescriptions. As the cataract grows worse, stronger glasses no longer improve sight, although holding objects nearer to the eye may help reading and close-up work. The pupil, which normally appears black, may undergo noticeable color changes and appear to be yellowish or white, says Peter Hersh, M.D., an assistant surgeon at Boston's Massachusetts Eye and Ear Infirmary.

Cataracts are typically detected through a medical eye examination. The usual test for visual acuity, the letter eye chart, may not, however, reflect the true nature of visual loss, says the American Academy of Ophthalmology. Other tests—which measure glare sensitivity, contrast sensitivity, night vision, color vision, and side or central vision—help nail down the diagnosis.

Because most cataracts associated with aging develop slowly, many patients may not notice their visual loss until it has become severe. Some cataracts remain small and never need treatment; others grow more quickly and progressively larger. Only when a cataract seriously interferes with normal activities is it time to consider surgery, doctors say. People who depend on their eyes for work, play and other activities may want their cataracts removed earlier than those whose needs are less demanding.

Some experts estimate that about 88 of every 100 persons receiving IOLs [intraocular lenses] will achieve 20/40 vision or better. (An individual with 20/40 vision can read letters on an eye chart from 20 feet away. While a person with normal 20/20 vision can read the chart from 40 feet away, 20/40 vision is good enough to get a driver's license in most states.) Among those who do not have other eye diseases, about 94 of 100 will achieve 20/40 vision.

SOURCE:
Hale, Ellen. "Lifting the Clouds of Cataracts." *FDA Consumer* (December 1989-January 1990): 28.

SURGERY

If you have cataracts, you needn't feel pressured into making an immediate decision about surgery. The typical cataract progresses slowly, and the decision to operate depends largely on how much the condition is affecting a person's life. People who have jobs or hobbies that require precision and good eyesight will need surgery early; others may prefer to wait.

Not too many years ago, cataract surgery was among the most feared operations for both patients and physicians. The procedure was tedious for the surgeon, uncomfortable for the patient and often produced less-than-satisfactory results. Patients had to spend up to two weeks in the hospital after the surgery, blindfolded and with their heads immobilized by heavy sandbags. Surgeons feared that even the slightest movement could ruin the outcome.

Today cataract surgery usually takes 30 to 60 minutes, thanks to advances in microsurgery and suturing. The procedure is done on an outpatient basis in virtually all instances—the patient arrives in the morning and goes home in the early afternoon.

The procedure itself involves a small incision directly into the eye. The clouded lens is removed, a plastic one inserted and the surgical opening closed. The surgery requires anesthesia around the eye, and some patients may receive a mild sedative to help them relax.

Though some patients can drive without difficulty after cataract surgery, it's a good idea to have someone else available to do the driving. The patient wears a patch for a day. Some people notice a mild, scratchy irritation, but most report no discomfort. Most patients can resume normal activities within a day to a week, but strenuous activity, especially heavy lifting, should be avoided for four to six weeks.

Occasionally, improvement in vision occurs almost immediately after cataract surgery, according to Dr. [Richard] Ruiz, [chairman of ophthalmology at The University of Texas Medical School at Houston], but more often the improvement occurs gradually over several months. It's important to note that a lens implant doesn't guarantee perfect vision. In fact, most people will continue to need glasses to correct either distance or near vision.

Although the majority of cataract operations are justified, some unwarranted procedures have caused permanent eye damage and blindness.

Therefore, if you're considering the surgery, use the following guidelines to help guard against an unnecessary lens implant:

- Go to an eye surgeon you know or one that your personal physician, family or friends recommend.
- Make sure the surgeon examines your eyes thoroughly before making a recommendation about surgery.
- If you have any doubts, get a second opinion.

Remember, cataracts progress slowly. Putting off the surgery does no harm. Even in people who are legally blind as a result of cataracts, lens implants can restore vision.

SOURCE:
"Cataract Surgery: When Is It Really Necessary?" *The University of Texas Lifetime Health Letter* 2, no. 6 (June 1990): 3.

* * *

When a cataract causes severe visual impairment, the decision to operate is an easy one. When impairment is moderate, the eye surgeon takes into consideration the patient's visual acuity and functional needs for near vision and distant vision. (Your tested eye is able to see objects, usually a letter, at 20 feet just as well as an eye with very good vision is able to see an object of the same size at the same distance of 20 feet. When the number on the bottom becomes larger, as in 20/100, it means poor vision in the tested eye. In this case, it means that you would need to move up to 20 feet in order to see a test object of the same size that a person with very good vision could see at 100 feet. [Definition courtesy of the American Academy of Ophthalmology, Inc.])

Although the decision to operate depends upon individual circumstances, as a general rule, a physician considers an operation when visual acuity is reduced to a level of 20/100 or 20/70. The surgeon may recommend an operation for individuals who have even better eyesight if their jobs or recreational activities require good vision. For example, an eye surgeon might suggest an operation for a jeweler, an artist, a librarian, or a craftsman who has only slight limitation of vision.

About the Operation

There are two fundamental ways of removing a cataract: the intracapsular method and the extracapsular method. In the intracapsular method, the eye surgeon removes the cataract and the capsule that surrounds the cloudy lens. The surgeon makes an incision where the cornea (the clear protective membrane covering the front of the eye) and the sclera (the white of the eye) meet. He or she carefully enters the front of the eye, gently pulls the iris out of the way, and attaches a freezing instrument (called a cryoprobe) to the capsule of the lens (cataract). The freezing probe creates an iceball that adheres to the capsule and allows the surgeon to slide the capsule and the lens out of the eye.

With the extracapsular technique, the surgeon does not remove the entire capsule. He or she opens the front of the capsule and by means of a special instrument, removes the hard, central nucleus of the lens and then sucks out the soft lens cortex. Although the extracapsular technique is becoming quite popular (nearly half of all cataract operations are done in this way), the eye surgeon will choose the procedure that is best suited for your condition and needs.

No matter which technique is used, the eye surgeon usually injects a local anesthetic to deaden the nerves around and within the eye. Such injections cause only mild discomfort during the operation; discomfort after the operation is easily controlled with mild pain-killers. It is equally acceptable for a general anesthetic to be used for the operation.

SOURCE:
American College of Surgeons. *When You Need an Operation: About Cataract Surgery in Adults.* n.d. pp. 2–3.

CONTACT LENSES AND LENS IMPLANTS

Because a cataract operation removes the lens of the eye, the eye can no longer focus. There are three ways in which the eye can be helped to focus again.

1. Cataract glasses. Cataract glasses are thick spectacles that may be given to some patients, particularly older people who are housebound or bedridden or those who have severe diabetes or chronic eye inflammations. The glasses are not as satisfactory for others, however, because magnification is high. Cataract glasses magnify objects to approximately 25 percent larger than normal, and people may be uncomfortable when glasses greatly magnify ordinary objects. Cataract glasses distort side vision. As a result, many people are distracted by the difference that exists between front and side vision.

Cataract glasses may be given to patients immediately after the operation. However, it takes about six weeks or more for the eye to recover sufficiently to allow patients to use the glasses in their routine activities.

2. Contact lenses. Contact lenses do not distort side vision and magnify objects only 5 percent larger than normal; consequently, they are preferable to glasses for many people who have had a cataract operation. Contact lenses are not trouble free, however. People have to learn how to put them in, take them out, and care for them in general.

A contact lens may be given to a patient four to six weeks after the operation if the eye is healing properly.

3. Lens implants. Nearly two-thirds of the patients who undergo cataract surgery have an artificial plastic lens implanted in the eye. The implant, which is slightly larger than the normal lens, is placed in the eye at the time of the cataract operation. If you receive an implant, you should have some degree of vision within a few days. However, you will not be able to see distant objects clearly until about two months after the operation. Even then you may need eyeglasses to read or to do close work.

Implants are being used more frequently because they eliminate the need to handle contact lenses or to deal with the visual discomfort of cataract glasses. However, not every patient can be considered a candidate for an implant. Generally speaking, people who are over age 55 and who do not have a major eye disease or severe diabetes are candidates for a lens implant.

SOURCE:
American College of Surgeons. *When You Need an Operation: About Cataract Surgery in Adults.* n.d. 3-5.

RECOVERING FROM THE OPERATION

If a patient is otherwise in good health, the chances are great that the operation will be performed on an outpatient basis, and the patient will be sent home on the same day. After the operation, your surgeon may suggest that you wear a patch over the affected eye for several days; the decision as to whether or not you will wear such a patch will be based on your doctor's assessment of your condition and your own preferences. You will be encouraged to wear a shield of some sort at night so that you cannot accidentally poke yourself in the eye.

Most people who develop cataracts will need an operation on the second eye at a later date. If the eye surgeon performs routine, traditional lens extraction, an operation on the second eye may be done a few weeks after the first operation. If implants are being placed in the eyes, the interval between the two operations may be as long as six months.

Whether you have cataract glasses, contact lenses, or lens implants, you occasionally may be bothered by bright sunlight. In places where there is more than a normal amount of sunlight, such as near a large body of water or in areas covered by snow, you may wish to wear dark glass to reduce glare.

A cataract operation is one of the safest procedures that is being performed today, and there are relatively few complications associated with it. Cataract operations are quite effective; they improve vision to some degree in approximately 98 percent of adult patients, providing that the retina and optic nerve are healthy.

SOURCE:
American College of Surgeons. *When You Need an Operation: About Cataract Surgery in Adults.* n.d. p. 5.

RESOURCES

PAMPHLETS

American Academy of Ophthalmology:

Eye Facts about Cataract Surgery. 1986. n.d.

American College of Surgeons:

When You Need an Operation: About Cataract Surgery in Infants and Children. n.d. 8 pp.

California Medical Association:

"Cataracts." *HealthTips* index 140. June 1989. 2 pp.

National Institute on Aging:

Aging and Your Eyes (Age Page). October 1987.

BOOKS

Cataracts: A Consumer's Guide to Choosing the Best Treatment. Washington, DC: Public Citizen's Health Research Group, 1981. 161 pp.

Maloney, William, Lincoln Grindle, and Donald Pearcy. *Consumer Guide to Modern Cataract Surgery.* Fallbrook, CA: Lasenda Publishers, 1986. 141 pp.

RELATED ARTICLES

"Cataracts: Surgery and Lens Implants Can Help Restore the Precious Gift of Eyesight." *Mayo Clinic Health Letter* 7 (February 1989): 2-3.

Donshik, Peter C., Stuart L. Fine, and others. "The Aging Eye: Thieves of Sight." *Patient Care* 23 (April 15, 1989): 38-48.

Liu, Ingrid Y., Jon White, and Andrea Z. LaCroix. "The Association of Age-Related Macular Degeneration and Lens Opacities in the Aged." *American Journal of Public Health* 79 (June 1989): 765-769.

Taylor, Hugh R., Sheila K. West, and others. "Effect of Ultraviolet Radiation on Cataract Formation." *The New England Journal of Medicine* 319, no. 22 (December 1, 1988): 1429-1433.

CEREBRAL PALSY

OVERVIEW

A general term for nonprogressive disorders of movement and posture resulting from damage to the brain in the later months of pregnancy, during birth, in the newborn period, or in early childhood.

A child with cerebral palsy may suffer from spastic paralysis (abnormal stiffness and contraction of groups of muscles), athetosis (involuntary writhing movements), or ataxia (loss of coordination and balance). The degree of disability is highly variable, ranging from slight clumsiness of hand movement and gait to complete immobility. Other nervous system disorders, such as hearing defects or epileptic seizures, may be present. Many affected children are also mentally retarded, although a proportion are of normal or high intelligence.

In the US about two to six babies per 1,000 develop cerebral palsy. There has only been a slight reduction in cases in the past 20 years.

In over 90 percent of cases the damage occurs before or at birth. Probably the most common cause is cerebral hypoxia (poor oxygen supply to the brain).

A maternal infection spreading to the baby within the uterus is an occasional cause. A rare cause is kernicterus, which results from an excess of bilirubin (bile pigment) in babies with hemolytic disease of the newborn. The baby is severely jaundiced, and the bile pigment damages the basal ganglia (nerve cell clusters in the brain concerned with control of movement).

Following birth, possible causes include encephalitis or meningitis (infections of the brain or its protective covering), or a head injury.

Often cerebral palsy is not recognized until well into the baby's first year. Sometimes, but not always, some of the infant's muscles are initially hypotonic (floppy), and the parents may notice that the baby in some way does not "feel right" when held. There may also be feeding difficulties.

Once the disability is apparent, most affected children fall into one of two groups—a spastic group, in which the muscles of one or more limbs are permanently contracted and stiff, thus making normal movements very difficult; and a smaller, athetoid group, characterized by involuntary writhing movements.

The diplegic child has delayed development in many movement skills and has difficulty learning to walk. In hemiplegia the limbs of the affected side grow slowly; there may be some sensory loss from the affected side of the body.

In quadriplegia, it may be difficult to know whether the child's arms or legs are the worst affected; mental retardation is usually severe. Often, the child never learns to walk.

The athetoid type of cerebral palsy results from damage to the basal ganglia, due either to birth asphyxia caused by hypoxia or to kernicterus.

Mental retardation, with an IQ below 70, occurs in about three quarters of all people with cerebral palsy, but the exceptions are important and occur particularly among athetoids; many athetoids and some diplegics are highly intelligent.

None of the various types of cerebral palsy is progressive (i.e., they do not worsen), but the features of the condition change as the child gets older, often for the better with patience and skilled treatment.

Parents of babies who are "at risk" from cerebral palsy—for example, babies born prematurely or during particularly difficult births—are generally encouraged to take the child more frequently for routine checkups by a physician, who will test with particular care for any abnormalities in the baby's muscle tone and reflexes, and for any delay in reaching various developmental milestones. The diagnosis may rely on a combination of abnormalities.

Although cerebral palsy is incurable, much can be done to help children affected by it. Abilities need to be recognized and developed to the full, as much stimulation as possible should be offered, and loving patience must always be shown.

Physical therapy is required to teach the child how to develop muscular control and maintain balance. This therapy is often given initially at a special school or clinic and then continued at home, possibly with the use of special equipment.

Inadequate speech can be helped greatly by speech therapy. For children who cannot speak at all, sophisticated techniques and devices have been developed to teach them how to communicate nonverbally.

Every attempt is made to place children with mild cerebral palsy in normal schools, but those who are severely affected need the special help available at schools for the physically and/or mentally handicapped.

Children with only moderate disability have a near-normal life expectancy and, with the help of social services, most of those who can move around and communicate effectively grow up to lead a relatively independent and normal life.

SOURCE:

Clayman, Charles B. "Cerebral Palsy." In *The American Medical Association Encyclopedia of Medicine*. New York: Random House, 1989. pp. 248–249.

CAUSES

Physicians have long assumed that lack of oxygen at birth is the main cause of cerebral palsy. But new evidence challenges this belief.

Cerebral palsy develops when the part of the brain controlling movement functions improperly. Its symptoms, which can range form clumsiness to immobility and mental retardation, emerge in early childhood. Lawsuits have blamed it on medical negligence during delivery, says Jack Shonkoff, M.D., at the University of Massachusetts in Worcester.

But the actual causes may occur much earlier. Last year, scientists in the California Birth Defects Monitoring Program in Emeryville and the School of Public Health at the University of California at Berkeley finished monitoring more than 19,000 pregnancies and births.

"Seventy-eight percent of the children with cerebral palsy had not suffered oxygen deprivation at birth," explains Claudine Torfs, Ph.D., who headed the research. "And the great majority of infants who had been oxygen-deprived did not have cerebral palsy."

The scientists linked other risk factors to the disorder, including some birth defects, low birth weight, abnormal fetal position and premature separation of the placenta. "This is evidence that babies with cerebral palsy had trouble long before labor and delivery—probably early in pregnancy," says Shonkoff.

SOURCE:

Baker, Sherry. "Palsy: Trauma in the Womb." *Health* (February 1991): 20.

TREATMENT

Early identification of cerebral palsy can lessen developmental problems and lead to appropriate treatment when it helps the most. Special educators and physicians have discovered that early intervention can make an important difference. Early intervention programs enlist parents and other family members in working with the child in specific activities. These activities, designed by a therapist, provide the child with the stimulation needed to overcome slower development which is part of cerebral palsy. Other forms of treatment of children with cerebral palsy may include speech and language therapy, occupational therapy, physical therapy, medical intervention and social services. Among the services the older child with cerebral palsy may need are: attendant care, continuing therapy, special education, counseling, vocational training, and recreation training. The services required will vary from person to person depending on the nature and severity of the handicap. Important advances have taken place in the last decade which have a great effect on the long term well-being of children born with cerebral palsy. Advanced technology is being applied to the needs of severely disabled persons with cerebral palsy, including biofeedback, computers and engineering devices. Technological innovations have been made in areas of speech and communication, self-care, and job adaptation. The future may bring even more significant applications.

SOURCE:

"Back to the Basics: Cerebral Palsy." *Pediatrics for Parents* (May 1989): 2.

RESOURCES

ORGANIZATIONS

American Academy of Cerebral Palsy and Developmental Medicine. 1910 Byrd Avenue, Suite 118, Richmond, VA 23230.

National Easter Seal Society. 70 E. Lake Street, Chicago, IL 60601.

United Cerebral Palsy Association. 7 Penn Plaza, Suite 804, New York, NY 10001.

BOOK
Finnie, Nancy. *Handling the Young Cerebral Palsied Child at Home.* New York: Dutton, 1989.

RELATED ARTICLES
Eden, Alvin N. "Cerebral Palsy and Cystic Fibrosis." *American Baby* 52 (June 1990): 14, 77.

Friedman, Mel, and Ellen Weiss. "What You Should Know about Cerebral Palsy." *Parents* (May 1991): 68–70.

Palmer, Frederick B., Bruce K. Shapiro, and others. "The Effects of Physical Therapy on Cerebral Palsy: A Controlled Trial in Infants with Spastic Diplegia." *The New England Journal of Medicine* 318 (March 31, 1988): 803–808.

Skolnick, Andrew. "New Ultrasound Evidence Appears to Link Prenatal Brain Damage, Cerebral Palsy." *JAMA* 265 (February 28, 1991): 948–949.

Torfs, Claudine P., Barbara J. van den Berg, and others. "Prenatal and Perinatal Factors in the Etiology of Cerebral Palsy." *Journal of Pediatrics* 116 (April 1990): 615–619.

CERVICAL CANCER

(*See also:* PAP SMEARS)

OVERVIEW

Invasive cervical cancer accounts for 2.5 percent of all cancers that afflict women in the United States. About 13,500 cases of invasive carcinoma of the cervix are diagnosed in the United States each year, while there are at least 50,000 new cases of a pre-invasive cancer known as carcinoma in situ where the cancer cells are confined to the surface skin of the cervix.

But since 1940, there has been a steady decrease in the incidence of carcinoma of the cervix because most women with no symptoms are screened with cervical and vaginal Pap smears. The probability at birth that a white woman will eventually develop cervical cancer dropped from 1.1 percent in 1975 to 0.7 percent in 1985. Similarly, for black women the probability dropped from 2.3 percent in 1975 to 1.6 percent in 1985.

Over 90 percent of cervical carcinomas start in the surface cells lining the cervix and are called squamous cell carcinoma. About 5 to 9 percent start in glandular tissue (adenocarcinoma). Adenocarcinomas are more difficult to diagnose, but they are treated the same way as squamous cell carcinomas and the survival rate, stage for stage, is similar.

There are several types of adenocarcinoma. About 60 percent are the endocervical cell type, 10 percent are each of endometrioid and clear cell carcinomas and 20 percent are adenosquamous carcinoma.

There are two rare types of cervical carcinoma known as small cell carcinoma and cervical sarcoma. Both have a poor prognosis.

Most scientists believe that cervical warts or pre-invasive cervical cancer may develop over a period of months or years after the cervix is infected with the human papilloma virus (HPV). This early tumor—known as mild dysplasia or cervical intraepithelial neoplasia (CIN) Grade 1—can progress to moderate dysplasia (CIN-2), then to severe dysplasia and carcinoma in situ (CIN-3) and eventually to invasive carcinoma. Most physicians believe that about two thirds of all cases of severe dysplasia progress to invasive cancer if left untreated. This transformation takes anywhere from 3 to 30 years, about 10 years on the average.

Once the cervical cancer becomes invasive, it can spread locally to the upper vagina and into the tissues surrounding the upper vagina and the cervix (the parametrium). Eventually it grows toward the pelvic sidewall, obstructing the tubes (ureters) that drain urine from the kidney to the bladder. It can also spread to the bladder and rectum.

Cervical tumor cells can invade the lymphatic system and spread to the lymph nodes in the pelvic wall. Eventually they may spread to the iliac lymph nodes higher in the pelvis, the aortic lymph nodes, the nodes above the collarbone and occasionally to the groin nodes.

Metastases can also spread through the bloodstream to the outer vagina, vulva, lungs, liver and brain. Invasion of the pelvic nerves is common in advanced cases. There may also be spread within the abdomen when the tumor penetrates the full thickness of the cervix.

There is much evidence that cervical carcinoma is venereal in origin. Most researchers believe that the human papilloma virus is either the cause or a strong cofactor in the development of pre-invasive and invasive carcinomas of the cervix, as well as pre-invasive and invasive squamous cell cancer of the vagina and vulva. Ninety to 95 percent of squamous cell carcinomas of the cervix contain human papilloma virus DNA.

The virus is a sexually transmitted disease. There are more than 50 types of human papilloma virus (HPV) that infect humans. Types 6 and 11 usually cause warts, while types 16, 18, 31 and 33 usually result in high-grade cervical dysplasia (CIN-2 and 3) and carcinomas. The virus infects the tissues of the lower genital tract and may produce obvious genital warts or mild, moderate or severe dysplasia and carcinoma in situ. Genital warts are associated with cervical, vaginal and vulvar dysplasia and invasive carcinoma in about 25 percent of cases.

SOURCE:
Stern, Jeffrey L. "Cervix." *In Everyone's Guide to Cancer Therapy*. Dollinger, Malin, Ernest H. Rosenbaum, and Greg Cable (eds.). Kansas City: Somerville House, 1991. pp. 277–279.

RISK FACTORS

More than 90% of all cervical cancers are squamous cell carcinomas, and researchers believe that this cancer is a sexually transmitted disease.

Numerous risk factors identified in the past, such as early or multiple pregnancies, first intercourse at an early age, or previous herpes, gonorrhea, or syphilis infection, all correlate directly with the overall number of male sexual partners to whom a woman has been exposed. The number of sexual partners, in turn, correlates with the likelihood that the woman has also acquired human papilloma virus (HPV), now believed to be the primary culprit. Other risk factors such as smoking cigarettes or use of birth control pills may also be involved as independent factors or cofactors in cancer risk, and so may DES exposure during fetal development (DES daughters).

Several factors can reduce the risk of cervical cancer a woman faces. In general, any steps to avoid sexually transmitted infection will reduce cervical cancer risk. Lower than average risk is associated with:

- First intercourse deferred until age 18 to 20 or older
- Intercourse with only one male partner
- Use of condoms
- Use of a diaphragm
- Use of spermicide

Circumcision and Jewish ethnicity, thought in the past to be protective factors, are now known to be unrelated to cancer risk except to the extent that they correlate with sexual monogamy and abstinence before marriage.

Factors associated with higher than average cancer risk are:

- Previous CIN (cervical intraepithelial neoplasia, also called dysplasia)
- Genital wart virus infection (some strains)
- Previous vulvar or vaginal cancer
- Exposure to a male whose previous partner(s) had cervical cancer or CIN
- Exposure to a sexual partner who has (or had) penile cancer
- Exposure to more than one male sexual partner (compared to the risk for a woman with one lifetime partner, two partners increase the risk 250%; six partners, 600%)
- Smoking cigarettes
- DES (diethylstilbestrol) exposure during fetal development
- Birth control pills used four years or more
- Previous herpes, gonorrhea, syphilis, or other sexually transmitted infections
- First intercourse before age 18 to 20
- First pregnancy before age 18 to 20

SOURCE:
Stewart, Felicia H., Felicia Guest, and others. *Understanding Your Body*. New York: Bantam, 1987. pp. 755–756.

DIAGNOSIS AND STAGING

If the doctor's inspection or the Pap smear shows any abnormality, a biopsy—the removal of a tiny amount of suspicious tissue—is usually done. Doctors use several methods to identify areas of suspicious tissue for biopsy. With the Schiller's test, iodine is applied to the surface of the cervix. Normal cells are stained by the iodine; areas not stained are then biopsied. Doctors may also use a colposcope, which magnifies the view of the cervix and vagina, to inspect a suspicious area more closely. If a vaginal infection is suspected as the cause of the abnormal smear, the smear may simply be repeated after treatment of the infection.

If the biopsy and pap smear results are abnormal, or if the two tests give conflicting results, larger tissue samples may be required for an accurate diagnosis. These are obtained most often by conization or dilatation and curettage (D and C). In a D and C, the cervix is dilated to permit insertion of a curette, a small instrument that gently scrapes material from the uterine lining.

Examination of tissue samples from biopsy, conization, or D and C may reveal dysplasia, carcinoma in situ, cervical cancer, or other diseases. If evidence of cancer is found, further tests are done to determine its extent. The most important of these tests is a more thorough pelvic examination, including inspection of the abdomen, vagina, and rectum. A doctor can often feel a tumor or detect tenderness caused by a tumor in these areas. Cancer spreads to distant parts of the body, most often to the lung, in only about 15 percent of cervical cancer patients. Staging is a system used to describe the degree to which the cancer has spread:

- **Stage 0:** Carcinoma in situ
- **Stage I:** Carcinoma confined to the cervix
- **Stage II:** Carcinoma extends beyond the cervix but not to the pelvic wall
- **Stage III:** Carcinoma extends to the pelvic wall

- **Stage IV:** Carcinoma extends beyond the pelvis or invades the bladder or rectum

Almost all cervical cancers are squamous cell carcinomas. Squamous cells are a type of epithelial cell; any cancer that originates in epithelial cells is called a carcinoma.

SOURCE:
National Cancer Institute. *Cancer of the Uterus: Research Report.* NIH Pub. No. 87-171. July 1987 pp. 5-6.

TREATMENT

The choice of treatment for cervical cancer depends on the patient's general condition and on the stage of the disease. In its early stages, cervical cancer is usually treated with surgery or radiation or a combination of the two. Chemotherapy (treatment with anticancer drugs) is often recommended for later stages of the disease.

Stage I cervical cancer can be effectively treated with either surgery or radiation therapy. Surgery is often selected in younger women because it preserves the hormone-producing function of the ovaries. Surgical treatment consists of a hysterectomy, the removal of the entire uterus, including the cervix. The two types of treatment are equally effective, with cure rates of 85 to 90 percent.

In older women, radiation may be selected because it is more easily tolerated than surgery, particularly if other medical problems are present. Surgery may also be used in combination with radiotherapy if the shape of the tumor in the cervix makes insertion of radioactive implants difficult.

Most patients in whom the disease has progressed beyond stage I are treated with radiotherapy alone. However, if the cancer has spread minimally to the vagina (early Stage II), surgery may be selected for patients who are young and in good general health. The surgical procedure most often used is the radical hysterectomy, involving removal of the upper part of the vagina and nearby tissues and lymph nodes as well as the uterus.

Radiation treatment usually consists of a combination of external and internal radiation. X-rays from a linear accelerator or gamma rays from a cobalt source may be beamed through the body to the tumor site. Treatments of this kind are usually given (on an outpatient basis) over a period of several weeks. Radiation may also be applied directly to the cervix by inserting, through the vagina, tiny metal cylinders containing a radioactive element, such as radium or cesium. The cylinders are usually left in place for 2 or 3 days. Patients receiving internal irradiation are hospitalized for several days.

If the cancer has spread extensively or has reappeared after initial treatment with surgery or radiation therapy, chemotherapy may be prescribed. In such cases, anticancer drugs frequently are injected into the bloodstream, often in an outpatient setting. There is currently no standard treatment for stage IV cervical cancer, but many new regimens are being evaluated in clinical trials. Several current studies are evaluating the effectiveness of various anticancer drugs, alone and in combination with other drugs and/or radiation. Drugs used in combination chemotherapy protocols, or research programs, include cisplatin (Platinol), bleomycin, mitomycin (Mitomycin-C), vincristine, methotrexate, and doxorubicin (Adriamycin), usually in combinations of two or three.

Other investigational treatments of cervical cancer include immunotherapy and the use of radiation sensitizers. Immunotherapy is the use of drugs that stimulate the body's immune system to fight off disease. In treating cervical cancer, the immunotherapeutic agent most often used is the bacterium *C. parvum*. Immunotherapy is usually given in combination with radiation or chemotherapy. Radiation sensitizers are drugs such as misonidazole and hydroxyurea which, when given before the administration of radiation, are believed to make cancerous cells more sensitive to the radiation.

SOURCE:
National Cancer Institute. *Cancer of the Uterus: Research Report.* NIH Pub. No. 87-171. July 1987. pp. 6-8.

PROGNOSIS

The overall 5-year arrest rate for squamous cell carcinoma or adenocarcinoma originating in the cervix is about 45% in the major clinics. Percentage arrest rates are inversely proportionate to the stage of cancer: stage 0, 99%; stage 1, 77%; stage II, 65%; stage III, 25%; stage IV, about 5%.

SOURCE:
Schroeder, Steven A., Marcus A. Krupp, and others (eds.). *Current Medical Diagnosis & Treatment 1992.* Norwalk, CT: Appleton & Lange, 1992. p. 563.

RESOURCES

ORGANIZATIONS

American Cancer Society. 261 Madison Ave., New York, NY 10016.

National Cancer Institute. Office of Cancer Communication, Building 31, Room 10A18, Bethesda, MD 20892.

PAMPHLETS

American Cancer Society:

Facts on Uterine Cancer. 1989.

National Cancer Institute:

What You Need to Know about Cancer of the Uterus. NIH Pub. No. 89-1562. 1989.

RELATED ARTICLES

O'Brien, David M., and Carmichael, John A. "Presurgical Prognostic Factors in Carcinoma of the Cervix, Stages IB and IIA." *American Journal of Obstetrics and Gynecology* 158, no. 2 (1988): 250-254.

"Understanding Cervical Cancer." *HealthTips* NWH-4 (March 1990): 1-2.

Van Pelt, Dina. "Racial Differences in Cervical Cancer." *Insight* 6, no. 21 (May 21 1990): 59.

CESAREAN SECTION

INCIDENCE

Half of the 934,000 cesarean sections performed in the U.S. in 1987 were unnecessary, costing the public an extra $1 billion and uncalculated increased in maternal morbidity, with no discernible benefit to neonatal outcome, according to a health watchdog group's findings.

The nation's 24.4% cesarean rate is double the optimal 12% suggested by obstetric experts, said Drs. Lynn Silver and Sidney Wolfe, coauthors of a report by the Public Citizen Health Research Group [HRG].

And the rate has quadrupled since 1970, reflecting obstetricians' disregard of a widely publicized 1980 NIH consensus statement that urged reins on the surgery, they noted. The single largest contributor to the rate is repeat section, despite the American College of Obstetricians and Gynecologists' 1982 guidelines that promote attempting vaginal delivery by most women who have had a previous section.

ACOG [American College of Obstetricians and Gynecologists], which published even stronger guidelines last year to discourage repeat procedures, declines, however, to "project the ideal percentage of C-sections for every hospital in the nation," said a spokeswoman. . . .

The association has not addressed the Health Research Group's recommendations for decreasing the surgery rate for breech presentation, dystocia, or fetal distress—or for decreasing financial incentives to do cesarean sections. But several third party payers adopted the HRG's suggestion that fees be the same for all deliveries.

The report documents cesarean section rates for 41 states and the District of Columbia that range from a low of 17.9% for Alabama to a high of 30.3% for the nation's capital, with no associated impact on perinatal mortality. Rates cited for 2,388 hospitals in 30 states range from zero to 53% of all deliveries at one Florida hospital, with no relation to hospital status as a low-risk or high-risk facility. And rates for individual Maryland physicians, listed by hospital and code number, range from zero to 57%, with no relation to the physician's number of deliveries.

Private, for-profit hospitals had the highest rates. State, local, and federal government hospitals had the lowest. Patients with the "best-paying insurance plans" had the highest rates.

SOURCE:
Pollner, F. "U.S. C-Section Rate Remains Twice what Experts Advise." *Medical World News* 30, no. 1 (February 27, 1989): 45.

DEFINITION

Cesarean childbirth, an operation to deliver a baby through an incision in the abdomen, can be traced back through history to Egypt in 3000 B.C. The procedure's name comes from a set of Roman laws, Lex Caesare, which in 715 B.C. mandated surgical removal of an unborn fetus upon death of the mother.

Until recent decades the operation usually had been used as a last resort because of a high rate of maternal complications and death. But with the availability of antibiotics to fight infection and the development of modern surgical techniques, the once high maternal mortality rate has dropped dramatically. As a result, the cesarean childbirth rate has increased dramatically. . . .

Cesarean childbirth is a major operation that actually involves a series of separate incisions in the mother. The skin, underlying muscles and abdomen are opened first and then the uterus is opened, allowing removal of the infant.

There are two main types of cesarean operations, each named according to the location and direction of the uterine incision:

- cervical—a transverse (horizontal) or vertical incision in the lower uterus, and
- classical—a vertical incision in the main body of the uterus.

Today, the low transverse cervical incision is used almost exclusively. It has the lowest incidence of hemorrhage during surgery as well as the least chance of rupturing in later pregnancies. Sometimes, because of fetal size (very large or very small) or position problems (breech or transverse), a low vertical cesarean may be performed.

In the classical operation, a vertical incision allows a greater opening and is used for fetal size or position problems and in some emergency situations. This approach involves more bleeding in surgery and a higher risk of abdominal infection. Although any uterine incision may rupture during a subsequent labor, the classical is more likely to do so and more likely to result in death for the mother and fetus than a cervical incision.

SOURCE:
National Institute of Child Health and Human Development. *Facts about Cesarean Childbirth.* n.d. pp. 2-3.

REASONS FOR HIGH INCIDENCE

An increased use of well-run birth centers may be one avenue toward reducing the alarmingly high number of cesarean deliveries in the U.S. That rate hovers around 24 percent, despite the evidence that:

- Cesareans are four times more risky than vaginal births, says the American College of Obstetricians and Gynecologists (*National Underwriter*, January 22, 1990).
- Between one-half and one-third of all C-sections are unwarranted, according to a study by Public Citizen (*Wall Street Journal*, January 27, 1989).
- Cesareans do not lower the rate of newborn death (*Public Citizen*).
- The cesarean rate could be dramatically lowered if more women were allowed a trial of vaginal birth after cesarean, also known as VBAC. Only 46 percent of all hospitals offer trial of labor to women who have had a previous C-section (*Statistical Bulletin*, October-December 1989), even though the American College of Obstetricians and Gynecologists issued guidelines in 1988 that recommended trials of VBAC.

Unless changes are made, the cesarean rate may reach 40 percent by the year 2000 (*Statistical Bulletin*). Unfortunately, no one has been able to rein in the runaway rate, despite recommendations made by medical specialty organizations such as the American College of Obstetricians and Gynecologists and Canada's Society of Obstetricians and Gynecologists. The problem is that guidelines don't change doctors' bad habits, according to a Canadian study on cesarean rates, because the inappropriate practices are sustained by "powerful nonscientific forces" (*New England Journal of Medicine*, November 9, 1989).

What are these powerful forces? Physicians claim that fear of malpractice litigation forces them to perform more cesarean surgery. Other experts suggest that physicians today have little experience with difficult vaginal births. Regional factors are also at play: C-section rates are highest in the Northeast and South and the lowest in the Midwest and West. Rates are lowest for small hospitals, and are lower for government hospitals than nonprofit or proprietary hospitals (*Statistical Bulletin*).

And then there's the siren song of the dollar. Doctors charge more for cesareans—68 percent more, according to a report in the February 2, 1990, *Journal of the American Medical Association*. A C-section is more likely when a private insurance company foots the bill (*Statistical Bulletin*), or when the woman comes from a wealthy family (*New England Journal of Medicine*, July 27, 1989).

SOURCE:
"Nurse-Midwives and Birth Centers: A Team That Lowers the Cesarean Rate." *People's Medical Society Newsletter* 9, no. 3 (June 1990): 6, 8.

VBAC—ONCE A C-SECTION, ALWAYS A C-SECTION?

In 1988, the American College of Obstetricians and Gynecologists (ACOG) issued guidelines for VBAC [Vaginal Birth After Cesarean] and, in effect, positioned VBAC as the preferred method of delivery instead of the alternative, unless there were contra-indications.

The ACOG opinion said that each hospital should develop its own VBAC protocols. It also urged that prospective VBAC mothers be counseled and encouraged to undergo trial labor if their previous uterine incision was low transverse (horizontal), even if failure of labor to progress was the reason for their first cesarean. The guidelines were based on studies reporting that repeat operations could be avoided 50 to 80 percent of the time for appropriate cases.

One of the world's widely recognized VBAC authorities and proponents, Dr. Bruce Flamm, is area research chairman for Kaiser-Permanente Medical Center in Riverside, CA. He is also assistant clinical professor of obstetrics and gynecology at the University of California, Irvine. In one of the largest retrospective studies ever reported, Flamm and colleagues examined data from 57,553 live births. Of the 4,929 women with prior C-sections, 1,776—about 36 percent—attempted VBAC.

Seventy-four percent were able to deliver vaginally. There was no maternal or perinatal death related to rupture of the uterine scar, the most feared complication of VBAC. Actually, reported maternal and perinatal death rates for VBAC are lower than for repeated C-sections. The risk of maternal mortality after C-section is due to greater chance of infection, hemorrhage and anesthesia complications. Prematurity is the primary risk to the infant.

SOURCE:
Aylsworth, J. "Unnecessary Cesarean Operations: Vaginal Birth After Cesarean (VBAC) vs. Repeat Cesarean Sections." *Priorities* (Spring 1990): 19–20.

SAFETY OF VBAC

From my personal experience with hundreds of "previous cesarean" mothers, I have come to the conclusion that for the majority of women normal birth after cesarean section is both safe and likely to succeed.

Cesarean section and normal birth after cesarean section may be controversial subjects, but some people go too far. For example, I've seen books that portray obstetricians as uncaring individuals who mercilessly seek any excuse to perform an operation. This type of vicious nonsense serves no purpose. However, it must be acknowledged that there are some obstetricians who, by distorting the risks of normal birth after cesarean section, continue to coerce women into unnecessary surgery. Neither these intractable doctors nor the irate childbirth activists who campaign against them can give a dispassionate view of birth after cesarean section. I'm convinced that the "truth" about the cesarean section controversy lies somewhere in between these two diametrically opposed points of view.

SOURCE:
Flamm, Bruce L. *Birth After Cesarean: The Medical Facts.* New York: Prentice Hall, 1990. p. xxi.

QUESTIONS TO ASK YOUR OBSTETRICIAN

Women selecting an obstetrician should ask him or her directly about the percentage of deliveries done by cesarean in the practice. Some authorities calculate that, on average, cesareans are necessary in only 12 to 14 percent of deliveries. New York's health department, in its forthcoming consumer booklet "Cesarean Birth and VBAC," steers prospective parents away from doctors and hospitals whose cesarean rates exceed 20 percent.

Also ask about the doctor's practice style. What approach does the obstetrician take to fetal monitoring, previous cesarean, breech presentation, and slow-moving labor? What circumstances require cesarean delivery? Are indications of fetal distress confirmed by a fetal scalp blood test? Is a second opinion sought before proceeding to all but emergency surgery? Must you have intravenous infusion during labor, or can you eat and drink lightly?

Ask also about the facility in which you'll deliver. Does it require a specific management plan, such as active management of labor? Does it offer a constant labor companion (or allow you to bring your own)? Is the staff open to nonmedical interventions, such as a warm shower?

Your practitioner's attitudes and temperament can also be crucial. If a physician or midwife is forthright, flexible, and willing to take your wishes into account, chances are you'll feel comfortable and work well with one another. Decisions about most cesareans are made at an emotional and stressful time. Preparing for the possibility in advance, laboring in a way that minimizes the likelihood, and working with someone you respect and trust is the best way to avoid an unnecessary cesarean.

SOURCE:
"Too Many Cesareans." *Consumer Reports* (February 1991): 126.

RESOURCES

ORGANIZATIONS

American College of Obstetricians and Gynecologists. 409 12th St. SW, Washington, DC 20024.

American Society for Psychoprophylaxis in Obstetrics / Lamaze. 1840 Wilson Blvd. Suite 204, Arlington, VA 22201.

Health Research Group. 2000 P Street NW, Washington, DC 20036.

International Childbirth Education Association. P.O. Box 20048, Minneapolis, MN 55420–0048.

BOOKS

Donovan, B. *The Cesarean Birth Experience: A Practical, Comprehensive, and Reassuring Guide for Parents and Professionals.* Boston: Beacon, 1986.

Jones, C. *Birth without Surgery: A Guide to Preventing Unnecessary Cesareans.* New York: Dodd, Mead, 1987.

Mitchell, K. and M. Nason. *Cesarean Birth: A Couple's Guide for Decision and Preparation.* Revised Edition. New York: Beaufort Books, 1985.

Richards, L. B. and others. *The Vaginal Birth after Cesarean Experience: Birth Stories by Parents and Professionals.* South Hadley, MA: Bergin & Garvey, 1987.

RELATED ARTICLES

Gould, J. B., B. Davey, and others. "Socioeconomic Differences in Rates of Cesarean Section." *The New England Journal of Medicine* 321, no. 4 (July 27, 1989): 233–239.

Jonas, H. S., and S. L. Dooley. "The Search for a Lower Cesarean Rate Goes On" (editorial). *JAMA* 262, no. 11 (September 15, 1989): 1512–1513.

"Once a Cesarean, Always a Cesarean?" *HealthTips* index WH–49 (July/August 1989).

Porreco, R. P. "Meeting the Challenge of the Rising Cesarean Birth Rate." *Obstetrics & Gynecology* 75, no. 1 (January 1990): 133–136.

Seiler, J. S. "The Demise of Vaginal Operative Obstetrics: A Suggested Plan for its Revival." *Obstetrics & Gynecology* 75, no. 4 (April 1990): 710-712.

Stafford, R. S. "Alternative Strategies for Controlling Rising Cesarean Section Rates." *JAMA* 263, no. 5 (February 2, 1990): 683-687.

"Unnecessary Cesarean Sections: How to Cure a National Epidemic." *Health Letter* 5, no. 3 (March 1989): 1–6.

CHEMOTHERAPY

DEFINITION

In modern usage, chemotherapy usually refers to the use of chemicals to destroy cancer cells on a selective basis. The cytotoxic agents used in cancer treatments generally function in the same manner as ionizing radiation; they do not kill the cancer cells directly but instead impair their ability to replicate. Most of the nearly 40 anticancer drugs commonly used act by interfering with DNA and RNA activities associated with cell division.

Chemotherapeutic agents are often used in combination with radiation treatments for their synergistic effect. A cytotoxic agent, for example, may be used to render a tumor cell more sensitive to the effects of radiation. Thus, by making the cancer cell more vulnerable to the effects of ionizing radiation, the cancer can be controlled with smaller doses of radiation than would be possible with radiation alone.

SOURCE:
Glanze, Walter D., Kenneth N. Anderson, and Lois E. Anderson (eds.). "Chemotherapy." In Mosby's *Medical, Nursing, & Allied Health Dictionary.* 3d ed. St. Louis: Mosby, 1990. p. 237.

OVERVIEW

Chemotherapy is the use of drugs or medications to treat disease. The term comes from two words that mean "chemical" and "treatment." Most people have had some type of chemotherapy for illness during their lives—for example, taking penicillin for an infection. Today, the word "chemotherapy" is used most often to describe a method of cancer treatment.

Cancer chemotherapy can consist of one drug or a group of drugs that work together (combination chemotherapy). A treatment plan that also includes surgery and/or radiation therapy is called combined modality treatment. In adjuvant chemotherapy, anticancer drugs are used after another treatment, to destroy any cancer cells that may remain after surgery or radiation therapy.

Chemotherapy has proven very effective in cancer treatment. In 1980, over 46,000 cancer patients were cured with the use of anticancer drugs, either alone or combined with radiation therapy and/or surgery.

Cancer cells grow in an uncontrolled manner, and they may break away from their original site and spread to other parts of the body. Anticancer drugs disrupt the cancer cells' ability to grow and multiply.

Chemotherapy may be given in several ways. Sometimes the drugs are used to obtain a local effect (for instance, in treating skin cancer). In other cases, chemotherapy is given to achieve a total-body (systemic) effect.

The best way to get the drug to the cancer site depends on the particular type of cancer and the drug or combination of drugs used. The medicine may be taken by mouth or injected into a muscle, or it may be given through a vein. Once in the blood, an anticancer drug is carried through the body to reach as many cancer cells as possible. How fast the cells are destroyed may vary with different medicines and different types of cancer.

Anticancer drugs can affect normal tissues also, because they act on any rapidly dividing cells in the body. The normal cells most likely to be affected are those in the bone marrow, gastrointestinal (GI) tract, reproductive system, and hair follicles. Most normal cells are able to recover quickly when the treatment is over.

SOURCE:
National Cancer Institute. *Chemotherapy and You.* NIH Publication No. 91-1136. June 1990, pp. 2–3.

SIDE EFFECTS

Whether you have side effects depends on the particular drug used and your individual response to it. There are more than 50 drugs used alone and in various combinations to treat the more than 100 types of cancer. Therefore, it is hard to predict whether a particular patient will have a specific side effect. In fact, you could notice a certain side effect after one treatment and not see the same effect the next time.

You should discuss possible side effects with your doctor, nurse, or pharmacist. You need to know what to expect from treatment and which side effects may need medical attention.

Some side effects of chemotherapy (for instance, fatigue and hair loss) may start in the early weeks of treatment and continue through its end. Others, such as nausea and vomiting, may occur for just a few hours right after a treatment. Most side effects of chemotherapy will gradually disappear once treatment is stopped and the healthy cells have a chance to grow normally. The unwanted effects of treatment can be unpleasant, but they must be measured against the medicine's ability to destroy the cancer.

People having chemotherapy can become discouraged because of the length of the treatment or the side effects that occur. If you begin to feel unhappy about your therapy or how it's progressing, talk to your doctor or nurse. It may be that your medication or the treatment schedule can be altered. Remember, though, that your doctor will not ask you to continue treatments unless the expected benefits outweigh the problems you may have.

Some side effects can decrease during treatment as your body adjusts to the therapy. However, you should remember that the time it takes to get over some of the troublesome side effects and regain energy varies from person to person. How soon you will feel better depends on many factors, including your condition and the kinds of medicines you've been taking.

SOURCE:
National Cancer Institute. *Chemotherapy and You*. NIH Publication No. 91-1136. June 1990, pp. 8-9.

ORAL COMPLICATIONS

One million Americans will develop cancer this year. For those having surgery, chemotherapy or irradiation, dental care—before, during and after treatment—is crucial, concludes an NIH consensus panel.

Though intensive therapy has made headway against the disease, treatment side effects have also increased, especially in the sensitive tissues of the mouth. It's estimated that as many as 400,000 cancer patients develop acute or chronic oral complications that not only affect treatment tolerance, but also interfere with the quality of life—even life itself.

Side effects include a variety of oral lesions and ulcers, as well as fungal, viral and bacterial infections. Gum disease, cavities, growth abnormalities and loss of bone, taste and protective saliva flow are also common.

To prevent and reduce oral problems, the NIH panel recommends every cancer patient have a comprehensive oral exam before therapy starts. If time permits, treat pre-existing dental problems aggressively, including gum disease, cavities, salivary gland disorders and poor oral hygiene. Tooth extractions and endodontic (root canal) treatment should be completed at least two weeks before therapy to reduce possible infection sites.

SOURCE:
Sears, Cathy. "Cancer's Second Strike: NIH Urges Well-Timed Dental Care to Combat Treatment Side Effects." *American Health* 8 (November 1989): 38.

RISK OF INFECTION

Most anticancer drugs affect the bone marrow, decreasing its ability to produce blood cells. The white blood cells produced in the bone marrow help to protect your body by fighting bacteria that cause infection. If the number of white cells in your blood is reduced, there is a higher risk of getting an infection.

If you have a reduced white cell count, it is very important that you try to prevent infection by taking the following steps:

- Wash your hands often during the day; be sure to wash them well before eating and after using the bathroom.
- Avoid crowds as well as people who have contagious illnesses such as chicken pox or flu.
- Do not tear or cut your nail cuticles. Use cuticle cream and remover instead.
- To prevent breaks in your mouth, avoid using a hard toothbrush or dental floss. Your doctor, nurse, or dentist can suggest ways to clean your mouth gently.
- To prevent breaks in your skin, use an electric shaver rather than a razor.
- Do not squeeze or scratch pimples.
- Take a warm shower every day, and lightly pat your skin dry rather than rubbing briskly.
- If your skin becomes dry and cracked, use lotion or oil to soften and heal it.
- If you do cut or scrape your skin, clean the area at once with warm water and soap.
- After each bowel movement, clean the rectal area gently but thoroughly. If there is irritation or if hemorrhoids are a problem, ask your doctor or nurse for advice.

SOURCE:
National Cancer Institute. *Chemotherapy and You*. NIH Publication No. 91-1136. June 1990, pp. 19-20.

CONTROL OF NAUSEA AND VOMITING

Drugs that bind to a specific neurotransmitter receptor appear able to control most cases of chemotherapy-induced nausea and vomiting with minimal side effects. Physicians familiar with these serotonin antagonists are hailing them as a significant advance.

"Their development is the first major step for treating emesis" in 10 years, said Dr. Steven Grunberg, and associate professor of medicine at the University of Southern California in Los Angeles. In addition, the drugs "will give us a better understanding of the process of nausea and vomiting," and they may lead to improved antiemetic treatments for other types of patients, he said.

The two agents that appear most advanced in testing are granisetron (Smith Kline Beecham), which is in phase 2 studies, and ondansetron (Zofran, Glaxo), the subject of several completed phase 2 tests. Glaxo applied to the FDA for an NDA [New Drug Approval] for ondansetron last October.

SOURCE:
Noler, Mitchel L. "Ranks of Antiemetics Expanding." *Medical World News* 31 (February 12, 1990): 30.

RESOURCES

ORGANIZATIONS
American Cancer Society. National Office, 4 East 35th St., New York, NY 10001. Or local chapters (check yellow pages).

National Cancer Institute. Office of Communications, Building 31, Room 10A2X, Bethesda, MD 20892.

BOOKS

Bruning, Nancy. *Coping with Chemotherapy*. New York: Doubleday/Dial, 1985. 317 pp.

Reich, Paul R. *The Facts about Chemotherapy: The Essential Guide for Cancer Patients and Their Families*. Fairfield, OH: Consumer Reports Books, 1990. 224 pp.

PAMPHLETS

National Cancer Institute, Office of Cancer Communications:

Eating Habits: Recipes and Tips for Better Nutrition During Cancer Treatment. NIH Pub. No. 88-2079. 1988.

Taking Time: Support for People with Cancer and the People who Care about Them. NIH Pub. No. 88-2059. 1988.

ADDITIONAL ARTICLES

"Cancer Chemotherapy." *The Medical Letter on Drugs and Therapeutics* 31, no. 793 (June 2, 1989): 49-56.

Evans, William E., and others. "Clinical Pharmacology of Cancer Chemotherapy in Children." *Pediatric Clinics of North America* 36, no. 5 (October 1989): 1199-1230.

Morrow, Gary R. "Chemotherapy-Related Nausea and Vomiting: Etiology and Management." *CA-Cancer Journal for Clinicians* 39, no. 2 (March/April 1989): 89-104.

Young, Robert C. "Mechanisms to Improve Chemotherapy Effectiveness." *Cancer* 65, no. 3, suppl. (February 1, 1990): 815-822.

CHIROPRACTIC

(*See also:* BACK PAIN)

OVERVIEW

Although chiropractic may have ancient roots, its theoretical framework was not formally laid down until the late 1800s. The founding father, a Canadian healer named Daniel David Palmer, was highly skilled in mesmerism, a precursor of modern hypnotherapy. Palmer believed in a "universal intelligence" by which all living matter was organized and governed, and he was fascinated by the possibility that human health could be understood accordingly.

One day in 1885 while Palmer was waiting for a client, the janitor of his office building walked by. Palmer called out to the man, Harvey Lillard, but to no avail—the man had been deaf for seventeen years. Palmer brought him in and noticed a small bump on the back of Lillard's neck. Intuitively, Palmer pushed the bump in. In his writings, Palmer noted that "he [Lillard] could not hear the racket of a wagon in the street or the ticking of a watch" and that after this "specific adjustment," Lillard could "hear as before" the horses on the cobblestone street below.

From this event Palmer deduced that the nervous system was the ultimate control mechanism of the living body, and that one's inner healing power—a dynamic expression of universal intelligence—depended on the unimpeded functioning of this system. He reasoned that even subtle misalignments of the spine, which he termed "subluxations," could have a significant impact on one's health. By manipulating Lillard's neck, Palmer had freed the spine for normal transmission of nerve impulses—in this case, the impulses that make hearing possible.

A subluxation, Palmer later reasoned, could affect any one of the thirty-one pairs of spinal nerves that travel to and from the brain through a series of openings in the vertebrae. A vertebra out of line with those above or below it would tend to obstruct the opening between them and cause an impingement, hence pressure or irritation, on surrounding nerves. By this mechanism, essential nerve messages to tissues were distorted, causing poor health in those corresponding areas. Since the nervous system regulates and controls all systems of the body—the digestive, respiratory, circulatory, immune, muscular, and eliminative systems—a subluxation could have far-reaching effects.

Depending also on the way the vertebrae are positioned, the effects of a subluxation could either decrease or increase the activity of nerves, producing a potentially dangerous decrease or increase in the activity of organs and systems supplied by those nerves. For instance, a sluggish liver or pancreas could indicate decreased nerve input, whereas an overactive heart or stomach could signify excessive nerve input. Irritated nerves—partly a consequence of poisons produced by ruptured nerve fibers and nerve roots—could accompany either tendency.

After nearly a century of development, chiropractic still holds the therapeutic role of the spine as central. "Like the drive shaft of a car, the spine is the directional source of human power and dominates all bodily functions," says George Harvey, D.C., a North Carolina-based chiropractor who has worked on spines for forty years. "The spinal cord connects brain to body, enabling the brain to control the body and mediate our health and vitality. When the spine is well-aligned, the rest of the body will follow."

A chiropractic "adjustment" is a calculated concussion of force delivered at a certain point at the right time along the spine to relieve pressure and irritation on nerves branching out from the spinal cord. (Some forms of accidental trauma may correct subluxations, but such fortuitous kinds of "adjustment" are probably very rare.) Chiropractic treatments can be quite potent and may even be detrimental; if applied in an unskilled manner, adjustments can just as easily become maladjustments.

SOURCE:
Mead, Mark N. "Chiropractic's New Wave: Controversial New Ideas, Tools, and Techniques are Transforming this Spine-Oriented Therapy." *East West Journal* 19 (November 1989): 65–66.

EVALUATION OF EFFECTIVENESS IN TREATING BACK PAIN

Some surprising results have emerged from a study published in the June 2 *BMJ* (formerly the *British Medical Journal*) that may provide some new clues to low back pain, a problem that affects 75 percent of us at some time in our lives and costs this country billions of dollars annually in medical care and lost productivity.

The British research involved looking at day-to-day experience (known as "pragmatic" investigation) instead of using placebos and other procedures not part of "real" life ("fastidious" investigation). From March 1986 to March 1989, the prestigious Epidemiology and Medical Care Unit of the British Medical Research Council in Harrow, Middlesex, England, studied more than 700 patients in 11 different towns or cities in England. In order to compare traditional medical care with chiropractic manipulation, patients were randomly assigned to either type of treatment, after researchers first determined by physical examination and x-ray that patients had no infections, nerve root injuries, bone abnormalities, etc., that would make chiropractic care potentially dangerous. The type of treatment given at either clinic was not decided in advance, but whatever the treatment, it was carefully recorded. The response to treatment was evaluated in terms of level of pain, weight of objects that could be lifted, and length of time the patient could remain comfortably in the sitting position.

Previous studies have usually shown that chiropractic treatment produced results for only a matter of hours after each session. This study showed that the 378 patients receiving chiropractic care tended to have better results after the first six months of treatment than the 339 treated in medical clinics. These better results continued during the next two years of follow-up. Because the study was "pragmatic," the researchers were not able to determine why the chiropractic treatment produced better results. It may have been chiropractic manipulation, or it may have been something else. It is interesting, however, that the chiropractic care lasted much longer (up to 30 weeks) than the medical care (up to 12 weeks) and involved 44 percent more sessions. It could thus be hypothesized that increased contact between patient and chiropractor (as compared with the lesser contact in the medical clinics) may have had something to do with the better results in the former.

The all-too-common complaint of medical patients is the brief time they are able to spend with the therapist. Given the uncertain causes of most low back pain, it may be less the actual treatment procedures, and more the manner that treatment is given, that affects the outcome.

SOURCE:
"Back to Basics: British Medical Council Research on Low Back Pain." *Medical Update* 14 (December 1990): 4–5.

* * *

A British study of 741 randomly assigned patients aged 18–65 that compared chiropractic treatment with hospital outpatient care (utilizing more conservative physiotherapeutic techniques) in the treatment of low back pain without nerve root involvement found that although there was no difference in outcomes in patients with no history of back pain, those with such a history who were treated by chiropractors (DCs) fared significantly better at 6, 12 and 24 month follow-ups. . . .

Comment: Chiropractic propagandists are overstating the findings of this study. Its design places great limitations on its generalizability.

First, this was a pragmatic study meaning that the types of therapies applied in the 11 (of each) participating hospital and chiropractic clinics was [sic] not controlled. A pragmatic study does not compare one therapy (99% of the DC [chiropractor]-treated subjects were manipulated compared to only 12% of hospital-treated) with another but compares treatment sites that consumers might select. This limits the value of the data. In fact, it is the type of design NCAHF [National Council Against Health Fraud, Inc.] President William Jarvis has long advocated as a starting point in testing the efficacy of chiropractic.

Second, the researchers excluded patients with contraindications (eg, nerve root involvement, weakened bones, structural abnormalities) to avoid harm. If DCs do not screen for these contraindications, the pragmatic patient population of DCs would differ from this study.

Third, chiropractic care was limited to a maximum of 10 treatments. This is less than DCs are apt to do when on their own.

Fourth, the chiropractic care in this study extended over a significantly longer time period (up to 30 weeks compared to a maximum of 12 weeks at hospitals) and involved 44% more sessions.

Fifth, chiropractic care was more expensive ($280 vs $190). This may have been compensated for by less work absenteeism following care.

Sixth, we have been unable to obtain information on the reliability and validity of the Oswestry [England] test. We would have preferred a performance test rather than a questionnaire as a method of observation.

Lastly, researchers know that treatment groups may vary significantly even when random assignment is employed, especially when numbers are below 1600 (hence, the importance of replication of research findings by others).

SOURCE:
"Chiropractic Care Found Better for Low Back Pain." *NCAHF Newsletter* 13 (SeptemberOctober- 1990): 5.

NCAHF POSITION PAPER ON CHIROPRACTIC

NCAHF [National Council Against Health Fraud, Inc.] believes that a health care delivery system as confused and poorly regulated as is chiropractic constitutes a major consumer health problem. The fact that its practitioners possess useful skills in manipulative therapy, and the apparent need for such skills, provide an opportunity for a constructive solution. The chiropractic problem is so broad-based that every segment of the community involved with health care, scientifically, economically, legally or educationally, must inject itself into the chiropractic controversy. Only a comprehensive approach to a solution has any hope of succeeding. For this reason, NCAHF makes the following recommendations:

1. As consumers you are largely at your own risk when choosing a practitioner of any kind because the law offers more protection to providers than consumers, therefore, choose health care practitioners carefully—particularly a chiropractor.

2. Distinguish between manipulative therapy per se and treatment based upon the specious chiropractic theory. Be alert to the fact that although manipulative therapy has distinct value in the treatment of back pain and may provide subjective relief in other chronic conditions, and chiropractors are educated and trained in manipulation, they represent but one source of this service. If you do choose a chiropractor ask him/her to work closely with your medical doctor.

3. Chiropractic theory is nonscientific, and most chiropractors have not been taught to practice on the basis of the same body of knowledge about health and disease recognized by health scientists around the world.

4. Understand that some chiropractic treatments involve considerable risk. Manipulation involving the rapid rotation of the head and neck or sudden movements have greater potential for injury than more conservative types of therapy. Do not submit to a "full spine" x-ray. This practice has doubtful diagnostic value, and the radiation exposure may have long range dangers.

5. Be aware that many chiropractors engage in nonscientific practices which can result in unnecessary expense. Also, nonscientific practitioners may delay the proper treatment of serious disorders causing excessive debility or needless death.

6. Beware of chiropractors who advertise about "danger signals that indicate the need for chiropractic care," make claims about cures, try to get patients to sign contracts for lengthy treatment, promote regular "preventive" adjustments, use scare tactics, or disparage conventional health care.

7. Demand that your legislative representative introduce and/or support laws that provide greater consumer protection in health care.

SOURCE:
National Council Against Health Fraud, Inc. *Position Paper on Chiropractic.* 1985. p. 3.

OPPOSITION OF THE AMERICAN MEDICAL ESTABLISHMENT

The U.S. District Court, Seventh Circuit, opinion on August 27, 1987 by Judge Susan Getzendanner stated that "the AMA and its officials instituted a boycott of chiropractors in the mid-1960's by informing AMA members that chiropractors were unscientific practitioners and it was unethical for a medical physician to associate with chiropractors. . . this conduct constituted a conspiracy among the AMA and its members and an unreasonable restraint of trade in violation of Section I of the Sherman Anti-Trust Act."

Judge Getzendanner wrote, ". . . the AMA has never acknowledged the lawlessness of its past conduct . . . there has never been public retraction of articles such as "The Right and Duty of Hospitals to Deny Chiropractors Access to Hospitals" . . . the systematic, long-term intent to destroy a licensed profession suggests that an injunction is appropriate in this case." Evidence in the case demonstrated that the AMA knew of scientific studies which implied that chiropractic care was twice as effective as medical care in relieving many painful conditions of the neck and back, as well as related musculoskeletal-neurological problems. There also was evidence that the AMA knew that chiropractic care of pregnant women greatly reduced the pain and suffering experienced by women during the months leading up to—and including—time of labor and delivery, without the need for chemical pain killers that could be harmful to both mother and child. . . .

Because Judge Getzendanner found the American Medical Association, the American College of Surgeons (ACS) and the American College of Radiologists (ACR) guilty of conspiring to destroy chiropractic, the AMA was permanently enjoined from "restricting, regulating or impeding or aiding and abetting others from restricting, regulating and impeding the freedom of any AMA member or any institution or hospital to make an individual decision as to whether or not that AMA member, institution or hospital shall professionally associate with chiropractors, chiropractic students or chiropractic institutions."

Just three days before the Court issued its injunction against the AMA, the co-defendants (the ACR and the ACS) reached a settlement with the chiropractic plaintiffs which ended the litigation against them. The ACR issued the following policy statement on inter-professional relations with chiropractors: "ACR declares that, except as provided by law, there are and should be no ethical or collective impediments to inter-professional association and cooperation between Doctors of Chiropractic and medical radiologists in any setting where such association may occur. . ."

In addition to its policy statement, the ACR agreed to pay $200,000 to help defray the legal expenses of the chiropractic plaintiffs. And the ACS agreed to pay $200,000 to the Kentuckiana Children's Center, a Louisville, Kentucky, facility for mentally and physically handicapped children founded and directed by Dr. Lorraine Golden, D.C. This chiropractor's dream of a multipurpose, inter-disciplinary children's center was severely impeded for 34 years by the actions of the medical profession which refused to cooperate with the Center in treating its more than 400 disadvantaged special children.

SOURCE:

Arthur, Patricia B. "Chiropractors' Victory against AMA." *The Doctor's People Newsletter* 2 (February 1989): 2–4.

RESOURCES

ORGANIZATIONS

American Chiropractic Association. 1701 Clarendon Blvd., Arlington, VA 22209.

Council on Chiropractic Education. 4401 Westown Parkway, Suite 120, West Des Moines, IA 50265.

International Chiropractors Association. 1901 L St. NW, Suite 800, Washington, DC 20036.

BOOK

Altman, Nathaniel. *Everybody's Guide to Chiropractic Health Care.* Los Angeles: Jeremy P. Tarcher, Inc., 1989.

RELATED ARTICLES

Cherkin, Dan, Frederick A. MacCornack, and Alfred O. Berg. "Family Physicians' Views of Chiropractors: Hostile or Hospitable?" *American Journal of Public Health* 79, no. 5 (May 1989): 636–637.

Meade, T. W., and others. "Low Back Pain of Mechanical Origin: Randomised Comparison of Chiropractic and Hospital Outpatient Treatment." *British Medical Journal* 300 (June 2, 1990): 1431–1437.

Walker, Mary. "Choosing a Chiropractor: A D.C.'s Approach May Range from Hands-On to High-Tech." *East West* (February 1991): 26–31.

CHLAMYDIA

(*See also:* GONORRHEA; PELVIC INFLAMMATORY DISEASE; SEXUALLY TRANSMITTED DISEASES; SYPHILIS)

OVERVIEW

Infections due to chlamydia ("kla-mid-ee-uh") are the most common sexually transmitted disease (STD) in the United States today, with an estimated 3 to 4 million new cases occurring each year. Pelvic inflammatory disease (PID), a serious complication of chlamydial infection, has recently emerged as a major cause of infertility among women of childbearing age. The organism can cause a broad range of infections in both men and women.

Chlamydial infections are caused by a bacterium, *Chlamydia trachomatis*. Among adults, these infections are transmitted only during vaginal or anal sexual contact with an infected partner. A mother may pass the infection to her newborn during delivery.

The early symptoms of chlamydial infection are usually mild; for this reason, it has sometimes been called "the silent STD." If symptoms occur, they usually appear within 1 to 3 weeks after exposure. One of every two infected women and one of every four infected men may have no symptoms whatsoever. As a result, the disease is often not diagnosed until complications develop.

In men, chlamydial infections cause about 40 percent of the cases of nongonococcal urethritis (NGU), an inflammation of the urinary tract. The most common symptoms of NGU are a discharge of mucus or pus from the penis; some men also notice pain when urinating. Pain or swelling in the scrotal area may be signs of epididymitis, an inflammation of a part of the male reproductive system located near the testicles.

Women with chlamydial infections may experience pain during urination, a vaginal discharge, or abdominal pain.

Chlamydial infection can also cause proctitis (inflamed rectum) and conjunctivitis (inflammation of the lining of the eye). Chlamydia bacteria have also been found in the throat. A particular strain of chlamydia causes an uncommon STD called lymphogranuloma venereum (LGV), which is characterized by swelling and inflammation of the lymph nodes in the groin. Other complications may follow if LGV is not treated at this stage.

Chlamydial infections are easily confused with gonorrhea because the symptoms of both diseases are similar, and they often occur together. Until recently, the only way to diagnose chlamydial infections was to take a sample of secretions from a patient's genital area and then grow any bacteria that are present into colonies to determine whether chlamydia is present. Although still widely used, this culture method often fails to detect chlamydial infections because chlamydia bacteria are not easily grown in a laboratory culture.

Within the past few years, scientists have developed several rapid tests for diagnosing chlamydial infections. Researchers supported by the National Institute of Allergy and Infectious Diseases (NIAID) have developed one such test. Rapid diagnostic tests use sophisticated techniques and a dye to detect the organism; they can be performed during a routine checkup; and results are available within 30 minutes. Many doctors recommend that all persons who have more than one sex partner, and especially women under age 35, be tested for chlamydial infection each year.

SOURCE:

National Institute of Allergy and Infectious Diseases. *Chlamydial Infections*. NIH Pub. No. 87-909B. August 1987. pp. 1–2.

CHLAMYDIA—AND PELVIC INFLAMMATORY DISEASE

The high risk that women with chlamydia will develop pelvic inflammatory disease (PID) lends a sense of urgency to the efforts to control chlamydia in the adolescent population. This risk is as much as 10 times higher in teens than in older women. Up to 26% of adolescent girls with chlamydia develop PID. Studies have shown that 45% of cases of PID are caused by chlamydia, compared with 36% for gonorrhea.

When a woman with chlamydia develops PID, the cost of treatment and long-term health risks increase. Patients face a 10% to 25% chance of scarring leading to infertility after one episode of PID, a 35% to 50% chance after two episodes, and the possibility of developing chronic PID.

SOURCE:
Stein, Ann P. "The Chlamydia Epidemic: Teenagers at Risk." In *Medical Aspects of Human Sexuality* (February 1991): 28.

DIAGNOSIS

Your clinician will suspect chlamydia if you have a typical chlamydial cervical discharge and if your cervix has red, swollen areas and seems friable (crumbly). Pap test results may also raise the suspicion of chlamydia. A Pap test, however, is not an accurate way to determine your diagnosis. Your clinician can confirm the diagnosis with laboratory tests such as culture, monoclonal antibody test, immunofluorescence, or enzyme immunoassay. (If these sound like expensive, sophisticated tests, they are. Because chlamydia is such a fastidious organism, fairly high technology is required to diagnose it successfully outside its normal environment.) Your clinician may also look for white blood cells in a sample of your discharge. Because gonorrhea often coexists with chlamydia your clinician will also collect a cervical discharge sample for a gonorrhea culture. If you also have gonorrhea, you will be treated for both infections at the same time.

SOURCE:
Stewart, Felicia H., Felicia Guest, and others (eds.). "Chlamydia (Chlamydia Trachomatis, Mucopurulent Cervicitis, Male Nongonococcal Urethritis)." *Understanding Your Body*. New York: Bantam, 1987. p. 485.

TREATMENT

When patients with cervicitis or urethritis test positive for chlamydia, treat with a seven-day course of tetracycline or doxycycline. If the patient is allergic to tetracycline or is pregnant, give erythromycin stearate. (Note: Erythromycin estolate is not recommended during pregnancy because of the increased risk of cholestatic hepatitis.)

In patients with PID, give a 14-day course of doxycycline plus cefoxitin or ceftriaxone adequate to treat gonorrhea. If the patient requires hospitalization (and many adolescents do), the doxycycline may be given intravenously, until the patient can take oral therapy.

When suspicion is high for gonorrhea or chlamydia at the initial visit, treatment decisions need to be made immediately to avoid further spread of the disease and risk to the patient. In this situation, if mucopurulent cervicitis is the primary finding, test for and treat both gonorrhea and chlamydia pending test results, since they commonly coexist. Patients with epididymitis should also be treated for both chlamydia and gonorrhea since culture is not possible.

Emphasize to the patient the importance of treating exposed partners. According to CDC guidelines, exposure to chlamydia mandates antibiotic treatment if testing is not available. If the patient has onset of symptoms within 30 days of contact with a partner who was chlamydia positive, the patient should be treated regardless of culture results.

SOURCE:
Stein, Ann P. "The Chlamydia Epidemic: Teenagers at Risk." *Medical Aspects of Human Sexuality*. (February 1991): 29, 32.

TREATMENT WITH MONODOX

In early 1991, Oclassen [Pharmaceuticals, Inc.] will also introduce Monodox (doxycycline monohydrate), a new oral antibiotic approved for treatment of the most prevalent STD, chlamydia. . . .

Chlamydial infections can usually be cured by antibiotics taken over a period of 7 to 10 days. The CDC recommends that uncomplicated chlamydial infections be treated with doxycycline—a derivative of tetracycline.

The majority of current therapies for chlamydial infections are based on doxycycline hyclate. In addition to the nausea and gastro-intestinal irritation which can occur from oral antibiotics, including doxycycline, the doxycycline hyclate formulation is reported to be one of the most common causes of the more serious side effect of esophageal ulceration.

Monodox is the U.S. brand name of a product containing doxycycline monohydrate. The monohydrate compound is virtually pH neutral (pH 5–6) compared to the more acidic (pH 2–3) doxycycline hyclate antibiotics currently available. In a preclinical study, the pH profile of the monohydrate demonstrated a reduced potential for esophageal ulceration.

"We believe Monodox represents an important improvement over existing therapies," said Tony DiTonno, vice president, marketing and sales for Oclassen. "Since our company specializes in drug therapies for sexually transmitted and dermatologic diseases, Monodox is an exciting acquisition for us."

SOURCE:
"New Treatments for Chlamydial Infections and Genital Warts." *NCI Cancer Weekly* (December 24, 1990): 6–8.

PREVENTION

Use of condoms by men and diaphragms by women can help limit the spread of chlamydia. However, medical authorities agree that the key to stopping the disease is better detection. Once it is identified, chlamydia can be cured quickly and painlessly with antibiotics.

Detection of chlamydia requires a test that is not part of a standard medical checkup. You have to ask for it. So stopping the disease is largely your responsibility. Sexually active people are at highest risk of getting the disease and therefore should discuss chlamydia with a physician. Pregnant women should too, since chlamydia can endanger them and their unborn children.

After the discussion, the physician may decide diagnostic testing is necessary. If so, test results can be obtained within 24 hours.

People who are being treated for another STD should also discuss chlamydia with a physician. Dual infections of chlamydia and gonorrhea are common. However, different drugs are required to treat the two diseases.

SOURCE:
Abbott Laboratories. *Chlamydia Is Not a Flower. It's a Sexually Transmitted Disease with Devastating Effects.* 1989. p. 3.

RESOURCES

RELATED ARTICLES

"Chlamydia: Cloak and Dagger." *Harvard Medical School Health Letter* (October 1988): 7-8.

"Chlamydia: Easy Come, Easy Go." *Mademoiselle* 97 (January 1991): 57.

"Fighting Chlamydia." *American Baby* (September 1990): 20.

Samuels, Sandra. "Chlamydia: Epidemic among America's Youth." *Medical Aspects of Human Sexuality* (December 1989): 16-23.

Schachter, Julius. "Chlamydial Infections." *The Western Journal of Medicine* 153 (November 1990): 523-524.

"Screening for Chlamydia in Pregnant Women." *American Family Physician* 42 (August 1990): 491-492.

CHOLESTEROL

(*See also:* FOOD/NUTRITION GUIDELINES)

OVERVIEW

Anyone can develop high blood cholesterol regardless of age, sex, race, or ethnic background. But, because there are no warning symptoms or signs, you are likely to be surprised at such a diagnosis. Don't be alarmed, but do take it seriously. Like high blood pressure, most people are unaware that their blood cholesterol levels are high until they learn it from their doctor. And, like high blood pressure, it is a potential threat to your health that you can do something about.

If you have just learned that you have high blood cholesterol, there are some important facts you need to know to protect your health. First, you need to find out what high blood cholesterol is, how high your level is, and what you can do to lower it. Then prepare to make some changes. Although these changes will depend on many factors considered by your doctor, modifying your diet is the preferred way to lower blood cholesterol. . . .

High blood cholesterol is one of the three major risk factors for coronary heart disease (cigarette smoking and high blood pressure are the other two). In other words, high blood cholesterol can significantly increase your risk of developing heart disease. Fortunately all three risk factors are "modifiable"; that is, you can do something about them. You can take steps to lower your cholesterol level and thus lower your risk for coronary heart disease.

High blood cholesterol occurs when there is too much cholesterol in your blood. Your cholesterol level is determined partly by your genetic makeup and the saturated fat and cholesterol in the foods you eat. Even if you didn't eat any cholesterol, your body would manufacture enough for its needs.

The risk of developing coronary heart disease increases as your blood cholesterol level rises. This is why it is so important that you have your blood cholesterol level measured. Currently, more than half of all adult Americans have blood cholesterol levels of 200 mg/dl or greater, which places them at an increased risk for coronary heart disease. Approximately 25 percent of the adult population 20 years of age or older has blood cholesterol levels that are considered "high," that is, 240 mg/dl or greater.

Your doctor will measure your level with a blood sample taken from your finger or your arm and will confirm this result with a second test if it is greater than 200 mg/dl. The following table can help you see how the results of your total blood cholesterol tests relate to your risk of developing coronary heart disease.

Desirable Cholesterol: Less than 200 mg/dl

Borderline-High Cholesterol: 200 to 239 mg/dl

High Cholesterol: 240 mg/dl and above

A blood cholesterol level of 240 mg/dl or greater is considered "high" blood cholesterol. But any level above 200 mg/dl, even in the "borderline-high" category, increases your risk for heart disease. If your blood cholesterol is 240 mg/dl or greater, you have more than twice the risk of someone whose cholesterol is 200 mg/dl, and you need medical attention and further testing.

When your high blood cholesterol level is combined with another major risk factor (either high blood pressure or cigarette smoking), your risk for coronary heart disease increases even further. For example, if your cholesterol level is in the "high" category and you have high blood pressure, your risk for coronary heart disease increases six times. If you also smoke, your risk increases more than 20-fold. Other factors that increase your risk for coronary heart disease include a family history of coronary heart disease before the age of 55, diabetes, vascular (blood vessel) disease, obesity, and being male. Whether your total blood cholesterol is in the "borderline-high" category or "high" category, you should make some changes in your diet to lower your level. More specifically, if your level is in the "borderline-high" category and you have coronary heart disease or two other risk factors for coronary heart disease or is in the "high" category, your physician will prescribe more aggressive treatment and follow your cholesterol levels more closely. If your cholesterol level is desirable, you should have your level checked again in 5 years and take steps to prevent it from rising. . . .

Most coronary heart disease is caused by atherosclerosis, which occurs when cholesterol, fat, and other substances build up in the walls of the arteries that supply blood to the heart. These deposits narrow the arteries and can slow or block the flow of blood. Among many things, blood carries a constant supply of oxygen to the heart. Without oxygen, heart muscle weakens, resulting in chest pain (angina), a heart attack (myocardial infarction), or even death. Atherosclerosis is a slow progressive disease that may start very early in life yet might not produce symptoms for many years. . . .

Lowering your high blood cholesterol level will slow fatty buildup in the walls of the arteries and reduce your risk of a heart attack and death caused by a heart attack. In fact, some studies have shown that, in adults with "high" blood cholesterol levels, for each 1 percent reduction in total cholesterol levels, there is a 2 percent reduction in the number of heart attacks. In other words, if you reduce your cholesterol level 15 percent, your risk of coronary heart disease could drop by 30 percent. . . .

In the United States, blood cholesterol levels in men and women start to rise at about age 20. Women's blood cholesterol levels prior to menopause (45–60 years) are lower than those of men of the same age. After menopause, however, the cholesterol level of women usually increases to a level higher than that of men. In men, blood cholesterol levels off around age 50 and the average blood cholesterol level declines slightly after age 50. Since the risk of coronary heart disease is especially high in the later decades of life, reducing blood cholesterol levels may be important in the elderly.

SOURCE:
National Heart, Lung and Blood Institute. *So You Have High Blood Cholesterol.* June 1989, pp. 1-7.

JOINT STATEMENT BY THE AMERICAN HEART ASSOCIATION AND NATIONAL HEART, LUNG, AND BLOOD INSTITUTE

Is High Serum Cholesterol a Risk Factor for Coronary Heart Disease?

Will Lowering Serum Cholesterol Help Prevent Coronary Heart Disease?

Strong scientific data provide positive answers to both of these questions. The evidence linking elevated serum cholesterol to CHD [Coronary Heart Disease] is overwhelming. Epidemiologic, clinical, genetic, and laboratory animal studies all indicate that high serum levels of cholesterol are causally related to coronary atherosclerosis and increased risk of CHD. The epidemiologic evidence includes comparisons among various populations and prospective studies within populations. In both types of studies, the predictive connection between serum cholesterol levels and future occurrence of CHD is continuous and positive throughout the range of cholesterol levels typically found in the United States. Moreover, in individuals with genetic forms of hypercholesterolemia, premature CHD commonly occurs even in the absence of other risk factors.

SOURCE:
Task Force on Cholesterol Issues, American Heart Association. "The Cholesterol Facts: A Summary of the Evidence Relating Dietary Fats, Serum Cholesterol, and Coronary Heart Disease. A Joint Statement by the American Heart Association and the National Heart, Lung, and Blood Institute." *Circulation* 81, no. 5 (May 1990): 1721–1722.

LDL AND HDL

LDL and HDL refer to two types of "lipoproteins." These are packages of cholesterol, fat, and protein that are made by the body to carry fat and cholesterol through the blood. They are not in the foods you eat.

LDLs are low density lipoproteins. They carry most of the cholesterol in the blood. If the level of LDL-cholesterol is elevated, cholesterol and fat can build up in the arteries contributing to atherosclerosis. This is why LDL-cholesterol is often called "bad cholesterol."

HDLs are high density lipoproteins. They contain only a small amount of cholesterol. HDLs are thought to carry cholesterol back to the liver. Thus HDLs help remove cholesterol from the blood, preventing the buildup of cholesterol in the walls of arteries. HDL-cholesterol is often called "good cholesterol."

If the average of your total cholesterol measurements is either "borderline-high" or "high," your doctor should ask you to return for another test. This test will show values for your LDL-cholesterol, HDL-cholesterol, and triglycerides. Your doctor will ask you to fast (except for water or black coffee) for 12 hours before the test.

LDL- and HDL-cholesterol levels more accurately predict your risk of coronary heart disease than a total cholesterol level alone. A *high* LDL-cholesterol level or a *low* HDL-cholesterol level increases your risk.

How Is My Total Blood Cholesterol Measured?

Cholesterol measurement requires a blood sample which may be drawn from a vein in your arm or taken by a fingerprick. If your first measurement is 200 mg/dL or greater, it should be rechecked with a second measurement on blood drawn from your arm. You do not have to fast for a total blood cholesterol measurement.

A second measurement is important. It helps your doctor decide what to do next. Your cholesterol level naturally changes over time. Also, lab errors can affect the number. A second measurement helps your doctor find your average number.

SOURCE:
National Heart, Lung, and Blood Institute. *Facts About Blood Cholesterol.* October 1990. p. 3.

OVERSTATEMENT OF CHOLESTEROL RISKS?

For the 60 million Americans with high blood-cholesterol levels, the federal government's National Cholesterol Education Program (NCEP) recommends a strict, medically supervised diet. If that doesn't help, then cholesterol-lowering drugs are often the next option. This massive anti-cholesterol effort is one of the largest medical interventions in the country's history. Yet now, earlier findings and recommendations about cholesterol are being seriously challenged.

Leading the assault are two new books: *Heart Failure* by journalist Thomas J. Moore, and *Balanced Nutrition: Beyond the Cholesterol Scare* by Dr. Fredrick Stare, a founder of the Harvard School of Public Health's Department of Nutrition, Dr. Robert Olson, professor of medicine at the State University of New York at Stony Brook, and Elizabeth Whelan, president of the American Council on Science and Health. Many of their views are supported in a September 7, 1989, article in *The New England Journal of Medicine* by Dr. Allan S. Brett of the Harvard Medical School. Among their assertions are the following:

- Cholesterol risks have been overstated. In the absence of cigarette smoking and high blood pressure, elevated cholesterol alone does not appear to be as serious a risk factor for heart disease as we have been led to believe.
- Low cholesterol, however, may have unanticipated adverse consequences, according to research Moore cites, including increased incidence of strokes and cancer.
- Lowering cholesterol through diet, Moore states, can be difficult and the results sometimes minimal.
- The benefits of cholesterol-lowering drugs have been exaggerated, and their side effects minimized or ignored. . . .

Brett, Moore, Stare and the other authors have raised important and challenging questions about cholesterol. If nothing else, these questions remind us that the human body is a complex machine with an uncanny instinct for defying simple answers. Because of that, there is ultimately one question that outweighs all others: What do we now know about cholesterol and its effect on our health? Here's a summary of the research:

1. Men. The evidence is overwhelming that men ages 25 to 55 are at high risk for coronary heart disease if their cholesterol level is 240 or above. While those with lower cholesterol readings have less risk, the possibility of disease increases with the addition of a risk factor, such as smoking or high blood pressure. If they have two additional risk factors, the prospect of getting coronary heart disease is significantly greater.

Research is limited on older men, ages 60 and over. While it is known that cholesterol levels increase as the body ages, there is conflicting evidence about whether these higher cholesterol levels place older people at greater risk for coronary heart disease.

While the dangers of low cholesterol are not as well documented as those for high cholesterol, the evidence suggests that young and middle-aged men with cholesterol levels below 160 are at low risk for coronary heart disease but may experience increased incidence of strokes and cancer. Some evidence suggests that cholesterol levels between 160 and 200 are the healthiest if there are no other risk factors present. However, this is by no means conclusive.

2. Women. Most cholesterol studies have focused on young and middle-aged men. However, there has been enough research to show that pre-menopausal women—even those with cholesterol levels above 240—seldom develop coronary heart disease unless they have additional risk factors.

Post-menopausal women with high cholesterol level develop coronary heart disease at roughly the same rate as middle-aged men with high cholesterol levels. However, as post-menopausal women grow older, the gap between their risk of heart disease and that of men their own age appears to narrow.

3. Low-cholesterol diets. The link between cholesterol levels in the blood and consumption of fatty and cholesterol-rich foods (pork, egg yolks, butter, etc.) appears to be less clear-cut than previously believed. However, the evidence remains powerful that a diet heavy in fatty and cholesterol-rich foods is unhealthful.

4. Cholesterol-lowering drugs. The long-term effects of most cholesterol-lowering drugs have not been determined. While many of these drugs succeed in lowering cholesterol—in some cases significantly—the evidence that they extend life is not conclusive.

Because of potential side effects, these drugs should be approached with caution and only when all other approaches fail. Any decision about taking them should be made in consultation with a physician and by carefully weighing the risks and benefits.

SOURCE:
Pekkanen, John. "New Questions about Cholesterol." *Reader's Digest* (April 1990): 103–104, 107–108.

DIETARY THERAPY

Whatever the reasons may be for your high blood cholesterol level—diet, heredity, or both—the treatment your doctor will prescribe first is diet. If your blood cholesterol level has not decreased sufficiently after carefully following the diet for 6 months, your doctor may consider adding cholesterol-lowering medication to your dietary treatment. Remember, diet is a very essential step in the treatment of high blood cholesterol. Cholesterol-lowering medications are more effective when combined with diet. Thus they are meant to supplement, not replace, a low-saturated fat, low-cholesterol diet.

The following are some guidelines for dietary changes to help you lower your blood cholesterol level. Your new diet is low in saturated fat and low in cholesterol and is adequate in all nutrients, including protein, carbohydrate, fat, vitamins, and minerals.

- Eat less high-fat (especially those high in saturated fat).
- Replace part of the saturated fat in your diet with unsaturated fat.
- Eat less high-cholesterol food.
- Choose foods high in complex carbohydrates (starch and fiber).
- Reduce your weight, if your are overweight.

There are two major types of dietary fat—saturated and unsaturated. Unsaturated fats are further classified as either polyunsaturated or monounsaturated fats. Together, saturated and unsaturated fats equal total fat. All foods containing fat contain a mixture of these fats.

One of the goals in your blood cholesterol-lowering diet is to eat less total fat, because this is an effective way to eat less saturated fat. Because fat is the richest source of calories, this will also help reduce the number of calories you eat every day. If you are overweight, weight loss is another important step in lowering blood cholesterol levels. If you are not overweight, be sure to replace the fat calories by eating more food high in complex carbohydrates.

Remember: When you decrease the amount of total fat you eat, you are likely to reduce the saturated fat and calories in you diet.

SOURCE:
National Heart, Lung, and Blood Institute. *Eating to Lower Your High Blood Cholesterol.* NIH Pub. No. 89-2920. June 1989. pp. 5-6.

REDUCED BY NIACIN

Niacin's ability to reduce cholesterol levels in the blood has long been recognized, but because it was a vitamin and cannot be patented, no drug company has bothered to test and promote it in the fight against coronary heart disease. But the current National Cholesterol Education Program, which aims to get every adult with high cholesterol identified and treated, has led some doctors to take a hard look at niacin.

Last December researchers from the University of Pennsylvania reported that niacin was the least costly medication available for reducing cholesterol levels. Niacin can achieve a 1 percent reduction in cholesterol for one-third to one-half the cost of other cholesterol-lowering drugs, they calculated.

Large doses of nicotinic acid—but not nicotinamide—lower the levels of two harmful fatty substances in the blood: low-density lipoprotein (LDL) cholesterol and triglycerides. As a further benefit, niacin therapy raises the protective form of cholesterol, called HDL (for high-density lipoprotein). Thus, drug doses of niacin may help cleanse coronary arteries of obstructing fatty deposits.

In a collaborative study financed by the National Heart, Lung and Blood Institute, more than 1,000 middle-aged men who had already suffered one heart attack took large doses of niacin for five years. Nine years after the study ended, they were found to be less likely to have died of a second heart attack. This benefit was seen despite a potentially serious side effect associated with niacin therapy: an increased incidence of abnormal heart rhythms.

SOURCE:
Brody, Jane E. "The Two Faces of Niacin: A Substance that Lowers Cholesterol Level, but Not Without Side Effects." *The New York Times* (March 7, 1991): B5.

USE OF PRESCRIPTION DRUGS

There are several medications your physician can prescribe to help you lower your blood cholesterol levels. The report issued by the National Cholesterol Education Program cited the bile acid sequestrants—cholestyramine and colestipol—and nicotinic acid as the drugs of first choice. The report underscored the effectiveness and the long-term safety of these drugs as demonstrated in research studies. The report also cited a new class of drug—HMG CoA reductase—which has demonstrated considerable effectiveness in lowering cholesterol levels. One drug in this class—Lovastatin—has been approved for use by the Food and Drug Administration. Because of its newness, long-term safety data has not yet been established. Other drugs cited in the report which were not considered as efficacious in lowering LDL-cholesterol as those mentioned above include gemfibrozil and probucol. All cholesterol-lowering medications should be taken only with the advice of and under the supervision of your physician.

SOURCE:
National Heart, Lung and Blood Institute. *So You Have High Blood Cholesterol.* June 1989. p. 24.

RESOURCES

ORGANIZATION

National Cholesterol Education Program. National Heart, Lung, and Blood Institute, Bethesda, MD 20892.

BOOKS

Cooper, Kenneth. *Controlling Cholesterol.* New York: Bantam, 1988.

Kowalski, Robert E. *The 8-Week Cholesterol Cure: How to Lower Your Blood Cholesterol by Up to 40 Percent Without Drugs or Deprivation.* New York: Harper, 1987.

RELATED ARTICLES

"Choice of Cholesterol-Lowering Drugs." *The Medical Letter On Drugs and Therapeutics* 33, no. 835 (January 11, 1991): 1-4.

"The Cholesterol Controversy." *Harvard Medical School Health Letter* 15, no. 2 (December 1989): 1-3.

"Cholesterol: The Numbers." *Harvard Medical School Health Letter* (March 1989): 4-8.

"How to Chop Down Sky-High Cholesterol." *Prevention* (February 1991): 38, 42, 44, 129-134.

LaRosa, John C. "At What Levels of Total Low- or High-Density Lipoprotein Cholesterol Should Diet/Drug Therapy Be Initiated? United States Guidelines." *The American Journal of Cardiology* 65, no. 12 (March 20, 1990): 7F-10F.

Liebman, Bonnie. "The HDL/Triglycerides Trap." *Nutrition Action Healthletter* (September 1990): 1, 5-7.

Nash, D. T. "Lowering Cholesterol Naturally." *Postgraduate Medicine* 87, no. 2 (February 1, 1990): 63-65, 68.

CHOOSING A PHYSICIAN

OVERVIEW

Board Certified. This is the gold standard when evaluating a doctor. After a residency, a doctor becomes eligible to take the certification examination given by the medical board that governs that field of practice. There are 23 boards recognized by the American Board of Medical Specialties (ABMS), the national umbrella of medical boards. They include the American Board of Internal Medicine (93,000 members), the American Board of Family Practice (37,000), and the American Board of Obstetrics and Gynecology (25,000). A "board-eligible" doctor has completed a residency and any other prerequisites for board certification, but has not yet taken—or not yet passed—the exam. Many boards discourage doctors from using the term because it can be misleading. Caution: There are more than a hundred boards that are not recognized by the ABMS even though their members may claim "board certification." Some of these boards are sincere. Others offer certification to any doctor who sends in a check.

Team Player. Doctors affiliated with hospitals, group medical practices or HMOs are often a safer bet than solo practitioners. The latter are less likely to remain up-to-date and, unlike doctors affiliated with organizations, they are not routinely evaluated by their peers or employers. The best doctors tend to teach full- or part-time at teaching hospitals or have patient-admitting privileges there. These physicians are the most likely to be highly respected by other doctors and to have cutting-edge medical knowledge.

Highly Trained. Doctors must complete four years at an accredited medical school and pass state exams in order to be licensed. Graduates of foreign medical schools (except those in Canada) must pass certain other examinations as well. Most doctors also complete a residency program—usually three to seven years of specialty training in a field such as internal medicine or family practice. Some now supplement their residency with a "postdoctoral" year or two focusing even more on a particular area. An internist, for example, may study heart disease or cancer. Be sure to ask what specific field a doctor's training was in. Not all states prevent a psychiatrist, say, from treating runner's knee. But clearly a doctor who followed an orthopedic residency with post-doctorate work in sports medicine would be a better choice.

Well Groomed. Most people make an intuitive link between taking good care of yourself and being able to look after others. A 1987 study that polled patients on physicians' attire found that patients—especially older, less well-off ones—wanted a doctor to convey an image of respect and authority. They applauded white coats, ties for male doctors and skirts for females; sportswear and blue jeans got a thumbs down. Many patients—and physicians—also believe a doctor should set a good example in health habits. "If a physician has an ashtray on the desk or is very fat, that would be a turn-off," says Craig Strafford, M.D., president of the 62-physician Holzer Clinic in Gallipolis, Ohio.

Conscientious. The rate of patients' compliance with doctors' instructions can be as low as 50%. For that reason, "It's important for the doctor to call, to ask how the patient is doing, to see if, for example, a medication needs changing," says family physician Dudley Phillips, M.D., chairman of the public relations committee of the American Academy of Family Practice. A good doctor also follows up on prevention advice. Discussions on weight loss, exercise or regulating high blood pressure should be ongoing, not just part of your initial visit.

Up-to-date. With the fast pace of medicine, well-trained doctors can end up giving second-rate care if they don't keep up—and keeping up is hard to do. It means reading journals, attending conferences and continuing-education courses, and interacting with peers in journal clubs, meetings and hospital and medical society committees, often after long days at the office or hospital.

Recertification is now required every 10 years by the boards of internal medicine and obstetrics and gynecology and every seven by the family-practice board. Some boards began requiring recertification only recently, so many doctors may not be recertified for quite a while. It's worth asking a doctor, especially one who is over age 55, when his or her last certification was.

Doesn't believe in magic. There are few quick fixes, even in modern-day medicine. A good doctor won't make big promises or offer magical treatments, says internist M. Boyd Shook, M.D., clinical assistant professor of medicine at the University of Oklahoma at Oklahoma City: "If a doctor claims that he's got an easy way for you to lose weight, keep your cholesterol down or your back from hurting, I think you should run like heck to another doctor."

Good communicator. Many patients think a pleasant bedside manner is the crucial quality in a physician. But though warmth and a caring attitude are important, a friendly doctor isn't necessarily as bright as his smile. Likewise, a doctor may be lousy at chit-chat but a brilliant diagnostician. What any excellent physician must have is a sharply honed ability to communicate medical info. So much good health care depends on patients ministering to themselves—particularly during pregnancy or with chronic conditions like asthma, hypertension or arthritis—that a doctor's role is often to help you understand self-treatment activities. He or she should make eye contact with you and listen intently to any complaints.

Beloved by Nurses. If you ask current or former patients about a physician's abilities, the opinion you get will likely be based on a sample size of one. Other doctors may also be subjective since they themselves may receive referrals for recommending each other. The most unbiased sources may be local hospital nurses. They rarely gain anything from recommending a particular doctor. "They can tell you who's good, who's sloppy, who's not up to date," says public-health expert John E. Kralewski, Ph.D., of the University of Minnesota at Minneapolis.

Hard to get at 4 A.M. Patients might rate high a doctor who promises to be available for emergencies 24 hours every day. But physicians need sleep just like the rest of us. It's far more important that a doctor have a trustworthy colleague covering on some nights and weekends than always be reachable himself. The back-up physician should be in the same specialty and located nearby.

A good doctor should, however, be available for emergencies or walk-ins during the day. Most doctors do put air in their daily schedules. For example, Dudley Phillips, M.D., schedules four patients an hour but leaves three visits open each day to accommodate the unexpected.

SOURCE:

Tanne, Janice Hopkins. "Making Doctor Right." *Health* 22, no. 9 (October 1990): 52–53.

EVALUATIVE DATA

Right now, despite the growing patients' rights movement and the wide interest in health issues, many people remain surprisingly unsavvy about evaluating a physician. According to a recent nationwide Gallup Poll commissioned by the American Medical Association, the number one criterion patients used in selecting their last new doctor was another patient's recommendation, not objective information about the doctor's skill. "Most people make better-informed decisions about buying a refrigerator than choosing a physician," says Tom Higgins, the founding editor of *HealthWeek*, a journal for health-care managers. But soon that may change. As both patients and large companies that foot the bill for their employees' health coverage become more concerned with the bottom line, they are demanding more objective measures for judging doctors. Soon, "medicine will be stripped of its mystique," Higgins says. The result, he wrote in a recent *Healthweek* editorial, "will be a landmark shift in power in American medicine, and it has already begun."...

At the moment, the average person hoping to assess a doctor's skill won't find much evidence that patient power is leading to more reliable information. There is still not much objective data on doctors available to patients. Last year, researchers Julia M. Reade, M.D., of Massachusetts General Hospital in Boston and Richard M. Ratzan, M.D., of the University of Connecticut School of Medicine in Farmington, set out to verify the credentials of doctors listed in a Connecticut yellow pages much the way a patient would. Their efforts were frequently stymied. For example, in the directory, some physicians described themselves as "board certified," meaning they had passed the qualifying exam administered by the medical board overseeing their specialty. But when Reade and Ratzan contacted the boards directly, they discovered that some of these organizations wouldn't comment to patients on physicians' membership status.

The researchers concluded: "Obtaining access to complete, up-to-date and verified information about physicians is all but impossible. The standard advice consumers are given about sources of information is inadequate." Since the study was released, the American Board of Medical Specialties (ABMS), the umbrella organization of American medical specialty boards, has begun offering a toll-free number, (800) 776-CERT, which patients can call to confirm a doctor's board certification.

SOURCE:

Silver, Nan. "How Good Is Your Doctor?" *Health* (October 1990): 49–50.

BOARD CERTIFICATION—MEANINGFUL OR MEANINGLESS?

For years consumers have considered specialty board certification to be one of the fundamental criteria of medical competency.

But is that necessarily so? According to recent reports in the medical literature, any group of physicians can set up a medical board and hand out board certifications. For consumers, that is worrisome news. It means that board certification is not necessarily a helpful signpost in the vast health care wilderness.

In theory, certification is designed to assure the public that a physician has met certain standards of knowledge, experience, and skills set by other medical professionals to ensure high-quality care in the specialty. Usually, this means that the certified doctor has education beyond that necessary to earn an M.D. or a D.O. and has passed a special written exam. In a sense, certification is a way for the medical profession to recognize those with specialized knowledge in a particular field of medicine (or to separate the wheat from the chaff).

In reality, not every branch of medicine has a specialty certification board. Nor is certification by itself a foolproof indicator of competence: A doctor may perform well on paper but flub up in actual practice. Also, the prerequisites for certification vary from board to board. For example, some boards give their "diplomates" (board-certified doctors) certificates that are valid for only seven to 10 years; doctors must go through a periodic reexamination and/or get additional education to remain board-certified. In contrast, other specialty boards never require recertification at all.

As is typical of the medical world, a bureaucracy has been established to operate and oversee the certification process. The American Board of Medical Specialties (ABMS) in Evanston, Illinois, is an organization that, in a sense, certifies the certification boards. It recognizes 23 specialty boards with 380,000 physician members and issues certificates in 31 specialties and 57 subspecialties. But not all specialty boards fall under the ABMS umbrella. An additional 105 medical specialty boards—often called self-designated specialty boards—don't have ABMS recognition.

It's this growth in specialty boards that is causing great debate in the medical world. As reported in *Hospitals* (August 5, 1989), some members of the medical profession (the American Board of Medical Specialties among them) claim that the proliferation of specialty boards "dilutes the core purpose of specialty certification: allowing the public to identify practitioners who have earned formal recognition of skill in a specific specialty area." As one Chicago hospital medical affairs director told that publication: "Specialty boards have become so confusing that they run the risk of becoming meaningless." These folks call for one standard of competency; in particular, the one established by ABMS.

SOURCE:
"Special Certification: Meaningful or Meaningless?" *People's Medical Society Newsletter* 8 (December 1989): 1.

THE PHYSICIAN-PATIENT RELATIONSHIP

It may be trite to emphasize that physicians need to approach patients not as "cases" or "diseases" but as individuals whose problems all too often transcend the complaints which bring them to the doctor. Most patients are anxious and frightened. Often they go to great ends to convince themselves that illness does not exist, or unconsciously they set up elaborate defenses to divert attention from the real problem that they perceive to be serious or life-threatening. Some patients use illness to gain attention or to serve as a crutch to extricate themselves from an emotionally stressful situation; some even feign physical illness. Whatever the patient's attitude, the physician needs to consider the terrain in which an illness occurs—in terms not only of the patients themselves but also of their families and social backgrounds. All too often medical workups and records fail to include essential information about the patient's origins, schooling, job, home and family, hopes and fears. Without this knowledge it is difficult for the physician to gain rapport with the patient or to develop insight into the patient's illness. Such a relationship must be based on thorough knowledge of the patient and on mutual trust and the ability to communicate with one another. . . .

The American Board of Internal Medicine has defined humanistic qualities as encompassing integrity, respect, and compassion. Availability, the expression of sincere concern, the willingness to take the time to explain all aspects of the patient's illness, and an attitude of being nonjudgmental with patients who have lifestyles, attitudes, and values different from those of the physician and which he or she may in some instances even find repugnant are just a few of the characteristics of the humane physician. Every physician will, at times, be challenged by patients who evoke strongly negative (and occasionally strongly positive) emotional responses. Physicians should be alert to their own reactions to such patients and situations and consciously monitor and control their behavior so that the patients' best interests remain the principal motivation for their actions at all times.

The famous statement of Dr. Francis Peabody is even more relevant today than when delivered more than half a century ago:

> *The significance of the intimate personal relationship between physician and patient cannot be too strongly emphasized, for in an extraordinarily large number of cases both the diagnosis and treatment are directly dependent on*

it. One of the essential qualities of the clinician is interest in humanity, for the secret of the care of the patient is in caring for the patient.

SOURCE:
Wilson, Jean D., and others (eds.). *Harrison's Principles of Internal Medicine.* 12th Ed. New York: McGraw-Hill, 1991. pp. 1, 2.

RESOURCES

BOOKS
American Board of Medical Specialties. *ABMS Compendium of Certified Medical Specialists.* 3d ed. 7 vols. Evanston, IL: American Board of Medical Specialties, 1990–1991.

American Medical Directory. *Directory of Physicians in the United States.* 32d ed. 4 vols. Chicago: American Medical Association, 1990.

Directory of Medical Specialists. 24th ed. 3 vols. Wilmette, IL: Marquis Who's Who, 1989–1990.

Jones, J. Alfred, and Gerald M. Phillips. *Communicating with Your Doctor.* Carbondale, IL: Southern Illinois University Press, 1988.

Simmons, Nicole, Phyllis McCarthy, and Sidney Wolfe. *6892 Questionable Doctors.* Washington, DC: Public Citizen Health Research Group, 1990.

Stutz, David R., and Bernard Feder. *The Savvy Patient: How to Be an Active Participant in Your Medical Care.* Fairfield, OH: Consumer Reports Books, 1990. 288 pp.

RELATED ARTICLES
Lipman, Marvin M. "When to Fire Your Doctor—and How to Find Another." *Consumer Reports Health Letter* (April 1990): 30–31.

Reade, Julia M., and Richard M. Ratzan. "Access to Information: Physicians' Credentials and Where You Can't Find Them." *New England Journal of Medicine* 321 (August 17, 1989): 466–468.

Sloane, Leonard. "Coping with a Change in Doctors: Finding a Compatible Doctor and Obtaining Medical Records Can Both Involve Time and Effort." *New York Times* (July 14, 1990).

CHRONIC FATIGUE SYNDROME

DEFINITION

The chronic Epstein-Barr virus syndrome is a poorly defined symptom complex characterized primarily by chronic or recurrent debilitating fatigue and various combinations of other symptoms, including sore throat, lymph node pain and tenderness, headache, myalgia, and arthralgias. Although the syndrome has received recent attention, and has been diagnosed in many patients, the chronic Epstein-Barr virus syndrome has not been defined consistently. Despite the name of the syndrome, both the diagnostic value of Epstein-Barr virus serologic tests and the proposed causal relationship between Epstein-Barr virus infection and patients who have been diagnosed with the chronic Epstein-Barr virus syndrome remain doubtful. We propose a new name for the chronic Epstein-Barr virus syndrome—the chronic fatigue syndrome—that more accurately describes this symptom complex as a syndrome of unknown cause characterized primarily by chronic fatigue. We also present a working definition for the chronic fatigue syndrome designed to improve the comparability and reproducibility of clinical research and epidemiologic studies, and to provide a rational basis for evaluating patients who have chronic fatigue of undetermined cause.

SOURCE:
Holmes, G. P., J. E. Kaplan, and others. "Chronic Fatigue Syndrome: A Working Case Definition." *Annals of Internal Medicine* 108, no. 3 (March 1988): 387–389.

OVERVIEW

Chronic fatigue syndrome began receiving widespread attention in the mid-1980's after reports of about 100 cases in the Lake Tahoe area of California. Questions immediately arose as to whether the ill-defined mix of symptoms amounted to a discrete disease at all, and if so, whether it was a new condition or was merely an old malady like the neurasthenia of the 1860's, since known by other names, including Icelandic disease.

Now that some of the dust has settled, chronic fatigue syndrome appears to be the same as what is called low natural killer cell syndrome in Japan and myalgic encephalomyelitis in England. In the United States, chronic fatigue syndrome has also been called Epstein-Barr virus syndrome, chronic mononucleosis and yuppie flu.

The debilitating, but seldom fatal condition seems to affect many more women than men, and adults more than children. The ailment often leaves victims fatigued for months, even years. It can cause nonspecific flu-like symptoms, including headaches, sore throats, swollen lymph nodes, fever and pain in the muscles and joints. It can cause an inability to think clearly and concentrate, memory loss, confusion, irritability, sleep disturbance and depression. There is no standard laboratory test yet available for giving a reliable diagnosis of chronic fatigue syndrome. Doctors must rely on sharp clinical intuition and criteria set by the Centers for Disease Control to judge whether a patient has the syndrome.

The lack of a clearly diagnostic test is highly frustrating for patients and health workers alike. Thus the ailment has sometimes become a faddish catch-all label for symptoms that cannot be otherwise explained.

In reports and in interviews, more than a dozen experts cited a trend in which many doctors have come to believe the syndrome is real, although most remain skeptical or are yet to be persuaded. Among those who are convinced that chronic fatigue syndrome is a real disease, three principal theories are being pursued. One is that any of a number of infections agents and possibly chemicals can provoke the immune system to counterattack and somehow keep it in a lasting state of activation. The immune system spurs production of cytokines, a family of powerful agents that gird up the immune system for fighting foreign substances. Among the known cytokines are interleukin and tumor necrosis factor, both of which are used in experimental cancer therapy. They are known from these experiments to cause side effects like fatigue, muscle aches and other generally short-lived symptoms of conventional viral infections known as the flu.

According to this theory, the victims of chronic fatigue are those who cannot get rid of common infectious agents the way most people do, perhaps because of genetic differences. The result is a permanently activated state in which the immune system stays in high drive, as if to combat a continuing viral infection.

The second theory is that chronic fatigue syndrome is caused by viruses that infect parts of the brain and resist detection by the standard diagnostic tests. New laboratory and diagnostic measures are being developed to explore this concept.

The third theory holds that the syndrome is primarily a muscle disease; the fatigue results secondarily from muscle dysfunction.

SOURCE:
Altman, Lawrence K. "Chronic Fatigue Syndrome Finally Gets Some Respect." *The New York Times* (December 4, 1990): B5, B9.

DIAGNOSTIC CRITERIA

Recently, there has been a renewed interest in people who suffer chronically from fatigue, weakness, decreased ability to concentrate, and poor memory. In some of these cases, tests for the Epstein-Barr virus have been positive, leading some physicians to diagnose chronic infectious mononucleosis.

A number of things can produce fatigue, weakness, and loss of memory, including stress, an unidentified disease, or a psychological condition such as depression. Experts have developed the term chronic fatigue syndrome to designate this vague group of symptoms. (A syndrome is simply a collection of symptoms.) No definite cause for the chronic fatigue syndrome has been found, although emotional and psychological factors may play a role. Usually, there is no underlying viral infection.

Certain criteria have been proposed that should be met before the diagnosis of chronic fatigue syndrome can be made. First, you must suffer from recent and extreme fatigue and weakness that has impaired your ability to work for 6 months. All other known diseases, infections, or psychiatric illnesses that might cause these symptoms must be ruled out. In addition, you must have six of the following criteria: 1) low-grade fever (99.5°F to 100.5°F) or chills; 2) sore throat; 3) painful lymph nodes in the neck or armpits; 4) general weakness; 5) prolonged fatigue following previously tolerated exercise; 6) generalized headaches; 7) unexplained muscle soreness; 8) pain that moves from one joint to another, without evidence of redness or swelling; 9) forgetfulness, irritability, and confusion; 10) sleep disturbance.

Finally, your physician must be able to identify the presence of two of the following physical signs: 1) low-grade fever (99.5°F to 100.5°F); 2) small, tender lymph nodes in the neck or armpits; 3) redness of the throat, without evidence of a bacterial infection.

For chronic fatigue syndrome, the symptoms are treated and allowed to run their course.

The key question is whether these symptoms represent a new disease or are a collection of complaints without clear cause. We think that this is not a new disease. Many people who claimed to have symptoms of fatigue underwent tests that showed they had been exposed to the Epstein-Barr virus. However, further analysis has shown that many people exposed to the Epstein-Barr virus are free of symptoms. And not all those who do say they have symptoms have been exposed to the virus.

The chronic fatigue syndrome is just that—a syndrome or collection of symptoms. In most cases, there is no underlying disease causing it.

SOURCE:
Mayo Clinic Family Health Book. New York: Morrow, 1990. p. 853.

SIGNS AND SYMPTOMS

Though no one has precise numbers, epidemiologists guess that 2 million to 5 million Americans have been stricken. The illness has spawned four national patients' organizations and some 400 local support groups. Officials at the Atlanta-based Centers for Disease Control (CDC), the federal agency responsible for tracking infectious disease, say they receive 1,000 to 2,000 calls about the condition every month. Dr. Jay Levy, a San Francisco AIDS researcher, calls it "the disease of the '90s."

The ailment goes by a range of different names. The British and Canadians know it as myalgic encephalomyelitis, or ME. The Japanese call it low natural killer cell syndrome. In this country, patients' groups call it chronic fatigue immune dysfunction syndrome (CFIDS), but it is generally known as chronic fatigue syndrome (CFS). Some of the common symptoms—fevers and lymph-node swelling, night sweats, persistent diarrhea, joint and muscle pain—have a disturbingly familiar ring. But unlike AIDS, this gray plague doesn't kill people, unless they take their lives in despair. It simply turns them into confused invalids. Many patients suffer mood swings or panic attacks and most develop a low-grade dementia.

Sleep disturbances are common, as are vision problems. Some sufferers lose their hair, or their fingerprints, or they develop acne for the first time. And though the illness sometimes lifts after a few hellish months, it can linger for years—or recede only to return.

Mounting evidence suggests that CFS is an immune-system disorder in which the body works frantically but inefficiently to control common viral infections. In a flurry of small studies, immunologists have found clear breaches in the body's defense system.

SOURCE:
"Chronic Fatigue Syndrome: A Modern Medical Mystery." *Newsweek* (November 12, 1990): 62, 64.

RESOURCES

ORGANIZATIONS

Chronic Fatigue and Immune Dysfunction Syndrome Association. P.O. Box 220398, Charlotte, NC 28222-0398.

Chronic Fatigue Immune Dysfunction Society. P.O. Box 230108, Portland, OR 97223.

National Chronic Fatigue Syndrome Association. 919 Scott Avenue, Kansas City, MO 66105.

BOOKS

Feiden, Karyn. *Hope and Help for Chronic Fatigue Syndrome: The Official Guide of the CFS/CFIDS Network.* New York: Prentice Hall, 1990.

Skoff J. A., and C. R. Pellegrino. *Chronic Fatigue Syndrome.* New York: Harper, 1988.

RELATED ARTICLES

"Chronic Fatigue—What Does It Mean?" *Harvard Medical School Health Letter* 14, no. 5 (March 1989): 1–3.

Goldenber, D. L., and others. "High Frequency of Fibromyalgia in Patients with Chronic Fatigue Seen in a Primary Care Practice." *Arthritis and Rheumatism* 33, no. 3 (March 1990): 381–387.

Koo, D. "Chronic Fatigue Syndrome: A Critical Appraisal of the Role of Epstein-Barr Virus." *Western Journal of Medicine* 150 (May 1989): 590–595.

Troiano, Linda R. "Tired All the Time? You Could Have CFS!" *Good Housekeeping* (January 1991): 165–166.

Zoler, M. L. "Taking the Syndrome Seriously: Chronic Fatigue." *Medical World News* (December 12, 1988): 33–41.

COLIC (INFANTILE)

OVERVIEW

Infants cry—it is their means of vocal expression. There is, however, a group of infants who are healthy but show irritability, crying and signs of discomfort to a greater extent than others. These infants have colic. As concisely described by Meadow and Smithells, colic is "a very common problem arising in early life and lasting, as a rule, not beyond the age of three months. An otherwise placid baby devotes one part of the day, most commonly between the 6 P.M. and the 10 P.M. feeds, to incessant crying. He may or may not stop when picked up, but certainly cries again if put down. Attention to feeds, warmth, wet nappies, etc., are unavailing."

Colic consists of recurrent paroxysms of apparent abdominal pain starting at about the second to the sixth week of life and usually ending by four months. These cycles last from three hours a day to 12 to 15 hours a day in severe cases. The child becomes hypertonic, sometimes alternating body posture from contracting into a little ball (thighs flexed up against the abdomen and arms drawn tightly inward), while beet red in coloration, to suddenly stretching out and stiffening almost spastically. Abdominal distention is common, as are flatus and borborygmus. Frequently, greenish mucoid stools are passed. The infant sucks with vigor, gulping formula and air; transient relief is achieved, then suddenly the infant is grasped by another episode of apparent gastrocolic cramping and pain, and begins to cry out again. The infant is commonly fretful and inconsolable, and makes piercing cries that wrench parents into despair. This is colic at its worst.

Some infants have spasmodic attacks that last only a few minutes; others appear to be in pain all day. The most common expression of colic, however, is evening fussiness after feeding. Infants with colic may have some gastroesophageal reflux but do not have vomiting, diarrhea, persistent abdominal distention or poor growth. The presence of these symptoms should prompt a search for a diagnosis other than colic.

Colic occurs in 20 to 30 percent of infants. Its cause remains unknown, but there are three popular hypotheses: exogenous antigens, abnormal gastrointestinal motility, and anxious mother-child interaction.

SOURCE:
Colon, A. R., and J. S. DiPalma. "Colic." *American Family Physician* 40, no. 6 (December, 1989): 122.

INFANT TEMPERAMENT AND BEHAVIOR

The fascination of colic for the researcher and thoughtful practitioner lies in its status as the earliest example of a behavior problem resulting from an incompatible interaction between characteristics of the infant and the environment. Thomas et al demonstrated more than 20 years ago how such a "poor fit" between normal variations in the child's temperament and parental management predisposed to behavior problems between ages 2 and 10 years even in the absence of preexisting abnormalities in either child or parent. According to current evidence, infants who cry excessively are normal but likely to more sensitive, more irritable, and less easily soothed than average. Parents often handle these infants inappropriately because of poor understanding or tolerance of the crying. Consequently, the amount of crying increases. Problems in the feedings, the infant's physical status, or the parents' emotional health may be present, but they need not be and usually are not.

We may not be able to change the infant's temperment but we can alter the outcome by influencing the parent-child interaction. What colicky babies usually need is more soothing and less stimulation. To accomplish this, parents are helped by a supportive relationship with a wise and sympathetic physician.

SOURCE:
Carey, William B. "Colic: Exasperating but Fascinating and Gratifying." *Pediatrics* 84, no. 3 (September, 1989): 568–569.

RELATIONSHIP TO MILK

No one knows what colic is, but a mother knows when her child has it. There are many proposed causes, but none have been proven. Commonly cited culprits are cow's milk and soy protein. In a breast-fed baby with colic, the mother's milk consumption has been cited as the cause.

Colic is just as likely in babies fed human milk as it is in those fed formula—about 20 percent. There is a higher incidence in babies given non-iron fortified formula. It's speculated this occurs because both parents and doctors often switch colicky babies to these formulas thinking the iron is part of the problem.

Studies looking for intestinal damage in infants with colic found none. If the signs and symptoms of colic were from malabsorption of milk proteins, some damage would occur. If a milk-fed infant develops signs of a true milk allergy, such as wheezing, rash, chronic runny nose, etc., then she may benefit from elimination of milk from her diet.

So where does this leave you, the mother of a colicky baby? Probably no better off than before, except now you know that milk or soy is most likely not the cause of the problem.

SOURCE:
Sagall, Richard J. "Milk Not to Blame." *Pediatrics for Parents* 9 (May, 1988): 6.

COPING

It's no joke. Nothing wears away at a parent's nerve like a baby's crying spells. Other harsh noises are merely annoying, but a baby's wailing is downright distressing, because it makes you feel so helpless, so frustrated, so inadequate as a parent.

That feeling is universal. All babies cry; it is natural, normal, even healthy—at least for baby. The toll it takes on your mental health is another matter. The guide that follows will help you understand why your baby cries, what you may be able to do about it, and how to hold on to what remains of your sanity when it seems as if the shrieking will never stop.

Colic is currently defined as a condition in which each day a baby has a crying period, normally around the same time, that cannot be attributed to any of the usual causes of discomfort. Although little is known about its cause, it afflicts about 20 percent of all babies in their first three months of life.

Although you can't cure your baby's colic, you can cope with it. Calming tactics that sometimes quiet colicky babies include:

- **Rhythmic motion.** Rock your child in a cradle or in your lap in a rocking chair; put her into a soft baby carrier that holds her close to your chest, and "wear" her around the house; take her for a ride in an elevator or in an auto (in her car seat).
- **Swaddling.** Wrap your baby snugly in a lightweight blanket. This will not only make him feel secure but will also inhibit the Moro reflex, his habit, when he is startled, of flinging his arms out and bringing them back. This involuntary movement can itself upset a colicky baby and make him cry.
- **Baby massage.** In this traditional Indian practice, "the baby is stroked in a continuous, flowing movement from head to foot, using light stroking and deeper massage," writes Sheila Kitzinger in *The Crying Baby* (Viking, 1989). For specifics turn to Vimala Schneider's *Infant Massage: A Handbook for Loving Parents* (Bantam, 1982).

SOURCE:
Arnott, Nancy. "How to Conquer Crying and Colic." *American Baby* (May, 1990): 71, 73, 75.

WHEN ALL ELSE FAILS. . .

There's no single, surefire way to calm a crying baby. There are, however, countless methods that parents have tried, all with some success. These include:

A lambskin—A cuddly cushion of wool can make a crib, car seat, or stroller cozier and help your baby fall asleep more easily.

Mirrors—Unbreakable reflective surfaces such as those that appear on many baby toys can often capture and hold a fussy infant's attention.

A baby carrier—This bears another mention, because it seems to succeed for two reasons. Even if the proximity to your body fails to quiet baby, the carrier frees your arms and lets you go anywhere without feeling that you're neglecting your fussy child.

SleepTight—The SleepTight Infant Soother consists of a vibration unit that mounts under the crib and a sound unit that attaches to the crib rail. Your pediatrician can tell you whether the SleepTight would be appropriate and useful in your baby's case (the device is not promoted directly to consumers).

Singing and/or dancing—A musical interlude can work wonders. Partner your baby by holding him up close or propped on your arm. Look into his eyes as you glide around the floor to the sound of your own vocal accompaniment or to recorded music.

Comfort sucking—Babies have strong sucking needs unrelated to their need for food; they simply find it comforting to hold something in their mouth. Offer the breast, a finger, or a pacifier.

Spring into action—Clutch baby securely against your chest, supporting her head. Stand on a mattress and slowly rock, shifting your weight from side to side.

White noise—Run the vacuum or blow dryer (set on cool) to provide a constant hum. If you can't take the din, try tapes of ocean waves or waterfalls.

Give it a spin—Strap baby into a car seat or infant seat, and secure it to the top of a washer or dryer. Start the machine, and stay by baby's side for the ride.

SOURCE:
Arnott, Nancy. "How to Conquer Crying and Colic." *American Baby* (May, 1990): 71, 73, 75.

RESOURCES

RELATED ARTICLES

Barr, Ronald G., Michael S. Kramer, and others. "Feeding and Temperament as Determinants of Early Infant Crying/Fussing Behavior." *Pediatrics* 84, no. 3 (September, 1989): 514-521.

Geertsma, M. Alex, and Jeffrey S. Hyams. "Colic—A Pain Syndrome of Infancy?" *Pediatric Clinics of North America* 36, no. 4 (August, 1989): 905-919.

Turkington, Carol. "24 Hours With a Colicky Baby." *American Baby* (November, 1990): 92-93, 95-97.

Verner, Gayle. "When Your Baby Won't Stop Crying." *Parents' Magazine* 65 (February, 1990): 82.

COLORECTAL CANCER

OVERVIEW

Cancers that develop in the cecum, colon, and rectum are known as colorectal cancers. Like other types of cancer, they can invade and destroy normal tissues and extend into surrounding structures. Also, cancer cells can break away from a primary tumor and metastasize, or spread, to other parts of the body through the lymphatic system or the bloodstream. When colorectal cancer cells spread, they most often travel to the liver. Cells that migrate to the liver or other organs can continue to divide abnormally and form secondary (metastatic) tumors. The cancer cells that form metastatic tumors in the liver, lungs, or elsewhere in the body have the same characteristics as the cells of the primary tumor. Although another organ is affected, the disease is still called colon cancer or rectal cancer. Methods used to treat the metastatic disease depend on the site and type of the primary (original) cancer and on the location and extent of the secondary tumors.

Most colorectal cancers are adenocarcinomas, which arise in the epithelial tissue, or lining, of the large bowel. . . .

The incidence of colorectal cancer in the United States is among the highest in the world. Cancers of the colon and rectum affect roughly 5 percent of Americans at some time in their lives. These cancers account for about 15 percent of all cancers diagnosed in this country. Only cancer of the lung and common skin cancers occur more frequently, and only lung cancer causes more deaths. It is estimated that 147,000 new cases of colorectal cancer (76,000 in women and 71,000 in men) were diagnosed in this country in 1988, with colon cancer affecting more than twice as many people as rectal cancer.

Colorectal cancer is rare in young people. Fewer than 6 percent of cases occur before the age of 50. Incidence increases markedly after age 50, continues to rise until age 75, and then tapers off. The average age at the time of diagnosis is 60.

SOURCE:

National Cancer Institute. *Cancer of the Colon and Rectum: Research Report*. NIH Pub. No. 88-95. March 1988. pp. 3-4.

POLYPS AND COLORECTAL CANCER

Sporadic (not inherited) intestinal polyps, or adenomas, are another risk factor. These polyps—chiefly those classified as adenomatous (or tubular), villous, and intermediate (or tubulovillous)—may become cancerous, particularly if they grow larger than an inch in diameter. These growths, which arise most often in the rectum and sigmoid colon, are different in their appearance, texture, microscopic characteristics, and potential for cancerous change. Adenomatous polyps are believed to occur in up to 15 percent of the adult population in the United States. Although these polyps usually do not cause symptoms, they can cause intermittent bleeding and, if they are large, can obstruct the passage of waste material. Invasive cancer develops in roughly 5 percent of adenomatous polyps. Villous polyps are less common, affecting fewer than 3 or 4 percent of the population. These growths bleed easily and may cause the passage of mucus with bowel movements. An estimated 40 percent become cancerous. Intermediate polyps are somewhat more common than the villous type; cancer develops in about 23 percent. The most common colorectal polyps, called hyperplastic polyps or hyperplastic mucosal tags, are harmless.

Scientists now believe that many—perhaps most—cancers of the large bowel arise from adenomatous, villous, and intermediate polyps. Removing these growths (polypectomy), often through a sigmoidoscope or colonoscope, is one way to prevent colorectal cancer. Also, because new polyps develop in nearly half of all patients who have had such growths removed, careful followup is necessary. An ongoing study is testing the possibility that vitamins C and E may reduce the recurrence rate of colorectal polyps. Thus far, however, research does not suggest that people should take vitamin supplements to try to prevent the growth of colorectal polyps.

SOURCE:
National Cancer Institute. *Cancer of the Colon and Rectum: Research Report.* NIH Pub. No. 88-95. March 1988. pp. 3-4.

DIETARY RISKS

With each new dietary study, eating seems to become less of a joyful experience and more of a risky business. The latest word follows that depressing pattern: Researchers announced that the chances of developing colon cancer appear to rise almost in direct proportion to the amount of red meat and animal fat that people consume. That left fearful Americans grappling with the question: Is it wise to eat any red meat at all?

Reporting in the *New England Journal of Medicine*, Harvard scientists found that women who had beef, lamb or pork as a daily main dish ran 2½ times the risk of developing colon cancer as did those who ate the meats less than once a month. One surprise: eating dairy products, which also tend to be high in animal fats, did not appear to increase the disease risk. The conclusions are drawn from a study of 88,751 nurses that was begun in 1980. The women filled out diet and medical questionnaires and were resurveyed at intervals over the next six years; 150 of the nurses developed colon cancer. The researchers believe their findings apply to men as well, though confirmation awaits the results of a parallel study.

SOURCE:
Toufexis, Anastasia. "Red Alert on Red Meat: The Link Between High-Fat Diets and Colon Cancer Gets Stronger." *Time* (December 24, 1990): 70.

SIGNS AND SYMPTOMS

The symptoms and signs associated with colorectal cancer are relatively nonspecific. Changes in the normal pattern of bowel habits should be viewed with suspicion, particularly in persons greater than 40 years old. The recent onset of persistent constipation, diarrhea, or tenesmus in an older patient should alert the physician to the possibility of an existing colonic neoplasm. The presence of cramping abdominal pain occurring with altered bowel habits may be indicative of tumor-related colonic obstruction. Colorectal cancer may also occur in the presence of, or mimic, acute diverticulitis.

Rectal bleeding, visible or occult, is commonly associated with colorectal cancer. The passage of bright red blood per rectum is most often seen with lesions of the rectosigmoid, but can be seen with cancer anywhere in the colon. Melenic stools may be observed in patients with right-sided lesions and occasionally with obstructing cancers. The presence of hypochromic, microcytic anemia in a male or postmenopausal female may be the only presenting signs of colorectal cancer and should prompt a thorough investigation.

SOURCE:
Fleishcher, David E., Stanley B. Goldberg, and others. "Detection and Surveillance of Colorectal Cancer." *JAMA* 261, no. 4 (January 27, 1989): 580-585. Copyright 1989, American Medical Association.

SIGMOIDOSCOPY

There are several different tests used to screen for colorectal cancer. When performed regularly, they can be life-saving. On the down side, certain of the tests can be uncomfortable and, for some people, embarrassing. The three primary screens for colorectal cancer are the digital rectal exam, the fecal occult blood test, and sigmoidoscopy.

You should have an annual digital rectal examination at age 40 and up, and annual testing of the stool for occult blood at age 50 and up. Also, a sigmoidoscopy—an examination of the lower colon using a thin, lighted tube inserted into the rectum—should be done at age 50 and again at 51; after that, if nothing is found, you should have one every three to five years.

Suspicious findings on any of these tests should lead your doctor to recommend a colonoscopy. Knowing what to expect from any of these procedures, and preparing for them properly, will make them more effective and, at the same time, lessen the inconvenience to you.

Flexible proctosigmoidoscopy is a quick procedure that requires no preparation, isn't particularly uncomfortable, and is by far the best method for detecting early colorectal cancers, finding about half of all tumors. Yet surveys have found that as few as 13% of people over 50 undergo the procedure. Some of this reticence is because these exams were formerly done—and are still done by some physicians—with what is known as a rigid sigmoidoscope. While safe and effective for viewing a small length of the colon, rigid sigmoidoscopic exams are indeed uncomfortable. The newer, flexible scopes are much more comfortable and, at three times the length of the rigid model, bring to view much more of the colon.

SOURCE:
"Colorectal Cancer: Early Detection is a Cure." *The Johns Hopkins Medical Letter* (March 1991): 5.

OCCULT BLOOD TEST

Some patients benefit from having their colorectal cancers and adenomas detected by fecal occult blood testing prior to the appearance of symptoms. However, evidence that periodic occult blood testing is able to reduce overall mortality is not yet available from well-designed, controlled trials. While informed opinion and results from uncontrolled studies suggest a potential benefit from occult blood screening, the high proportion of false-positive test results with unavoidable attendant risks, together with problems of patient compliance, mandate caution in the development of any recommendations.

Although testing the stool for occult blood is an imperfect way to detect colorectal cancers and adenomas, no other more cost-effective, acceptable alternative has been identified and generally accepted based on rules of scientific evidence. There is insufficient evidence to suggest that practitioners who currently are recommending occult blood screening for patients older than 45 or 50 years change that practice. On the other hand, there is insufficient evidence to suggest adoption of occult blood screening in those settings where it is not currently being employed. There is a stronger a priori argument for screening subjects with a family history of colorectal cancer in a first-order relative.

SOURCE:
U.S. Preventive Services Task Force. "Occult Blood Screening for Colorectal Cancer." *JAMA* 261, no. 4 (January 27, 1989): 592. Copyright 1989, American Medical Association.

STAGING

Once cancer has been diagnosed, other tests help determine the extent of the disease (staging), so that appropriate treatment can be planned.

Several staging systems have been used for colorectal cancer. The Dukes system, developed over 40 years ago and later modified, is widely used by both clinicians and researchers. It divides colorectal cancers into several stages.

- Stage A refers to carcinoma in situ, a small cancer in the mucosa that has not spread; the cancer cells have not reached the submucosa, where lymph and blood vessels are located;
- Stage B1 tumors extend through the submucosa into the muscularis externa;
- Stage B2 describes tumors that penetrate through the bowel wall;
- Stage C means that regional lymph nodes are involved; and
- Stage D indicates that the disease has spread to other organs.

SOURCE:
National Cancer Institute. *Cancer of the Colon and Rectum: Research Report.* NIH Pub. No. 88-95. March 1988. pp. 14-15.

TREATMENT

There are three main ways to treat cancer of the colon and rectum: surgery, radiation therapy, and chemotherapy. Another method, called immunotherapy, is now being studied in clinical trials. The doctor may use just one method or combine them. The decision is based on the patient's individual needs. In some cases, the patient may be referred to specialists in the different kinds of cancer treatment.

The standard treatment for most colon and rectal cancers is surgery. The kind of operation will depend mostly on the location and size of the tumor. Some of the operations are described below.

The surgeon may be able to remove only the part of the bowel that contains the cancer and then join the healthy sections together. This operation is called a bowel resection. Often, it is all that is needed.

During surgery, the lymph nodes near the tumor are also removed. One of the ways that cancer spreads through the body is by way of the lymph system. The surgeon removes the lymph nodes to check if cancer cells are present in them. This information is important in planning future treatment.

If the cancer is blocking the bowel, a procedure called a colostomy may be needed. For this surgery, the cancerous bowel is removed and the surgeon creates an opening in the abdomen (called a stoma) for the body's wastes to be removed, bypassing the lower colon and rectum. A colostomy may be temporary or permanent.

- A temporary colostomy is done to let the lower colon and rectum heal. When the area has healed, a second operation is done to close the stoma. Normal bowel functions are regained.
- A permanent colostomy is needed when the entire lower rectum is removed. Only about 15 percent of patients with colorectal cancer need a permanent colostomy.

After surgery for a colostomy, a special bag called an appliance is attached to the stoma to collect waste matter. The appliance does not show under most clothing. While in the hospital, the patient may see an enterostomal therapist, a trained health care worker who teaches patients with a colostomy how to care for the stoma and appliance.

In radiation therapy (also called x-ray therapy, radiotherapy, cobalt treatment, or irradiation), high-energy rays are used to stop the cancer cells from growing and multiplying. Radiation therapy is sometimes used before surgery to shrink the tumor. More often, it is used after surgery to destroy any cancer cells that may remain, or to relieve pain. Radiation therapy is given in hospitals, clinics, or private offices. Most patients can have radiation therapy as outpatients.

The use of drugs to treat cancer is called chemotherapy. Adjuvant therapy is the use of drugs following primary treatment if there is reason to suspect that cancer cells remain in the body after surgery or radiation therapy.

Anticancer drugs may also be used when there are signs that the cancer has spread.

The various kinds of drugs used to treat cancer are given to patients in different ways: by mouth, or by injection into a muscle, an artery, or a vein. The drugs travel through the bloodstream to almost every area of the body.

Depending on which drugs are used, the patient may need to stay in the hospital for a few days so that the effects of the drugs can be watched. From then on, the patient may be given chemotherapy as an outpatient, or at home. Chemotherapy is most often given in cycles—a treatment period, followed by a rest period, then another treatment, and so on.

Because cancer can spread, the treatments used against this disease must be powerful. It is rarely possible to limit the effects of radiation or chemotherapy so that only cancer cells are destroyed. Some healthy cells may be damaged at the same time. For this reason, patients may have unpleasant side effects. Patients having radiation therapy may have skin reactions (redness or dryness) in the area being treated, and they may be unusually tired. In addition, patients may have diarrhea, nausea, or vomiting. Radiation to any part of the pelvic area may also cause side effects in the reproductive organs (such as infertility or impotence).

The side effects of chemotherapy depend on the drugs that are given and the response of the patient. Chemotherapy commonly affects hair cells, blood-forming cells, and the cells lining the digestive tract. As a result, patients may have side effects such as hair loss, lowered blood counts, nausea, or vomiting. Most side effects end after the treatment is over.

SOURCE:
National Cancer Institute. *What You Need To Know about Cancer of the Colon and Rectum.* NIH Pub. No. 90-1552. November 1990. pp. 7-10.

CHEMOTHERAPY

An advisory panel of the U.S. National Institutes of Health has recommended a chemotherapy for stage III colon cancer patients who undergo surgery that involves a combination of 5-fluorouracil (5-FU) and levamisole.

The therapy had been tested by the U.S. National Cancer Institute in a clinical trial of 1,300 patients that ended [in 1989]. The committee said that 5-FU and levamisole appeared to reduce cancer recurrence by 41 percent and reduce mortality by 33 percent. "Overall survival percentages at 3½ years were estimated to be 71 percent vs. 55 percent for the control group," the report says, while side effects "were well tolerated."

"Many, many answers still need to come in before we are even close to winning the battle once someone is diagnosed with colon or rectal cancer," cautions Dr. Glenn Steel Jr., of Harvard University, who chaired the panel. He says it is not understood how levamisole reduces cancer recurrence.

The panel recommends surgery alone for stage I patients, citing an 80 to 90 percent five-year survival rate. It urges chemotherapy and radiation for stages II and III, while calling for additional drug trials to assess treatment combinations.

SOURCE:
Cooper, Mike. "Drug Combination Endorsed for Colon Cancer Patients." *NCI Cancer Weekly* (May 7, 1990): 5-6.

GENETIC ORIGINS

Five months after they identified a gene that they thought might set off colon cancer, researchers now say another gene is almost certainly the true initiator of the disease. The newly discovered gene sits right next door on the chromosome to the other gene, and it has all the telltale defects that the previous candidate had lacked.

"This is the gold standard we were waiting for," said Dr. Raymond L. White of the University of Utah, who helped find both colon cancer genes.

The newly detected gene should fulfill the promise raised by the first contender, that of allowing doctors to detect a colon tumor at the earliest possible stage, when it is easily excised through surgery.

The gene will also permit doctors to identify those with an inborn predisposition to colon cancer, a propensity thought to account for at least 20 percent of all colon cancer cases and possibly many more. People found to carry the defective gene could then be screened with heightened diligence.

"This is a major milestone in colorectal cancer research that will echo around the world," said Dr. Henry T. Lynch, a colon cancer specialist at Creighton University School of Medicine in Omaha. "I haven't done too well in treating patients with advanced colon cancer, and neither have any of my colleagues. The most important thing is to detect the cancer early, when it's at a curable stage, and that's what this work is all about."

SOURCE:
Angier, Natalie. "Doctors Link Gene to Colon Cancer." *The New York Times* (August 9, 1991): A8.

RESOURCES

ORGANIZATIONS

American Cancer Society. 1599 Clifton Road NE, Atlanta, GA 30329. Or local affiliate.

National Cancer Institute. Office of Cancer Communications, Building 31, 9000 Rockville Pike, Bethesda MD 20892.

United Ostomy Association. 36 Executive Park, Suite 120, Irvine, CA 92714.

RELATED ARTICLES

Day, Donald. "Battling Colon Cancer: Fiber, Calcium, Check-ups and New Drugs Join the Cause." *American Health* (March 1990): 17–18.

Farley, Patrick C., and Kenneth H. McFaden. "Colorectal Cancer: Are Adjuvant Therapies Beneficial?" *Postgraduate Medicine* 84, no. 6 (November 1, 1988): 175–183.

Guiteras, G. Patrick. "Colorectal Cancer Screening." *Executive Health Report* (February 1991): 2–3.

Guthrie, James F., and others. "On the Alert for Colorectal Cancer." *Patient Care* (April 30, 1989): 19–27.

Kolata, Gina. "Animal Fat Is Tied to Colon Cancer: Largest Study of Diet in U.S. Backs Long-Held Theory." *The New York Times* (December 13, 1990): A1, A16.

Steele, Glenn, Jr., T. S. Ravikumar, and Peter N. Benotti. "New Surgical Treatments for Recurrent Colorectal Cancer." *Cancer* 65, no. 3, suppl. (February 1, 1990): 723–730.

U.S. Preventive Services Task Force. "Screening for Colorectal Cancer." *American Family Physician* 40, no. 5 (November 1989): 119-125.

Wexner, Stephen. "The Early Detection of Colon Cancer." *Priorities* (Spring 1991): 25–26.

COMMON COLD

OVERVIEW

Everyone has had a cold. Sometime or other you have had a runny nose with sneezing, watery eyes, headache, sore throat and fever. Occasionally, you may experience hoarseness and coughing. The cold usually begins with a watery discharge from the nose that soon thickens and has a yellow to green color. Medical science, for all its achievements, does not yet have a cure for the common cold.

The common cold is a minor illness caused by one of as many as 200 different kinds of viruses. These viruses can also cause laryngitis or bronchitis by infecting either the larynx ("voice box") or the bronchial tubes in the lungs. Infections are spread from one person to another by hand-to-hand contact or by a cough or a sneeze that sprays many virus particles into the air. Good hygiene and common sense can limit the spread of the cold. Cover your nose and mouth when you cough or sneeze. Use disposable tissues (not handkerchiefs) and wash your hands often.

If you stay at home you may protect others from the spread of your infection. The best advice for treatment of a common cold is directed towards control of the symptoms and comfort of the patient. A typical common cold will last three to four days. A mild secondary bacterial infection often prolongs this to a week or longer. One should rest in a room with adequate moisture and a comfortable temperature. The body can best heal itself if it is neither too hot nor too cold. A vaporizer or humidifier can be used to increase moisture (the nose functions best with the humidity at 70%). If your cold lasts more than seven days or if you develop a fever higher than 102 degrees Fahrenheit, an ear infection, laryngitis or bronchitis, you should see your doctor.

You may get temporary relief with aspirin, acetaminophen, or various over-the-counter cold, cough, "sinus" tablets, syrups or nasal sprays. (Most nasal sprays should not be used for more than seven days since prolonged use can lead to dependency.) Use these carefully and read directions. Children should not be given aspirin because of its relation to Reye Syndrome. Drink lots of water and other non-alcoholic liquids. A person in good health who becomes the victim of a cold does not usually need to see a doctor. These viruses do not respond to antibiotics. Severe infections may require medical care and prescription medication. If you have asthma, or frequent onset of either bronchitis or ear infections, you should see your doctor at the first sign of a head cold. If you have a very high temperature and pains all over your body you may have influenza.

SOURCE:

California Medical Association. "The Common Cold." *HealthTips* index 72 (October 1989): 1–2.

TRANSMISSION

The set of symptoms we call a cold may be caused by one of more than a hundred different types of rhinovirus. The large number of different strains makes the chances of a vaccine being developed slight. Rhinovirus grows well at relatively low temperatures, such as those found in the nose. This is why it's rarely found in the trachea or lungs.

There are many misconceptions about how people get a cold. Kissing, sneezing, or coughing, even directly into someone's face, will not transmit a cold. A handshake is the most effective way to give someone your cold. It's easy for a child with a cold to pick the virus up on his hands. All he has to do is touch his nose or eyes and he has the virus on his hands. Anyone who touches his hands can pick up the virus. If the recipient touches his eyes or nose, the virus can set up shop and cause a cold. Rhinovirus can survive for about three hours on a doorknob or formica surface.

One way to prevent hand-to-hand transmission is with a virucidal (kills viruses) agent, such as iodine. Unfortunately, this is somewhat impractical and can stain hands. There is now a tissue impregnated with an antiviral agent. It helps, but doesn't eliminate all of the virus.

So when your child gets a cold, keep his hands clean and well washed. And every one in the family should do the same. But don't feel defeated if, despite your best efforts, someone else in the family gets a cold.

SOURCE:
"The Cold Facts." *Pediatrics for Parents* 10, no. 1 (September 1989): 7.

COMMON COLD—AND VITAMIN C

Is this the C season? "Most colds can be prevented or largely ameliorated by control of the diet. . . . The dietary substance that is involved is vitamin C. . . . At the first sign that a cold is developing . . . begin the treatment by swallowing one or two 500-mg tablets." So wrote Nobelist Linus Pauling back in 1970. And since publication of his book *Vitamin C and the Common Cold,* that nutrient has become the single most popular supplement on the market. A third of the U.S. population takes it.

Yet despite the current fashion to heed Dr. Pauling's advice, scientists have never proved the efficacy of his treatment plan, which amounts to taking eight to 17 times the Recommended Dietary Allowance of 60 milligrams all at once. And while the combined results of eight studies show that people who took vitamin C had only about one tenth of a cold less each year than those who did not, the difference is "far from statistically significant" according to the *American Journal of Medicine.* What's more, the association between vitamin C and lessened severity of cold symptoms appears to be due largely to the power of suggestion. That is, even people who thought they were taking vitamin C but were actually given a placebo said they felt better.

Sniffles aside, there are other reasons not to self-prescribe vitamin C supplements. One is that large doses can cause diarrhea. In addition, anyone who regularly takes megadoses of vitamin C and then stops abruptly may end up with a condition called rebound scurvy, in which the body grows so accustomed to overdoses of C that when it goes back to receiving what is normally an adequate amount it reacts by producing scurvy-like symptoms such as bleeding gums, inability to heal wounds, and rough, dry skin. To be sure, incidences of rebound scurvy are uncommon, but they do occur, both in adults and in infants born to mothers who take high-dose vitamin C supplements during pregnancy.

In the latest investigation of the effects of too much vitamin C, researchers at the U.S. Department of Agriculture's Western Human Nutrition Research Center in San Francisco administered two diets to a small group of men, one containing the RDA of 60 milligrams and the other, 10 times the RDA (which, by the way, you can get in a single pill bought virtually anywhere). The result: The men were more likely to have sensitive gums after going off the high-vitamin C diet. For that reason, the scientists suggest that people who are used to taking large doses of vitamin C should wean themselves gradually. Cutting back to a pill every other day, for instance, would be prudent.

Ironically, it has been found that people who take vitamin C supplements are often the very ones who are already getting adequate amounts in their food. That's understandable, since it's one of the easiest nutrients to get plenty of in the diet. Just one small orange, one red pepper, one half cup of Brussels sprouts or broccoli, or one grapefruit provides 100 percent of the RDA.

SOURCE:
"Is This the C Season?" *Tufts University Diet and Nutrition Letter* 6, no. 1 (December 1988): 1.

COLD MEDICATIONS

Most cold sufferers experience nasal congestion, caused by swelling of the mucous membranes in the nose. Decongestants can ease that problem. They constrict dilated blood vessels, shrinking the swollen tissue and opening nasal passages. The result is freer breathing, better drainage, and a reduced feeling of stuffiness.

There are two kinds of decongestants: topical (sprays and drops) and oral (tablets and caplets). Each has advantages and drawbacks.

Topical decongestants are more effective than oral ones. A recent study, for example, showed that the topical ingredient oxymetazoline produced four times as much decongestion as oral use of pseudoephedrine, the ingredient in Sudafed and several other oral products. The topical remedy also worked faster, producing improvement within five minutes versus 30 to 60 minutes for the oral decongestant.

Most standard topical decongestants—Dristan, Sinex, Neo-Synephrine II—use phenylephrine hydrochloride as their active ingredient. Newer, longer-acting products, such as Afrin, Duration, and Neo-Synephrine II, contain oxymetazoline or xylometazoline.

The drawback of topical decongestants is that overuse can lead to "rebound congestion," stuffiness worse than the original problem. Each application produces an initial decongestant effect and then some irritation and inflammation, which tends to go unnoticed. But if the drug is used frequently, the delayed effects begin to predominate. The more you use the product, the more irritated, inflamed, and blocked up your nasal passages become. Eventually, treatment may require the use of oral or topical steroid drugs to break the cycle. Accordingly, topical decongestants should be used sparingly, and only for a few days.

Probably the best time to use a topical decongestant is before bed, to help insure a good night's sleep. Another good time is first thing in the morning, when nasal passages tend to be stuffiest.

In contrast to topical decongestants, oral ones can be taken daily for up to a week. They can be used alone or along with a topical product, serving as maintenance therapy to reduce the need for the topical decongestant.

Oral decongestants don't produce rebound congestion, but they can cause other side effects, such as mouth dryness or interference with sleep (if taken shortly before bedtime). Potentially more serious are blood-pressure elevations that can occur with their use.

The oral decongestant most likely to raise blood pressure is phenylpropanolamine (PPA). It's widely used in shotgun cold remedies (Alka-Seltzer Plus, Contac, Dimetapp, and Dristan Capsules among others). In addition, it's the active ingredient in all diet pills, such as Appedrine, Dexatrim, and Dietac. . . .

About 25 percent of people with colds get headaches, 10 percent have muscle pain, and 1 percent run mild fevers. All these symptoms respond well to the three standard nonprescription pain relievers: aspirin, acetaminophen, or ibuprofen.

Aspirin and acetaminophen can be found in many shotgun cold remedies. But it's cheaper to buy the straight pain reliever—if you don't already have some on hand. . . .

One caution about pain relievers: Children with cold symptoms shouldn't take aspirin. Studies have shown a strong link between aspirin and Reye's syndrome, a rare but potentially fatal illness that strikes children and teenagers. The studies found that victims of Reye's syndrome often had been given aspirin for flu-like symptoms or chicken pox. Colds are different from flu, but distinguishing a bad cold from mild flu isn't easy. To be on the safe side, give children acetaminophen for the aches or pains of a cold. . . .

A sore throat is often the first symptom of a cold. It affects about half of all cold sufferers, who can choose from a legion of lozenges, sprays, and mouthwashes to soothe the pain.

The FDA considers seven ingredients effective in relieving or dulling sore-throat irritation: benzocaine, benzyl alcohol, dyclonine hydrochloride, hexylresorcinol, menthol, phenol compounds, and salicyl alcohol. Brands with sufficient amounts of these ingredients include Chloraseptic Sore Throat lozenges and spray, Oracin, Spec-T Sore Throat Anesthetic Lozenges, and Sucrets.

SOURCE:
"Cold Remedies: Which Ones Work Best?" *Consumer Reports* 54 (January 1989): 9, 10.

WHEN YOU HAVE MORE THAN A COLD

Seek medical help when any of the following occur:

- A high fever greater than 101°F (38.3°C) accompanied by shaking chills and coughing up thick phlegm (especially if greenish or foul-smelling).
- Sharp chest pain when you take a deep breath.
- Cold-like symptoms which do not improve after seven days.
- Coughing up of blood.
- Any significant throat pain in a child.
- A painful throat in addition to any of the following:

  1) Pus (yellowish-white spots) on the tonsils or the throat.

  2) Fever greater than 101°F or 38.3°C.

  3) Swollen or tender glands or bumps in the front of the neck.

  4) Exposure to someone who has a documented case of "strep" throat.

  5) A rash during or after a sore throat.

  6) A history of rheumatic fever, rheumatic heart disease, kidney disease, or chronic lung disease such as emphysema or chronic bronchitis.

SOURCE:
"Colds: How to Treat Them." *Health Letter* 6, no. 12 (December 1990): 5.

ANTIVIRAL THERAPY—INTERFERON

There is good news and bad news. The good news is that nose drops and nasal sprays containing interferons show promise. Interferons, natural substances produced by infected human cells, cause antiviral proteins to form in noninfected cells. These proteins inhibit the growth of many different viruses. Advanced genetic engineering has lowered the cost of producing purified interferon. At high doses given over the length of a cold season, these interferon-containing products are proven to prevent rhinovirus infection.

The bad news is two-fold. First, a list of side effects—from nasal stuffiness and blood-tinged nasal mucus to ulcerations on the lining of the nose—are reported by about 25% or users within a few weeks of beginning use. Generally, these side effects relate to dose. The higher, more effective doses cause the greatest problem; the best-tolerated low doses do the least amount of good. In addition, the long-term usefulness and safety of this general method remain unclear.

The risk of catching a cold is especially high immediately after another family member becomes ill. So an alternative approach that has been tested is a shorter, one-week course of nasal interferon for exposed family members. Testing proved this reduces the likelihood of developing a cold, and also has a lower rate of side effects. Unfortunately, the benefit of this treatment appears limited to rhinovirus colds and does not seem to stop other virus-caused colds.

Second on the bad news list is that interferon sprays and drops are not yet FDA-approved for this use. Although they are available to treat other, more severe illness, doctors cannot prescribe them as yet to prevent rhinovirus colds.

Other antiviral agents are being investigated, however, so new products are on the horizon.

SOURCE:
"Interferons: Future Hope." *Executive Health Report* 27, no. 1 (October 1990): 5.

RESOURCES

PAMPHLET
National Institute of Allergy and Infectious Diseases: *The Common Cold.* NIH Pub. No. 85-107. October 1985.

RELATED ARTICLES
Cohn, J. P. "Here Come the Bugs." *FDA Consumer* 22 (November 1988): 6-10.

Curley, F. J., Irwin, R. S., and others. "Cough and the Common Cold." *American Review of Respiratory Diseases* 138 (1988): 305-311.

Glezen, W. P., and others. "Closing in on the Common Cold?" *Patient Care* 24, no. 1 (January 15, 1990): 189-197, 200.

"Making Headway Against the Common Cold." *Consumer Reports Health Letter* 2, no. 12 (December 1990): 89-91.

O'Brien, M. B. "Washing Away Colds." *Pediatrics for Parents* (September 1988): 6.

"Panel Says Antihistamines Useless for Colds." *Medical World News* 29 (February 8, 1988): 37.

Trebo, R. "The Cold War Heats Up: Scientists Block First Step in Viral Invasion." *American Health* 8 (November 1989): 12.

CONSTIPATION

(*See also:* DIARRHEA; IRRITABLE BOWEL SYNDROME)

OVERVIEW

As many as 13 percent of adult Americans describe themselves as affected by constipation, including a quarter of those aged 60 and older. And while not a major health threat, constipation can result in discomfort and what Dr. Steven Castle, a physician at the Veterans Administration Medical Center in West Los Angeles who has written on constipation, calls a diminished "sense of well-being."

A wide variety of diseases can cause constipation, including diabetes, Parkinson's and thyroid dysfunction. Many common drugs can also cause constipation, including high blood pressure or heart disease medications, antacids, and antidepressants. Because this list of drugs is so large, one of the first treatment steps Dr. Castle recommends for anyone suffering from constipation is to review with a physician the necessity of any drug you may be taking (including non-prescription drugs) and to discontinue those which are not necessary and to consider non-constipating alternatives for those which are.

More often than not, however, a problem with constipation can't be traced to a specific cause. Rather, the cause is apt to be what Dr. Castle describes as an interplay between various long-term habits and a possible physiological predisposition. For treating constipation of this sort, Dr. Castle recommends a multi-step approach.

A Five-Step Approach

1) Avoid laxatives. Laxatives, notes Dr. Castle, tend to be advertised as "safe and gentle." Perhaps in response to such advertising, sales of laxatives in the U.S. increase every year and now exceed half a billion dollars annually. Moreover, some experts estimate that up to 15 percent of Americans misuse or abuse laxatives. Most should not be used for more than 1 or 2 weeks, yet there are numerous reports of people who use laxatives regularly despite having daily or more frequent bowel movements.

The problem with this is that many laxatives—particularly those known as "stimulant" or "irritant" laxatives—are far from innocuous. These laxatives work by stimulating muscle contractions in the colon. Over time, however, they can produce nerve damage, loss of muscle tone, and, paradoxically, constipation. There are no good numbers on the subject, but Castle and other experts believe long-term use of stimulant or irritant laxatives is a major cause of constipation.

2) Improve bowel habits. Wastes in the colon are moved forward as a result of coordinated muscle contractions which tend to occur naturally after meals and in the morning. For most people these contractions generate an urge to have a bowel movement. However, some people may ignore or suppress these urges. This may be due to time constraints, social discomfort, or lack of facilities. But whatever the reason, the result can be a reduced ability to recognize the urge to defecate and a corresponding failure to take advantage of periods when it is most naturally conducive to do so.

To address this, Dr. Castle recommends setting aside time in the mornings and perhaps after meals in a "relaxed environment" for the purpose of having a bowel movement. Doing so routinely can help reestablish the link between periods when bowel movements are most likely to occur naturally, awareness of the urge to defecate, and an appropriate response.

3) Fluid and fiber. In Australia constipation is considered a "summer disease" because it occurs most commonly when the weather is hot and people are dehydrated. Feces are composed primarily of water and an adequate water intake will help ensure softer, easier to pass stools. Dr. Castle recommends at least 8 to 10 glasses of fluid per day but cautions that this total should not include caffeine- or alcohol-containing beverages, which cause the loss of more water than they provide.

Fiber, particularly in the form of wheat bran, is widely considered something of a cure-all for constipation. Yet there is surprisingly little good scientific evidence for support this belief. Indeed, many studies show that people who are constipated eat as much, if not more, fiber than those who are not constipated. And one recent analysis of 20 different studies examining the effects of bran concluded that there was "no justification" for the claim that bran could return constipated people to a pattern of normal bowel movements.

Nonetheless, fiber may be of help to some people. For this reason physicians generally recommend that people who are constipated increase their fiber consumption to see if this has a beneficial effect. The best sources of fiber for this purpose are bran and whole-grain breads and cereals. However, psyllium-based laxatives such as Metamucil may also be of help. These laxatives work by increasing stool bulk and softness and can be used for extended periods without the drawbacks of other laxatives.

4) Exercise. People who are constipated tend to be less physically active than those who are not. Because exercise helps stimulate muscle contractions in the colon, experts recommend that people affected by constipation try to increase the amount of exercise they receive. A morning walk, says Dr. Castle, is ideal for this purpose.

5) A one-month trial. For otherwise healthy people, the steps recommended here should in most cases produce an improvement within days to weeks. If during this period there is a need for more immediate relief, Dr. Castle recommends glycerin suppositories rather than stimulant or irritant laxatives.

If there has been no improvement after a month, it is probably wise to see a doctor.

SOURCE:

Shepherd, Steven. "Constipation: Laxatives Are Rarely the Answer." *Executive Health Report* (October 1990): 2-3.

CAUSES

First of all, it should be understood that constipation is a symptom, not a disease. Like a fever, it can be caused by many different conditions. Most people have experienced an occasional brief bout of constipation that has corrected itself with diet and time. The following is a list of some of the most common causes.

- **Imaginary Constipation.** This is very common and results from misconceptions about what is normal and what is not. If recognized early enough, this type of constipation can be "cured" by informing the sufferer that the frequency of his or her bowel movements is normal.
- **Irritable Bowel Syndrome (IBS).** Also known as "spastic colon," IBS is one of the most common causes of constipation in the United States. Some people develop spasms of the colon which delay the speed with which the contents of the intestine move through the digestive tract and lead to constipation.
- **Bad Bowel Habits.** A person can initiate a cycle of constipation by ignoring the urge to defecate. Some people do this to avoid using public toilets, others because they are "too busy." After a period of time a person may stop feeling the urge. This leads to progressive constipation.
- **Laxative Abuse.** People who habitually take laxatives become dependent upon them. They may require increasing dosages until, finally, the intestine becomes insensitive and fails to work properly.
- **Travel.** People often experience constipation when traveling long distances. Why this is so is not known but may relate to changes in life style, schedule, diet, and drinking water.
- **Hormonal (Gland) Disturbances.** Certain hormonal disturbances such as an underactive thyroid gland, can produce constipation.
- **Pregnancy.** It is well known that pregnancy can cause constipation. The basis may be partly mechanical, in that the pressure of the heavy womb compresses the intestine, and may be partly hormonal due to changes in the glands of the body during pregnancy.
- **Fissures and Hemorrhoids.** Painful conditions of the anus can produce a spasm of the anal sphincter, which aggravates constipation.
- **Other Diseases.** A large number of diseases that affect the body tissues (such as scleroderma or lupus) and certain neurological or muscular diseases (such as multiple sclerosis, Parkinson's disease, and stroke) can be responsible for constipation.
- **Loss of Body Salts.** The loss of body salts through the kidneys or through vomiting or diarrhea is another cause of constipation.
- **Mechanical Compression.** Scarring, inflammation around diverticula, tumors, and cancer can produce mechanical compression of the intestines and result in constipation.
- **Nerve Damage.** Injuries to the spinal cord and tumors pressing on the spinal cord may produce constipation by affecting the nerves that lead to the intestine.
- **Medications.** A large number of medications can cause constipation. These include pain medications (especially narcotics), antacids that contain aluminum, antispasmodic drugs, antidepressant drugs, tranquilizers, iron supplements, and anticonvulsants (for epilepsy).
- **Poor Diet.** A factor in the development of constipation may be the shift away from high-fiber foods (vegetables, fruits, whole grains) to foods that are high in animal fats (meats, dairy products, eggs) and refined sugar (rich desserts and other sweets) but low in fiber. Some studies have suggested that high-fiber

diets result in larger stools, more frequent bowel movements, and therefore less constipation.

SOURCE:
Schuster, Marvin. National Digestive Diseases Information Clearinghouse. *What is Constipation?* NIH Pub. No. 86-2754. February 1986.

REMEDIES

What Treatment Is Available for Constipation?

Prevention is the best treatment. The first step is to understand that normal frequency varies widely, from three movements a day to three a week. It is important to know what is normal for you so that you can avoid developing a laxative habit by treating constipation that does not really exist. If a laxative habit does exist, substitute milder laxatives for stronger ones, and, then, gradually withdraw the milder ones.

If an underlying disorder is causing constipation, treatment should be directed toward the specific cause. For example, if an underactive thyroid is causing constipation, thyroid extract may help.

Instead of relying upon laxatives and enemas, eat a well-balanced diet that includes unprocessed bran, whole wheat bread, and prunes and prune juice. Bowel habits are also important; set aside sufficient time after breakfast or dinner, or after morning coffee, to allow for undisturbed visits to the toilet. And never ignore the urge to defecate.

To stimulate intestinal activity, drink plenty of fluids and exercise regularly. Special exercises may be necessary to tone up abdominal muscles after pregnancy or whenever abdominal muscles are lax.

If it becomes necessary to take laxatives or suppositories, they should not be used for longer than 2 or 3 weeks without the advice of a doctor. Different laxatives act on different portions of the intestine. For example, some stimulate the small intestine, whereas others stimulate the colon. Different types of constipation require different medications, depending upon the underlying cause. Remember, your doctor is best qualified to determine when a laxative is needed and which type is best.

Above all, it is necessary to recognize that a successful treatment program requires persistent effort and time. Constipation does not come on overnight and it is not reasonable to expect that it can be relieved overnight.

SOURCE:
Schuster, Marvin. National Digestive Diseases Information Clearinghouse. *What Is Constipation?* NIH Pub. No. 86-2754. February 1986.

BENEFITS OF DIETARY FIBER

Constipation is primarily a colonic problem. In the colon fibre increases stool bulk, holds water, and also acts as a substrate for colonic microflora, further increasing stool bulk by increasing bacterial, water, and slat content and producing hydrogen, methane, and other gases that augment the bulking effect. It decreases transit time, reduces intracolonic pressure, and produces a softer stool. All these effects are beneficial in relieving constipation, but the evidence comes mainly from studies on normal colons. An additional 20g/day of bran increases faecal weight by 127% and decreases mean transit time by 41%. The same quantity of cabbage, carrot, or apple fibre produces a smaller but similar effect. Large particles of bran give significantly greater increases in stool weight and water content with significantly shorter transit times than finely ground bran. Raw bran is more effective than processed bran. Transit time is reduced by fibre most noticeably in those with slow intestinal transit and may increase in those with naturally rapid transit. Meta-analysis suggests that the same effects of bran in healthy controls are also found in patients with the irritable bowel syndrome, diverticular disease, and chronic constipation. Constipated patients, however, have lower stool weights and slower transit than normal subjects whether they take bran or not.

High fibre diets can help relieve constipation naturally in almost all patients, including those with the irritable bowel syndrome. The benefits may be limited by poor tolerance and by dietary inflexibility, particularly in elderly people for whom supplements may be better than changing eating habits. Fibre intake should probably be mixed and increased gradually over weeks or even months. Wheat bran is most effective in relieving constipation, though it is less palatable and often poorly tolerated by those used to a refined diet.

SOURCE:
Taylor, Rodney. "Management of Constipation." *British Medical Journal* 300 (April 21, 1990): 1063-1064.

RESOURCES

ORGANIZATION
National Digestive Diseases Information Clearinghouse. Box NDDIC, Bethesda, MD 20892.

PAMPHLET
Proctor and Gamble. *Constipation: What You Can Do About It.* April, 1986.

RELATED ARTICLES

Cerrato, Paul L. "Is America Really Constipated?" *RN* (May, 1989): 81-82, 84, 86, 88.

Cummings, Mike. "Overuse Hazardous: Laxatives Rarely Needed." *FDA Consumer* (April, 1991): 33-35.

Donatelle, Edward. "Constipation: Pathophysiology and Treatment." *American Family Physician* 42, no. 5 (November, 1990): 1335.

Shepherd, Steven. "Constipation: Laxatives Are Rarely the Answer." *Executive Health Report* (October, 1990): 22-23.

Tremaine, William J. "Chronic Constipation: Causes and Management." *Hospital Practice* (April 30, 1990): 89-90, 92, 95-96, 99-100.

CONTRACEPTION

OVERVIEW

In the U.S. today, the most popular forms of birth control are those that are most removed from the sex act. In more than 50 percent of marriages where contraception is practiced, one of the partners has been sterilized, in about two-thirds of the cases the woman. Of all women of childbearing age (fifteen to forty-four), married and single, 24 percent rely on sterilization for birth control. The next most common method is the pill (19 percent), followed by the condom (9 percent), the diaphragm (4 percent), natural birth control, withdrawal, and the intrauterine device (1 percent each). (The remaining 41 percent use no method.) The IUD used to be near the top of the list, but has fallen into disfavor because of the health risks it presents to women and the resulting lawsuits filed against IUD manufacturers.

To determine which methods are the most effective at preventing pregnancy, there are two failure rates to consider for each method. The first is the likelihood of getting pregnant if you use the method correctly every time. The second is the likelihood of getting pregnant if you use it about as diligently as the average person. The second rate may be a better approximation of how you will fare, unless you are an unusually motivated and disciplined person who is going to insert your diaphragm with just the right amount of spermicidal jelly every time. Effectiveness statistics indicate that the safest methods—natural birth control, the diaphragm, the condom, and other barrier methods—require the most diligence. Unless used with care, these methods can allow pregnancy to occur more often than the invasive technologies—the pill, hormonal implants, the IUD, and sterilization.

If a method is not acceptable to a woman, however, it's going to fail no matter how effective it looks on paper. The pill and the IUD may have high effectiveness rates, but 50 percent of women quit using them during the first year because of adverse reactions such as cramps and excessive bleeding. Some of those women become pregnant before finding another mode of contraception, but those pregnancies are not reflected in the pill's and the IUD's effectiveness rate statistics.

In choosing a method, people should also examine their attitudes about sex, says Norsigian. Referring to those people who reject the condom and the diaphragm and choose contraceptives that are separate from the sex act, such as the pill and the IUD, Norsigian says, "I think we've reached the point where some methods are often not well used because of a complex array of social problems. Sex is screaming at us in the media but people have not found a way to talk about it. Some women don't want to touch themselves to put in a diaphragm." American teenagers, especially, don't want to spoil a romantic moment by putting on a condom, says Norsigian.

Finally, you shouldn't think about contraception without considering sexually transmitted diseases. "STDs should be first and foremost in people's minds in a way that they never have been before," says Norsigian. Unless you're in a longterm monogamous relationship, in which you are absolutely sure that your partner is faithful, you should take precautions against STDs. And even when you know your partner is monogamous, you should still be careful. "Sometimes people are carrying diseases from previous relationships and don't know it," Norsigian points out. "There's always that chance."

In case you think it's worth taking that chance, consider these facts: AIDS will kill you. Papilloma, the virus that induces genital warts, and herpes are permanent. Once a virus gets into your system, it never goes out, says Felicia Guest, co-author of *Contraceptive Technology* (Irvington Publishers, 1989) and a specialist in sexually transmitted diseases. It may become dormant, but it never leaves your body. You are condemned to cope with it forever. Other STDs may not be permanent but they can cause a great deal of pain and leave you permanently infertile.

SOURCE:
Bruce, Gene. "A Woman's Guide to Birth Control." *East West* 20 (November 1990): 62.

ORAL CONTRACEPTIVES

On October 26, 1989 the Food and Drug Administration's Fertility and Maternal Health Drugs Committee advised that the upper age limit for oral contraceptive use be removed. The Committee emphasized that this recommendation applied only to healthy, non-smoking women. Formerly, the Committee recommended that smokers not use the birth control pill past the age of 35 and non-smokers could continue taking the pill until age 40.

The National Women's Health Network testified against eliminating the age limit and we advise our members to adhere to the old rules. The Committee made its decision in an absence of scientific data; by relying on dangerous assumptions, it has approved of what amounts to experimentation on older women.

The birth control pills used today have much lower dosages of hormones than the prototypes of thirty years ago. Studies that linked oral contraceptives to thromboembolic disorders (abnormal blood-clotting that can result in strokes, heart attacks, and blood clots to the lung) and other medical conditions were based on studies of the high-dose pills. The recommendations of an age limit were based on the unacceptably high rate of pill-related illness and death in older women. . . .

The Committee's reasoning is that low-dose pills are safer than high-dose pills. There is a difference, however, between safer and safe; there is insufficient data available on women who have only taken the low-dose pill. Population planners and many physicians think that the low-dose pills are completely harmless and in fact have beneficial effects in terms of protecting against ovarian cancer, endometrial cancer, and anemia. While it is true that high-dose pills have protective effects against ovarian cancer and endometrial cancer, there is no evidence that the low-dose pills have the same protective effect! There are no data to support the claim that pills in current use have all the positive effects and none of the negative effects of higher-dose pills.

SOURCE:
Fugh-Berman, Adriane. "Should Women Over Forty Take the Pill?" *Network News* (January-February 1990): 4.

ORAL CONTRACEPTIVES—RISKS

Contrary to popular opinion, using birth control is safer and healthier than not using it, according to a report released today.

"The average woman who has ever used the pill is less likely to get cancer and die as a result before age 55 than a woman who has never used the pill," the report said.

When the risk of death is set against deaths prevented, using contraception, including the pill, saves 120 to 150 lives per 100,000 women, the report said. Contraception also prevents about 1,500 hospitalizations per 100,000 women per year, it said.

Figures published today by the Alan Guttmacher Institute indicate that on balance the protective effects of contraception—including prevention of at least two kinds of cancer, endometriosis, pelvic inflammatory disease and, of course, the health hazards of pregnancy—far outweigh the danger of its side effects.

The only doubtful case is that of breast cancer. Over all, it appears that the pill prevents breast cancer. But some studies have shown that women in their 30s and early 40s who have used the pill for many years may have an increased incidence of cancer. At the same time, women in their late 40s and early 50s who have been long-term users have fewer breast cancers than those who have never used the pill.

SOURCE:
Hilts, Philip. "Birth Control Safer Than Unprotected Sex." *New York Times* (April 23, 1991): B8(N).

CONTRACEPTIVE SPONGE

A relative newcomer to the array of contraceptive products available without a prescription, the contraceptive sponge was first marketed in 1983. It is made of polyurethane and contains the spermicide nonoxynol-9. Its effectiveness is 80 percent to 87 percent. Before intercourse, the sponge is inserted into the vagina to cover the cervix, forming both a physical and chemical barrier to sperm. It should be left in place for at least six hours after intercourse. The sponge may be left in place up to 24 hours and is still effective if intercourse is repeated during that time. It should be discarded after use.

As with spermicides, a small percentage of users may experience irritation or allergic reactions from use of contraceptive sponges.

There have also been reports of difficulty in removing the sponge and of its fragmenting in the vagina. A woman who experiences such problems should contact her physician.

There have been a few cases of the rare but potentially fatal illness called toxic shock syndrome (TSS) among women using contraceptive sponges. However, the rate is very low—less than one TSS case per 3 million sponges used. And women can minimize this already low risk by carefully following the directions on the leaflet accompanying the product.

SOURCE:
Willis, Judith Levine. *Comparing Contraceptives*. DHHS Pub. No. (FDA) 89-1123. March 1989. pp. 1-2.

CONTRACEPTIVE IMPLANTS (NORPLANT)

The perfect contraceptive may never exist, but something more convenient and reliable than anything else on the market in this country has recently been approved for sale. Known as Norplant, the new product consist of six tiny capsules that a doctor inserts under the skin of a woman's upper arm, using a local anesthetic. These capsules release a constant low flow of levonorgestrel, a synthetic form of progesterone. This hormone prevents ovulation and thickens the cervical mucus, impeding the passage of sperm into the uterus. The implant is painless once in place and usually invisible. It works for five years and is 99% effective (the failure rate of the Pill is 3%; of the diaphragm, up to 20%). Easily removed by a doctor, Norplant does not affect fertility after it is removed—a woman who decides to become pregnant will return to her original fertility level as soon as she stops using Norplant. The device is already in use in 17 other countries and has undergone clinical trials for 20 years.

Norplant appears to have side effects similar to those of the Pill. In a five-years clinical trial in San Francisco involving 205 women, a majority reported menstrual changes such as prolonged bleeding or spotting between period. Headaches and mood changes were also cited. Wyeth-Ayerst, the manufacturer of Norplant, states that 27% of users experienced prolonged menstrual periods and 17% reported spotting. Some women [experience] more than one reaction. However, side effects usually disappear in six to twelve months. Most women in the San Francisco study expressed satisfaction with Norplant and said they would continue using it or would ask for it again. Although some women who can't take estrogen may be able to use Norplant, smokers, hypertensive, women with severe liver disease, and those with blood clotting disorders should use some other form of contraception.

SOURCE:
"A New Choice." *University of California, Berkeley Wellness Letter* 7 (March 1991): 2-3. Excerpted from *The University of California, Berkeley Wellness Letter,* Copyright Health Letter Associates, 1991.

RESOURCES

ORGANIZATIONS

Alan Guttmacher Institute. 111 Fifth Ave., New York, NY 10003.

National Women's Health Network. 1325 G Street NW, Washington, DC 20005.

Planned Parenthood Foundation of America. 810 Seventh Ave., New York, NY 10014.

PAMPHLETS

American College of Obstetricians and Gynecologists, Patient Education Pamphlets:

Barrier Methods of Contraception. Pub. no. AP022. n.d.

Contraception: Which Method for You? Pub. no. AP005. n.d.

Family Planning by Periodic Abstinence. Pub. no. AP024. n.d.

Oral Contraceptives. Pub. no. AP021. n.d.

California Medical Association:

"Barrier Methods: Familiar, Safe Contraceptives." *HealthTips* index WH-10 (April 1990): 2 pp.

"Family Planning." *HealthTips* index WH-21. 1986.

Do It Now Foundation:

Preg-Not: A Modern Guide to the Pill and Other Contraceptives. 1988. 20 pp.

Food and Drug Administration (FDA):

Comparing Contraceptives. DHHS Pub. No. (FDA) 85-1123. 1985.

BOOK

Silber, Sherman J. *How NOT To Get Pregnant: Your Guide to Simple, Reliable Contraception*. New York: Scribner's, 1987. 323 pp.

RELATED ARTICLES

Burns, Elizabeth A., and others. "Which Barrier Contraceptive for Whom?" *Patient Care* (September 30, 1988): 109-123.

Cadden, Vivian. "The Five-Year Contraceptive: Is It Right for You?" *McCall's* (March 1991): 62, 64, 68.

Jimenez, Sherry L. M. "10 Myths about Birth Control." *American Baby* (December 1990): 37, 43-44.

Prendergast, Alan. "Beyond the Pill: The Search for a Male Contraceptive Illuminates the Need for New Forms of Birth Control." *American Health* (October 1990): 37-44.

Segal, Marian. "Norplant: Birth Control at Arm's Reach." *FDA Consumer* (May 1991): 9-11.

CRACK/COCAINE

(*See also:* DRUG ABUSE)

OVERVIEW

Fifteen years ago nobody thought cocaine was addictive because it produced few withdrawal symptoms. Today scientists consider it one of the most addictive drugs in existence because of the intense cravings it creates. The more you take, the more you want—and the more it takes from you. Laboratory rats given a choice between cocaine, food, and water will starve themselves to get more and more doses of the drug. Similarly, people will spend their paychecks, abandon their families and ruin their health in pursuit of cocaine highs.

More than 25 million people in the United States have tried cocaine. Ten million are regular users; 5 million suffer serious problems related to their use; 1 million are addicted. Every day 5,000 Americans try cocaine for the first time. Twenty percent of those who continue to use it will end up addicted.

Cocaine, derived from the leaves of the South American coca plant, comes in several different forms. Coca paste, the first product extracted from the plant, is widely used in South America, usually added to and smoked in tobacco or marijuana cigarettes. Cocaine hydrochloride, the form most common in the United States, is a white powder that is sold by the gram (1/28th of an ounce), half-gram, or quarter gram in paper packets called "bindles." Cocaine powder is inhaled through the nose ("snorted") from tiny spoons, rolled-up dollar bills, or straws. It can also be mixed with water and injected.

Freebase, a purified form of cocaine that is smoked in a water pipe, results from the process of applying ether, baking soda, or other solvents to cocaine powder and heating the mixture. This process separates the pure cocaine from most of the hydrochloride salt base and removes some, but not all, of the cutting agents—local anesthetics, sugars, and stimulants—that dealers add to cocaine to enhance their profits. Using the highly volatile ether makes the conversion process especially risky—comedian Richard Pryor set his clothes on fire and nearly died in a freebase accident in 1980.

Crack is freebase that comes in ready-to-smoke chunks or "rocks," saving users the time and trouble of converting the drug to smokable form and making it easier for them to carry and use. Crack rocks are sold in small vials, folding papers, or foil packets. In some areas crack comes in 3-inch sticks with ridges known as "french fries." Crack is usually smoked in a water pipe. Some users apply it to tobacco or marijuana cigarettes known as "fry daddies."

Cocaine is a central nervous system stimulant and local anesthetic. It constricts blood vessels; increases temperature, heart rate, and blood pressure; depresses appetite; and numbs any tissue it touches. Its attributes as an anesthetic and vasoconstrictor ideally suit it to surgery involving the nose, throat, larynx, and lower respiratory passages. But street users take coke for its stimulant effects. Snorting the drug produces a mild high; injecting or smoking it brings on an intense high that users describe as orgasmic.

Cocaine gets to the brain quickly, gives users a brief rush of euphoria, and wears off within an hour. Inhaled intranasally, it reaches its peak effects in 15 minutes; injected, in 5 minutes; smoked, in 15 seconds. At low doses it enhances sexual desire and makes users feel alert, energetic, outgoing, and self-confident. They experience a sense of power and mental clarity. Many believe the drug improves performance in all areas of life. At high doses or with ongoing use, cocaine begins to have less pleasurable effects.

Snorters experience an incessantly runny nose, bloody nose, sores inside the nostrils, and sometimes a perforated septum—a tiny hole in the nasal membrane. IV users put themselves and their spouses or partners at risk of hepatitis, AIDS, and other diseases. Smokers can seriously damage their lungs. They often feel pain in their chest and throat and cough up black phlegm. Other side effects of heavy cocaine use include sweats, tremors, twitching, racing heart, weight loss, malnutrition, sexual dysfunction, anxiety, panic, insomnia, paranoia, auditory or visual hallucinations, "coke bugs" (the sensation of bugs crawling over the skin), psychosis, coma, strokes, seizures, liver damage, heart failure, and respiratory arrest. Sudden death can occur in otherwise healthy people. In a process known as "kindling," regular users can become supersensitive to cocaine and overdose after ingesting a very small amount. In 1986, sports stars Len Bias and Don Rogers died of cocaine overdoses.

Cocaine use inevitably creates a high-low syndrome. Its short-lived high is always followed by depression and craving because the drug depletes the brain's supply of natural chemicals such as norepinephrine and dopamine. Regular users, especially smokers, tend to binge on coke for days at a time—or until they run out of coke or money—doing small amounts of the drug every ten or fifteen minutes in an effort to keep the high constant. But the high is so brief that it is impossible for anyone to ever do enough coke to sustain it. Most users take cocaine in combination with other drugs. They use depressants like alcohol and tranquilizers, or marijuana (which acts as a depressant), to induce sleep or relax their taut nerves. Such polydrug use further entrenches the high-low syndrome. The more cocaine you take, the more anxious you get, the more alcohol you drink to calm down, the less high you feel from cocaine, the more cocaine you do. It's a vicious cycle.

SOURCE:
Yoder, Barbara. *The Recovery Resource Book.* New York: Simon & Schuster, 1990. pp. 204–206.

CHRONIC INTOXICATION

Chronic, persistent and regular use of cocaine by any route of administration has identifiable and characteristic consequences. Chronic use can produce virtually any psychiatric disorder (e.g., affective disorder, schizophrenia and personality disturbances). Withdrawal from chronic cocaine use also has a predictable and typical protracted course.

With chronic use, some of the acute effects of intoxication wane and become less intense and of shorter duration. The intensity and duration of euphoria actually lessen with the development of tolerance. Most cocaine addicts state that their initial trial of cocaine produced the greatest euphoria. Euphoria diminishes with further cocaine use over months and years. The addict continues a futile chase for the initial high. In addition, the user experiences less euphoria with successive doses within a short time, such as a binge over hours. Escalation of continued use with diminishing euphoric effects emphasizes the mystery of addictive behavior.

Other effects that accompany repeated cocaine use, such as anxiety and depression, increase to an alarming degree. The addict may experience profound depression with sensations of helplessness, hopelessness and suicidal ideation. A pervasive paranoia is persistently felt by the addict and is punctuated by distressing paranoid delusions in which the addict believes other are "spying on him" or "out to get him." Derogatory auditory and bizarre visual hallucinations are less commonly present in the chronic user. Insomnia, depressed appetite and intense anxiety combine to produce fatigue and eventual exhaustion. When not severely intoxicated, the addict is typically irritable, suspicious, anxious, dysphoric and guarded.

The libido is depressed and sexual performance is impaired, with impotence in males and inorgasmia in females. Males have difficulty with erections and ejaculations, whereas females are sexually unresponsive.

Muscular twitches, tremors and weakness are common in chronic users. Eventually, malnutrition and weight loss occur. Nasal ulcers, nasal bleeding and chronic sinusitis are almost inevitable consequences of chronic intranasal use.

SOURCE:
Miller, Norman S., Mark S. Gold, and Robert L. Millman. "Cocaine." *American Family Physician* 39, no. 2 (February 1989): 117–118.

TREATMENT OF COCAINE ADDICTION

Experts agree that the goals of treating cocaine addiction are to (a) break the cycle of binges and then (b) prevent relapse.

Binge cycles are perpetuated by several factors. In order for treatment to be successful, programs must address all of these factors:

Avoid the depression associated with cocaine withdrawal—This is managed in many ways, including combinations of individual, group, and family therapy. Anti-depressants can be added for severe depression.

Restrict supplies—There are many strategies to make cocaine unavailable. Some specialists recommend that families control all of the user's funds. Many programs insist on routine urine testing for cocaine. Some patients will find it impossible to stay away from cocaine despite a variety of creative efforts. These patients may need temporary hospitalization to eliminate any possibility of acquiring more drug.

Avoid cues which trigger cocaine cravings and lead to relapse—It is now suspected that chronic cocaine use may be associated with, and in fact may produce, subtle changes in the brain. These changes may well be responsible for the acute cravings and subsequent relapses so often suffered by cocaine addicts. Scientists know that the slightest environmental cue or the need to enjoy simple pleasures can trigger cocaine cravings and lead to relapse. Therapists should determine which cues trigger cocaine cravings for each patient, and help the patient avoid them entirely.

Avoiding cues may be as dramatic as selling a car from which all cocaine transactions took place, to simply avoiding parties with certain friends. Therapists should also be aware of the possibility that the patient may be suffering from an inability to feel pleasure which can last for months.

Some patients find it impossible to resist their powerful cocaine cravings. Researchers are evaluating various medications for their effectiveness in reducing craving and promoting abstention, but they are all still experimental. Some of the drugs being investigated include: (1) buprenorphine, a pain-killer, which works with cocaine addiction, (2) desipramine, an anti-depressant, which has reduced cravings and promoted abstention in many difficult-to-treat patients, (3) flupenthixol, an anti-psychotic, which acts as an anti-depressant and promotes abstinence for an average of 24 weeks and (4) carbamazapine, an anti-seizure drug, which may help reduce cocaine craving and stem seizures brought on by chronic use. . . .

Long term treatment focuses on helping the patient build a full and satisfying life without cocaine. In particular, therapists help patients develop strategies for dealing with a lifetime of stresses which could trigger relapse.

SOURCE:
American Council on Science and Health. *Cocaine: Facts and Dangers*. April 1990. pp. 32–33.

WITHDRAWAL PROBLEMS

One of the major problems in cocaine abuse is the development of tolerance and psychologic dependence. When drug use is stopped, the individual often experiences withdrawal symptoms, such as depression, muscle tremors, headache, ravenous hunger and change in sleep patterns.

Withdrawal symptoms usually occur within 24 to 48 hours of the last dose of cocaine, and they may last seven to ten days. At present, there is no specific treatment for these symptoms. A variety of therapies have been partially successful and are still under investigation.

Since cocaine causes an increase in adrenergic and dopaminergic activities, treatment of withdrawal symptoms is related to increasing the activities of these neurotransmitters. Desipramine (Norpramin, Pertofrane), which blocks the reuptake of norepinephrine, may be the drug of choice for the treatment of depression and sleep disturbances associated with cocaine withdrawal. Bromocriptine (Parlodel), a dopamine receptor agonist, increases central dopaminergic neurotransmission.

Bromocriptine, 0.625 mg given orally four times daily, produces a rapid decrease in psychiatric symptoms. Administered in a single dose of 1.25 mg, bromocriptine has been found to decrease the craving for cocaine. Drugs such as lithium, methylphenidate (Ritalin) and other antidepressants are still experimental for this purpose.

Like alcoholics, cocaine addicts require intensive psychologic support. Groups such as Narcotics Anonymous can be effective for cooperative patients.

SOURCE:
DiGregorio, G. John. "Cocaine Update: Abuse and Therapy." *American Family Physician* 41, no. 1 (January 1990): 250.

RESOURCES

ORGANIZATIONS
American Council for Drug Education. 204 Monroe St., Rockville, MD 20850.

Hazelden Foundation. Box 11, Center City, MN 55012.

National Clearinghouse for Alcohol and Drug Information. P.O. Box 2345, Rockville, MD 20852.

PAMPHLETS
National Institute on Drug Abuse:

Cocaine/Crack: The Big Lie. 1989. 9 pp.

When Cocaine Affects Someone You Love. 1989. 11 pp.

BOOKS

Baum, Joanne. *One Step Over the Line: A No-Nonsense Guide to Recognizing and Treating Cocaine Dependency*. New York: Harper & Row, 1985.

Gold, Mark. *800-COCAINE*. New York: Bantam, 1984.

Johanson, Chris-Ellyn. *Cocaine: A New Epidemic*. New York: Chelsea House, 1986. 107 pp.

Weiss, Roger D., and Steven M. Mirin. *Cocaine*. Washington, DC: American Psychiatric Press, 1987. 178 pp.

RELATED ARTICLES

Bouknight, LeClaire Green, and Reynard R. Bouknight. "Cocaine—A Particularly Addictive Drug." *Postgraduate Medicine* 83, no. 4 (March 1988): 115–118, 121–122, 124, 131.

Hannan, Deborah J., and Alan G. Adler. "Crack Abuse: Do You Know Enough about It?" *Postgraduate Medicine* 88, no. 1 (July 1990): 141–143, 146–147.

Pike, Ronald F. "Cocaine Withdrawal: An Effective Three-Drug Regimen." *Postgraduate Medicine* 85, no. 4 (March 1989): 115–116, 121.

CYSTIC FIBROSIS

OVERVIEW

Cystic fibrosis is the commonest inherited, potentially fatal disease among Caucasians, especially those of North European descent. . . .

Cystic fibrosis strikes with varying degrees of severity. It involves an inability to move salt or sodium chloride (particularly the chloride part) and water through the channels in cells that line certain organs. The flawed chloride transport and consequent dryness of cell surfaces result in abnormally thick secretions that hamper the normal function of organs such as the lungs, sweat glands, intestine, and pancreas. The lung defect usually poses the greatest danger because thick, sticky mucus plugs the airways and leads to frequent respiratory infections. Many CF sufferers find life a constant battle against bacterial infections. Digestion may also be impeded because thick secretions obstruct the ducts, slow the flow and deplete the supply of pancreatic enzymes. The lack of digestive enzymes hinders food absorption, leading to malnutrition and fatty stools. People with pancreatic insufficiency must take many pills daily to prevent under-nourishment.

The first comprehensive report of the disease in 1936 described it as "cystic fibrosis of the pancreas" because the thick mucus that blocks the flow of secretions causes scarring or fibrosis of the pancreas. However the pancreatic problem isn't usually the most dangerous aspect of CF, nor is the pancreas always seriously affected. (About 15 percent of patients are classed as pancreas sufficient.) Nonetheless, the term cystic fibrosis has largely stuck; in a few countries it's called mucoviscidosis. In the 1960s it became clear that the basic defect is faulty salt transport and that the sweat of CF sufferers is unusually salty. The sweat test, which detects the elevated salt content, has become the standard diagnostic tool for CF.

During the 1980s, scientists recognized chloride transport as the primary flaw. And in 1985, thanks largely to the work of researchers at Toronto's Hospital for Sick Children, the gene responsible for CF was located on human chromosome number seven. In 1989, the molecular code of the gene (the sequence of chemical units in DNA) was accurately described. From that, scientists deduced the structure of the protein controlled by the gene—now named CFTR (TR stands for transmembrane conductance regulator). Recent work suggests that the CFTR protein resides in the so-called apical membrane of affected cells and probably plays some crucial part in regulating chloride movement through cell surfaces.

CF treatment has gradually improved, prolonging survival so that some now live well into their 40s. Many who reach adulthood lead near-normal lives—depending on the degree of organ damage. Whereas in 1960 only about four percent of children born with CF lived beyond their teens, almost 80 percent now reach adulthood, the current age of survival averaging 26 years. However, most sufferers need lifelong medication to combat lung infections and assist digestion. The 1990s will probably see clarification of the CF defect—the precise functional flaw (how salt regulation goes wrong)—development of more effective treatment and the establishment of comprehensive carrier screening tests.

SOURCE:

"Gene Discovery Brings Cystic Fibrosis Cure Closer." *Health News* (December 1990): 5.

INHERITANCE OF CF GENES

Every child receives a chromosome 7 from the mother and a chromosome 7 from the father to make a complete chromosome 7 pair. In the case where both parents are CF carriers, their child may receive a CF gene from each parent, from only one parent, or from neither parent.

It is when a child inherits two CF genes—one from the mother and one from the father—that he or she actually inherits cystic fibrosis.

This type of inheritance pattern is called autosomal recessive. In simpler terms, this means that a child must inherit a "double dose" of the CF gene in order to be affected. In the case of a carrier, where there is only one CF gene, the normal gene makes up for the effects of the CF gene, and the CF gene is recessive.

In summary, there are three possible combinations or inheritance patterns of the chromosome 7 pair, which indicate whether a child inherits cystic fibrosis, is a carrier, or is a non-carrier.

Even when both parents are carriers of the CF gene, their children will not automatically inherit CF. The CF gene will be carried by one-half of the father's sperm and by one-half of the mother's eggs. If, by chance, both the sperm and the egg involved in conception carry the gene for CF, the child will inherit two CF genes and thus will have CF. (In this case, both the chromosomes of the child's chromosome 7 pair will carry the CF gene.)

SOURCE:
Cystic Fibrosis Foundation. *The Genetics of Cystic Fibrosis.* Pub. no. OMD-09. pp. 5–6.

GENETIC SCREENING

The discovery and cloning of the gene sets the stage for development of CF carrier tests. There is however a vigorous debate as to whether or not widespread, universal screening for CF carriers should be performed on the population before all the existing mutations are known. Since all the 60 CF mutations reported to date only add up to 85 percent of the possible gene errors, mass screening done now would miss some CF carriers. While the benefit of identifying carriers (one in 25 people) is clear, most experts argue against widescale screening until at least 95 per cent of the possible CF mutations are known. (Some biotechnology companies have already developed CF carrier test kits and are prepared to start commercial testing, even though such tests would miss some carriers.)

In known CF families, where the particular mutation has been characterized, carrier screening is already widely done. Before the gene discovery, parents only became alerted to the possibility of having a child with CF if they'd already had one or more affected children. Now, carriers can be detected with reasonable accuracy in CF families. And genetic tests on unborn babies (examining cells removed from the chorionic villi or amniotic fluid around the fetus) permit prenatal diagnosis as early as two months after conception. The DNA from fetal cells can be examined to see if the fetus carries any known mutation. If the flawed gene sequence is found, the fetus has CF and the parents can decide whether or not to terminate the pregnancy.

SOURCE:
"Gene Discovery Brings Cystic Fibrosis Cure Closer." *Health News* (December 1990): 7.

NEW TREATMENTS

With the unveiling of two promising treatments, some surprising molecular insights, and the apparent success of a gene therapy experiment, researchers last week boosted their already upbeat sense that they are winning the war against cystic fibrosis (CF).

The new reports augment a wave of optimism that began 18 months ago, when scientists found the faulty gene that causes the inherited disease. Striking one in 2,500 U.S. infants, CF causes mucus to accumulate inside the lungs, providing a rich environment for fatal lung infections in the first few decades of life.

Researchers described the new treatments, which seek to prevent lung infections and improve pulmonary function, at a conference in Bethesda, Md., sponsored by the National Heart, Lung, and Blood Institute (NHLBI) and the Cystic Fibrosis Foundation. One approach takes aim at a problematic enzyme called neutrophil elastase, secreted in massive amounts by well-intentioned but over-stimulated white blood cells in the lungs of CF patients. At high concentrations, the enzyme damages lung tissues and suppresses anti-bacterial immune responses.

NHLBI pulmonary specialists Noel G. McElvaney and Ronald G. Crystal led tests of a neutrophil-elastase-destroying enzyme called alpha-1 antitrypsin in 24 patients. Inhaled as an aerosol twice daily for one week, alpha-1 antitrypsin lowered neutrophil elastase levels in the lungs and improved the ability of white blood cells there to kill lung-infecting bacteria. Details of the treatment, which caused no noticeable side effects, appear in the Feb. 16 [1991] *Lancet.*

A second novel treatment targets another CF complication. Large numbers of white blood cells die while ridding the lungs of bacteria. As the cells break down, they dump their DNA into the lungs where it accumulates and clogs bronchial passages. To help clear the lungs, scientists are experimenting with twice daily inhalations of a genetically engineered, DNA-destroying enzyme called human DNase.

In a study of 24 CF patients receiving DNase for six days, the enzyme significantly improved lung function while leaving DNA inside living cells unharmed, says NHLBI's Richard C. Hubbard. Researchers at NHLBI and at the University of Washington in Seattle plan larger trials to determine optimal dosages of the enzyme.

SOURCE:

Weiss, Rick. "Cystic Fibrosis Treatments Promising." *Science News* 139 (March 2, 1991): 132.

RESOURCES

ORGANIZATION

Cystic Fibrosis Foundation. 6931 Arlington Road, Bethesda, MD 20814. (800) FIGHT-CF or (301) 951-4422 (in MD).

PAMPHLETS

California Medical Education and Research Foundation:

"Cystic Fibrosis." *HealthTips* index 358 (November 1988): 2 pp.

Cystic Fibrosis Foundation:

Cystic Fibrosis: A Summary of Symptoms, Diagnosis and Treatment. 1984.

ADDITIONAL ARTICLES

Cystic Fibrosis: "Toward the Ultimate Therapy" (editorial). *The Lancet* (November 17, 1990): 1224–1225.

Seligmann, Jean. "Curing Cystic Fibrosis? Genes Convert Sick Cells." *Newsweek* (October 1, 1990): 64.

Wilfond, Benjamin S. and Norman Fost. "The Cystic Fibrosis Gene: Medical and Social Implications for Heterozygote Detection." *JAMA* 263, no. 20 (May 23–30, 1990): 2777–2783.

CYSTITIS

(*See also:* URINARY TRACT INFECTIONS)

OVERVIEW

Urinary tract infections are second only to respiratory infections when it comes to bacterial problems that plague mankind—or, more commonly, womankind. The National Kidney Foundation estimates that 10–20% of women have had at least one urinary tract infection (also called UTI or cystitis), and 80% of this group has had them recurrently. Fortunately, researchers have uncovered several clues to this troublesome infection and developed new approaches to treatment and prevention.

Cystitis is an inflammation of the bladder. Although some cases are due to fungus or a virus, most are caused by one of several types of bacteria. The most common, *E(sherichia) coli*, accounts for about 90% of all UTI's. The classic symptoms include a frequent, urgent need to urinate and a painful burning sensation (called dysuria) upon urination. Lower back pain, pelvic pressure and urine that is cloudy or blood-tinged are other tell-tale symptoms. If left unchecked, cystitis can spread upward to the kidneys (called ascending UTI), where it brings on fever and chills and can be much more serious.

Although they do occur in men, UTI's are often viewed as a woman's problem. "Plain and simple, UTI's are more common in women because their urethras (the passage from which urine exits the bladder) are so much shorter," explains Michael Palumbo, M.D. of the New York University School of Medicine. "This makes it easier for bacteria to get from outside into the bladder."

E. coli normally live in the intestine and bowel without causing any disruption, but once they make their way to the bladder, the trouble begins. "Bacteria tend to live better in warm, moist places," says Dr. Palumbo, "so the area around the urethra is a common breeding site." Most typically, a woman develops a UTI if she has been sexually active (hence the moniker "honeymoon cystitis"), or has been careless with her hygiene habits (for example, wiping from back to front after a bowel movement).

Why do some women seem to develop UTI's more easily than others? Some experts say genetics may be the key, since research has shown that women with certain blood antigens (called the Lewis groups) are more susceptible to cystitis. The cells that line their urinary tracts seem to have far more receptors to which bacteria can adhere. Others may lack glycosaminoglycan, a substance found on the surface of the bladder that is inhospitable to bacteria. Another possible cause for recurrent infections is an ill-fitting diaphragm: If it's too big, it pushes against the neck of the bladder, interfering with normal body function and resulting in a backup of urine, which serves as a breeding ground for bacteria.

SOURCE:

Gagliardi, Nancy. "A New Look at Cystitis." *Weight Watchers Women's Health and Fitness News* (December 1990): 4–5.

TREATMENT

The majority of lower urinary tract infections are caused by *Escherichia coli*, with *Staphylococcus saprophyticus* the second most common cause of infection. Other organisms can be present, but they are unusual in otherwise healthy women with uncomplicated infections. Most strains of *E. coli* that cause cystitis are susceptible to all antibiotics in the concentrations achievable in the urine.

In otherwise healthy women with uncomplicated infections, single-dose antibiotic therapy is sufficient and is associated with far fewer side effects and costs than longer courses of treatment. Certain patients, however, are not good candidates for single-dose therapy. Patients should not be given single-dose therapy if they are pregnant, diabetic or elderly. Unsuspected upper urinary tract infection may be present in a significant number of these patients, and a ten- to 14-day course of antibiotics should be given. . . .

Ampicillin (Amcill, Omnipen, Polycillin, etc.), amoxicillin (Amoxil, Polymox, Trimox, etc.) and trimethoprim-sulfamethoxazole (Bactrim, Septra) have been the most extensively evaluated drugs for single-dose regimens, with the majority of studies suggesting that trimethoprim-sulfamethoxazole is preferable. However, other antibiotics in a large single dose will also eradicate most urinary pathogens.

All patients treated with single courses of antibiotics should have follow-up cultures. These cultures can be performed in a cost-efficient manner with a urine dipslide either at the physician's office or by the patient at home. A positive dipslide should be sent to a microbiology laboratory for identification of the organism and sensitivity testing. With proper selection of patients for single-dose therapy, approximately 80 to 90 percent of patients will be cured and only a few post-treatment microbiology laboratory evaluations will need to be done. Patients who have positive cultures after single-dose therapy should be assumed to have upper urinary tract disease and should be treated for 14 days.

Because of failure rates of up to 20 percent with single-dose therapy, many clinicians are now treating uncomplicated infections with a three-day course of antibiotics. Three-day regimens of trimethoprim-sulfamethoxazole or norfloxacin (Noroxin) have given excellent results, and the incidence of side effects is as low as with single-dose treatment. Data on this duration of treatment are not sufficient to permit definite recommendations, but three-day regimens appear promising. As with single-dose therapy, candidates for three-day therapy must be carefully chosen to exclude those with a high probability of upper tract infection.

SOURCE:

Johnson, Mary Anne G. "Urinary Tract Infections in Women." *American Family Physician* 41 (February, 1990): 566-567.

INTERSTITIAL CYSTITIS

If you have heard of cystitis, you probably know it as a urinary tract infection that's easily cured by taking an antibiotic. However, doctors are becoming increasingly aware of another kind of cystitis that's not as simple to treat. Some symptoms resemble those of a bacterial infection—pelvic pain and a frequent, intense urge to urinate—but interstitial cystitis (IC) is not caused by bacteria. Rather, it's a chronic inflammation of the bladder wall. Symptoms can range from mild but annoying to downright miserable. Although there's no cure for IC, it is treatable. And sometimes the condition temporarily disappears on its own.

In the past, IC was regarded as a rare disease, affecting fewer than 100,000 Americans, most of them elderly women. Some researchers now judge that number to be as high as 500,000. Although the condition is most commonly diagnosed among women in their 20s and 30s, about 10 percent of sufferers are men, and it can strike at any age.

Doctors are just beginning to get a handle on many aspects of IC: its causes, treatments and impact on people's lives. Much of this knowledge can be credited to the Interstitial Cystitis Association (ICA), which in 1987 conducted a national survey that estimated the prevalence of IC. These results were widely publicized among the general public as well as doctors. The message—that IC causes considerable suffering in a significant number of people—eventually spread to funding groups. Soon research money began to trickle in. . . .

People who suspect they have IC should see a urologist, who specializes in diseases of the kidney and bladder. He or she will first order tests to be sure a urinary tract or vaginal infection isn't causing discomfort. The next step is a cystoscopy, which is performed in a hospital with the patient under general anesthesia. The urologist may perform a biopsy during cystoscopy to rule out the rare possibility of bladder cancer or precancer.

Just getting a diagnosis can be a great relief, says Debra Slade, the executive director of ICA. And treatment can help alleviate IC symptoms—in some cases eliminating them entirely—in about 80 to 90 percent of all cases, according to Hanno.

Therapy ranges from filling the bladder with a solution that calms inflammation to taking oral drugs that are thought to plug the holes in the bladder lining. Because the various treatments, which are explained here, aren't equally effective in everyone, doctors often utilize a trial-and-error approach. Some people may only need one course of treatment, but many IC sufferers require therapy periodically throughout their lives, says Dr. Alan J. Wein, professor and chairman, division of urology, Hospital of the University of Pennsylvania in Philadelphia.

Bladder distention—When doctors noticed that cystoscopy can improve symptoms, bladder inflation was elevated from diagnosis to treatment status. About 30 percent of patients report relief after the procedure, which stretches the bladder and may temporarily shut down pain receptors. (Paradoxically, it may do this by damaging nerve endings in the bladder lining.) In some cases, repeating distension periodically can control IC.

DMSO (dimethyl sulfoxide)—Once considered a fringe arthritis therapy, the chemical has gained respectability since doctors realized that when placed in the bladder, it reduces pain and inflammation about 70 percent of the time. Dr. Stanley Jacob, Gerlinger professor of surgery at Oregon Health Sciences University in Portland, one of the first doctors who tried DMSO for IC in the 1960s, thinks it works by quelling tissue-damaging substances called free radicals, believed to be one cause of pain and inflammation.

Most people respond after four to six treatments, given every two weeks, usually in a urologist's office. A catheter carries DMSO into the bladder, where it remains for about 15 minutes. Sometimes other drugs, such as steroids, are added to the chemical mix. . . .

Oral medications—A wide range of drugs have been used to treat symptoms, including steroids, antihistamines, antispasmodics, muscle relaxants—even aspirin—with conflicting results. As researchers become more familiar with the physical changes that IC produces, though, they are narrowing their focus. Here are three promising drugs:

Amitriptyline (brand name: Elavil), the most widely used IC medication, is an antidepressant with the fortunate side effect of pain relief. Many who don't respond to DMSO or distention are helped by this drug, says Hanno, especially those who are bothered more by pain than by urgency. (Some can't tolerate the drowsiness and sluggish feeling the drug causes, though.) Amitriptyline is still considered experimental for IC.

Sodium pentosan polysulfate (brand name: Elmiron), which is in use in Europe, may win FDA approval as early as this year, making it the first oral medication specifically targeted for IC. With a chemical makeup that resembles the bladder lining, Elmiron is thought to coat and protect the bladder wall. About 40 percent of people who take the drug report significant relief, with few side effects, says [Dr. C. Lowell] Parsons [professor of surgery/urology at the University of California at San Diego].

Nalmefene, now in the early testing stages, appears to work by blocking the relaease of pain-causing histamines, which may accumulate in the bladder area in people with IC. The drug was effective in more than half of people tested, according to a preliminary trial that will be reported at this month's meeting of the American Urological Association.

SOURCE:

Mosedale, Laura. "Embattled Bladders." *Health* (May 1990): 40-41, 78.

RESOURCES

ORGANIZATION

Interstitial Cystitis Association. P.O. Box 1533, Madison Square Station, New York, NY 10159.

PAMPHLET

Norwich Eaton Pharmaceuticals, Inc. Lieter, Elliot. *Cystitis: How You Can Help Control It.* Pub. No. 2080-74. February, 1987.

BOOKS

Chalke, Rebecca, and Kristene E. Whitmore. *Overcoming Bladder Disorders.* Fairfield, OH: Consumer Reports Books, 1990.

Gillespie, Larrian, and Sandra Blakeslee. *You Don't Have to Live With Cystitis!* New York: Rawson, 1986.

Schrotenboer, Kathryn, and Sue Berkman. *The Woman Doctor's Guide to Overcoming Cystitis.* New York: New American Library/Plume, 1987.

Shreve, Caroline. *Cystitis: The New Approach.* Rochester, VT: Thorson Publishing Group, 1986.

RELATED ARTICLES

Corriere, Joseph N., Philip M. Hanno, and others. "Cystitis: Evolving Standard of Care." *Patient Care* 22 (February 29, 1988): 33.

Greengard, Samuel. "Bladder Fire: Women Band Together to Fight Interstitial Cystitis." *American Health* 8 (June, 1989): 20.

Levine, David Z. "Interstitial Cystitis: An Overlooked Cause of Pelvic Pain." *Postgraduate Medicine* 88, no. 1 (July, 1990): 101-102, 107, 109.

"Painful Bladder Diseases: Interstitial or Abacterial Cystitis?" *The Lancet* (February 13, 1988): 337-338.

DENTAL IMPLANTS

OVERVIEW

There are millions of Americans who do endure the hassles of dentures. A 1985–1986 survey by the National Institute for Dental Research found that Americans 65 and older had lost an average of 10 teeth, and those 35 to 64 had an average of nine teeth missing. Four out of 10 (42 percent) of Americans 65 and older have lost all their teeth, as have 4 percent of those 35 to 65 years of age.

Ordinary dentures, generally made of plastic, are custom-fitted to match and adhere to the upper or lower jaw or made to clamp on to remaining teeth with metal supports or bridges.

But today there are dental implants, which add a method of attaching the denture with metal anchors directly and permanently to the jaw bone with no need to ever be removed by the wearer.

Dental scientists have discovered materials that will bond with bone and withstand the pressure created by biting and chewing. The bonding process is called "endosseous [within the bone] integration." Refined surgical techniques and follow-up have reduced the likelihood of the implant loosening, breaking, or being rejected by the body.

As many as 100,000 Americans will undergo surgery to be fitted with dental implants by 1992, according to a report of a June 1988 National Institutes of Health consensus development conference on dental implants. That compares with an estimated 24,500 implants done before 1985.

At least 10,000 dentists implant dental prostheses today, compared to 1,000 or so five years ago, the conference report stated. Dental implants are now being done at a rate of about 6,000 to 7,500 a year, adds Paul J. Mentag, a dentist and assistant professor of prosthodontics at the University of Detroit.

"We have the ability to functionally and aesthetically rehabilitate the oral invalid to a state of excellent dental health," says Paul H.J. Krogh, a Washington, D.C. oral and maxillofacial (jaw) surgeon and president of the Academy of Osseointegration, which represents 1,150 oral surgeons, other dental professionals, assistants, technicians, physicians and scientists.

"Not every patient is a candidate for implants," cautions the American Dental Association (ADA), headquartered in Chicago, which represent 146,000 dental professionals and students.

ADA points out there is no substitute for natural teeth, that implants will never function as well as the real thing. And the association's position is that implants are not suggested for cosmetic purposes alone.

"The best implant is a natural tooth," echoes Albert Guckes, a prosthodontic consultant at the dental clinic of the National Institute of Dental Research, Bethesda, MD. "With today's technology we can salvage badly damaged teeth, and that's the way to go," he says.

ADA says an individual's decision whether or not to have a dental implant should be made only after a careful examination and consultation with the person's dentist. A second professional opinion can add perspective.

If you are thinking of having dental implants, consider the following:

- Determine if it is possible to save your own teeth.
- Will you be able to keep the schedule required for implant surgery and follow-up? Some implants require many visits and a second stage of surgery. It

may take as long as four to six months before the implant is completed.

- Know what to expect in the way of pain, soreness, and possible long-term restrictions to your diet. You also may have to wear temporary devices.
- Will you be able to follow special oral hygiene instructions and maintain a schedule of regular dental checkups that may go on for years?
- Your body might reject the implant after a few months or a few years. Are you prepared to accept that possibility?
- Medical risks are inherent in implant surgery, just as in any surgical procedure. In implant surgery, risks include sinus perforation, local and systemic infection, and paresthesias (abnormal or impaired skin sensation). . . .

Four general designs of devices are in use in implant dentistry today. The two most frequently used, according to Barry E. Sands, biomedical engineer at the [FDA] Center for Devices and Radiological Health, are:

- **One-and two-stage cylindrical implants.** These are inserted directly into holes drilled into the jawbone as sockets for screws to anchor a single false tooth, groups of false teeth, or entire rows of replacements. In two-stage implants, the cylinder is fitted into the bone and the gum is sutured closed over the device until the area heals and the device bonds to the bone around it. Then the surgical site is reopened to allow abutments to be placed in the cylinders, and the prosthesis is attached.
- **Blade types.** Shaped to fit channels cut lengthwise into the jaw bone, blades have openings to accept bone regrowth through their framework. Tiered vanes above the gum line allow attachment of the prosthesis, which is generally done at the same time as the surgery.

The other types of devices—pin- and tooth-shaped—are less frequently implanted today and are generally used only for replacing individual teeth.

Most implant hardware in use today is made from titanium alloys. Coatings of calcium phosphates, carbon compounds, and titanium are sometimes added to promote successful bonding of the implant to bone. However, the coatings have not been shown to improve the bonding of the implant to bone, according to Sands.

SOURCE:

Modeland, Vern. "Dental Implants: The Latest in False Teeth." *FDA Consumer* 22 (December 1988-January 1989): 13.

RISKS

There are at least three areas in which the assessment of patient risk should be considered, including risks associated with the surgery and/or anesthesia, psychological risks, and medical risks. Risks associated with the surgical procedure may include inadvertent perforation of the nasal sinus, local and systemic infection, and nerve injury. Before surgery a medical history should be taken to evaluate the history of the presenting problem and chief complaints. A review of the current status of the patient's organ systems should be made.

Children need special consideration, given long-term morbidity concerns, requirements of growth, manual dexterity, and coping skills.

Psychological stressors and motivational factors have been shown to influence patient response to surgery and long-term compliance with oral hygiene maintenance. These stressors include both familial and social environmental factors such as job satisfaction, financial status, and health concerns. Specific mental conditions may require psychological intervention to assist with patient cooperation and outcome satisfaction. Individuals with excessive neurotic concerns, depression, anxiety, and specific medical fears or previous negative medical or dental experiences should be appropriately evaluated. Relative contraindications include individuals with psychotic symptomatology, especially requiring psychotropic medication, and somatization disorders or chronic pain complaints where medical symptoms are exhibited in the absence of organic evidence. Tobacco use, alcohol, or drug dependency may interfere with good nutrition or compliance requirements.

Temporary conditions that may result from implant placement may include pain and swelling, speech problems, and gingivitis. Long-term problems may include nerve injury, local bone loss exacerbation, hyperplasias, local or systemic bacterial infection, and infectious endocarditis in susceptible individuals, including those with body part replacement. Existing natural dentition may be compromised.

Factors related to prediction of health risks need to be continuously assessed before the surgical decision, after implantation, during the temporary waiting period, following the loading period, and at 6-month intervals throughout the followup period. Reliable and valid standardized measurements sensitive to both psychological and physical factors should be used in clinical prospective studies to enhance comparison across studies.

SOURCE:

Dental Implants. National Institutes of Health Consensus Development Conference Statement 7, no. 3 (June 15, 1988): 5.

SELECTING A QUALIFIED PRACTITIONER

Selecting the right dentist or dental team is a must. Dot Olsen of Staten Island, NY, can't stop smiling: She's had dental implants—artificial teeth attached to metal anchors inserted into her jawbone—for three years and loves the results.

But as Olsen discovered, implant therapy isn't simple or quick (about six months for her), nor is it for everyone.

She required further surgery for an additional implant, and many of her friends have had painful or unsuccessful experiences. Olsen believes selecting the right dentist is the key to finding your way through the implant maze. Absolutely, say leading implant experts.

"Misperceptions abound about implant therapy, " says Dr. Paul Schnitman, chairman of implant dentistry at Harvard. "Consumers don't fully understand what's involved—and dentists have different opinions about treatment."

Reason: The demand for implants has simply out-paced dental training. The high-tech advances and the deluge of makers' claims for 50 different implant types are daunting.

The lack of regulatory controls adds to the confusion. Unlike oral surgery, for example, implant therapy lacks specialty status. There are no national standards for patient care or even dentists' training. Thus, implant dentistry has had an erratic track record, according to the FDA.

To deal with the confusion, the FDA is bringing research standards into line for class III bone-integrated (endosseous) implants. By 1992, their makers must back up their safety claims with costly studies. Some manufacturers are appealing the classification.

But the government can't help consumers with a crucial step in treatment: selecting a qualified practitioner from among the 20,000 general dentists, periodontists, oral surgeons and prosthodontists (bridge experts) trained largely by implant manufacturers. This group includes a small subset of several hundred dentists who have met the tough guidelines set by the American Academy of Implant Dentistry (AAID), which wants specialty status for implant technology.

Whatever a dentist's other credentials, leading experts, including former AAID president Dr. Ronald Evasic, advise patients to look specifically for dentists with a "learning curve that goes up in implants."

SOURCE:

Sears, Cathy. "Boning Up on Implants: Selecting the Right Dentist or Dental Team Is a Must." *American Health* 9 (July-August 1990): 32.

RESOURCES

ORGANIZATIONS

American Academy of Implant Dentistry. 6900 Grove Road, Thorofare, NJ 08086.

American Academy of Periodontology. 211 E. Chicago Ave, #114, Chicago, IL 60611.

American Dental Association. 211 E. Chicago Ave., Chicago, IL 60611.

National Institute of Dental Research. NIH Building 30, Bethesda, MD 20892.

PAMPHLET

American Academy of Periodontology:

Dental Implants: Are They Right for You. 1989.

ADDITIONAL ARTICLES

"Dental Implants: How Good They Are, How Long They Last." *Johns Hopkins Medical Letter* (March 1989): 2.

Holland, Lisa. "Dental Implants." *Good Housekeeping* (January 1990): 158.

Langer, Burton. "Dental Implants Used for Periodontal Patients." *Journal of the American Dental Association* (October 1990): 505-508.

Smith, Dale E., and George A. Zarb. "Criteria for Success of Osseointegrated Endosseous Implants." *Journal of Prosthetic Dentistry* 62, no. 5 (November 1989): 567-572.

DEPRESSION

OVERVIEW

During any 6-month period, 9 million American adults suffer from a depressive illness. The cost in human suffering cannot be estimated. Depressive illnesses often interfere with normal functioning and cause pain and suffering not only to those who have a disorder, but also to those who care about them. Serious depression can destroy family life as well as the life of the ill person.

Possible the saddest fact about depression is that much of this suffering is unnecessary. Most people with a depressive illness do not seek treatment, although the great majority—even those with the severest disorders—can be helped. Thanks to years of fruitful research, the medications and psychosocial therapies that ease the pain of depression are at hand. . . .

Depressive disorders come in different forms, just as do other illnesses, such as heart disease. Within [the three most prevalent] types there are variations in the number of symptoms, their severity, and persistence.

Major depression is manifested by a combination of symptoms that interfere with the ability to work, sleep, eat, and enjoy once pleasurable activities. These disabling episodes of depression can occur once, twice, or several times in a lifetime.

A less severe type of depression, dysthymia, involves long-term, chronic symptoms that do not disable, but keep you from functioning at "full steam" or from feeling good. Sometimes people with dysthymia also experience major depressive episodes.

Another type is bipolar disorder, formerly called manic-depressive illness. Not nearly as prevalent as other forms of depressive disorders, bipolar disorder involves cycles of depression and elation or mania. Sometimes the mood switches are dramatic and rapid, but most often they are gradual. When in the depressed cycle, you can have any or all of the symptoms of a depressive disorder. When in the manic cycle, any or all [manic] symptoms may be experienced. Mania often affects thinking, judgment, and social behavior in ways that cause serious problems and embarrassment. For example, unwise business or financial decisions may be made when an individual is in a manic phase. Bipolar disorder is often a chronic recurring condition.

SOURCE:
National Institute of Mental Health, Office of Scientific Information. *Plain Talk About Depression*. DHHS Pub. No. (ADM) 89-1639. 1989, p. 1.

SIGNS AND SYMPTOMS

The term "depression" can be confusing since it's often used to describe normal emotional reactions. At the same time, the illness may be hard to recognize because its symptoms may be so easily attributed to other causes. People tend to deny the existence of depression by saying things like, "She has a right to be depressed! Look at what she's gone through." This attitude fails to recognize that people can go through tremendous hardships and stress without developing depression, and that those who do fall victim can and should seek treatment.

Nearly everyone suffering from depression has pervasive feelings of sadness, helplessness, hopelessness and irritability. In addition, professional help should be sought if you or someone you know has had four or more of the following symptoms continually for more than two weeks:

- Noticeable change of appetite, with either significant weight loss or weight gain, though not dieting.

- Noticeable change in sleeping pattern, such as fitful sleep, inability to sleep or sleeping too much.
- Loss of interest and pleasure in activities formerly enjoyed.
- Loss of energy, fatigue.
- Feelings of worthlessness.
- Persistent feelings of hopelessness.
- Feelings of inappropriate guilt.
- Inability to concentrate or think, indecisiveness.
- Recurring thoughts of death or suicide, wishing to die, or attempting suicide.
- Melancholia (defined as overwhelming feelings of sadness and grief), accompanied by waking at least two hours earlier than normal in the morning, feeling more depressed in the morning and moving significantly more slowly.
- Disturbed thinking, a symptom developed by some severely depressed persons.

For many victims of depression, these mental and physical feelings seem to follow them night and day, appear to have no end in sight and cannot be alleviated by happy events or good news. Some people are so disabled by feelings of despair that they cannot even build up the energy to call a doctor. If someone else calls for them, they may refuse to go because they are so hopeless that they think there's no point to it.

SOURCE:
American Psychiatric Association. *Let's Talk Facts About Depression.* 1988. pp. 1-3.

CAUSES

The cause of depression is elusive—and it is clear that successful treatment must take into account the whole fabric of a person's life, not just a single thread. While there is speculation that a complex interweaving of biology, personality, and inadequate or inappropriate coping strategies that a person has developed over the course of a lifetime leads to depression, there is no evidence that any of these alone can cause mood disorders.

It is thought that a disruption in the normal interplay between certain chemicals in brain cells and the neurotransmitters (substances that facilitate the passage of impulses from one nerve cell to another) plays an important part in the onset of clinical depression. Depression also runs in families (although some experts assert that this is due to a learned coping style rather than a genetic trait). Studies of identical twins, for example, show that if one twin suffers from depression, there is a 50-to-90% chance that the other twin will, too. A 1987 study seemed to find a single gene from manic-depression that ran through six generations of an Amish family—but follow-up analyses have since raised serious doubts as to whether any single gene could account for any kind of depression.

Since not every pair of identical twins suffers from the same mood disorders, psychological factors presumably come into play also. Traumas such as the loss of a parent during childhood, repeated low-level stressors, rejections, and failures may contribute. And certain personality types—people with low self-esteem or who tend to be dependent on others—are more vulnerable to depression.

Finally, some cases are rooted in underlying medical conditions: stroke, thyroid disorders, hepatitis, viral pneumonia, or cancer. Other cases are induced by medication, including barbiturates, tranquilizers, heart drugs, hormones, blood pressure medication, pain killers, arthritis drugs, and even some antibiotics. The depression disappears when the medication is stopped. Depression can also be related to chronic alcohol use.

SOURCE:
"Depression: Lifting the Cloud." *The Johns Hopkins Medical Letter: Health After 50* (November 1990): 4-5.

TREATMENT—ANTIDEPRESSANTS

There are more than 20 antidepressant drugs currently available. They work by modifying the levels of specific neurotransmitters in the brain. Because a variety of drugs target different neurotransmitters, and because imbalances of these neurotransmitters can vary from patient to patient, some drugs may be more effective than others for any individual. Sometimes a combination of drugs is best.

- Tricyclic antidepressants (named for the three-ring chain in their chemical structure) or TCAs, such as Pamelor, Norpramin, and Pertofrane, are the preferred drugs for initial treatment. They have been in use since 1957—so their degree of safety is well-known.

Because of the number of TCAs available, your physician may well try several different ones to find the one that has the fewest side effects for you. Though some patients begin to feel better in as little as a week, full benefit may take as long as six weeks.

- Monoamine oxidase inhibitors—or MAOIs—such as Nardil and Parnate, are the second line of drugs tried if TCAs prove ineffective. MAOI users must restrict their diet to avoid sudden potentially life-threatening jumps in blood pressure. Forbidden foods include: smoked meat, aged cheese, pickled fish, red wine, and yogurts with active cultures.
- Lithium carbonate (such as Eskalith or Lithobid) is very effective in the treatment of bipolar mood disorder, and sometimes helpful for people who have only depressive episodes, especially if the drug is added to a TCA.
- Among other drugs now in use are Desyrel, Xanax (which may be useful for moderate depression, though it leads to physical dependence in a significant minority of patients and so is ordinarily only used as a

bridge medication until traditional antidepressants begin to work), and Prozac.

SOURCE:
"Depression: Lifting the Cloud." *The Johns Hopkins Medical Letter: Health After 50* (November 1990): 5.

TREATMENT—SECOND GENERATION ANTIDEPRESSANTS

Second-generation nontricyclic antidepressants, which include bupropion (Wellbutrin), fluoxetine (Prozac) and trazodone (Desyrel), have become popular because they are associated with a low incidence of side effects and are better tolerated than tricyclic agents. These drugs are minimally anticholinergic, induce minimal orthostatic change in blood pressure (excluding trazodone) and have a safe cardiovascular profile. They are also less sedating than tricyclic antidepressants and usually are not associated with iatrogenic weight gain. The advantages of the second-generation agents are most significant in medically ill and/or geriatric patients, who may demonstrate a lower tolerance for tricyclic antidepressants.

SOURCE:
Tollepson, Gary D. "Recognition and Treatment of Major Depression." *American Family Physician* 42, no. 5, (suppl.) (November 1990): 65S.

TREATMENT—PROZAC (FLUOXETINE)

Doctors have reported two more cases of suicidal behavior and suicidal fantasies that they believe can only be explained by the effects of the widely publicized antidepressant drug Prozac.

The new cases were described in a letter in [the February 7, 1991] issue of *The New England Journal of Medicine*. The physicians said the two cases differed from previous published reports of suicidal behavior linked to Prozac because the two patients had never before shown signs of wanting to kill themselves.

But Eli Lilly and Company of Indianapolis, the maker of Prozac, as well as many other physicians, vehemently deny that there is any scientific merit to the charge that the medication can prompt suicidal or violent acts. The company argues that its product is, in fact, less likely to make patients suicidal than other antidepressants.

Prozac, the commercial form of the compound fluoxetine, is already the center of a sharp legal and medical dispute. More than 50 lawsuits have been filed nationwide against Lilly. . . .

Many physicians are dismayed by the lawsuits and bad publicity, and they argue that the medication is being unfairly maligned. Prozac was introduced only three and a half years ago but is now among the most widely prescribed antidepressant drugs, accounting for about 20 percent of the market, or 6.1 million prescriptions, in 1989, the last year for which figures are available.

The vast majority of physicians have said the drug is one of the best medications in its category. It is able to match the older antidepressants in relieving the symptoms of the mental disease 60 percent to 80 percent of the time, they said, but does not touch off many of the debilitating side effects caused by the traditional antidepressant drugs, like extreme dizziness, weight gain, and high blood pressure.

SOURCE:
Angier, Natalie. "Suicidal Behavior Tied Again to Drug." *New York Times* (February 7, 1991): B7(N).

* * *

Although the evidence of an association between Prozac and suicide is not conclusive, careful medical supervision of patients on Prozac is clearly warranted. So too is warning patients and their families of the possibility that Prozac may induce intense, overpowering suicidal thoughts in some patients, even if they are taking it for problems other than depression. To get this important information to the public, the Health Research Group petitioned the Food and Drug Administration in April 1991 to put the following prominent box warning on Prozac's label. This information would then appear in the *Physician's Desk Reference.*

Warning: A small minority of persons taking Prozac (fluoxetine) have experienced intense, violent, suicidal thoughts, agitation and impulsivity. Some of the people involved had no prior history of depression or suicidal thoughts, and were being treated with fluoxetine for other problems (e.g. obsessive-compulsive disorder). Whether development of such symptoms is coincidental or drug-related is still under investigation. Prozac should only be used under careful medical supervision, and patients are advised to alert relatives and friends to their use of Prozac and the risk of suicidal obsession.

SOURCE:
"The Dangers of Prozac." *Public Citizen Health Research Group Health Letter* (May 1991): 9.

TREATMENT—LITHIUM

The medication lithium carbonate was introduced for the treatment of mania and bipolar affective disorder in the early 1950's. It has a powerful mood stabilizing effect and can be used safely. It is not a sedative, but prevents extremes of mood, either high or low.

Lithium's main benefit lies in the prevention of episodes and in treating an episode after it has occurred. Manic and depressive attacks occur less frequently and are less severe when lithium is taken regularly. Individuals with recurring manic-depressive (bipolar) and some forms of recurring depressive (unipolar) illness are often treated with lithium. When taken regularly and at a correct dosage, there is no sedation or other effects on awareness or mental functioning.

A medical evaluation including medical history, physical examination, and simple laboratory tests of blood and urine are needed. Because lithium is almost entirely eliminated from the body by the kidneys, laboratory tests of kidney function are done before starting lithium and at regular intervals thereafter. Tests of thyroid function are also advised since lithium may occasionally cause goiter (a harmless, treatable enlargement of the thyroid gland) or a mild decrease in thyroid function (hypothyroidism). A blood test of the level of thyroid hormones is usually done at regular intervals.

There is a simple, inexpensive blood test to measure the level of lithium in the blood, so the correct dosage can be precisely determined for each patient.

SOURCE:
National Alliance for the Mentally Ill. *Mood Disorders: Depression and Manic Depression.* n.d. p. 8.

PSYCHOTHERAPY

A number of structured, time-limited behavioral psychotherapies are available for the treatment of depression. These strategies are effective in reducing signs and symptoms in ambulatory patients with nonpsychotic major depression.

Psychotherapy is more likely to be beneficial if the current episode of major depression has been present for less than one year, if the patient has a history of good interepisode recovery, if the patient does not have a significant personality disorder, if the physical illness is not severe, and if the patient has a negative history for psychosis and bipolar disorder. For patients in whom pharmacotherapy alone has not been fully effective, a combined approach using psychotherapy and drug therapy may be useful.

SOURCE:
Tollepson, Gary D. "Recognition and Treatment of Major Depression." *American Family Physician* 42, no. 5, (suppl.) (November 1990): 68S–69S.

RESOURCES

ORGANIZATIONS

National Alliance for the Mentally Ill. 1901 North Fort Myer Drive, Suite 500, Arlington, VA 22209. (703) 524-7600.

National Depressive and Manic Depressive Association. Merchandise Mart, Box 3395, Chicago, IL 60654. (312) 939-2442.

National Foundation for Depressive Illness. 245 Seventh Avenue, 5th Floor, New York, NY 10001. (212) 620-7637 or 1(800)248-4344.

National Institute of Mental Health. Parklawn Building 15C-05, 5600 Fishers Lane, Rockville, MD 20857. (301) 443-4513.

National Mental Health Association. 1201 Prince Street, Alexandria, VA 22314-2971. (703) 684-7722.

PAMPHLETS

American Psychiatric Association:

Manic-Depressive Disorder. 1990.

National Alliance for the Mentally Ill:

Mood Disorders: Depression and Manic Depression. n.d. 12 pp.

National Institute of Mental Health, Public Inquiries Branch:

Bipolar Disorder: Manic-Depressive Illness. ADM 89-1009. 1989.

Depression/Awareness, Recognition, and Treatment (Fact Sheet). OM 88-4034. 1987.

Depressive Disorders: Treatments Bring New Hope. ADM 89-1491. 1989. 25 pp.

Helpful Facts about Depressive Disorders ADM 87-1536. 1987. 8 pp.

When a Friend Is Depressed: A Guide for Teenagers. OM 88-4036. 1988. 3 pp.

National Mental Health Association:

Adolescent Depression. 1986.

Depression: What You Should Know about It. 1988. 5 pp.

BOOKS

Ericksen, Corey. *Depression Is Curable.* Clackamas, OR: Rainbow Press, 1986. 84 pp.

Gold, Mark S. *The Good News about Depression: Cures and Treatments in the New Age of Psychiatry.* New York: Villard, 1987. 328 pp.

Klerman, Gerald. *Suicide and Depression Among Adolescents and Young Adults.* Washington, DC: American Psychiatric Press, Inc., 1986.

Papolos, Demitri, and Janice Papolos. *Overcoming Depression.* New York: Harper & Row, 1987. 319 pp.

Slagel, Priscilla. *The Way Up from Down: A Safe New Program that Relieves Low Moods and Depression with Amino Acids and Vitamin Supplements.* New York: Random House, 1987. 254 pp.

RELATED ARTICLES

Bacani-Oropilla, Teresita, and Steven B. Lippmann. "Chronic Depression: Issues in Long-Term Management." *Postgraduate Medicine* 85, no. 2 (February 1, 1989): 171–175.

"Beating Depression." *U.S. News & World Report* (March 5, 1990): 48–56.

Cohn, Jay, Wayne Katon, and Elliott Richelson, II. "Choosing the Right Antidepressant." *Patient Care* 24 (July 15, 1990): 88–101.

Feinberg, Michael. "Buproprion: New Therapy for Depression." *American Family Physician* 41, no. 6 (June 1990): 1787–1790.

Grady, Denise. "Wonder Drug, Killer Drug." *American Health* (October 1990): 60–65.

"The Promise of Prozac." *Newsweek* (March 26, 1990): 38–41.

"Prozac: A 'Wonder Drug' or Cause for Worry?" *Mayo Clinic Health Letter* (June 1991): 5–6.

Teicher, Martin H., Carol Glod, and Jonathan O. Cole. "Emergence of Intense Suicidal Preoccupation during Fluoxetine Treatment." *American Journal of Psychiatry* 147, no. 2 (February 1990): 207–210.

DIABETES

OVERVIEW

A complex disorder of carbohydrate, fat, and protein metabolism that is primarily a result of a relative or complete lack of insulin secretion by the beta cells of the pancreas or of defects of the insulin receptors. The disease is often familial but may be acquired, such as in Cushing's syndrome, as a result of the administration of excessive glucocorticoid. The various forms of diabetes have been organized into a series of categories developed by the National Diabetes Data Group of the National Institutes of Health. Type I diabetes in this classification scheme includes patients dependent upon insulin to prevent ketosis. The category is also known as the insulin-dependent diabetes mellitus (IDDM) subclass. This group was previously called juvenile-onset diabetes, brittle diabetes, or ketosis-prone diabetes. Patients with Type II, or non-insulin-dependent diabetes mellitus (NIDDM), are those previously designated as having maturity-onset diabetes, adult-onset diabetes, ketosis-resistant diabetes, or stable diabetes. Type II patients are further subdivided into obese NIDDM and nonobese NIDDM groups. Those with gestational diabetes (GDM), usually identified as Type III, are in a separate subclass composed of women who developed glucose intolerance in association with pregnancy. Type IV, also identified as Other Types of Diabetes, includes patients whose diabetes is associated with a pancreatic disease, hormonal changes, adverse effects of drugs, or genetic or other anomalies. A fifth subclass, the impaired glucose tolerance (IGT) group, includes persons whose plasma glucose levels are abnormal although not sufficiently beyond the normal range to be diagnosed as diabetic. . . .

The onset of diabetes mellitus is sudden in children and usually insidious in non-insulin-dependent diabetes mellitus (type II). Characteristically, the course is progressive and includes polyuria, polydipsia, weight loss, polyphagia, hyperglycemia, and glycosuria. The eyes, kidneys, nervous system, skin, and circulatory system may be affected, infections are common, and atherosclerosis often develops. In childhood and in the Type I, advanced stage of the disease, when no endogenous insulin is being secreted, ketoacidosis is a constant danger. The diagnosis is confirmed by glucose-tolerance tests, history, and urinalysis.

SOURCE:

"Diabetes Mellitus." In *Mosby's Medical, Nursing, and Allied Health Dictionary*. 3rd Edition. St. Louis: Mosby, 1990. pp. 361–362.

USE OF INSULIN

Insulin is a hormone produced in the pancreas, a gland located behind the stomach. Insulin is necessary for a process called metabolism by which digested foods are turned into the energy your body needs. Without insulin, glucose, a form of sugar produced when starches and sugars are digested, cannot be properly used. Instead, glucose builds up in the bloodstream and spills into the urine showing as "sugar in the urine." . . .

People with Type I (insulin dependent or juvenile) diabetes do not produce the insulin their bodies need. In order to supply the insulin needed to burn glucose for energy, insulin must be taken by injection every day. . . .

Until recently, insulin came only from the pancreases of cows and pigs, with pork insulin more closely duplicating human insulin. While beef, pork and beef-pork combinations are still widely used, there are now two types of "human" insulins available: semisynthetic (made by converting pork insulin to a form identical to human) and recombinant (made using genetic engineering). These are becoming more popular because of their purity and ability to be absorbed more quickly into the bloodstream. . . .

Different types of insulin work for different periods of time. The numbers shown here are only averages. The onset (how long it takes to reach the bloodstream to begin lowering the blood sugar), peaking (how long it takes to reach maximum strength) and duration (how long it continues to lower the blood sugar) of insulin activity vary somewhat from person to person, and even from day to day for the same person.

- Rapid or Regular Activity: Onset is within half an hour and activity peaks during a 2–5 hour period. It remains in the blood-stream for about 8 to 16 hours. These fast-acting, short-lasting insulins are useful in special cases: accidents, minor surgery or illnesses which cause the diabetes to go out of control, or whenever insulin requirements change rapidly for any reason. These are also being used more and more in combination with a long-acting insulin or alone prior to meals and at bedtime.
- Semilente: A special type of short-acting insulin that takes 1–2 hours for onset, peaks 3 to 8 hours after injection, and lasts 10–16 hours.
- Intermediate-Acting: Reaching the bloodstream 90 minutes after injection, intermediate-acting insulin peaks 4 to 12 hours later and lasts in the blood for about 24 hours. There are two varieties of this type of insulin: Lente (called L) and NPH (called N).
- Long-Acting: These insulins, which take 4 to 6 hours for onset, are at maximum strength 14 to 24 hours after injection, lasting 36 hours in the bloodstream. Long-acting insulin is referred to as U, for Ultralente.

SOURCE:

Juvenile Diabetes Foundation. *Information about Insulin*. December 1990. pp. 1, 3.

DIABETIC EMERGENCIES—HYPOGLYCEMIA AND HYPERGLYCEMIA

As you regulate your blood glucose and keep your diabetes record, there are two problems that you need to be able to recognize and treat: hypoglycemia and hyperglycemia. The first, hypoglycemia or an insulin reaction, can happen if you are taking insulin or oral medications.

Hypoglycemia means low blood glucose. This reaction happens when there is not enough glucose in your blood.

The most common causes of hypoglycemia are:

- too much insulin
- too much exercise
- not enough food

A hypoglycemic reaction comes on very suddenly. It often happens at the time when insulin action is at its peak, during or after strenuous exercise, or when a meal is delayed. Most people learn to recognize their own symptoms of an insulin reaction.

If you start feeling any symptoms or if you think your blood glucose may be too low, the best way to be sure is to check your blood level using a blood glucose test strip. If your blood glucose is less than 70 mg/dl, then you are probably having a hypoglycemic reaction.

Some symptoms that you may notice are:

- sweating, weakness, anxiety, trembling, fast heartbeat
- inability to think straight, irritability, grouchiness
- hunger
- headache
- sleepiness

If untreated, low blood glucose can lead to confusion, coma or convulsions.

Hypoglycemia comes on rather quickly, usually within minutes. If you have a hypoglycemic reaction, you should treat it immediately by eating some form of carbohydrate (sugar). You need to have something like glucose tablets or sugar cubes with you at all times to take at the first sign of a reaction. Your body needs fast-acting sugar at that time.

After you have an insulin reaction, you need to think about why the reaction happened. Perhaps your meal was late, you got too much exercise, or you took your medication at a different time. Very often, reactions can be avoided by closely following your treatment plan.

Contact your physician or nurse for further advice if you are having insulin reactions more than once a week, or if you can't identify the cause of your insulin reactions.

The second problem that you need to be aware of is hyperglycemia or high blood glucose. The signs of high blood glucose may be the same as the symptoms you had when you learned you had diabetes. These include:

- blood glucose over 240 mg/dl
- more urine output than usual
- increased thirst
- dry skin and mouth
- decreased appetite, nausea or vomiting
- fatigue, drowsiness, or no energy

Hyperglycemia usually occurs slowly, over several hours or days. It may be caused by:

- not taking enough insulin
- an illness (such as a cold or flu)
- an infection
- eating too much
- stress
- certain medications

If symptoms of hyperglycemia occur:

1. Take your usual insulin dose. DO NOT SKIP IT!

2. Keep eating your meals.

3. Test your blood for glucose and your urine for ketones every two hours.

4. CONTACT YOUR DOCTOR OR NURSE FOR ADVICE.

In people with Type I diabetes, untreated hyperglycemia may lead to a build-up of ketones (ketoacids) in the bloodstream. The kidneys try to get rid of the ketones by spilling them into the urine. As the blood glucose and ketones (ketoacids) rise higher and higher, large amounts of glucose, ketones, and water are lost through the kidneys. You can detect ketones in your urine by testing your urine with ketone test strips. Test your urine for ketones whenever your blood glucose level is 300 mg/dl or higher.

If left untreated, this process results in dehydration, thirst, low blood pressure, high blood glucose and ketoacidosis. This is a life-threatening event which must be treated immediately.

SOURCE:
Barnett, Carol, and Martha M. Funnell. *Life with Diabetes: Diabetes Defined.* Ann Arbor, MI: Michigan Diabetes Research Center, University of Michigan, 1987. pp. 15-17.

PANCREAS TRANSPLANTS

There have been several approaches to transplantation used to provide healthy insulin producing cells to the person with Type I diabetes. Two approaches use whole pancreases (obtained from cadavers) or segments of pancreases (which can be donated by a living person). A third, highly experimental approach has been to transplant insulin-producing cells (obtained primarily from cadavers).

Finding adequate numbers of donors presents a challenge, not only in diabetes but also in other organ transplant areas (such as kidney, heart and liver transplants). There are many more potential recipients waiting for transplants than there are donors.

There is serious concern about placing the donor of a pancreas segment at risk for future development of diabetes. Scientists are studying this problem at the present time.

One area that shows great promise is the transplantation of insulin-producing islet cells. Scientists are working on methods to pretreat cells with ultraviolet rays before they are transplanted, to protect them against rejection.

Other scientists are working on placing these cells inside plastic bubbles or membranes to protect them. At the present time, most medical centers doing transplants will do these procedures on persons with diabetes who also are having kidney transplants because of kidney failure related to diabetes. Since the recipients of kidney transplants must have anti-rejection treatment anyway, they are not at increased risk when they take these potentially toxic drugs after implantation of a whole or partial pancreas or islet cells.

If your pancreas is not functioning properly, one of the ways to handle this problem is to replace it. Transplanting healthy, functioning organs (whole, partial or cells only) is one approach. The other approach is to create an artificial (man-made) pancreas.

The closest thing to an artificial pancreas that scientists have developed is an "open loop" insulin infusion pump. This device is called "open loop" because the person using it must instruct the pump to release a specific amount of insulin. The user must measure his or her own blood glucose levels and instruct the pump to deliver the appropriate amounts of insulin based on these measurements.

SOURCE:
Beaser, Richard S., Gordon C. Weir, and Joan Hill. "Diabetes Research Update." *Diabetes in the News* 10 (January-February 1991): 9-10.

DIABETIC RETINOPATHY

If you are among the 10 million people in the United States who have diabetes—or if someone close to you has this disease—you should know that diabetes can affect the eyes and cause visual impairment. . . .

Diabetic retinopathy is a potentially serious eye disease caused by diabetes. It affects the retina—the light-sensitive tissue at the back of the eye that transmits visual messages to the brain. Damage to this delicate tissue may result in visual impairment or blindness.

Diabetic retinopathy begins with a slight deterioration in the small blood vessels of the retina. Portions of the vessel walls balloon outward and fluid starts to leak from the vessels into the surrounding retinal tissue. Generally, these initial changes in the retina cause no visual symptoms. However, they can be detected by an eye specialist who is trained to recognize subtle signs of retinal disease.

In many people with diabetic retinopathy, the disease remains mild and never causes visual problems. But in some individuals, continued leakage from the retinal blood vessels leads to macular edema. This is a build-up of fluid in the macula—the part of the retina responsible for the sharp, clear vision used in reading and driving. When critical areas of the macula become swollen with excess fluid, vision may be so badly blurred that these activities become difficult or impossible.

Some people with diabetes develop an even more sight-threatening condition called proliferative retinopathy. It may occur in people who have macular edema, but also can develop in those who don't. In proliferative retinopathy, abnormal new blood vessels grow on the surface of the retina. These fragile new vessels can easily rupture and bleed into the middle of the eye, blocking vision. Scar tissue also may form near the retina, ultimately detaching it from the back of the eye. Severe visual loss, even permanent blindness, may result. But this happens in only a small minority of people with diabetes.

SOURCE:
National Eye Institute. *Diabetic Retinopathy*. November 1990. pp 1–2.

DIABETIC DIET—AMERICAN DIABETES ASSOCIATION RECOMMENDATION

The American Diabetes Foundation's recommended diet is spelled out in "Nutritional Recommendations and Principles for Individuals with Diabetes Mellitus: 1986," published in the January/February 1987 issue of *Diabetes Care*. These recommendations call for a diet that contains:

- Ideally, up to 55 to 60 percent of calories from carbohydrates. These carbohydrates should be mainly complex carbohydrates and naturally occurring sugars, like those in milk and fruits.
- 0.8 gram of protein per kilogram of body weight. This is about 54 grams for a 150-pound person.
- Less than 30 percent of calories from fat. Unsaturated fats (vegetable oils or margarine) are preferable to saturated fat (meats and dairy products).
- Up to 40 grams per day of fiber, particularly the soluble form of fiber found in beans, oat products, and fruits.
- Less than 1,000 milligrams of sodium per 1,000 calories, not to exceed 3,000 milligrams of sodium per day. 1,000 milligrams of sodium is equal to about 2,500 milligrams of salt (about ½ teaspoon).
- Less than 300 milligrams of cholesterol per day.

In deciding whether an advertised food would be appropriate for your diet, read the label carefully. Some label terms have definitions set by the Food and Drug Administration (FDA). Others are used loosely and may not tell much about the product. Here are commonly used label terms and what they mean:

- Low-calorie foods can have no more than 40 calories per serving and 0.4 calories per gram.
- Reduced-calorie products have at least one-third fewer calories than a regular product.
- Diet or dietetic. A product that is labeled "diet" or "dietetic" must meet the standards for low-calorie or reduced-calorie food or make a claim of special dietary usefulness.
- Sugarless, sugar-free, or no-sugar. Products labeled "sugar-free" may contain certain sweeteners, such as xylitol or the sugar alcohol sorbitol, that have as many calories as table sugar (sucrose). These foods may raise your blood-glucose levels less than sucrose, but they contain the same number of calories and must be factored into your meal plan. Because consumers have a right to expect that something labeled "sugar-free" is low or reduced in calories, the label must alert them if this is not the case. A product sweetened with a calorie-containing sweetener like sorbitol must carry a warning such as "Not a reduced-calorie food" or "Not for weight control."
- No added salt means that no salt has been added in the preparation of the product. What is naturally in a product will still be there.
- Sodium labeling has precise definitions. Sodium-free means less than 5 milligrams of sodium per serving. Very low sodium means less than 35 milligrams per serving. Low sodium is less than 140 milligrams per serving.
- Light and lite do not have precise definitions. Generally, if a light product is intended for weight loss, it must meet the requirements for low- or reduced-calorie foods.

In addition to looking for these specific terms, be sure to check the nutrition labeling on a product. Any product that makes nutritional claims must have a nutrition label listing how many calories and how much protein, carbohydrate, and fat are in a serving. The nutritional label must also tell the U.S. Recommended Daily Allowance of protein and seven specified vitamins and minerals.

SOURCE:
"Nutrition Notes." *Diabetes Forecast* (March 1990): 12–13. Reproduced with permission from *Diabetes Forecast*, March 1990.

RESOURCES

ORGANIZATIONS

American Diabetes Foundation. National Service Center, P.O. Box 25757, 1660 Duke St., Alexandria, VA 22313.

National Diabetes Information Clearinghouse. P.O. Box NDIC, Bethesda, MD 20892.

University of Michigan Diabetes Research and Training Center. S2310 Old Main Hospital, 1500 East Medical Center Drive, Ann Arbor, MI 48109.

PAMPHLETS

American Diabetes Association:

Adults: Diabetes and You. 1989. 44 pp.

Children: Diabetes and You. 1987. 16 pp.

Seniors: Diabetes and You. 1987. 40 pp.

What You Need to Know about Diabetes. 1989. 6 pp.

California Medical Association:

"Self-Blood Glucose Monitoring for Diabetics." *HealthTips* index 448 (February 1990): 2 pp.

Juvenile Diabetes Foundation International:

Monitoring Your Blood Sugar. n.d. 4 pp.

What You Should Know about Juvenile (Insulin-Dependent) Diabetes. 1983. 9 pp.

National Institute of Arthritis, Diabetes & Digestive & Kidney Diseases:

Insulin Dependent Diabetes. NIH Pub. No. 90-2098. 1990. 21 pp.

Non-Insulin Dependent Diabetes. NIH Pub. No. 87-241. 1987.

BOOKS

American Diabetes Association. *Diabetes in the Family.* Revised editions. Englewood Cliffs, NJ: Prentice-Hall, 1987. 190 pp.

American Diabetes Association, and American Dietetic Association. *Family Cookbook.* Volume III. Englewood Cliffs, NJ: Prentice-Hall, 1987. 434 pp.

Krall, Leo P., and Richard S. Beaser. *Joslin Diabetes Manual.* 12th edition. Philadelphia: Lea & Febiger, 1989. 406 pp.

RELATED ARTICLES

Bantle, John P. "The Dietary Treatment of Diabetes Mellitus." *Medical Clinics of North America* 72, no. 6 (November 1988): 1285-1299.

Bohannon, Nancy J. V. "Diabetes in the Elderly: A Unique Set of Management Challenges." *Postgraduate Medicine* 84, no. 5 (October 1988): 283-295.

Molitch, Mark E. "Diabetes Mellitus: Control and Complications." *Postgraduate Medicine* 85, no. 4 (March 1989): 182-194.

Nash, J. Madeleine. "A Slow, Savage Killer: Scientists Are Battling High Blood Sugar, the Overlooked Affliction That Strikes Millions." *Time* (November 26, 1990): 52-54.

Soon-Shiong, Patrick, and Robert P. Lanza. "Pancreas and Islet-Cell Transplantation: Potential Cure for Diabetes." *Postgraduate Medicine* 87, no. 8 (June 1990): 133-134, 139-140.

"Transplantation or Insulin." *The Lancet* 335, no. 8702 (June 9, 1990): 1371-1372.

DIARRHEA

(*See also:* CONSTIPATION; IRRITABLE BOWEL SYNDROME)

OVERVIEW

Most people have frequent, watery bowel movements for 1 or 2 days each year. This change from the usual pattern of stools is recognized as diarrhea and called by many different names. Symptoms commonly disappear in a short time, and the only important effect is that water and salts are lost from the body. For most people, the episode is more an inconvenience than an illness. But sometimes diarrhea lasts for weeks or months, and then it can be an indication of major disease. This more serious form of diarrhea may be accompanied by blood, mucus, or undigested food in the stools. The disease causing diarrhea may also produce fever, abdominal cramps, weight loss, nausea, and/or vomiting. So, we should try to separate the mild and short-lived episodes of diarrhea from continuous and severe diarrhea with these other features.

A hundred or more different diseases can cause diarrhea. Fortunately, most of the severe causes are rare and the most common form is the one that affects most of us for a few days each year. It is due to a simple infection usually caused by a virus. The more serious causes include ulcerative colitis (when blood is usually present in the stools), regional ileitis (Crohn's disease), some forms of intestinal cancer (when pain and weight loss might also be present), and some disorders of the intestine that lead to poor digestion of food. "Nervous diarrhea," which is part of the irritable bowel syndrome (IBS), is very common and often shows up briefly when we face the stress of a term paper or a job interview. However, some people suffer nervous stress fairly constantly and may have continuous diarrhea because of it. We shall not consider nervous diarrhea, ulcerative colitis, or cancer any further in this fact sheet.

The common illness, which may last several days, often called "intestinal flu," is often due to one of a number of viruses that infect the bowel, making it weep fluid. The excess of fluid in the bowel leads to liquid stools. The inflammation may also be associated with cramping abdominal pain, nausea, and vomiting.

Other common infectious diarrheas may be caused by bacteria. These bacteria irritate the bowel and make it pour out fluid. The inflammation may also be associated with cramping abdominal pain. "Travelers' diarrhea" is due to particular bacteria common in certain areas of the world. People living in these areas are usually well adjusted to the bacteria, but people who are new arrivals are susceptible to these bacterial infections. Although most infectious diarrheas are brief illnesses, some do not go away after a few days. More serious forms can be caused by microbes other than bacteria, such as amoebae and giardia, that can become established in the bowel and cause problems that persist for weeks or months. Contaminated food or water, public swimming pools, and communal hot tubs are possible sources of these infections.

Mild forms are very common and insignificant, apart from minor discomforts and perhaps the loss of a few days from work. Nevertheless, mild gastrointestinal upsets are among the most common reasons for absences from work and are costly to society because of this. Between one-quarter and one-half of visitors to foreign countries develop travelers' diarrhea; most episodes are mild. However, infectious diarrhea can have serious consequences in certain persons. Young infants, very old people, or those who have major illnesses can be seriously weakened by even a minor infection. Simple infectious diarrhea is still a major killer in underdeveloped countries, where infections of the bowel are estimated to cause millions of deaths annually among infants.

SOURCE:
National Digestive Diseases Information Clearinghouse. Phillips, Sidney F. *Diarrhea: Infections and Other Causes.* NIH Pub. No. 86-2749. 1985. pp. 1-2.

CAUSED BY ANTIBIOTICS

Antibiotics save lives, but they can also cause serious illness. As many as 20% of patients who take them develop diarrhea, occasionally accompanied by colitis and sometimes by pseudomembranous colitis (PMC), a life threatening superinfection.

Nearly every antibiotic can cause diarrhea. It's more than likely to happen, however, with oral or multiple antibiotic therapy. The most common culprits are clindamycin, ampicillin, the cephalosporins, and the aminoglycosides (excluding parenteral gentamycin and tobramycin).

Symptoms may begin within hours of the first dose or may not show up for weeks after the patient finishes the course of therapy. Neither dosage nor duration of treatment predicts the occurrence of diarrhea.

What it is [that] antibiotics do to cause diarrhea hasn't been firmly established. They may irritate the intestinal mucosa directly, reducing its absorption capacity and increasing motility, or they may work indirectly, by promoting overgrowths of pathogens that produce irritating toxins. Antibiotics are also known to kill lactobacilli, bacteroides, and other anaerobes that protect the intestine against harmful bacteria such as *Clostridium difficile, Shigella, Salmonella, Staphylococcus,* and *Yersinia.*

In some cases, patients do not develop antibiotic-associated diarrhea even though their stool cultures show overgrowths of *C. difficile* and other pathogens. Newborns, in fact, frequently have similar overgrowths with no symptoms at all; a glycoprotein found in breast milk, it's believed, may protect their mucosa against toxins.

A recent study suggests that a non-pathogenic yeast, *Saccharomyces boulardii,* may have some prophylactic value. Patients who took the yeast before starting antibiotic therapy were less likely to develop diarrhea than those who received a placebo. Eating yogurt or other products containing live lactobacilli also helps some people.

SOURCE:
Rowland, Marie A. "When Drug Therapy Causes Diarrhea." *RN* 52 (December 1989): 32.

SELF-TREATMENT

Adult patients with acute, nonspecific diarrhea should be advised to decrease their activity until they feel better or the diarrhea resolves. Adequate hydration is extremely important. The patient should be encouraged to take clear liquids, such as ginger ale, decaffeinated cola, decaffeinated tea, broth, Gatorade, and gelatin for the first 24 hours or until the vomiting and diarrhea stop. The patient should be encouraged to drink two to three liters of fluid a day, because most complications associated with diarrhea result from the loss of fluids and electrolytes.

During the next 24 hours, the patient may eat bland foods, such as cooked cereals, rice, soup, bread, crackers, baked potatoes, eggs, or applesauce. Fruits, vegetables, fried or spicy foods, bran, candy, and caffeinated and alcoholic beverages should be avoided. The patient may progress to his or her regular diet after two or three days.

The symptoms of acute, nonspecific diarrhea may be controlled with over-the-counter medications. Loperamide, a recently marketed antidiarrheal agent, helps decrease the frequency of loose bowel movements. Loperamide normalizes bowel motility and prolongs the transit time of intestinal contents. In addition, loperamide enhances absorption and reduces secretion, thereby diminishing the loss of fluids and electrolytes.

Bismuth subsalicylate is often used for the treatment of travelers' diarrhea. However, a large volume of bismuth subsalicylate is usually required for efficacy.

Whereas kaolin and pectin have been used since ancient times for diarrhea, well-controlled studies documenting their clinical efficacy are lacking.

Parents of an infant who has acute diarrhea should be warned to watch for significant fever. Fever alone may not be cause for concern, but may be significant in relation to other symptoms that may be present, such as vomiting and dehydration. Parents should monitor the infant's rectal temperature several times a day. Good hygiene is important to avoid contaminating other family members (parents should wash their hands after handling the infant and before preparing food).

The child should be closely observed for signs and symptoms of dehydration. For the first 24 hours, the child should receive only clear liquids. Osmotically balanced fluids such as Lytren (Mead Johnson Nutritionals) or Pedialyte (Ross Laboratories) can be obtained at a pharmacy or grocery store.

SOURCE:
Brownlee, H. James., Jr. "Family Practitioner's Guide to Patient Self-Treatment of Acute Diarrhea." *American Journal of Medicine* 88 (suppl. 6A) (June 20, 1990): 6A-27S-6A-29S.

TRAVELERS' DIARRHEA

All travelers from industrialized countries going to developing countries quickly develop a rapid, dramatic change in their intestinal flora. These new organisms often include the potential enteric pathogens. Those who develop diarrhea have ingested an inoculum of virulent organisms sufficiently large to overcome individual defense mechanisms, resulting in symptoms. . . .

TD is usually a mild, self-limited disorder, with complete recovery even in the absence of therapy; hence, therapy should be considered optional.

1. Fluids should be taken as described above.

2. If rapid relief of symptoms is desired after one or two unformed stools accompanied by cramps, nausea, or malaise, diphenoxylate [Lomotil] or loperamide may be taken. An alternative is to start bismuth subsalicylate (1 oz every 30 minutes for eight doses). Although this regimen decreases the number of stools and increases their consistency, the beneficial activity of bismuth subsalicylate is somewhat slower than that of antimotility drugs.

3. If it is important to shorten the course or decrease the severity of moderate to severe TD, antimicrobial agents may be taken. After three or more loose stools with symptoms, consideration can be given to a short course of TMP/SMX [Trimethoprim/Sulfamethoxazole—Bactrim] or TMP alone or doxycycline.

4. A small percentage of travelers have persisting diarrhea with serious fluid loss, fever, and blood or mucus in the stools. This suggests that a more serious illness is involved, and such individuals should seek medical attention.

In conclusion, travelers to areas of high risk should obtain an antimotility drug or bismuth subsalicylate for milder forms of TD, and an antimicrobial agent (TMP/SMX or TMP alone or doxycycline) for more severe TD. Advice concerning side effects of these drugs and various aspects of hygiene and dietary precautions should be obtained. By obtaining the proper drugs in advance, the beleaguered traveler might avoid buying over-the-counter drugs abroad with potentially dangerous ingredients.

SOURCE:

NIH Office of Medical Applications of Research. "Travelers' Diarrhea." *NIH Consensus Development Conference Statement* 5, no. 8. n.d. pp. 2, 4–5.

RESOURCES

ORGANIZATION

National Digestive Disease Information Clearinghouse. Box NDDIC, Bethesda, MD 20892.

RELATED ARTICLES

"Advice for Travelers." *The Medical Letter on Drugs and Therapeutics*. 32, no. 815 (April 6, 1990): 33–36.

Avery, Mary Ellen and John D. Snyder. "Oral Therapy for Acute Diarrhea." *New England Journal of Medicine* 323, no. 13 (September 27, 1990): 891–894.

Cohn, Jeffrey P. and Dori Stehlin. "Preventing 'Turista' and Other Travelers' Ailments." *FDA Consumer* 25 (March 1991): 24–27.

Dukes, George E. "Over-the-Counter Antidiarrheal Medications Used for the Self-Treatment of Acute Nonspecific Diarrhea." *American Journal of Medicine* 88 (suppl. 6A) (June 20, 1990): 6A-24S - 6A-26S.

Ross, Phillip E. "Competition Promises More Options for Diarrhea Treatment." *New York Times* (March 30, 1989).

DIETARY FATS

(*See also:* FOOD/NUTRITION GUIDELINES)

OVERVIEW

Heart disease is a chronic disease. It takes years to develop symptoms. There is no single cause, but we recognize many factors that increase the risk for its development. After years of research into the reasons for rapid development of atherosclerosis, most scientists agree on two of these. First, high levels of low-density lipoproteins (LDL higher than 160 milligrams per deciliter [mg/dl]) increase the risk. Second, low levels of high-density lipoproteins (HDL lower than 40 mg/dl) increase the risk as well.

Saturated fat, the "heavy" in any number of other health problems, is implicated in heart disease, as well, because of its effect of raising the level of LDL cholesterol in the blood. A person's LDL cholesterol depends primarily on his or her liver's ability to remove LDL from the bloodstream. To do this job effectively requires the presence of receptors on the outside of cells. The number of LDL receptors in the liver appears to decline when diets are high in saturated fat (greater than 7% to 10% of total calories). Hence, if you need to lower your LDL cholesterol to decrease your risk of heart disease, avoid saturated fats.

Sources of saturated fats are usually easy to identify: they tend to be animal fats and other fats that are hard at room temperature. This includes the liquid dairy fat in milk and cream. In addition to animal fats, palm and coconut oils are high saturated fat culprits. Vegetable oils, liquid at room temperatures, have mostly unsaturated fats—monounsaturated (canola oil and olive oil) and polyunsaturated (corn oil, peanut oil, soybean oil, safflower oil, and sunflower oil). Both monounsaturated and polyunsaturated fats are excellent dietary substitutes for saturated fat. Research . . . has shown corn and safflower oil to have the best results in reducing blood cholesterol levels. Research in other laboratories supports the use of the other vegetable oils. Actually, every vegetable oil is a mixture of all three types of fats. We classify an oil based on its predominant fat content. Corn oil and soybean oil are often the least expensive and are therefore highly cost-effective.

Currently about 15% of the calories Americans eat come from saturated fat. Cutting down to the recommended 7% to 10% is not that hard, but it does take some commitment to making changes. . . Your major focus should be on the foods in your diet that contribute most to your saturated fat intake. In the average American diet, the following foods account for much of our intake of saturated fat:

Hamburgers and cheeseburgers. Response: broil the meat and leave off the cheese (omit bacon as well).

Whole milk. Response: switch to 2%, 1%, ½%, or skim milk; the lower the fat the better.

Cheese (excluding cottage). Response: use low-fat varieties like mozzarella and limit intake. Some new diet cheeses are also low in saturated fat; nevertheless, limited intake is advised.

Beef steaks, roasts. Response: roast, bake, or broil these. Trim fat well before cooking and at the table.

Hot dogs, ham, lunch meats. Response: eat hot dogs sparingly and choose lean varieties of ham and other lean lunch meats, such as turkey, tuna, and chicken.

Doughnuts, cakes, and cookies. Response: at home make these with liquid vegetable oils. With cookies, make sheet cookies, as the oil substitution causes cookies to spread. Frost cakes with 7-minute icing, powdered sugar, fruit glazes, or scant amounts of regular frosting. When away from home, seek out the new fat-free cake varieties, omit frosting (or most of it), and limit intake of baked goods made with shortening or butter.

Lowering saturated fat intake is more important than reducing dietary cholesterol in reducing LDL levels. Only about 25% of people are able to lower their LDL cholesterol level much by eating less cholesterol than we usually eat. Most people show only a minimal effect, or no effect at all. However, almost everyone who lowers saturated fat intake can lower an elevated serum cholesterol level about 10% to 20%, especially if he or she is currently eating the typical American diet high in saturated fats.

The bottom line is that anyone with a high LDL cholesterol level should be concerned about heart disease. To minimize your risk, learn how to reduce saturated fat intake.

SOURCE:
Wardlaw, Gordon. "Reducing Saturated Fat Helps Lower Cholesterol." *Healthline* (July 1990): 11–12.

CLASSIFICATION OF OILS

Vegetable oils are made up of a mixture of compounds called fatty acids. Individually, the fatty acids are known as saturated, polyunsaturated or monounsaturated, depending on their chemical structures. When more than one-third of the fatty acids in an oil are saturated, then the oil itself is considered to be a saturated oil. When less than one-third of the fatty acids are saturated, the oil is considered unsaturated. Unsaturated oils are then further classified into polyunsaturated and monounsaturated, depending on which type predominates.

Saturated Oils. Oils containing primarily saturated fatty acids raise blood cholesterol levels, and are the least heart-healthy. The majority of saturated fats like lard, beef tallow or butterfat come from animals. A few saturated fats, however, come from plants, namely the tropical oils—coconut, palm and palm kernel. While these tropical oils contain no cholesterol (all vegetable oils and plant food are cholesterol-free), they do raise cholesterol in the blood. In fact, saturated fats in the diet are more potent raisers of blood cholesterol than cholesterol-containing foods.

Although not available in supermarkets as bottled cooking oils, tropical oils, until recently, have been widely used in processed foods such as cookies, cakes, pastries and nondairy creamers. Food manufacturers have used them because they're less expensive than soybean oil, have a long shelf life and, according to manufacturers, consumers like the taste they impart to foods in cooking.

Now, however, consumers are demanding that the highly saturated oils be removed from products. So, many manufacturers have switched from tropical oils to partially hydrogenated soybean oils. It's a step in the right direction. Though tropical oils never constituted a high percentage of our fat intake (about 1 to 2 percent), the trend to reformulate products without them is welcome.

Current Advice: Limit saturated fat to less than 10% of total calories (or one-third of fat intake).

SOURCE:
Helm, Janet. "EN's Guide to Heart-Healthy Oils." *Environmental Nutrition* 12 (August 1989): 1–2.

CALCULATING FAT CONTENT

To make sure that no more than 30 percent of total calories come from fat, all anyone needs to do is figure out the average number of calories in the foods eaten daily, take 30 percent of that average, and then divide by 9 to determine how many grams of fat will squeeze into the particular figure arrived at. The formula becomes clearer with an example. Take 39-year-old Carol. She has been trying in a casual way to follow a low-fat diet for some time simply as a matter of principle but now realizes it's something she's going to have to get serious about; she has just gone for her first physical in many years and has learned that she has high blood cholesterol. Carol is at an advantage since, as an on-again, off-again dieter, she has learned the approximate number of calories in most of the items she eats and already knows that she takes in about 1,800 calories a day. Her next step is to figure out 30 percent of 1,800, which is accomplished by multiplying 1,800 by .30 for a total of 540. In other words, she has 540 calories a day to "spend" on fat. The question now becomes how many grams of fat can "fit" into 540 calories. Since each gram comes to 9 calories, all she has to do is divide 540 by 9 for a total of 60 grams. Sixty grams may not sound like much. After all, it takes about 28 grams to make one ounce, and that means Carol is allowed only a drop more than 2 ounces of fat a day. But depending on the foods she chooses, she can do extremely well. In fact, the less fat she eats, the more food she can fit into her 1,800-calorie plan.

Why? When you cut out fat, you cut out the greatest single source of calories in the diet. Consider that two Hostess Ding Dongs and one large plum weigh the same amount—75 grams—but 20 of the Ding Dongs' grams come from fat, and just half a gram of fat is in the plum. That difference is a large part of the reason that Ding Dongs contain 345 calories and the plum, only 41. Another way of putting it is that even if you ate eight times the weight of the Ding Dongs in plums, you'd still be taking in only 4 grams of fat and 328 calories, 17 fewer than the 345-calorie Ding Dong total. It's the same with grains, which are also quite low in fat. It would take three slices of whole-wheat bread to make the weight of the Ding Dongs, but since each slice has only about one gram of fat, the calorie count subsequently comes out comparatively low—183 calories or 61 calories a slice. Indeed, even five slices of whole-wheat bread—an amount few people would eat in a day, let alone one sitting—contain just 5 grams of fat and fewer than 345 calories. None of this is to say that a Ding Dong—or two—should forever be off-limits. It does mean, however, that if you ought to be consuming in the neighborhood of 60 grams of fat a day and one of the items you choose contains 20 of those grams, you are using up a third of your fat "allowance" right there and will surely go over the prudent fat and calorie limit you have set for yourself if you do that too many times.

It should be fairly easy at this point to determine the maximum number of grams of fat to be eaten in a day—60 for the 1,800-calorie woman, 67 for the 2,000-calorie man, 50 for the 1,500 calorie dieter, and so on. But there is still the problem of knowing how many grams of fat are in each food consumed. Many items do not carry nutrition labels, so there is no way of learning their fat content by looking at the package.

SOURCE:
"What Is a Gram of Fat . . . and How Many Should You Eat?" *Tufts University Diet and Nutrition Letter* 7 (October 1989): 5–7.

DIETARY FATS—LINKED TO HEART DISEASE

Because people with high blood cholesterol have a high rate of heart disease, because a low-fat diet can reduce blood cholesterol levels, and because "the magnitude of the problem posed by elevated blood cholesterol levels is very clear," NCEP [National Cholesterol Education Program] on Feb. 27 [1990] recommended that all Americans over 2 reduce the saturated fat and cholesterol content of their diets.

FDA, along with a coalition of 39 federal agencies and health organizations, endorsed the recommendation. F. Edward Scarbrough, Ph.D., acting director of FDA's office of nutrition and food sciences, points out that disease may develop from many years of eating a diet high in saturated fat and that dietary habits are established long before an individual is diagnosed with coronary heart disease. "Eating a healthy diet makes good disease prevention sense in general," says Scarbrough.

Good disease prevention, according to the new NCEP recommendations, includes a diet containing:

- less than 10 percent of total calories from saturated fatty acids
- an average of 30 percent of total calories or less from all fat
- total calories necessary to reach or maintain a desirable body weight
- less than 300 milligrams of cholesterol per day

According to the report, the major decrease in total fat should be in calories from saturated fatty acids. Saturated fat raises blood cholesterol more than anything else in the diet, even more than dietary cholesterol. Saturated fats usually are solid at room temperature. They are present in largest amounts in animal products such as butter, cheese and meat. (Whole milk, which has a relatively high saturated fat content—5.1 grams in 8 ounces—is one exception to this guideline.)

SOURCE:
Blumenthal, David. "Making Sense of the Cholesterol Controversy." *FDA Consumer* 24 (June 1990): 14.

RESOURCES

RELATED ARTICLES

Drewnowski, Adam. "The New Fat Replacements: A Strategy for Reducing Fat Consumption." *Postgraduate Medicine* 87, no. 6 (May 1, 1990): 111–114, 117–118, 121.

Green, Michael H. "A Perspective on Dietary Fats, Plasma Cholesterol and Atherosclerosis." *Nutrition Today* 24 (June 1989): 6–8.

Kleiner, Susan M. "Tropical vs. Hydrogenated Oils." *Executive Health Report* 26 (August 1990): 7.

Shields, Jo Ellen, and Eleanor Young. "Fat in Fast Foods—Evolving Changes." *Nutrition Today* (March/April 1990): 32–35.

Task Force on Cholesterol Issues, American Heart Association. "The Cholesterol Facts. A Summary of the Evidence Relating Dietary Fats, Serum Cholesterol, and Coronary Heart Disease." *Circulation* 81, no. 5 (May 1990): 1721–1733.

Trevisan, Maurizio, and others. "Consumption of Olive Oil, Butter, and Vegetable Oils and Coronary Heart Disease Risk Factors." *JAMA* 263, no. 5 (February 2, 1990): 688–692.

DIETARY FIBER

(*See also:* FOOD/NUTRITION GUIDELINES)

OVERVIEW

For almost a generation, dietary fiber has been a household word and has carried a remarkably persuasive aura of disease prevention. Both the public and cereal companies have taken up dietary fiber with great enthusiasm. Consumers can now rate breakfast cereals by the amount of fiber listed on the box and take particular note if the cereal contains oat bran, a source of soluble fiber thought to be of particular merit. What is truth and what is fiction about dietary fiber?

Fiber is present in all plant foods that have had no more than a minimum of processing. Thus, our ancestors consumed considerable amounts of fiber, since their diet was composed of coarse foods little altered by technology. When the milling of wheat produced a white flour almost devoid of roughage or bran, there were rebels who decried this diminution of what nature had provided. One of these rebels was a New England clergyman named Sylvester Graham. His name is now affixed to graham crackers and graham flour, both foodstuffs with a high fiber content. Graham was a fervent, widely traveled speaker who advocated eating home-baked bread made of coarse, unsifted flour and, among other things, the use of a hard mattress and cold showers, which he regarded as reasonable prescriptions for a healthy life.

In the modern era, however, we owe much of the public and scientific interest in dietary fiber to two medical missionaries working at Makerere Medical College in Kampala, Uganda. They were Dr. Denis Burkitt and Dr. H. C. Trowell, both astute observers of the epidemiology of human disease who achieved fame apart from their views on dietary fiber. Burkitt discovered Burkitt's lymphoma, and Trowell described an important disease of infant malnutrition, kwashiorkor. They also noted the rarity of many "Western" diseases in the Africans whom they treated. Their patients did not have coronary heart disease, hypertension, diabetes, or, in particular, certain common gastrointestinal disorders such as constipation, diverticulitis, hemorrhoids, appendicitis, cancer of the large bowel, or hiatal hernia. Trowell and Burkitt developed the "fiber hypothesis": these diseases did not occur in Africans because their diet contained much roughage that had been purified out of the Western diet. Burkitt, in particular, spoke widely in this country before medical audiences about the importance of dietary fiber and abundant stools. One maxim attributed to him (and paraphrased here) should be noted by those concerned about the cost of medical care: the size and frequency of the stools of a population are inversely proportional to the number of hospital visits. A high-fiber diet, he believed, might prevent many of the Western diseases rarely seen in sub-Saharan Africa, where the diet was rich in relatively unprocessed plant foods.

A high-fiber diet is now widely accepted as treatment for patients with constipation, diverticulitis, or hemorrhoids. The link to the prevention of coronary heart disease rests largely on the possible effects of dietary fiber on plasma lipid levels. Such effects may be mediated by the promotion of bile-acid excretion in the stool or by the blockage of cholesterol absorption. Some dietary fibers do bind bile acids and thus may have a cholesterol-lowering effect similar to that of the bile-acid-sequestrant drugs.

It is important now to put the fiber hypothesis into perspective. Most therapeutic low-cholesterol, low-saturated-fat diets call for the replacement of dietary saturated fat and cholesterol-rich foods with carbohydrates containing starch and fiber. One could use a variety of starchy carbohydrates, such as rice, potatoes, pasta, bread, beans, any one of many cereal products, including oat bran, and fruits and vegetables—all of which would provide the wide range of choices necessary in any program of dietary change.

Perhaps even more important are the beneficial gastrointestinal effects of a diet high in fiber. Besides preventing constipation, hemorrhoids, and possibly diverticulitis, dietary fiber may have a role in preventing cancer of the large bowel, which is rapidly becoming the most common cancer in the United States. Colon cancers have been prevented in laboratory animals by dietary fiber, and there is good reason for supposing that potential carcinogens in the intestinal contents would be diluted, bound, and more rapidly passed out of the system by a diet high in fiber. However, much remains to be learned.

SOURCE:
Connor, William E. "Dietary Fiber—Nostrum or Critical Nutrient?" (editorial). *The New England Journal of Medicine* 322 (3) (January 18, 1990): 193–195.

RECOMMENDED INTAKE

Information on levels of dietary fiber intakes in the US population is very limited, and available only for adults. Data have been derived using a variety of measurement methods (diet records, food disappearance, experimental diets, etc.) and are based on a variety of methods of food analysis. There is no single, universally acceptable method for determining total dietary fiber. Analytic procedures may yield dietary fiber values for a single food that differ by 100%. Currently, US food composition tables give values for "crude fiber." The procedures for determining crude fiber destroy all the soluble fiber fraction and variable amounts of insoluble fiber. Thus, total dietary fiber content, the sum of soluble and insoluble fibers, is greatly underestimated. . . .

The ideal dietary fiber intake has not been defined; a Recommended Dietary Allowance for dietary fiber has not been established. However, there is general agreement that dietary fiber is part of a healthful diet. The advice concerning dietary fiber, "eat foods with adequate starch and fiber," given in Dietary Guidelines for Americans seems reasonable. An adequate amount of dietary fiber can be obtained by choosing several servings daily from a variety of fiber-rich foods such as whole-grain breads and cereals, fruits, vegetables, legumes, and nuts.

When fiber intake is increased significnatly, gas, intestinal distension, and diarrhea may occur. These side effects are caused by bacterial fermentation of fiber with release of volatile fatty acids, hydrogen, carbon dioxide, and methane. Dietary fiber intake should be increased gradually along with adequate fluid intake so the gastrointestinal tract can adjust to the change. The gastrointestinal distrubances associated with initial fiber ingestion should subside within 24 to 48 hours.

Very large intakes of fiber have been reported to cause colon obstruction. This is far more likely to occur with improper use of fiber supplements and laxatives than with fiber-rich foods. When fiber intakes are increased, it is important to increase the intake of liquids.

Fiber may interfere with the absorption of some minerals. However, this does not seem to pose a problem for people with adequate nutrient intakes. Moderate levels of fiber intake are unlikely to cause nutrient deficiencies. Consumption of fiber from a wide variety of food sources is recommended to decrease possible adverse effects from increased consumption of fiber.

SOURCE:
Council on Scientific Affairs. "Dietary Fiber and Health." *JAMA* 262, no. 4 (July 28, 1989): 542–546. Copyright 1989, American Medical Association.

EFFECTS ON CONSTIPATION

Constipation is primarily a colonic problem. In the colon fibre increases stool bulk, holds water, and also acts as a substrate for colonic microflora, further increasing stool bulk by increasing bacterial, water, and salt content and producing hydrogen, methane, and other gases that augment the bulking effect. It decreases transit time, reduces intracolonic pressure, and produces a softer stool. All these effects are beneficial in relieving constipation, but the evidence comes mainly from studies on normal colons. An additional 20 g/day of bran increases faecal weight by 127% and decreases mean transit time by 41%. The same quantity of cabbage, carrot, or apple fibre produces a smaller but similar effect. Large particles of bran give significantly greater increases in stool weight and water content with significantly shorter transit times than finely ground bran. Raw bran is more effective than processed bran. Transit time is reduced by fibre most noticeably in those with slow intestinal transit and may increase in those with naturally rapid transit.

SOURCE:
Taylor, Rodney. "Management of Constipation: High Fibre Diets Work." *British Medical Journal* 300, no. 6731 (April 21, 1990): 1063–1064.

LIPID LOWERING EFFECTS

Oat bran has recently received much attention as a means of lowering cholesterol levels. Oat bran may be consumed as cooked hot cereal, muffins and bread, or it may be sprinkled on other foods. This type of fiber is usually well tolerated. The most common problem is finding a way to consume enough oat bran each day to lower cholesterol. Oat bran muffins, which may be eaten for breakfast and for snacks, offer a practical solution to this problem.

The lipid-lowering effect of water-soluble fiber is dose-related. When an adequate amount of water-soluble fiber is consumed each day, a 10 to 20 percent reduction in cholesterol may be expected. A reasonable initial approach for a patient with hypercholesterolemia would be to follow the National Cholesterol Education Program's Step One Diet and increase daily consumption of water-soluble dietary fiber. This approach may result in palatable, effective and less expensive treatment program for a large number of patients with hypercholesterolemia.

SOURCE:
Nuovo, James. "Use of Dietary Fiber to Lower Cholesterol." *American Family Physician* 39, no. 4: 140.

PROTECTION AGAINST COLORECTAL CANCER

A new study offers the best evidence to date that diet high in insoluble fiber—the kind found especially in wheat bran and whole grains—may protect against cancer of the colon and rectum, the second leading cause of cancer deaths in the U.S. The evidence about fiber's role has until now come mostly from research showing that in countries where people eat lots of fiber, colon cancer is relatively rare. Animal studies have also found that fiber can reduce the risk of colon cancer. But now scientists at New York Hospital-Cornell Medical Center have shown that wheat bran can have a direct effect in people who have precancerous polyps.

The four-year-long study followed 58 men and women at very high risk because of an inherited condition characterized by the continuing development of numerous polyps in the colon and rectum starting early in life. Over time such polyps gradually enlarge and become malignant. Half the subjects had their regular diet supplemented by a wheat-bran cereal high in insoluble fiber (they ate a total of 22.4 grams of fiber a day); the others were given a low-fiber look-alike cereal (they ate an average of 12.2 grams of fiber a day, about as much as the average American). During the study neither the researchers nor the subjects knew who was eating which cereal. Over the course of the study, polyps were more likely to have shrunk both in size and number in the people on the high-fiber cereal.

The researchers also found that subjects given daily supplements of vitamins C and E—which have been suggested as protectors against colon and rectal cancer—derived no additional benefit.

No one knows exactly how fiber may protect against this cancer, but there are several likely mechanisms. It may move food faster through the bowel, thus decreasing exposure of the bowel wall to potential carcinogens. And fiber may dilute carcinogens or possibly bind or inactivate them in some way. Though this study looked at a select group at very high risk for cancer, the researchers believe that the findings apply to everyone.

SOURCE:
"The Anticancer Fiber. (Insoluble Fiber in Wheat Bran)." *The University of California, Berkeley Wellness Letter* 6 (December, 1989): 2. Excerpted from *The University of California, Berkeley Wellness Letter,* Copyright Health Letter Associates, 1989.

RESOURCES:

ORGANIZATIONS

American Dietetic Association. 208 S. LaSalle St., Suite 1100, Chicago, IL 60604.

National Cancer Institute. NIH Bldg. 31, 9000 Rockville Pike, Bethesda, MD 20892.

U.S. Department of Agriculture. Human Nutrition Information Service, 6506 Belcrest Rd., Hyattsville, MD 20782.

PAMPHLETS

U.S. Department of Agriculture:

Dietary Fiber. (Good Sources of Nutrients). January, 1990.

U.S. Department of Agriculture and U.S. Department of Health and Human Services:

"Nutrition and Your Health: Dietary Guidelines for Americans." *Home and Garden Bulletin.* no. 232. 1990. 27 pp.

BOOKS

National Academy of Sciences, National Research Council, Food and Nutrition Board. *Diet and Health: Implications for Reducing Chronic Disease Risk.* Washington: National Academy Press, 1989. 749 pp.

U.S. Department of Health and Human Services, Public Health Service. *The Surgeon General's Report on Nutrition and Health.* DHHS (PHS) Pub. No. 88-50215. Washington D.C.: U.S. Government Printing Office, 1988. 712 pp.

RELATED ARTICLES

Gorman, Mary Ann, and Carol Bowman. "Position of the American Dietetic Association: Health Implications of Dietary Fiber—Techincal Support Paper." *Journal of the American Dietetic Association* 88, no. 2 (February 1988): 217-221.

Heaton, K. W. "Dietary Fiber." *British Medical Journal* 300 (June 9, 1990): 1479-80.

Kritchevsky, David. "Dietary Fiber Revisited." *British Medical Journal* 300 (July 1990): 13-14.

"Oat Bran for Lowering Blood Lipids." *The Medical Letter on Drugs and Therapeutics* 300, no. 780 (December 2, 1988): 111-112.

DILATION AND CURETTAGE (D&C)

(*See also:* UTERINE FIBROIDS)

OVERVIEW

Dilation and Curettage (D&C) is a very common surgical operation performed on many women each year. It is often used to diagnose or treat abnormal bleeding from the uterus. It can also provide important information about whether a woman has cancer of the uterus. . . .

Dilation means stretching the opening of the cervix with special instruments to make it wider. Once the opening of the cervix is enlarged, another instrument is inserted into the uterus to loosen and remove the lining of the uterus. This is called curettage. It can be done with an instrument called a curette, or by suction applied through a tube, called suction curettage. After a D&C is performed, an new lining will build up in the uterus during the next menstrual cycle. . . .

A D&C is often done when a woman has heavy or prolonged menstrual periods or bleeding between periods. These menstrual irregularities have many different causes, one of which is hormone imbalance. Hormone imbalance leads to a thickening of the lining of the uterus and sometimes causes irregular or prolonged bleeding. This condition can occur at any age but is more common in young women just starting to menstruate and older women before menopause.

Bleeding from the uterus can also be caused by certain types of growths, most of which are not cancerous. Polyps are growths that are attached by a stem or stalk usually to the lining of the uterus or to the cervix. Those inside the uterus can usually be removed by a D&C. Leiomyomas (fibroids) are tumors that grow from the cells that make up the uterine muscle. They are rarely cancerous. Although they can cause bleeding and cramping, there are often no symptoms. A doctor can detect some of these tumors with D&C, but another operation may have to be done to remove the tumor.

Bleeding may also be a sign of cancer of the endometrium. Women over age 40 have a higher risk of endometrial cancer. A D&C or another procedure, called endometrial biopsy, is often performed when a woman over 40 has abnormal vaginal bleeding, especially after menopause. . . .

A D&C is a brief operation. First the doctor carefully examines the reproductive organs in the pelvic area of the body for any unusual changes. Then the walls of the vagina are separated with a speculum, as in a routine vaginal exam, so the doctor can see the cervix. The cervix is held in place with an instrument similar to a clamp. To dilate the cervix, a series of tapered rods of increasing widths are inserted into the opening of the cervix. Under the pressure of these rods, the walls of the cervix are gently widened. An instrument called a curette is then passed into the uterus. This instrument is used to scrape the walls of the uterus. Pieces of the lining of the uterus are loosened and removed. These will be sent to a laboratory to be examined under a microscope. A sample of the lining can also be removed from the uterus by applying suction through a slender tube.

SOURCE:

American College of Obstetricians and Gynecologists. *Dilation and Curettage (D&C).* 1989. pp. 1–5.

RISKS

What are the risks? First, any surgery using general anesthesia carries some risks—ranging in severity from the mild discomfort of nausea to the possibility of cardiac arrest and death. In addition, several complications are specific to the D & C:

- Perforation of the wall of the uterus is not rare. The uterus is an internal organ that must be explored from an external opening. Thus the operating field is necessarily limited, and the surgeon cannot view the site of the surgery, the uterus itself. The operation is risky because the instruments used to perform the procedure—cervical dilators to enlarge the opening and curettes to spoon out the contents—are sharp and relatively pointed. Women who subsequently undergo abdominal surgery are sometimes found to have uterine scars indicating that an unrecognized perforation had taken place. Although perforation may not cause major aftereffects, any accidental entry into the abdominal cavity is a potentially serious event. Infection, internal bleeding, and damage to the bladder and intestine can occur.
- Excessive bleeding is another hazard of a D & C. When bleeding cannot be controlled by any other means, an emergency hysterectomy must be performed. Though rare, to a woman who has not fulfilled her reproductive desires, this is an especially unfortunate consequence of this "minor" surgery.
- Infection is a risk of any invasive procedure. In young women, infection can damage the fallopian tubes, which are critical for pregnancy and childbearing.
- Scarring of the uterine lining, an infrequently occurring problem known as Asherman's syndrome, is another result of repeated or overly vigorous D & Cs.

SOURCE:

Keyser, H. H. "All About D & Cs: What You (and a Million Other Women) Should Know Before Consenting to this 'Simple' Operation." *Prevention* (May 1988): 76–77.

ALTERNATIVES

Depending on the reason D & C is being considered, an endometrial biopsy or a vacuum scraping procedure may be reasonable options.

Endometrial biopsy is commonly used in evaluating fertility problems or bleeding problems experienced by young women when the main goal is to assess the hormone response of the uterine lining. Endometrial biopsy is like a miniature D & C. Little or no cervical dilation is required and the curet or scraper that is used is very narrow so it can pass through the undilated cervical canal. It is possible in most cases to obtain a few shreds of uterine lining satisfactory for microscopic evaluation using this technique.

A local anesthetic to temporarily block nerves in the cervix and the base of the uterus is commonly used for endometrial biopsy. The anesthetic, however, does not completely eliminate pain, and fairly intense cramping during each scrape is likely. Extensive or thorough scraping, therefore, may not be possible.

Vacuum scraping with a local anesthetic is also feasible as an office procedure. Instead of a metal curet, a slender plastic tube attached to a vacuum is inserted through the cervical canal and scraped along the uterine lining to obtain the strands of lining tissue needed. Several types of vacuum equipment are available for this purpose; some use vacuum created by an electric vacuum pump and some use a large, hand-held syringe as a vacuum source. Vacuum probably permits a more thorough scraping of the lining surface with less discomfort than endometrial biopsy, and is more comparable to D & C in its goals. Studies of vacuum scraping accuracy show that it is comparable to D & C in its ability to detect uterine cancer, but may not be as useful in detecting and removing uterine lining polyps.

The choice between endometrial biopsy, vacuum scraping, and D & C with anesthesia depends on your feelings about possible discomfort and anesthesia risk, as well as financial and medical considerations. D & C is essentially painless with general anesthesia, but may cost as much as $1,000 more than office procedure options. General anesthesia also involves greater risk than local anesthesia, and complication rates after D & C from bleeding, infection, and perforation are somewhat higher than rates after an office vacuum procedure or endometrial biopsy. In comparing risks, however, it is important to remember that the vacuum scraping patients studied were probably younger and healthier overall than D & C patients; the D & C may have been chosen because of extremely heavy bleeding, a very tight cervical canal, or a strong suspicion of cancer.

Neither D & C nor vacuum scraping can provide absolute assurance that uterine cancer is not present. They are among the best techniques available, but small areas of abnormal lining could be missed. If bleeding problems persist after an initial D & C or vacuum procedure, follow-up and further evaluation will be essential. The procedure may need to be repeated periodically until your problems are resolved.

SOURCE:

Stewart, F. H., F. Guest, and others. *Understanding Your Body: Every Woman's Guide to a Lifetime of Health*. New York: Bantam, 1987. pp. 842–843.

RESOURCES

ORGANIZATION

American College of Obstetricians and Gynecologists. 409 12th St. SW, Washington, DC 20024-2188.

RELATED ARTICLES

Gimpelson, R. J., and H. O. Rappold. "A Comparative Study Between Panoramic Hysteroscopy with Directed Biopsies and Dilation and Curettage: A Review of 276 Cases." *American Journal of Obstetrics and Gynecology* 158, no. 3 (March 1988): 489–492.

Hammond, R. H., and P. G. Saunders. "Diagnostic Role of Dilatation and Curettage in the Management of Abnormal Premenopausal Bleeding." *British Journal of Obstetrics and Gynecology* 96 (April 1989): 496–500.

DOWN SYNDROME

(*See also:* PRENATAL TESTING)

OVERVIEW

Down syndrome, the most common genetic birth defect associated with mental retardation, occurs equally across all races and levels of society. The effects of the disorder on physical and mental development are severe and are expressed throughout the life span. The individual's family is also affected emotionally, economically and socially. . . .

Down syndrome is a combination of physical abnormalities and mental retardation characterized by a genetic defect in chromosome pair 21. All normal cells in the human body, except ova and sperm cells, have 46 chromosomes—44 autosomes and two sex chromosomes. Normal reproductive cells contain 23 chromosomes—22 autosomes and one sex chromosome.

In all other (nonreproductive) body cells, chromosomes occur in pairs. The 22 pairs of autosomes are identified by number while the remaining pair of sex chromosomes is designated XX for females or XY for males. Each autosome appears identical to its partner, but each pair is different in its genetic content, and frequently in appearance, from all other pairs.

The genetic defect associated with Down syndrome is the presence of extra material on the chromosome pair designated 21. Although other genetic disorders may be associated with an extra chromosome, only Down syndrome is characterized by extra chromosome 21 material. The forms in which this extra material can appear are classified as:

Trisomy 21—the presence of three rather than the normal pair of chromosomes designated as 21. The genetic abnormality most frequently associated with Down syndrome (95 percent of all cases), trisomy 21, results from an error in cell division during the development of the egg or sperm, or during fertilization.

Translocation—an interchange of chromosomes or parts of chromosomes which may result in a mismatched pair. Children with translocation Down syndrome, which occurs in about four percent of the cases, have an extra number 21 chromosome which has broken and become attached to another chromosome. In certain cases, a person can carry a broken chromosome 21 without showing any symptoms of Down syndrome because the correct amount of genetic material is there, even though some of it is out of place. Normally, children receive one chromosome of pair 21 from each parent. However, a parent with a translocation can pass on his or her normal chromosome 21 plus the translocated chromosome 21, giving the child too much genetic material for chromosome 21.

Mosaicism—a very rare form of Down syndrome, appearing in about one percent of individuals with the disorder. Affected persons have cells with different chromosome counts (for example, 46 in some cells and 47 in others). Mosaicism is not carried in the parents' chromosomes; it is accidental, resulting from an error in cell division of the fertilized egg. Since only some of their cells have an abnormal number of chromosomes, babies with mosaic Down syndrome may have only some of the features of the disorder.

The distinct physical characteristics of Down syndrome include slanting eyes; slightly protruding lips; small ears; slightly protruding tongue; short hands, feet and trunk; and sometimes, an unusual crease on the palm of the infant's hand. Congenital heart defects are common and mystagmus (involuntary movement of the eyes), enlarged liver and spleen also occur. In 99 percent of cases, there is mild to severe mental retardation.

SOURCE:

National Institute of Child Health and Human Development. *Facts about Down Syndrome*. Annual 1984. pp. 1–3.

CHROMOSOME TESTING

Amniocentesis is the most common prenatal test for diagnosing chromosome abnormalities. Doctors traditionally perform amniocentesis between the fifteenth and eighteenth weeks of pregnancy. This timing is a function of the availability of the fluid, the time required for cell culture and analysis, and the ability to safely perform therapeutic abortion of necessary.

In recent years, the test has been done between the tenth and fourteenth weeks of pregnancy, apparently without any more risk than traditional amniocentesis. The amount of cells extracted from early amniocentesis procedures, however, is low, leading to a low rate of successful cell culture.

Before the test itself, the patient meets with a genetic counselor to discuss details of the procedure, as well as implications of the results. The counselor also assesses the patient's history. The patient must also sign an informed consent form, acknowledging that she has been apprised of the procedure's risk.

During the test, the doctor applies a local anesthetic to an area of the mother's abdomen, and then inserts a hypodermic-like needle. Using an ultrasound monitor for guidance, he positions the needle away from the baby, and withdraws about 20 cubic centimeters of the amniotic fluid that surrounds the fetus. The fluid contains fetal urine, as well as skin cells.

Technicians grow the cells in the laboratory and examine their chromosomes. The chromosome pattern can predict the infant's health and sex. Because of the time it takes to grow skin cells and evaluate chromosome patterns, it usually takes about four weeks to get the results.

Is amniocentesis risk-free? About one to two percent of women experience vaginal spotting or some minimal leakage of amniotic fluid, but these conditions disappear on their own. Uterine infection is also possible, but extremely rare. The risk of miscarriage due to the procedure, thanks to the use of high-quality ultrasound, is less than one percent.

SOURCE:
Kazilimani, Esther. "The Precautions of Prenatal Testing." *Priorities* (Winter 1990): 22.

GENETIC COUNSELING

Once parents have a child with Down syndrome, there is an increased risk of having another child with Down syndrome in future pregnancies. If the child's chromosome analysis reveals trisomy 21, the risk of recurrence is approximately one in a hundred. If, however, the child has translocation Down syndrome and one of the parents is a translocation carrier, the risk increases markedly. The actual risk of having another child with Down syndrome will depend on the type of translocation and whether the translocation is carried by either the father or the mother. Most genetic counselors and physicians suggest, and parents often request, amniocentesis in pregnancies following the birth of a child with Down syndrome. Amniocentesis is also recommended to pregnant women age 35 years and older because of the increased risk of having a child with Down syndrome. During amniocentesis, a small amount of fluid which surrounds the unborn baby is withdrawn from the amniotic sac. Examination of the cultured cells from the amniotic fluid will show whether the mother is carrying a baby with normal or abnormal chromosomes.

SOURCE:
National Down Syndrome Congress. *Down Syndrome.* 1988. p. 10.

TREATMENT—CELL THERAPY

Cell therapy is an unconventional treatment that has been used for a variety of conditions, including Down syndrome. The administration of freeze-dried or lyophilized cells derived from fetal tissues of vertebrate animals (specifically sheep and rabbits) has been suggested as a treatment for Down syndrome by several investigators. This alternative, unconventional therapy has also been administered in Europe to persons without Down syndrome to improve well-being and to enhance longevity. It has been used for a wide range of conditions, including heart disease, circulatory failure, infertility, cancers, and mental illness. The protocols for the use of cell therapy vary depending on the practitioner, but all preparations are originally derived from living animal tissue.

Cell therapy has been used to treat as many as 5,000,000 individuals with a variety of illnesses and conditions. Sicca cell therapy is one form of therapy that is being used in some countries for the treatment of Down syndrome. Because this therapy is not available in the United States, some families have traveled to Germany for treatment, and an increasing number of persons have received lyophilized material sent by mail from other countries to the United States. Although interest in cell therapy among US families of children with Down syndrome has been increasing, sicca cell treatments are not legally available in the United States under Federal Drug Agency regulations.

The sicca cell regimen for Down syndrome is purported to result in improvement of a number of functions, including IQ, motor skills, social behavior, height, immunologic functioning, language skills, and memory. . . .

In our retrospective study of 190 persons with Down syndrome, 11% of parents involved their children in a program of cell therapy. Although no studies of cell therapy have been done in the United States, investigators in England and Germany found no evidence that cell therapy for Down syndrome improves a child's development or effectively alters growth.

SOURCE:
Van Dyke, Don C., David J. Lang, and others. "Cell Therapy in Children with Down Syndrome: A Retrospective Study." *Pediatrics* 85, no. 1 (January 1990): 79.

RESOURCES

ORGANIZATIONS

March of Dimes Birth Defects Foundation. 1275 Mamaroneck Ave., White Plains, NY 10605.

National Down Syndrome Congress. 1800 Dempster St., Park Ridge, IL 60068.

National Down Syndrome Society. 141 Fifth Ave., New York, NY 10010.

Parents of Down Syndrome Children. c/o Montgomery County Assn. for Retarded Citizens, 11600 Nabel St., Rockville, MD 20852.

Support Organization for Trisomy 18/13 (SOFT). 3648 W. Valley West Dr., West Jordan, UT 84088.

PAMPHLET

March of Dimes Birth Defects Foundation:

Down Syndrome. October 1985. 2 pp.

BOOK

Stray-Gundersen, Karen (ed.). *Babies with Down Syndrome: A New Parent's Guide*. Kensington, MD: Woodbine House, 1986. 242 pp.

RELATED ARTICLES

Baird, Patricia A., and Adele D. Sadovnick. *The Lancet* 2, no. 8269 (December 10, 1988): 1354–1356.

"Cell Therapy in Children with Down Syndrome." *Child Health Alert* (July 1990): 4–5.

"Declining Mortality from Down Syndrome: No Cause for Complacency (editorial)." *The Lancet* 335 (April 14, 1990): 888–889.

Heins, Henry C. "What Causes Down Syndrome?" *American Baby* (April 1991): 18, 82–83.

Wright, Janice. "Down Syndrome: Mapping Chromosome 21." *American Baby* (February 1990): 18.

DRUG ABUSE

(*See also:* ALCOHOLISM; CRACK/COCAINE)

OVERVIEW

The United States has the highest rate of illicit drug use of any industrialized country in the world. In 1962 less than 4 percent of the population over the age of 12 had ever used illegal drugs. By 1985 at least 33 percent—70 million people—had experimented with them and 23 million people used them regularly. Today almost 80 percent of young people in their mid-twenties have tried illegal drugs. There are half a million heroin addicts in this country, 1 million cocaine addicts, 3 million marijuana addicts, and many millions more who are disabled by chronic drug use. These substances claim the lives of more than 6,000 Americans each year. They cost us $34 billion annually in crimes, accidents, lost work time, and health-care services.

People have been using drugs since the beginning of civilization, often with good intentions: to improve their sense of well-being, to be relieved of physical ailments, to enhance their spiritual lives. Six thousand years ago the Sumerians called opium "joy." Five thousand years ago the Chinese and other cultures found medicinal uses for marijuana. Three thousand years ago the Aztec and Toltec Indians incorporated peyote buttons into their religious ceremonies. In these ancient cultures drugs had specific uses and were limited to socially important rituals and practices. Today we rely on drugs to cure all that ails us: anxiety, stress-related aches and pains, spiritual emptiness. We have hundreds of over-the-counter and prescription drugs—and, if we're so inclined, a few dozen illegal substances—to choose from. And we don't confine our use to culturally significant ceremonies. We use drugs liberally, wherever and whenever we please.

Drugs come in and out of style as readily as the clothes we wear, and for some of the same reasons: media attention, cost, availability, and positive or negative experience associated with their use. The US drug problem first escalated in the mid-1960s, when young people attempting to expand their consciousness discovered LSD. In 1968 methamphetamine was the hot new drug, and stimulant psychosis turned the street scene violent. The increase in the use of uppers led to an increase in the use of downers—alcohol and barbiturates—as speed freaks attempted to counteract the effects of their drug of choice. Heroin became the big problem in ensuing years. By the end of 1970 30,000 American soldiers in Vietnam were addicted to heroin and two a day were dying from overdoses. In the early 1970s drug use moved out of the counterculture and into the culture at large. People smoked pot almost as openly as they drank beer. Housewives popped tranquilizers like candy. Executives turned from coffee to cocaine to get them through the day.

Illegal drug use began a long, gradual decline in the mid-1970s. Marijuana use among young people peaked in 1978, PCP in 1979, LSD in 1980, and amphetamines in 1982. Cocaine use among high school seniors, college students, and young adults declined for the first time in 1987. Despite this decrease illicit drugs—especially marijuana, cocaine, and stimulants—remain popular. The current high rate of stimulant use means a high rate of depressant use, just as it did in the 1960s. Heroin use is also on the rise—not in the general population, but among cocaine users who take a heroin-cocaine solution intravenously. Smokeable forms of all drugs are gaining popularity, leading more and more people to get addicted. People who wouldn't think of injecting drugs have no fear of smoking them, and smoke delivers the same level of chemicals to the brain as intravenous injection.

Illegal drug use does not reflect a perverse moral failing. Rather it mirrors the anxiety of modern life. While we dream of a utopian world in which everyone can just say no to drugs, our whole social structure pushes us toward substances that we hope will help us escape our pain: aspirin, alcohol, tranquilizers. For many people illegal drugs are the next logical choice for self-medication. Unfortunately, regular use can lead to dependence, because many of these substances are inherently addictive.

In the past 20 years scientists have made great progress in understanding how drugs work in the brain. They have discovered that individual drugs bind to specific receptor sites on nerve cells, sites that are designed to facilitate the body's natural stress-reducing and painkilling chemicals called neurotransmitters. For instance, nicotine fits like a key into a lock at the site where the neurotransmitter acetylcholine binds, while LSD fits into the site where serotonin binds. When too much of a drug gets into the brain, the body reduces the number of receptor sites. Therefore the drug loses some of its effectiveness, a condition known as tolerance, and the user is compelled to take more and more of it. Addiction thus occurs as a result of the way the drug alters the brain. For this reason scientists regard drug addiction as a biological disorder. They define it as a disease characterized by compulsion, loss of control, and continued use in spite of adverse consequences.

Most scientists believe it's not the fear of withdrawal but the seeking of pleasure that perpetuates addiction. Laboratory tests reveal that animals will endure great pain and exert enormous effort to get drugs. Rats will ignore foot shocks to keep getting cocaine, and monkeys will press a lever up to four thousand times to get just one dose of it. People, like laboratory animals, display similar compulsions. They will lie, cheat, steal, bet, and give up their jobs to get their drugs of choice. They'll risk exposure to the AIDS virus, lose their ability to function, ruin relationships with family and friends, undermine their children's health, starve themselves. This destructive behavior bears witness to the power of addictive disease. The erosion of values fills addicts with overwhelming guilt and shame, feelings that perpetuate drug-seeking behavior: They use drugs not only satisfy physiological urges but also to blot out their emotional pain.

Family members are usually the first to identify alarming signs of addiction: increasing family conflicts; paraphernalia found in the house; and the addict's frequent absences from work or school, trouble with the law, and memory blackouts. Confronting the addict usually leads to frustration, as he or she responds with denial and hostility. Trying to prevent the addict from using causes further resentment. As they attempt to control a situation that is out of control, family members themselves begin to behave compulsively. They need the support of peers and the help of a professional counselor to sort through the chaotic feelings, loss of trust, and sense of hopelessness that arise from living with addiction. With the help of other people who understand addictive disease, families can learn how to enjoy life again—whether or not the addict quits using. As they begin to take care of themselves, they will have more energy and understanding to deal effectively with family issues. They may also have a positive influence on the addict, helping him or her to recognize the problem.

That's the first step to recovery for addicts—acknowledging the addiction. Giving up drugs, including alcohol, is the next step. Some drugs produce minimal withdrawal symptoms, and addicts can wean themselves off them with little trouble. Other drugs—barbiturates, tranquilizers, and heroin—can cause intense discomfort. Detoxification from these drugs and any others whose withdrawal symptoms are protracted or painful should be medically supervised.

Once the drugs have been eliminated, addicts need to learn a whole new way of life. Most relapses occur in the first few months of abstinence, so during this time it's important to focus exclusively on recovery. Newly abstinent addicts need to give up drug-using associates. Those who live in neighborhoods where drug use is rampant are at particular risk. Addicts who participate in a Twelve-Step program such as Narcotic Anonymous develop supportive friendships with other recovering people. They also learn a philosophy that can help them improve their family relationships and get along in the world without drugs. Eighty percent of addicts who stay clean and sober for one year with the support of a Twelve-Step program maintain sobriety for at least five years.

People who give up illegal drugs cut a lot of unnecessary risk and tension out of their lives. They no longer have to fear getting busted for possession or losing a job because of a positive drug test. They don't have to worry about getting the money for their next fix, rock, or pill, and they don't have to waste energy trying to look clean when they're using. They can stop associating with unsavory characters and quit aligning themselves with a system of greed and violence. Through abstinence they can resign from the rat race and rejoin the human race. Recovery brings them many gifts, not the least of which are the simple peace of sobriety and the welcome renewal of self-respect.

SOURCE:

Yoder, Barbara. "Street Drugs." In *The Recovery Resource Book*. New York: Simon & Schuster, 1990. pp. 184–186.

MARIJUANA (POT)

Marijuana is still by far the most extensively used illicit drug. According to the latest survey (1985) almost 62 million Americans have tried marijuana in their lifetime and 20 million used the drug in the past year. Current use of marijuana decreased from 20 million in 1982 to 19 million in 1985 for the 12 and older population. Among employed 20–40 year olds, 16 percent reported using marijuana at least once in the past month. Starting in 1979 there has been a gradual decline in marijuana use among high school seniors. Marijuana use peaked in 1978 when almost 11 percent of high school seniors reported daily or almost daily use and has gradually declined to 2.7 percent in 1988.

A 1985 NIDA [National Institute on Drug Abuse] survey of clients admitted to drug abuse treatment programs shows that one in seven clients reported marijuana as their primary drug of abuse, second only to heroin.

The National Institute on Drug Abuse has supported extensive research into the effects of marijuana. Findings from several of these studies follow.

Significant progress has been made recently by several NIDA grantees in determining how marijuana acts on the brain. Several animal studies have focused attention on the hippocampus, the major component of the brain's limbic system that is crucial for learning, memory, and the integration of sensory experiences with emotions and motivation. Taken together, these results may provide the first clue to the mechanisms underlying marijuana induced euphoria and loss of memory and provide definitive evidence for a toxic effect of marijuana on brain nerve cells.

Researchers have found that THC, the psychoactive ingredient in marijuana, changes the way in which sensory information gets into and is acted on by the hippocampus. Studies have found that the information processing system and the activity of the neurons and nerve fibers are altered. Investigations have also shown that THC exerts an action directly on a part of the brain that scientists believe may underlie memory.

Two other studies found evidence that chronic THC exposure damages and destroys nerve cells and causes other pathological changes in the brain. The loss of cells appears to be similar to the loss seen with normal aging. This raises many concerns among which is that mild functional losses due to aging may interact with the effects of marijuana in an additive fashion, possibly placing long-term marijuana users at risk for serious or premature memory disorders as they age.

Scientists at the University of California, Los Angeles, found that the daily use of 1 to 3 marijuana joints appears to produce approximately the same lung damage and potential cancer risk as smoking 5 times as many cigarettes. The study results suggest that the way smokers inhale marijuana, in addition to its chemical composition, increases the adverse physical effects. The same lung cancer risks associated with tobacco also apply to marijuana users even though they smoke far less. The study findings refute the argument that marijuana is safer than tobacco because users only smoke a few joints a day.

Recent findings indicate that smoking marijuana while shooting up cocaine has the potential to cause severe increases in heart rate and blood pressure. Each drug alone produced cardiovascular effects. When they were combined, the effects were greater and lasted longer. The heart beat of the subjects in the study increased 29 beats per minute with marijuana alone and 32 beats per minute with cocaine alone. When the drugs were given together, the heart rate increased by 49 beats per minute and persisted for a longer time. The drugs were given with the subjects sitting quietly. In normal circumstances, an individual may smoke marijuana and inject cocaine and then do something physically stressful; they [then] may significantly increase risks of overload to the cardiovascular system.

The first controlled study in women on the acute effects of marijuana has shown that smoking a single marijuana cigarette after ovulation decreases the plasma level of one of the hormones essential for normal reproductive functioning. The luteinizing hormone is essential for implantation of the fertilized egg in the uterus. A single dose of marijuana during the luteal phase of the menstrual cycle suppressed the level of the hormone, suggesting the possibility that chronic use of marijuana may adversely effect reproductive functioning in women.

A study recently examined 1023 trauma patients admitted to the shock trauma unit at the Maryland Institute for Emergency Medical Services in Baltimore.

This unit received only the most seriously injured accident victims directly from the scene of the injury. This study found that one-third of all admitted patients had detectable levels of marijuana in their blood, indicating use of marijuana within two to four hours prior to admission to the unit. The study also found that four out of every ten persons 30 years or younger were under the influence of marijuana at the time of the accident.

A series of in depth case studies by a research team at the Center for Psychosocial Studies in New York City found that adults who smoked marijuana daily believed it helped them function better, improving self-awareness and relationships with others. In reality, the drug served as a buffer enabling users to tolerate problems, rather than make changes that might increase their satisfaction with life. The study indicated that these subjects used marijuana to avoid dealing with their difficulties and the avoidance inevitably made their problems worse. The most striking observation is the discrepancy between what study participants say and what is actually going on. Although users believed the drug enhanced understanding of themselves, it actually served as a barrier against self awareness.

SOURCE:
National Institute on Drug Abuse. *Marijuana Update* May 1989. pp. 1–3.

HALLUCINOGENS, PSYCHEDELICS, AND PCP

Hallucinogens, or psychedelics, are drugs that affect a person's perceptions, sensations, thinking, self-awareness, and emotions. Hallucinogens include such drugs as LSD, mescaline, psilocybin, and DMT. Some hallucinogens come from natural sources, such as mescaline from the peyote cactus. Others, such as LSD, are synthetic or manufactured.

PCP is sometimes considered an hallucinogen because it has some of the same effects. However, it does not fit easily into any one drug category because it also can relieve pain or act as a stimulant.

LSD is manufactured from lysergic acid which is found in ergot, a fungus that grows on rye and other grains. LSD was discovered in 1938 and is one of the most potent mood-changing chemicals. It is odorless, colorless, and tasteless. LSD is sold on the street in tablets, capsules, or occasionally in liquid form. It is usually taken by mouth but sometimes is injected. Often it is added to absorbent paper, such as blotter paper, and divided into small decorated squares, with each square representing one dose.

Mescaline comes from the peyote cactus and although it is not as strong as LSD, its effects are similar. Mescaline is usually smoked or swallowed in the form of capsules or tablets.

Psilocybin comes from certain mushrooms. It is sold in tablet or capsule form so people can swallow it. The mushrooms themselves, fresh or dried, may be eaten. DMT is another psychedelic drug that acts like LSD. Its effects begin almost immediately and last for 30-60 minutes.

The effects of psychedelics are unpredictable. It depends on the amount taken, the user's personality, mood, expectations, and the surroundings in which the drug is used. Usually, the user feels the first effects of the drug 30-90 minutes after taking it. The physical effects include dilated pupils, higher body temperature, increased heart rate and blood pressure, sweating, loss of appetite, sleeplessness, dry mouth, and tremors.

Sensations and feelings change too. The user may feel several different emotions at once or swing rapidly from one emotion to another. The person's sense of time and self change. Sensations may seem to "cross over," giving the user the feeling of "hearing" colors and "seeing" sounds. All of these changes can be frightening and can cause panic.

Having a bad psychological reaction to LSD and similar drugs is common. The scary sensations may last a few minutes or several hours and be mildly frightening or terrifying. The user may experience panic, confusion, suspiciousness, anxiety, feelings of helplessness, and loss of control. Sometimes taking a hallucinogen such as LSD can unmask mental or emotional problems that were previously unknown to the user. Flashbacks, in which the person experiences a drug's effects without having to take the drug again, can occur.

Research has shown some changes in the mental functions of heavy users of LSD, but they are not present in all cases. Heavy users sometimes develop signs of organic brain damage, such as impaired memory and attention span, mental confusion, and difficulty with abstract thinking. These signs may be strong or they may be subtle. It is not yet known whether such mental changes are permanent or if they disappear when LSD use is stopped.

PCP (phencyclidine) is most often called "angel dust." It was first developed as an anesthetic in the 1950s. However, it was taken off the market for human use because it sometimes caused hallucinations.

PCP is available in a number of forms. It can be a pure, white crystal-like powder, or a tablet or capsule. It can be swallowed, smoked, sniffed, or injected. PCP is sometimes sprinkled on marijuana or parsley and smoked.

Although PCP is illegal, it is easily manufactured. It is often sold as mescaline, THC, or other drugs. Sometimes it may not even be PCP, but a lethal by-product of the drug. Users can never be sure what they are buying since it is manufactured illegally.

Effects depend on how much is taken, the way it is used, and the individual. Effects include increased heart rate and blood pressure, flushing, sweating, dizziness, and numbness. When large doses are taken, effects include drowsiness, convulsions, and coma. Taking large amounts of PCP can also cause death from repeated convulsions, heart and lung failure, or ruptured blood vessels in the brain.

PCP can produce violent or bizarre behavior in people who are not normally that way. This behavior can lead to death from drownings, burns, falls (sometimes from high places), and automobile accidents. Regular PCP use affects memory, perception, concentration, and judgment. Users may show signs of paranoia, fearfulness, and anxiety. During these times, some users may become aggressive while others may withdraw and have difficulty communicating. A temporary mental disturbance, or a disturbance of the user's thought processes (a PCP psychosis) may last for days or weeks. Long-term PCP users report memory and speech difficulties, as well as hearing voices or sounds which do not exist.

Users find it difficult to describe and predict the effects of the drug. For some users, PCP in small amounts acts as a stimulant, speeding up body functions. For many users, PCP changes how users see their own bodies and things around them. Speech, muscle coordination, and vision are affected; senses of touch and pain are dulled; and body movements are slowed. Time seems to "space out."

SOURCE:
National Institute on Drug Abuse. *Hallucinogens and PCP.* DHHS Pub. No. (ADM) 86-1306. 1986. pp. 1-5.

SEDATIVE-HYPNOTICS

Sedatives-hypnotics are drugs which depress or slow down the body's functions. Often these drugs are referred to as tranquilizers and sleeping pills or sometimes just as sedatives. Their effects range from calming down anxious people to promoting sleep. Both tranquilizers and sleeping pills can have either effect, depending on how much is taken. At high doses or when they are abused, many of these drugs can even cause unconsciousness and death.

Barbiturates and benzodiazepines are the two major categories of sedative-hypnotics. The drugs in each of these groups are similar in chemical structure. Some well known barbiturates are secobarbital (Seconal) and pentobarbital (Nembutal). Diazepam (Valium), chlordiazepoxide (Librium), and chlorazepate (Tranxene) are examples of benzodiazepines.

A few sedative-hypnotics do not fit in either category. They include methaqualone (Quaalude), ethchlorvynol (Placidyl), chloral hydrate (Noctec) and mebrobamate (Miltown).

All of these drugs can be dangerous when they are not taken according to a physician's instructions.

[Sedative-hypnotics] can cause both physical and psychological dependence. Regular use over a long period of time may result in tolerance, which means people have to take larger and larger doses to get the same effects. When regular users stop using large doses of these drugs suddenly, they may develop physical withdrawal symptoms ranging from restlessness, insomnia and anxiety, to convulsions and death. When users become psychologically dependent, they feel as if they need the drug to function. Finding and using the drug becomes the main focus in life.

Taken together, alcohol and sedative-hypnotics can kill. The use of barbiturates and other sedative-hypnotics with other drugs that slow down the body, such as alcohol, multiplies their effects and greatly increases the risk of death. Overdose deaths can occur when barbiturates and alcohol are used together, either deliberately or accidentally.

Babies born to mothers who abuse sedatives during their pregnancy may be physically dependent on the drugs and show withdrawal symptoms shortly after they are born. Their symptoms may include breathing problems, feeding difficulties, disturbed sleep, sweating, irritability, and fever. Many sedative-hypnotics pass through the placenta easily and have caused birth defects and behavioral problems in babies born to women who have abused these drugs during their pregnancy.

Barbiturates are often called "barbs" and "downers." Barbiturates that are commonly abused include amobarbital (Amytal), pentobarbital (Nembutal), and secobarbital (Seconal). These drugs are sold in capsules and tablets or sometimes in a liquid form or suppositories.

The effects of barbiturates are, in many ways, similar to the effects of alcohol. Small amounts produce calmness and relax muscles. Somewhat larger doses can cause slurred speech, staggering gait, poor judgment, and slow, uncertain reflexes. These effects make it dangerous to drive a car or operate machinery. Large doses can cause unconsciousness and death.

Barbiturate overdose is a factor in nearly one-third of all reported drug-related deaths. These include suicides and accidental drug poisonings. Accidental deaths sometimes occur when a user takes one dose, becomes confused and unintentionally takes additional or larger doses. With barbiturates there is less difference between the amount that produces sleep and the amount that kills. Furthermore, barbiturate withdrawal can be more serious than heroin withdrawal.

All the other sedative-hypnotics can be abused, including the benzodiazepines. Diazepam (Valium), chlordiazepoxide (Librium), and chlorazepate (Tranxene) are examples of benzodiazepines. These drugs are also sold on the streets as downers. As with the barbiturates, tolerance and dependence can develop if benzodiazepines are taken regularly in high doses over prolonged periods of time.

Other sedative-hypnotics which are abused include glutethimide (Doriden), ethchlorvynol (Placidyl), and methaqualone (Sopor, Quaalude).

Methaqualone ("Sopors," "ludes") was originally prescribed to reduce anxiety during the day and as a sleeping aid. It is one of the most commonly abused drugs and can cause both physical and psychological dependence. The dangers from abusing methaqualone include: injury or death from car accidents caused by faulty judgment and drowsiness, and convulsions, coma, and death from overdose.

[Sedative-hypnotic "look-alikes"] are pills manufactured to look like real sedative-hypnotics and mimic their effects. Sometimes look-alikes contain over-the-counter drugs such as antihistamines and decongestants, which tend to cause drowsiness. The negative effects can include nausea, stomach cramps, lack of coordination, temporary memory loss, becoming out of touch with the surroundings, and anxious behavior.

SOURCE:
National Institute on Drug Abuse. *Sedative-Hypnotics*. DHHS Pub. No. (ADM) 86-1309. 1986. pp. 1-4.

OPIATES

Opiates, sometimes referred to as narcotics, are a group of drugs which are used medically to relieve pain, but also have a high potential for abuse. Some opiates come from a resin taken from the seed pod of the Asian poppy. This group of drugs includes opium, morphine, heroin, and codeine. Other opiates, such as meperidine (Demerol), are synthesized or manufactured.

Opium appears as dark brown chunks or as a powder and is usually smoked or eaten. Heroin can be a white or brownish powder which is usually dissolved in water and then injected. Most street preparations of heroin are diluted, or "cut," with other substances such as sugar or quinine. Other opiates come in a variety of forms including capsules, tablets, syrups, solutions, and suppositories.

Heroin ("junk," "smack") accounts for 90 percent of the opiate abuse in the United States. Sometimes opiates with legal medicinal uses also are abused. They include morphine, meperidine, paregoric (which contains opium), and cough syrups that contain codeine.

Opiates tend to relax the user. When they are injected, the user feels an immediate "rush." Other initial and unpleasant effects include restlessness, nausea, and vomiting. The user may go "on the nod," going back and forth from feeling alert to drowsy. With very large doses, the user cannot be awakened, pupils become smaller, and the skin becomes cold, moist, and bluish in color. Breathing slows down and death may occur.

Dependence is likely, especially if a person uses a lot of the drug or even uses it occasionally over a long period of time. When a person becomes dependent, finding and using the drug often becomes the main focus in life. As more and more of the drug is used over time, larger amounts are needed to get the same effects. This is called tolerance.

The physical dangers depend on the specific opiate used, its source, the dose, and the way it is used. Most of the dangers are caused by using too much of a drug, the use of unsterile needles, contamination of the drug itself, or combining the drug with other substances. Over time, opiate users may develop infections of the heart lining and valves, skin abscesses, and congested lungs. Infections from unsterile solutions, syringes, and needles can cause illnesses such as liver disease, tetanus, and serum hepatitis.

When an opiate-dependent person stops taking the drug, withdrawal usually begins within 4–6 hours after the last dose. Withdrawal symptoms include uneasiness, diarrhea, abdominal cramps, chills, sweating, nausea, and runny nose and eyes. The intensity of these symptoms depends on how much was taken, how often, and for how long. Withdrawal symptoms for most opiates are stronger approximately 24–72 hours after they begin and subside within 7–10 days. Sometimes symptoms such as sleeplessness and drug craving can last for months.

Researchers estimate that nearly half of the women who are dependent on opiates suffer anemia, heart disease, diabetes, pneumonia, or hepatitis during pregnancy and childbirth. They have more spontaneous abortions, breech deliveries, caesarean sections, premature births, and stillbirths. Infants born to these women often have withdrawal symptoms which may last several weeks or months. Many of these babies die.

The four basic approaches to drug abuse treatment are: detoxification (supervised withdrawal from drug dependence, either with or without medication) in a hospital or as an outpatient; therapeutic communities where patients live in a highly structured drug free environment and are encouraged to help themselves; outpatient drug-free programs which emphasize various forms of counseling as the main treatment; and methadone maintenance which uses methadone, a substitute for heroin, on a daily basis to help people lead productive lives while still in treatment.

Methadone, a synthetic or manufactured drug, does not produce the same "high" as illegal drugs such as heroin, but does prevent withdrawal and the craving to use other opiates. It often is a successful treatment for opiate dependence because it breaks the cycle of dependence on illegal drugs such as heroin. When patients are receiving methadone in treatment, they are not inclined to seek and buy illegal drugs on the street, activities which are often associated with crime. Patients in methadone maintenance programs also receive counseling, vocational training, and education to help them reach the ultimate goal of a drug-free normal life.

Narcotic antagonists are drugs which block the "high" and other effects of opiates without creating physical dependence or producing a "high" of their own. They are extremely useful in treating opiate overdoses and may prove useful in the treatment of opiate dependence.

SOURCE:

National Institute on Drug Abuse. *Opiates*. DHHS Pub. No. (ADM) 86–1308. 1986. pp. 1-5.

RESOURCES

ORGANIZATIONS

Do It Now Foundation. P.O. Box 2116, Phoenix, AZ 85036.

National Clearinghouse for Alcohol and Drug Information (NCADI). P.O. Box 2345, Rockville, MD 20852.

National Institute on Drug Abuse. 5600 Fishers Lane, Rockville, MD 20857.

PAMPHLETS

Do It Now Foundation:

Barbiturates—the Oblivion Express. DIN 111. 1986.

Drugs of Abuse—an Introduction to Their Actions and Their Potential Hazards. DIN 203. 1986.

National Clearinghouse for Alcohol and Drug Information:

Designer Drugs. CAP10. 1986. 2 pp.

Heroin. CAP 11. 1986. 4 pp.

MDMA/Ecstasy. CAP13. 1985. 2 pp.

BOOKS

Mothner, Ira, and Alan Weitz. *How to Get Off Drugs*. Fireside, 1984. 270 pp.

Seymour, Richard B., and David E. Smith. *Drugfree: A Unique, Positive Approach to Staying Off Alcohol and Other Drugs*. Facts on File, 1987. 271 pp.

RELATED ARTICLES

"Drug Abuse in the United States: Strategies for Prevention." *JAMA* 265, no. 16 (April 24, 1991): 2102-2107.

Franklin, Deborah. "Hooked, not Hooked: Why Isn't Everyone an Addict." In *Health* (November/December 1990): 39-52.

"How to Beat Drugs." *U.S. News and World Report* 107 (September 11, 1989): 69.

Schnoll, Sidney H., and Lori D. Karan. "Substance Abuse." *JAMA* 263 (May 16, 1990): 2682-2683.

Wilford, Bonnie B. "Abuse of Prescription Drugs." *The Western Journal of Medicine* 152 (May 1990): 609-612.

EATING DISORDERS

(*See also:* OBESITY; WEIGHT CONTROL DIETS)

OVERVIEW

People of all races can develop bulimia and anorexia, but the vast majority of patients are white, which may reflect socioeconomic, rather than racial, factors. Yet the illnesses are not restricted to females with certain occupational or educational backgrounds. What causes the illnesses and why they occur primarily in females are unknown.

The disorders are obsessive—that is, most victims can't stop their self-destructive behavior without professional medical help. Left untreated, either disorder can become chronic and can result in severe health damage, even death. . . .

Ordinarily, bulimia begins between ages 17 and 25. However, because many bulimics are deeply ashamed of their bingeing and purging and therefore keep these activities a guarded secret, an actual diagnosis may not be made until a patient is well into her 30s or 40s. In *Cosmopolitan* (January 1985), for example, Jane Fonda revealed that she had been a secret bulimic from age 12 until her recovery at age 35—bingeing and purging as much as 20 times a day.

Bulimia usually begins in conjunction with a diet. But once the binge-purge cycle becomes established, it can get out of control. Some bulimics may be somewhat underweight and a few may be obese, but most tend to keep a nearly normal weight. In many, the menstrual cycle becomes irregular. Sexual interest may diminish. Bulimics may exhibit impulsive behaviors such as shoplifting and alcohol and drug abuse. Many appear to be healthy and successful, perfectionists at whatever they do. Actually, most bulimics have very low self-esteem and are often depressed.

Binges may last eight hours and result in an intake of 20,000 calories (that's roughly 210 brownies, or 5½ layer cakes, or 18 dozen macaroons). One study, however, showed the average binge to be slightly less than 1¼ hours and slightly more than 3,400 calories (an entire pecan pie, for instance). Most binges are carried out in secret. Bulimics often spend $50 or more a day on food and may even steal (food or money) to support the obsession.

To lose the gained weight, the bulimic begins purging, which may include using laxatives—from 50 to 100 or more tablets at one time—or diuretics (drugs to increase urination) or self-induced vomiting caused by gagging, using an emetic (a chemical substance that causes vomiting), or simply mentally willing the action. Between binges, the person may fast or exercise excessively.

Bulimia's binge-purge cycle can be devastating to health in a number of ways. It can upset the body's balance of electrolytes—such as sodium, magnesium, potassium and calcium—which can cause fatigue, seizures, muscle cramps, irregular heartbeat, and decreased bone density, which can lead to osteoporosis. Repeated vomiting can damage the esophagus and stomach, cause the salivary glands to swell, make the gums recede, and erode tooth enamel. In some cases, all of the teeth must be pulled prematurely because of the constant wash by gastric acid. Other effects may be rashes, broken blood vessels in the cheeks, and swelling around the eyes, ankles and feet. For diabetics, bingeing on high-carbohydrate foods and sweets is particularly hazardous, since their bodies cannot properly metabolize the starches and sugars.

SOURCE:

Farley, Dixie. "Eating Disorders. When Thinness Becomes an Obsession." *FDA Consumer* (May 1986): 20–21.

ANOREXIA NERVOSA

The individual with anorexia nervosa is usually someone of normal or slightly above normal weight who starts on an "innocent" diet and eventually begins suppressing hunger sensations to the point of self-starvation. There is frequently a history of someone in the patient's family who is a dieter, overweight, or focused on staying slim and fit. Although the illness is most common among teenage or young adult women it can also affect males, preadolescents, older adults, and individuals from different ethnic and cultural backgrounds. Classic anorectics starve themselves to skeletal thinness, losing more than 15 percent (not infrequently 25–35%) of their original body weight. This dramatic weight loss is usually accompanied by an intense fear of gaining weight or becoming obese that does not diminish as weight loss progresses. Other characteristics of the disorder include a distorted body-image (indicated by the individual's claims of being fat even when emaciated), a refusal to maintain body weight over minimum normal weight for age and height, and the loss of menstrual periods.

The causes of anorexia nervosa are unknown. The widespread emphasis on diets and the desirability of thinness in our society certainly contribute to its high incidence, and psychological factors play an important role in its development.

SOURCE:
California Medical Association. *HealthTips* index 435 (July/August 1989): 1.

SIGNS AND DANGER SIGNALS

Eating disorders may be prevented or more readily treated if they are detected early. A person who has several of the following signs may be developing or has already developed an eating disorder.

Anorexia

The individual:

- has lost a great deal of weight in a relatively short period.
- continues to diet although bone-thin.
- reaches diet goal and immediately sets another goal for further weight loss.
- remains dissatisfied with appearance, claiming to feel fat, even after reaching weight-loss goal.
- prefers dieting in isolation to joining a diet group.
- loses monthly menstrual periods.
- develops unusual interest in food.
- develops strange eating rituals and eats small amounts of food, e.g., cuts food into tiny pieces or measures everything before eating extremely small amounts.
- becomes a secret eater.
- becomes obsessive about exercising.
- appears depressed much of the time.
- begins to binge and purge (see below).

Bulimia

The individual:

- binges regularly (eats large amounts of food over a short period of time).
- purges regularly (forces vomiting and/or uses drugs to stimulate vomiting, bowel movements, and urination).
- diets and exercises often, but maintains or regains weight.
- becomes a secret eater.
- eats enormous amounts of food at one sitting, but does not gain weight.
- disappears into the bathroom for long periods of time to induce vomiting.
- abuses drugs or alcohol, or steals regularly.
- appears depressed much of the time.
- has swollen neck glands.
- has scars on the back of hands from forced vomiting.

SOURCE:
National Institute of Mental Health. *Useful Information on Anorexia Nervosa & Bulimia.* DHHS Pub. No. (ADM) 87-1514. 1987. p. v.

DIAGNOSIS

Telltale physical signs:

A few key physical signs may help diagnose anorexia and bulimia in their early stages. Suspect an eating disorder when the body fat content is less than 22% by skin fold measurement. Carotenemia, acrocyanosis of the hands and feet, and brittle nails may be the result of bizarre eating habits. Parotid gland enlargement, tooth erosion, swollen gums, oral lacerations, and subconjunctival hematoma suggest bulimia. Examine the hands for signs of self induced vomiting—calluses or tooth marks, for example. Weight loss accompanied by signs of malnutrition is a clue to anorexia. Closely examine the eyes, neck, teeth, throat, and hands when you have reason to suspect bulimia. When a patient's weight loss raises the possibility of early anorexia, use calipers to measure skin fold fat of the biceps, triceps, and subscapular areas; follow the caliper manufacturer's guidelines to determine whether the body fat content is below 22%. Look for other evidence of malnutrition. The anorectic's diet, though meager, often consists largely of carrots and other vegetables containing [Beta]-carotene and may result in carotenemia, perhaps severe enough to make the skin yellow. You might note acrocyanosis of the feet and hands. The nails may be brittle and dry. You may find cardiac arrhythmia, especially if the patient has been abusing diet pills or laxatives.

Many obese patients have symptoms of bulimia, and many more have experimented with purging. It is most often the normal-weight bulimic who has lost control of her eating behaviors, however. But regardless of weight or weight fluctuation, the purging behavior causes nutritional deficiencies and physical complications. Closely examine the head, eyes, neck, throat, and hands. Painless parotid enlargement is a key diagnostic clue. Also, look for subconjunctival hematoma and swollen submandibular glands. Subconjunctival hematoma in bulimics is probably related to repeated episodes of forceful vomiting. The etiology of glandular enlargement, however, is not completely understood.

Examine the oral cavity. The bulimic patient appears at first to have poor oral hygiene. On closer scrutiny, you may find attrition and erosion of the teeth—the consequences of repeated vomiting. Boggy, ulcerative, and bleeding gingivae are common. The patient may have oral abrasions, lacerations, and contusions from inserting foreign objects to induce vomiting; acidic vomitus can cause further irritation. Inspect the tongue for glossitis, which may indicate a riboflavin deficiency. Ask the patient whether she has had a dry mouth or burning tongue, which might be a symptom of nicotinic acid deficiency.

Inspect the hands for clues to self-induced vomiting. Skin flaps, calluses, or tooth marks on the dorsal surface are the hallmarks.

SOURCE:
Edelstein, Carole K., Paul Haskew, and Janet P. Kramer. "Early Clues to Anorexia and Bulimia." *Patient Care* 23 (August 15, 1989): 155–163.

TREATMENT

AN and BN require a multidimensional approach to treatment, addressing all contributing factors. The initial step is to return eating to a more normal pattern. For bulimic patients, this stage involves cessation of bingeing, purging and dieting behaviors. For patients with AN, it involves reducing the patient's fears of a normal body weight by a process of gradual weight restoration. Strategies include encouragement and support, use of psychoeducational groups and materials, and medication to reduce the anxiety associated with eating. Some form of nutritional supplementation may be required, which may range from food or nutrient supplements to nasogastric or intravenous feeding of AN patients in extreme low-weight states. While nutritional rehabilitation alone is insufficient, treatments which do not address the effects of disordered eating and weight, or which collude with dieting behaviors by giving permission to eat minimal quantities of food by avoiding certain food groups, are unlikely to be effective.

Efforts to address significant psychological factors in the illness must proceed hand-in-hand with the return of good physical health. Individual psychological disturbance can be addressed initially by examining the abnormal cognitive distortions that underlie and support the illness behaviors. Assisting the patient to identify underlying affective states, thus allowing the development of alternate coping mechanisms for stress and reducing the need to monitor self-esteem by external cues, is ultimately helpful. Family involvement may be beneficial, especially in the younger age group. Such involvement should be aimed at encouraging the family to become more knowledgeable about the disease and to feel less helpless, rather than engaging the family in family therapy, at least initially.

A stepped approach to therapy has been found to be valuable for some patients with BN. A significant minority of bulimic patients will respond well to a minimal intervention, such as a few group sessions of a psychoeducational nature, providing basic information about the illness, consultation with a dietitian-nutritionist, and support to cope with any weight change that may occur. Patients who do not respond to such an approach may benefit from outpatient group therapy focusing on abnormal eating or outpatient individual psychotherapeutic treatment of a multidimensional nature. Patients who continue to be symptomatic may then be referred for more intensive treatment, either in a day hospital or an inpatient unit. The most resistant patients can be referred to a center dedicated to the treatment of these illnesses.

Medication may be useful in certain specific circumstances. Some patients with BN will respond to antidepressant medication in usual therapeutic doses with a marked reduction in bingeing. There is, however, no true "antianorexia" drug.

SOURCE:
Woodside, D. B. and P. E. Garfinkel. "An Overview of the Eating Disorders Anorexia Nervosa and Bulimia Nervosa." *Nutrition Today* 24 (June 1989): 27–29.

USE OF ANTIDEPRESSANTS

Antidepressant medication is useful in the treatment of bulimia nervosa, whether or not it is accompanied by major depression. Double-blind studies have demonstrated the efficacy of antidepressant agents in reducing the symptoms of bingeing and purging. The remission of the binge-purge behavior is probably due not merely to the treatment of an underlying depression but rather to a complex set of interactions involving the medication's effects on various neurotransmitters and central receptors.

It is generally recommended that therapy begin with a tricyclic antidepressant such as imipramine (Janimine, Tofranil) or desipramine (Norpramin, Pertofrane) at a low dosage (e.g., 50 mg per day). Patients should be advised of the more common side effects, which include dry mouth, constipation and postural dizziness. The dosage should be slowly increased by 50-mg increments every three to four days, until a daily dose of 150 mg is achieved. After the patient remains at that dosage level for one week, the serum drug concentration should be measured. The lower end of the therapeutic range for desipramine is 166 ng per mL and for imipramine, 180 ng per mL. To assure an adequate trial, patients should be maintained at these serum levels for at least three to four weeks. A decreased urge to binge generally occurs several weeks before any modification in the bingeing behavior.

SOURCE:

Giannini, A. James, Michael Newman, and others. "Anorexia and Bulimia." *American Family Physician* 41, no. 4 (April 1990): 1175.

RESOURCES

ORGANIZATIONS

American Anorexia/Bulimia Association, Inc. 133 Cedar Lane, Teaneck, NJ 07666.

Center for the Study of Anorexia and Bulimia. 1 West 91st St., New York, NY 10024.

National Anorexic Aid Society, Inc. P.O. Box 29461, Columbus, OH 43229.

National Association of Anorexia Nervosa and Associated Disorders. P.O. Box 7, Highland Park, IL 60035.

National Institute of Mental Health. Eating Disorders Program, Building 10, Room 3S231, Bethesda, MD 20892.

PAMPHLET

National Institute of Mental Health, Public Inquiries Branch:

Facts About Anorexia Nervosa. National Institute of Child Health and Human Development. November 1990. 7 pp.

BOOKS

Hirschman, Jane R., and Carol H. Munter. *Overcoming Overeating.* Reading, MA: Addison-Wesley, 1988.

Pope, Hamim G., and James I. Hudson. *New Hope for Binge Eaters: Advances in Understanding and Treatment.* New York: Harper/Coliphon, 1985.

Siegel, Michelle, and others. *Surviving an Eating Disorder—New Perspectives and Strategies for Family and Friends.* New York: Harper, 1988.

Vredevelt, Pam, and Joyce Whitman. *Walking a Thin Line—Anorexia and Bulimia: The Battle Can Be Won.* Portland, OR: Mulranomal Press, 1985.

ADDITIONAL ARTICLES

"Anorexia Nervosa: Obsession with Thinness." *Mayo Clinic Nutrition Letter* (April 1989): 2–3.

Comerci, George D. "Medical Complications of Anorexia Nervosa and Bulimia Nervosa." *Medical Clinics of North America* 74, no. 5 (September 1990): 1293–1310.

Cornelius, Coleman. "Portraits of Hope." *Shape* (April 1991): 80–106.

Mickley, Diane W. "Eating Disorders." *Hospital Practice* 23 (November 30, 1988): 58–62, 67–69, 73–74, 77–79.

Olsen-Noll, Cynthia G., and Michael F. Bosworth. "Anorexia and Weight Loss in the Elderly: Causes Range from Loose Dentures to Debilitating Illness." *Postgraduate Medicine* 85, no. 3 (February 15, 1989): 140–144.

Patton, George. "The Course of Anorexia Nervosa: About One in 30 Die, and Half Recover Fully After Six Years." *British Medical Journal* 299 (July 15, 1989): 139–140.

Price, William A. "Pharmacologic Management of Eating Disorders." *American Family Physician* 37, no. 5 (May 1988): 157–162.

Shepherd, Steven. "Recognizing Anorexia and Bulimia." *Executive Health Report* (August 1990): 2–3.

ENDOMETRIOSIS

(*See also:* MENSTRUATION)

DEFINITION

Endometriosis is a condition in which tissue that looks and acts like endometrial tissue is found in places other than the lining of the uterus. It occurs at menstruation when normal endometrial tissue backs up with menstrual blood through the fallopian tubes and then implants and grows in other places such as:

- Ovaries
- Tubes
- Outer surface of the uterus
- Bowel
- Other pelvic structures

Endometriosis may also develop on body tissues located anywhere in the abdomen; these tissues respond to the cycle of changes brought on by the female hormones just as the endometrium normally responds in the uterus. Thus, at the end of every cycle, when the hormones cause the uterus to shed its endometrial lining, endometrial tissue growing outside the uterus will break apart and bleed.

Unlike menstrual fluid from the uterus, which is discharged freely out of the body during menstruation, blood from the abnormal tissue has no place to go. Body tissues respond to this menstrual-type bleeding by

- Surrounding it with inflammation (tissue that becomes red, swollen, and painful around the area)
- Trying to absorb it back into the circulatory (blood) system

This monthly inflammation subsides when the bleeding ends (at the same time normal menstrual bleeding ends), and scar tissue is produced around the area. This pattern occurs in the same cycle as the menstrual cycle: month after month, patches of endometriosis are triggered by the female hormones to menstruate blood; the blood is absorbed by the surrounding, inflamed area; and scar tissue forms. Endometriosis may also cause adhesions: abnormal tissue growth that binds organs together.

Sometimes a patch of endometriosis is surrounded by enough scar tissue to cut off its blood supply; such tissue can no longer respond completely to the hormones. This is called a burned-out plaque of endometriosis. Other patches may rupture, or burst, during menstruation and spread their contents to other pelvic areas, causing new spots of endometriosis to develop. Thus, the condition may become gradually worse with time, although symptoms may come and go.

SOURCE:
American College of Obstetricians and Gynecologists. *Important Facts about Endometriosis.* September 1986. pp. 3–4.

OVERVIEW

Endometriosis affects at least five million women in their reproductive years. The name comes from the word "endometrium," which refers to the tissue that lines the inside of the uterus and builds up and sheds each month in the menstrual cycle. In endometriosis, endometrial tissue is found outside of the uterus developing into what are called implants or growths.

The most common locations of the endometrial growths are in the abdomen, involving the ovaries, fallopian tubes, the ligaments supporting the uterus, the area between the vagina and the rectum, the outer surface of the uterus, and the lining of the pelvic cavity. The intestines, rectum, bladder, cervix, vagina, and vulva are also sometimes involved. Endometrial growths are also sometimes found in other parts of the body, but this is uncommon.

The most frequent symptom of endometriosis is pain before and during menstrual periods. In some women, the pain is ceaseless and can make them unable to carry out the normal activities of life. Other symptoms can include pain during or after sexual activity, heavy or irregular bleeding, fatigue, pain with bowel movements at the time of the period and bladder problems. Endometriosis is a leading cause of infertility.

Any of these symptoms should lead a woman to see a competent doctor. (Any sense that your symptoms are not being taken seriously—a common problem because physicians were taught as recently as the early 1980s that these symptoms originate in the mind or in mental or emotional conflict—should cause you to seek a different doctor). Diagnosis of endometriosis requires confirmation by a laparoscopy. This is a relatively minor surgical procedure done under anesthesia. A laparoscope (a thin tube with a light in it) is inserted into an incision made in the patient's abdomen. By moving the laparoscope around, the surgeon can check the condition of the abdominal organs and determine if endometriosis is present.

The most common treatments for endometriosis include the use of hormones or surgical removal and cauterization of the growths. A new surgical technique being used is laser laparoscopy, in which a laser is used through the laparoscope to destroy growths. Patients are generally advised not to postpone pregnancy if they do plan to have children. However, pregnancy is not a cure for endometriosis, as was once thought. In many women, pregnancy does cause a temporary remission of symptoms. Radical surgery, involving hysterectomy and removal of the ovaries, as well as the endometrial growths, may become necessary in some long-standing and especially troublesome cases.

Prior to 1980, many physicians and researchers tended to dismiss endometriosis as being "just another women's problem." Then a Milwaukee writer and film-maker, Mary Lou Ballweg, started the Endometriosis Association. The idea was born from her own pain and suffering. Ms. Ballweg had endured endometriosis for many years and had finally undergone radical surgery.

SOURCE:

"Endometriosis Association Helps Women Cope with Baffling Disease." *The Network News* 15 (March-April 1990): 1–2.

TREATMENT

Since the growth of endometriotic tissue is dependent on sex hormones, hormonal therapy is often the first line of attack against the disease. Such therapies involve the use of high- and low-dose birth control pills, progestin (a synthetic hormone found in birth control pills), GnRH agonists or the synthetic male hormone Danocrine. These treatments, which typically are given in six-month courses, suppress the hormonal functions responsible for the buildup of endometriotic tissue and produce a pseudopregnancy (birth control pills and progestin) or pseudomenopause (GnRH agonists), or inhibit ovulation (Danocrine). According to David L. Olive, M.D., medical director of the Center for Reproductive Medicine at Humana Women's Hospital in San Antonio, all of the treatments appear equally effective in reducing the pain and amount of unwanted tissue growth. Hormonal therapy, however, is usually not an end in itself. Surgery is still often needed because endometriosis recurs, pain returns and fertility doesn't usually improve.

A major drawback of hormonal therapies is their extensive side effects. Progestin and birth control pills may produce bleeding between periods, nausea, headaches, weight gain and depression. GnRH agonists bring on the signs of menopause, including loss of bone mass. Danocrine's side effects often include severe depression, acne, weight gain, increased muscle, decreased breast size, enlargement of the clitoris and excessive facial hair growth. The adverse effects of progestin, birth control pills and GnRH agonists go away when the drugs are discontinued; the "masculinizing" effects of Danocrine often do not.

Recent research has brought about a number of advances in treatment:

New hormonal agents: The big news in endometriosis treatment is the approval of Synarel, a nasal spray, and Depo-Lupron, a once-a-month injectable drug. Both are hormone blockers that suppress ovarian function as effectively as Danocrine does, with more tolerable side effects that abate when therapy ends. The most dangerous, but reversible, side effect—loss of bone mass—places a woman at risk for osteoporosis. Other common side effects include hot flashes, vaginal dryness, headaches and a worsening of symptoms during the first month of treatment.

Therapeutic laparoscopy: Five years ago women would have required major abdominal surgery (called laparotomy) to remove endometriotic tissue; now surgeons can diagnose the disease, but also treat 80 percent of cases through the laparoscope. They can zap the tissue with lasers, cut it out with scissors or burn it away.

With laparoscopy, there's no hospital stay, which is one of its main advantages over other surgical options. It's also less painful and the recuperation is a few days versus a month. And the laparoscopy improves fertility rates, even more so than abdominal surgery, because it leaves fewer scars. This is important because growths tend to come back, and multiple surgeries are not uncommon.

If the tissue growth is extensive or laparoscopy and drugs fail to reduce pain and/or produce a pregnancy, laparotomy is still usually considered. The good news is that hysterectomy—in the past a common treatment for endometriosis—now often isn't.

SOURCE:
Monson, Nancy. "Endometriosis Update." *Glamour* (April 1991): 84, 88.

TREATMENT—USE OF NAFARELIN NASAL SPRAY

A prescription nasal spray to relieve the symptoms of endometriosis has been approved by FDA. Endometriosis is a sometimes disabling disease of the reproductive organs affecting as many as 5 million women of child-bearing age.

The drug, nafarelin acetate, works by suppressing menstruation. It will be marketed under the trade name Synarel by Syntex Corp.

Endometriosis is a condition in which tissue that is normally shed from the lining of the uterus (the endometrium) during menstruation attaches to other organs, particularly in the pelvic area.

These endometrial implants can bleed during the menstrual cycle, sometimes causing pelvic pain, severe menstrual cramps, heavy or irregular menstrual bleeding, and low back pain. . . .

Nafarelin acetate works indirectly to treat endometriosis by suppressing pituitary gland hormones (including estrogen) that regulate ovulation and menstruation.

The drug does not cure endometriosis, but by suppressing the menstrual cycle it can alleviate its symptoms and cause the endometrial implants to shrink or stop growing.

The new drug has not been shown effective for treating infertility associated with endometriosis.

Of 247 women treated with the drug for six months, 85 percent showed a partial or complete reduction in the size of implants. Six months after treatment was discontinued, symptoms reappeared in half who had experienced relief.

Use of nafarelin acetate for longer than six months is not recommended because the shutdown of estrogen may cause a small amount of bone loss. FDA advises women at risk of osteoporosis to discuss with their doctors the risks and benefits of using the drug.

Other side effects associated with nafarelin acetate include hot flashes, decreased libido, vaginal dryness, headaches, and nasal irritation.

SOURCE:
"Nasal Spray for Endometriosis." *FDA Consumer 24* (May 1990): 4.

ENDOMETRIOSIS—AND INFERTILITY

At its most severe, endometriosis clearly impedes conception. Implants can cover the ovary, preventing release of eggs. Adhesions can distort the anatomy of the fallopian tubes, thus interfering with fertilization of the egg or transport of the newly formed embryo to the uterus. Endometriosis this serious (classified as stage III or IV) is often treated in the hope of restoring fertility. Surgery to remove all detectable implants and adhesions is followed by hormonal therapy.

After treatment, about 40% of affected women will still be unable to conceive. They may then wish to consider assisted means of fertilization. Such methods involve surgically harvesting eggs from the woman. For in vitro fertilization and embryo transfer (IV-ET), the eggs are fertilized in the laboratory with the man's sperm; the resulting embryo is placed in the woman's uterus. In gamete intrafallopian transfer (GIFT), both eggs and sperm are transferred to the woman's fallopian tube for fertilization.

Whether milder forms of endometriosis (stages I and II) impair fertility is not known and is somewhat controversial. Endometriosis is definitely more common among infertile women than in the general population—at least ten times more so. Yet it is not at all clear whether endometriosis causes infertility or is only an associated finding. Women with mild endometriosis do not appear to be less fertile than women without the condition. Despite the uncertainty, though, some patients with no other known cause of infertility elect to have treatment in the hope of improving their chances.

How could endometriosis that doesn't physically block the ovaries or tubes cause infertility? Much research related to this question is under way. Endometriosis causes inflammation in the pelvis, increases the amount of fluid, and draws inflammatory cells into the region. These cells could harm eggs or sperm by directly attacking them or by releasing damaging enzymes and other substances.

SOURCE:
"Endometriosis and Infertility." *Harvard Health Letter* (June 1991): 6.

RESOURCES

ORGANIZATIONS
American Fertility Society. 2140 11th Ave. S, Suite 200, Birmingham, AL 35205.

Endometriosis Association. 8585 N. 76th Place, Milwaukee, WI 53223.

National Women's Health Network. 1325 G St. NW, Washington, DC 20005.

PAMPHLET
Winthrop Pharmaceuticals. *Understanding Endometriosis*. 1987. 14 pp.

BOOKS
Breitkopf, Lyle J., and Marion Gordon Bakoulis. *Coping with Endometriosis*. Englewood Cliffs, NJ: Prentice-Hall, 1988. 189 pp.

Lauerson, Niels H., and Constance de Swaan. *The Endometriosis Answer Book: New Hope, New Help*. New York: Rawson, 1988. 255 pp.

Weinstein, Kate. *Living with Endometriosis: How to Cope with the Physical and Emotional Challenges*. Reading, MA: Addison-Wesley, 1987. 313 pp.

RELATED ARTICLES

Barbieri, Robert L. "Comparison of the Pharmacology of Nafarelin and Danazol." *American Journal of Obstetrics and Gynecology* 162 (February 1990): 581-585.

Barlow, David H. "Nafarelin in the Treatment of Infertility Caused by Endometriosis." *American Journal of Obstetrics and Gynecology* 162 (February 1990): 576-579.

Kulpa, Pat. "Dealing with Endometriosis." *Shape* (December 1990): 36-37.

Shaw, Robert W. "Nafarelin in the Treatment of Pelvic Pain Caused by Endometriosis." *American Journal of Obstetrics and Gynecology* 162 (February 1990): 574-576.

EPILEPSY

OVERVIEW

There are many forms of epilepsy, each with its own characteristic symptoms. Whatever its form, the disease is caused by a problem in communication between the brain's nerve cells. Normally, such cells communicate with one another by sending tiny electrical signals back and forth. In someone with epilepsy, the signals from one group of nerve cells occasionally become too strong; so strong that they overwhelm neighboring parts of the brain. It is this sudden, excessive electrical discharge that causes the basic symptom of epilepsy, which is called an epileptic seizure, fit, or convulsion.

It is not yet known what causes the brain's communication system to misfire in this fashion, or why such events recur in some people. Exhaustive research, including the testing of great numbers of epileptics, has shown that roughly two out of three epileptics have no identifiable structural abnormality in the brain, that is, there is nothing that is visibly wrong. The epilepsy of the remaining one-third can generally be traced back to an underlying problem such as brain damage at birth, severe head injury, or brain-tissue infection. Occasionally the condition may be caused by a brain tumor. This is especially likely when the epilepsy appears for the first time in adulthood.

The basic symptom of epilepsy is a brief, abnormal phase of behavior commonly known as a seizure, fit, or convulsion. It is important to realize that a single such episode does not indicate that you have epilepsy. By definition, epileptic seizures recur. There are many forms of the disease, but two major types are petit mal and grand mal.

Petit mal epilepsy is a disease of childhood that does not usually persist past late adolescence. A child may have this form of epilepsy if, from time to time, he or she suddenly stops whatever activity is going on and stares blankly around for a few seconds (sometimes up to half a minute). During the blank interval, known as a petit mal seizure, the child is unaware of what is happening. There may be a slight jerking movement of the head or an arm, but petit mal seizures do not generally involve falling to the ground. When the seizure ends, the child often does not realize that the brief blank spell has occurred. Such children are sometimes thought simply to be "day dreamers."

The most characteristic symptom of grand mal epilepsy is a much more dramatic seizure. The person falls to the ground unconscious. Then the entire body stiffens. Next it twitches or jerks uncontrollably. This may last for several minutes and is usually followed by a period of deep sleep or mental confusion. During a seizure some people lose bladder control and pass urine freely. In many cases the person gets a warning of an impending seizure by having certain strange sensations before losing consciousness. Any such warning is known as an aura, and an aura can occur just prior to the occurrence of the seizure or as much as several hours before it strikes. It may consist of nothing but a sense of tension or some other ill-defined feeling, but some epileptics have quite specific auras such as an impression of smelling unpleasant odors or hearing peculiar sounds, distorted vision, or an odd bodily sensation, particularly in the stomach. Many epileptics learn to recognize their special aura, and this may give them time to avoid accidents when they become unconscious.

Other types of epilepsy are much less common than petit and grand mal. Two additional types are called focal epilepsy and temporal lobe epilepsy. A person with focal epilepsy does not necessarily lose consciousness; the seizure begins with uncontrollable twitching of a small part of the body, and the twitch gradually spreads.

The thumb of one hand, for instance, may start to jerk, followed by a jerking of the entire arm and then of the rest of that side of the body, after which there may be a more generalized seizure of the entire body. A person with temporal lobe epilepsy is likely to have an aura lasting only a few seconds. Then, without being aware of it, he or she does something entirely out of character, such as becoming suddenly angry, laughing for no apparent reason, or interrupting normal activity with some sort of bizarre behavior. Strange, chewing movements of the mouth are apt to occur throughout any such episode.

SOURCE:

Epilepsy. The American Medical Association Family Medical Guide. New York: Random House, 1987. pp. 289–291.

FIRST AID

First aid for a generalized tonic clonic (grand mal) seizure is basically very simple, and is designed to protect the safety of the person until the seizure stops naturally by itself. These are the key things to remember:

1. Keep calm and reassure other people who may be nearby.

2. Clear the area around the person of anything hard or sharp.

3. Loosen ties or anything round the neck that may make breathing difficult.

4. Put something flat and soft, like a folded jacket, under the head.

5. Turn him gently onto his side. This will help keep the airway clear. Do not try to force his mouth open with any hard implement or with fingers. It is not true that a person having a seizure can swallow his tongue, and efforts to hold the tongue down can injure teeth or jaw.

6. Don't hold the person down or try to stop his movements.

7. Don't attempt artificial respiration except in the unlikely event that a person does not start breathing again after the seizure has stopped.

8. Stay with the person until the seizure ends naturally.

9. Be friendly and reassuring as consciousness returns.

10. Offer to call a taxi, friend or relative to help the person get home if he seems confused or unable to get home by himself.

These steps apply only to a brief, uncomplicated seizure in someone who has epilepsy and who regains consciousness after the shaking has stopped. If this does not happen, if the seizures do *not* stop after about five minutes, or if another seizure begins shortly after the first, or if the seizure is of unknown cause or occurs in a person who is diabetic, injured, or pregnant, the safest course is to call for emergency medical assistance.

If someone has a different type of seizure, a complex partial seizure that produces confusion, and periods of dazed behavior in which consciousness is altered and communication blocked, the best course of action is to reassure others, keep calm, don't grab hold or restrain, guide gently away from hazards and remain with the person until he or she if fully aware of the surroundings once again.

SOURCE

Questions and Answers about Epilepsy. Epilepsy Foundation of America. 1985. 16 pp. Also from updates received from the Foundation, February 11, 1992.

PREVENTION OF SEIZURES

Years ago a diagnosis of epilepsy was more or less a guarantee that seizures would continue to take place in the future. But fortunately things are different today, and there are ways to prevent subsequent seizures. In many cases these methods are so successful that people go for years with complete seizure control.

Epileptic seizures can be prevented by:

- Regular use of anti-seizure medication
- Removal of brain tissue where seizures take place
- Special diet to produce a change in body chemistry
- Avoidance of special conditions known to trigger seizures in susceptible people.

Of the methods listed above, drug therapy is by far the most often used, and is almost always the method that is tried first.

A number of medications to prevent epileptic seizures are currently approved for use in the U.S., and of these, the following six are used most frequently:

Phenytoin (Dilantin), phenobarbital, ethosuximide (Zarontin), primidone (Mysoline), valproic acid (Depakene), and carbamazepine (Tegretol).

When taken regularly as prescribed, medication can prevent seizures in about half of all cases, and produce improvement in about 30 percent. The remaining patients do not get much relief from existing medications.

Removal of brain tissue

When drugs fail to prevent seizures, surgery may be an option.

Surgery for epilepsy is most likely to be successful when the seizures begin in one fairly small part of the brain that can be removed without affecting speech or memory or some other important brain function.

Although surgery is not used as often as drug therapy, the results are similar—about 70 percent of the patients getting either full or greatly improved control of seizures, and the rest having only slight improvement or none at all. Some people who have surgery may still have to take seizure medication afterwards.

Special diet

There is no proof at the present time that special doses of vitamins or trace metals or special foods will have any positive effect on epilepsy, except in rare cases where the underlying cause is vitamin deficiency. The only diet that has been successful in preventing seizures is one that is very high in fats. It is used in only a very small number of cases when all other methods of controlling seizures have failed. Like other therapies for epilepsy, it has to be prescribed by a doctor and monitored closely.

Avoiding seizure triggers

In a small number of cases it is possible to identify a certain action or event that will always produce seizures in sensitive people. These seizure "triggers" include flickering lights, breathing very quickly and deeply, and even, in very rare cases, reading or hearing a certain sound or piece of music.

One way to prevent seizures, once these causes have been identified, is to avoid the triggering circumstance as much as possible (although sometimes gradual exposure to the triggering situation in a controlled environment may reduce the sensitivity).

Loss of sleep, extreme fatigue, even emotional stress may also trigger seizures in susceptible people. The best way to prevent the reaction is to follow basic rules of good health—plenty of sleep, plenty of exercise, and a healthy diet.

SOURCE:
Epilepsy Foundation of America. *Preventing Epilepsy*. 1983. pp 14–15. Also from updates received from the Foundation, February 11, 1992.

ANTICONVULSANT DRUG THERAPY

Anticonvulsant therapy is the treatment of choice for most patients with epilepsy. Try one drug at a time. Gradually add a second drug to the regimen only if therapy with one of the agents indicated for the patient's seizure type fails. Refer the patient for neurologic evaluation if seizures are refractory to one-drug therapy. Consider withdrawing anticonvulsant medication only when patients have been seizure-free for 3–5 years and show no abnormality during physical and neurologic examination.

Treating partial seizures: Choose among carbamazepine, phenobarbital, phenytoin sodium and primidone to treat partial seizures—those beginning focally. Carbamazepine, phenobarbital, phenytoin sodium and primidone to treat partial seizures—those beginning focally. Carbamazepine is a good choice for children, since it does not cause the hyperactivity or sedation that can occur with phenobarbital and primidone or the adverse cosmetic effects sometimes associated with phenytoin. Add methsuximide, clorazepate dipotassium, or valproic acid if combinations of the first-line drugs are not effective.

When managing generalized seizures: Treat absence seizures with either ethosuximide or valproic acid. Treat the patient who also has tonic-clonic seizures with valproic acid alone. If either drug fails separately, treat with both. Treat generalized tonic-clonic seizures with carbamazepine, phenytoin sodium, or valproic acid. For myoclonic seizures, use valproic acid, and then try clonazepam, phenobarbital, phenytoin, and methsuximide. For atonic seizures, try valproic acid, phenytoin, carbamazepine, and ethosuximide in turn.

Pregnant women with epilepsy have a slightly higher risk of maternal and fetal complications than women who do not have the disorder. Neurologists advise that pregnant women with epilepsy continue to take anticonvulsants: Breakthrough seizures may be more dangerous to the baby than possible problems associated with the anticonvulsants. Help prevent loss of seizure control during pregnancy by adjusting drug dosages carefully and monitoring anticonvulsant serum levels.

SOURCE:
Dreifuss, F. E., Gallagher, B. B., and others. "Epilepsy: Management by Medication." *Patient Care* 22, no. 15 (April 15, 1988): 52.

SURGERY

Epilepsy is common. About 10% of all Americans will have at least one seizure at some time. Many people have one or a few attacks and then never have another one. For those with recurrent seizures, about 70% are satisfactorily controlled with antiepileptic drugs. Of the 150,000 people who develop epilepsy each year, 10% to 20% prove to have "medically intractable epilepsy." Many of these patients and their families have to deal with a chronic disorder that impairs the quality of life for all concerned.

Brain surgery is an alternative treatment if antiepileptic drugs fail, and it is being used more often. Several centers have reported success, and increasing numbers of patients are being referred for surgery, including many children. Improved technology has made it possible to identify more accurately where seizures originate in the brain (epileptic regions), and advances in surgery have made operative management safer. As a result, investigators have estimated that 2000 to 5000 new patients in the United states might be candidates for operations each year, compared with the present annual rate of about 500.

There is no precise definition of intractable epilepsy. Among the considerations are seizure frequency, seizure type, severity of attacks, and impact on quality of life. Before seizures are deemed intractable it is necessary to ascertain that the correct drugs have been used in the correct amounts. Complex partial seizures are more likely to be intractable than tonoclonic or other common forms of epilepsy. In uncontrolled complex partial seizures, the frequency of seizures varies from fewer than once a week to five or more each day. The clinical manifestations also vary in different patients. Some are not apparent to anyone but the patient; others disrupt daily activities and are socially embarrassing. If a patient falls during seizures that occur only a few times a year, repeated injuries and trips to emergency departments can make life miserable. Even one seizure a year may disqualify a person from having a driver's license. Disability is also influenced by the reaction of the patient's family, friends, teachers, or employers—all have an impact on what is judged severe enough to warrant consideration of surgical therapy.

There are other reasons to consider surgical therapy. For instance, repeated seizures may have adverse effects on the brain, leading to progressive cerebral degeneration and more severe clinical handicaps. Long-term use of antiepileptic drugs may cause toxic syndromes and may also have adverse effects on learning, scholastic achievement, development, and job performance. . . .

Before a patient is considered for surgery, evaluation should be sufficient to ensure the following:

- Nonepileptic attacks have been excluded and epilepsy is, in fact, present. Cardiogenic syncope, psychogenic seizures, and other nonepileptic states can closely mimic epileptic attacks.
- The epileptic seizure type and syndrome have been clarified. Primary and secondary epilepsies, partial seizures, and tonoclonic seizures respond to different antiepileptic drugs and different surgical procedures.
- Diagnostic tests have been performed to define a metabolic or structural cause of the epileptic attacks.
- The patient has had a reasonable trial of the appropriate antiepileptic drugs with adequate monitoring of compliance and the effects of the treatment.
- The patient and family have received detailed information about the specific seizure disorder, available drug treatments and side effects, and alternative treatments such as surgery.

If, after this evaluation, seizures prove to be intractable or drug treatment is unsatisfactory, appropriate patients should be referred to an epilepsy center to be evaluated for surgery. Referrals should be made as soon as it is clear that medical treatment is unlikely to result in further benefit. Early referrals may prevent the development of chronic psychosocial and physical problems that result from uncontrolled seizures.

Coexisting disorders may affect the decision to operate; they may include severe psychiatric disorders, profound developmental retardation, or progressive neurodegenerative diseases. After the initial evaluation and a full unsuccessful trial of medical therapy, surgery may be considered. Patients with partial seizures and secondarily generalized seizures (attacks that begin locally and spread to both sides of the brain) are potential candidates. Secondarily generalized seizures may take the form of atonic, tonic, or tonic-clonic attacks. Patients with seizures and childhood hemiplegia may also benefit from surgery. Patients with the following seizure types are potential candidates: complex partial seizures of temporal lobe origin or other focal seizures; generalized, atonic, akinetic, or myoclonic seizures; and partial seizures with childhood hemiplegia.

SOURCE:

NIH Consensus Conference. "Surgery for Epilepsy." *JAMA* 264 (August 8, 1990): 729, 733.

RESOURCES

ORGANIZATION

Epilepsy Foundation of America. 4531 Garden City Drive, Landover, MD 20785.

PAMPHLETS

CIBA-GEIGY:

Growing Up with Epilepsy: A Guide for Teenagers. 1985. 14 pp.

Cleveland Clinic Foundation:

Epilepsy. 1989. 16 pp.

Epilepsy Foundation of America:

Questions and Answers about Epilepsy. 1987. 16 pp.

A Patient's Guide to Medical Tests Used in Diagnosis and Treatment of Seizure Disorders. 1985. 7 pp.

A Patient's Guide to Medical Treatment of Childhood and Adult Seizure Disorders. 1986. 8 pp.

RELATED ARTICLES

Chadwick, D. "Diagnosis of Epilepsy." *The Lancet* 336 (August 4, 1990): 291–295.

Gram, L. "Epileptic Seizures and Syndromes." *The Lancet* 336 (July 21, 1990): 161–164.

Rylance, G. W. "Treatment of Epilepsy and Febrile Convulsions in Children." *The Lancet* 336 (August 25, 1990): 488–491.

Smith, J. R., H. F. Flanigin, and others. "Surgical Management of Epilepsy." *Southern Medical Journal* 82, no. 6 (June 1989): 736–742.

"Surgery for Epilepsy." *Mayo Clinic Health Letter* 9, no. 4 (April 1991): 1–2.

Sussman, Neil M. "Could It Be Epilepsy?" *Healthline* (April 1991): 10.

Tallis, R. "Epilepsy in Old Age." *The Lancet* 336 (August 4, 1990): 295–296.

Vining, E. P. G. "Educational, Social, and Life-Long Effects of Epilepsy." *Pediatric Clinics of North America* 36, no. 2 (April 1989): 449–461.

Wallace, S. "Childhood Epileptic Syndromes." *The Lancet* 336 (August 25, 1990): 486–488.

ESTROGEN REPLACEMENT THERAPY

(*See also:* MENOPAUSE; OSTEOPOROSIS)

OVERVIEW

For many women, the amount of estrogen produced by the ovaries decreases at about age 45–50. This decline, which is not noticed by most women, goes on for several years. As women get older the decline in estrogen levels becomes greater. This drop eventually causes the menstrual period to become less frequent and then stop. Menopause occurs when a woman no longer has her periods.

The decreased level of estrogen may also be responsible for the uncomfortable symptoms of menopause. Women may experience hot flashes, mood swings or depression and a decline in vaginal lubrication. The symptoms vary from woman to woman; some have no unpleasant effects while others find them very severe and require medical attention.

Osteoporosis, or bone loss, is another effect of reduced estrogen levels after menopause. Estrogen, calcium and exercise are needed to build and maintain bone. In women, bone density increases until age 30–35. The process of losing bone mass increases after menopause. Bone slowly loses calcium and becomes more brittle. As a result, a woman in her older years is more likely to have bone fractures.

The changes of menopause can be prevented by giving replacement estrogen in place of the estrogen that is no longer made by the body. This is called estrogen replacement therapy (ERT). The decision to begin ERT depends on a woman's medical history, symptoms and risk of bone loss. Not all women going through menopause need additional estrogen. With ERT, hot flashes occur less often and are less severe. It can also help in relieving vaginal dryness and discomfort. An important benefit of ERT is that it reduces the risk of coronary heart disease. If given shortly after menopause, estrogen replacement can also help prevent further bone loss. The amount of estrogen needed to reduce or prevent the symptoms of menopause varies from woman to woman. If estrogen is taken to guard against osteoporosis, long-term therapy is needed. When therapy ends, bone loss begins again.

Estrogen can be prescribed in pill form or as a cream or ointment for use in the vagina. It can also be applied as a skin patch. If a woman needs to take estrogen, her physician will explain how it should be taken. Like many medications, estrogen carries with it some degree of risk. When taken alone, it may be linked to cancer of the endometrium (lining of the uterus) and this risk may increase when large doses are taken for many years. For this reason, the lowest possible doses of estrogen that are still effective are used, and a synthetic form of the hormone progesterone is added. When given along with estrogen, progesterone can protect against endometrial cancer.

The benefits and risks of long-term estrogen use should be weighed and discussed by each patient and her physician. About 10 percent of the women receiving ERT experience minor side effects. These include swollen breasts, nausea, vaginal discharge, headaches, fluid retention and weight gain. A small percentage of women may show an increase in blood pressure while on ERT. In general, women who have had breast cancer should not take estrogen replacement. Those who have migraine headaches, diabetes, asthma or a history of blood clots or active liver disease may also be advised not to undergo ERT. These can often be controlled, however, even in patients taking estrogens. The major benefits are preventing osteoporosis and heart disease.

Women taking estrogen should follow instructions carefully and must be checked regularly by a physician. He/she should be notified about any unexpected vaginal bleeding. Not all women consider the benefits of ERT to be worth the risks. Eating a balanced diet wtih enough calcium, getting enough exercise and not smoking cigarettes can reduce the rate of bone loss.

SOURCE:
California Medical Association. "Estrogen." *HealthTips* index WH-54 (February 1990): 1-2.

RISKS

Many gynecologists now believe it [estrogen replacement therapy] should be taken by the majority of menopausal women. The recommendation has become so indiscriminate that we know of at least one instance in which a doctor suggested it to a woman with a known family history of breast cancer. ("It can be detected at an early, curable stage," was his overly optimistic reasoning.) ERT is increasingly promoted like a vitamin regimen that will ensure healthy old age. It is true that many of the established risks of ERT have been blunted by the reduction in dosage, and its five- to 14-fold risk of uterine cancer (after only two years of use) has been theoretically resolved by the addition of progestin, the synthetic version of another female hormone called progesterone. But even this has not been firmly established. The possibility of an ERT-induced breast cancer refuses to go away and the addition of progestin presents new uncertainties because little is known about its long-term effects.

It is ironic that "medical management" should be on the verge of an upswing after some researchers found the extent of menopause's multiple health risks to be highly inflated. The negative medical attitude toward menopause was attributed to numerous studies with an overrepresentation of women who had their ovaries removed. Surgical menopause is abrupt, drastic, and known to be associated with more severe mental and physical symptoms.

The decision to embark upon ERT should be based on findings from published studies. But virtually all the studies involved participants taking ERT in a very different way than is currently recommended. Much has changed over the last two decades, both in terms of dosage and its combination with progestin. In addition, women themselves have changed. It is quite possible that women now approaching menopause are healthier than their predecessors. They are likely to be more physically fit and to have benefited from improved knowledge of what constitutes a healthful diet. Even without ERT, they may reach advanced age with a lower rate of hip fracture and heart disease.

SOURCE:
Center for Medical Consumers. "Postmenopausal Hormone Therapy: Weighing the Risks and Benefits." *HealthFacts* 16, no. 144 (May 1991): 1, 3.

* * *

We now generally consider that the benefits of estrogen replacement therapy far outweigh its risks. To avoid the problems associated with estrogen deficiency, women should begin a lifelong course of estrogen replacement therapy during the perimenopausal period.

Estrogen replacement therapy should be considered for all postmenopausal women. The goals of estrogen replacement therapy are to minimize the benign symptoms and to reverse the predictable osteoporosis and atherosclerotic heart disease that can accompany estrogen deficiency. In this way we hope to reduce the high morbidity, mortality, and health care costs associated with the sequelae of untreated menopause.

SOURCE:
Mishell, Daniel R., Jr. "Estrogen Replacement Therapy: An Overview." *American Journal of Obstetrics and Gynecology* 161, no. 6, part 2 (December 1989): 1826.

RELATION TO BREAST CANCER

Researchers reporting in the November 28, 1990 *Journal of the American Medical Association* analyzed data collected between 1976 and 1986 from women aged 30 to 55 years old. The results suggest that women who now use estrogen replacements face a slightly higher risk of breast cancer than women who don't use estrogen, or who once did but have discontinued its use.

If you are taking estrogen supplements, should you discard them? We don't think so. The benefits far outweigh the minimal risks.

"This one study suggesting a tiny increase (in risk for breast cancer) is one of many studies that show little or no significant correlation between the use of estrogen and development of breast cancer," says Richard Sheldon, a Mayo Clinic obstetrician/gynecologist.

Estrogen replacement therapy give postmenopausal women relief from their No. 1 complaint—hot flashes. The hormone also protects against osteoporosis by slowing the loss of bone minerals after menopause begins.

Dr. Sheldon emphasizes that the risk of developing breast cancer from using estrogen is small. And there is an excellent screening test for breast cancer—the mammogram.

SOURCE:
"Estrogen Replacement Therapy: Is It Linked to Breast Cancer?" *Mayo Clinic Health Letter* (May 1991): 7.

RELATION TO HEART DISEASE

Several large studies conclude that postmenopausal women who take estrogen supplements may receive an added benefit—a lower risk of cardiovascular disease.

In one study, more than 32,000 postmenopausal nurses, who were currently using estrogen, experienced a 70 percent reduction in their risk of coronary disease.

Low doses of estrogens may protect against fatal and nonfatal heart attacks by lowering low-density lipoprotein

(LDL, the "bad" form) cholesterol and raising high-density lipoprotein (HDL, "good") cholesterol.

Estrogen replacement therapy also does not increase blood pressure directly, or the risk of stroke or thromboembolism.

If you have high total blood pressure or diabetes, or if you smoke cigarettes or are overweight, estrogen continues to be protective. But having these cardiovascular risk factors reduces estrogen's helpful effects.

SOURCE:
"Estrogen and Heart Disease." *Mayo Clinic Health Letter* 9, no. 5 (May 1991): 7.

RELATION TO OSTEOPOROSIS

There is little argument that the best documented benefit of ERT [estrogen replacement therapy] is reducing the rate of postmenopausal bone loss, thereby reducing the risk of fracture in later years. Immediate evidence of benefit can be demonstrated in randomized clinical trials by comparing bone loss, measured by single or dual photon absorptiometry, in estrogen- versus placebo-treated women. The inference that delayed bone loss reduces subsequent fracture risk is supported by case-control studies of fracture patients, in whom the estimated relative risk associated with estrogen use for 4 or more years is approximately 50 percent.

SOURCE:
Barrett-Connor, Elizabeth L. "The Risks and Benefits of Long-Term Estrogen Replacement Therapy." *Public Health Reports Supplements* (September-October 1988): 62.

RESOURCES

PAMPHLETS
American College of Obstetricians and Gynecologists:

Estrogen Use. 1988.

American Council on Science and Health:

Postmenopausal Estrogen Therapy: A Report by the American Council on Science and Health. 1984. 16 p.

Wyeth-Ayerest Laboratories:

What You Should Know about Estrogen Deficiency and Osteoporosis. 1990.

BOOKS
Nachtigall, Lila, and Joan Heilman. *Estrogen: The Facts Can Change Your Life*. New York: Harper, 1986. 205 pp.

Stewart, Felicia, and others. "Menopause." In *Understanding Your Body: Every Woman's Guide to Gynecology and Health*. New York: Bantam, 1987. pp. 587–626.

Utian, Wulf H., and Ruth S. Jacobowitz. *Managing Your Menopause*. New York: Prentice Hall, 1990.

RELATED ARTICLES
Barbo, Dorothy. "Estrogen—Benefits and Risks." *Healthline* (March 1990): 5.

Barrett-Connor, Elizabeth. "Postmenopausal Estrogen Replacement and Breast Cancer." *The New England Journal of Medicine* 321, no. 5 (August 3, 1989): 319–320.

Bergkvist, Leif, Adami Hans-Olov, and others. "The Risk of Breast Cancer After Estrogen and Estrogen-Progestin Replacement." *The New England Journal of Medicine*. 321, no. 5 (August 3, 1989): 293–297.

Farley, Dixie. "Estrogens." *FDA Consumer* (November 1990): 38–40.

Ferguson, Kristi J., Curtis Hoegh, and Susan Johnson. "Estrogen Replacement Therapy: A Survey of Women's Knowledge and Attitudes." *Archives of Internal Medicine* 149 (January 1989): 133–136.

Genant, Harry K., David J. Baylink, and J. C. Gallagher. "Estrogens in the Prevention of Osteoporosis in Postmenopausal Women." *American Journal of Obstetrics and Gynecology* 161, no. 6, part 2 (December 1989): 1842–1846.

Miller, Valery T., and others. "ERT: Weighing the Risks and Benefits." *Patient Care* 24 (June 15, 1990): 30–43.

Nachtigall, Lila. "Enhancing Patient Compliance with Hormone Replacement Therapy." *Obstetrics and Gynecology* 75, no. 4 (suppl.) (April 1990): 77S–80S.

Ross, Ronald R., Annlia Paganini-Hill, and others. "Cardiovascular Benefits of Estrogen Replacement Therapy." *American Journal of Obstetrics and Gynecology* 160, no. 5, part 2 (May 1989): 1301–1306.

EXERCISE

OVERVIEW

Only one older person out of four exercises regularly or maintains anything like the level of physical activity recommended by specialists on aging. Yet study after study shows the positive health effects of regular physical activity—even for the very old.

Exercising for a half hour twice a week significantly increased the health and mobility of men and women with serious chronic ailments in a program and study conducted by University of Michigan public health specialists. All participants were deemed at high risk for placement in nursing homes.

Most of the 75 men and women in the study were overweight and had never exercised regularly. All but a few were over 75 years of age.

Arthritis, hypertension, heart disease and diabetes were among the health problems—all of them worsened by inactivity—that the men and women in the study suffered from. Many reported at least three chronic health problems, the University of Michigan School of Public Health researchers said.

The exercises employed were gentle and easy to master. They included neck and shoulder rolls, spinal twists and side stretches, arm and leg flexes and extensions, and pelvis rocks. While seated on chairs, participants leaned backward and forward to flex abdominal muscles. Slow deep-breathing exercises were also part of the routine.

Even minor physical improvement often made major differences in the participants' functioning, the researchers said.

Participants said they could "get around and move faster" or "felt less stiff in the joints" or "had more energy and were able to walk longer distances." One woman said she could hold her cards better. Another said, "It has helped lift my spirits."

Another study suggests that moderate exercise may be important in preventing and delaying the onset of heart disease in older persons.

Heart disease occurred later and less frequently in the group of older persons who exercised than in the non-exercising control group in a two-year study conducted by the Medical College of Pennsylvania. A total of 184 persons were included in the trial, all of them healthy non-exercisers previously.

About 800,000 Americans over age 65 die annually from major cardiovascular diseases, the nation's leading cause of death.

The medical college estimates that about 27 percent of older Americans exercise regularly. A 1990 goal of 50 percent has been set by the U.S. Public Health Service (PHS) for all ages of the population.

At Duke University Medical Center, supervised exercise programs play a key role in intercepting the downward health spiral of persons suffering from chronic lung disease such as emphysema, bronchitis and asthma. "Many people with chronic lung disease descend to their level of breathlessness," said Neil MacIntyre, M.D., director of Duke's Comprehensive Pulmonary Rehabilitation Program. "When they feel breathless, they reduce their activity even more, which in turn lowers their level of breathlessness. It's a vicious downhill cycle. But if you can intercept the downward spiral and increase the level of activity, their breathlessness becomes less noticeable and easier to cope with," he said. At the conclusion of the hospital-based program, each patient gets an individual exercise "prescription" to follow at home, building on the progress achieved in the program.

About two-thirds of the patients in the Duke program maintained or increased their functional abilities, and their scores on psychological tests stayed the same or increased, MacIntyre said. The report covered about 400 patients.

Dramatic differences in death rates have been found between physically fit women with blood pressure below 120 and women in the lowest physical fitness level with diastolic resting blood pressure above 140, in research reported in the *Journal of the American Medical Association*.

The relative death risk of women in the group with the highest blood pressure and lowest fitness is rated 43.4 times greater—4,338 percent higher—than for the high-fitness, low blood pressure group. The study was based on data from more than 13,000 women, and it was published in the November 3, 1989 issue of the *Journal*.

Older people who engage in active exercise one or more hours a day have about half the risk of hip fracture as older people who exercise less than a half hour daily or not at all. This was among the findings of a University of Southern California study begun in 1981, of the lifestyle practices of 13,649 men and women living in Leisure World, a retirement community in Laguna Hills, Calif.

The findings on hip fractures, which were 40 percent less likely in women who did active exercise daily, were reported in the January 1991 issue of *Epidemiology*. Identified as active exercise were such activities as swimming, biking, tennis, jogging, vigorous walking, dancing and indoor exercise programs. Less vigorous activities such as golfing, gardening and household chores don't substantially reduce the risk of hip fractures, the findings suggest.

Evaluation of other risk factors showed that cigarette smokers had a significantly increased risk of hip fracture (which disappeared in ex-smokers) and that women who were taking estrogen had a lower risk of fracture.

The Public Health Service recommends regular physical exercise not only as heart disease and cancer prevention but also in delaying the onset [of] or preventing hypertension, obesity, osteoporosis, diabetes and some mental health problems. It may also reduce the incidence of stroke and help to maintain the mobility and independence of older people, the PHS's Office of Disease Prevention and Health Promotion states.

Aerobic exercise improved cardiorespiratory fitness, lowered cholesterol and increased bone mineral content in older men and women studied in 1989 by Duke University Medical Center and the North Carolina Spine Center.

Participants did aerobics for 60 minutes three times a week over a four-month period. At the end of the study the participants reported that they had more energy and endurance and were sleeping better. They also reported better family relations, better sex life, less loneliness, improved mood and greater self-confidence.

Although most older people are able to participate, to some extent, in a structured, progressive exercise program, they should have a physical examination before beginning, advises Richard Lampman, director of the University of Michigan Medical Center's Cardiac Fitness and Exercise Research program. The examination should include a stress test or exercise tolerance test to gauge current level of fitness, and an evaluation of medication being used to determine whether they should be altered to allow for increased activity levels. Blood testing for glucose and cholesterol levels should also be part of the comprehensive examination.

SOURCE:

Aging. U.S. Department of Health and Human Services. No. 362. 1991. Reprinted in: "Exercise Isn't Just for Fun." *Public Citizen Health Research Group Health Letter* (August 1991): 8–9.

PLANNING A PERSONAL EXERCISE PROGRAM

The decision to carry out a physical fitness program cannot be taken lightly. It requires a lifelong commitment of time and effort. Exercise must become one of those things that you do without question, like bathing and brushing your teeth. Unless you are convinced of the benefits of fitness and the risks of unfitness, you will not succeed.

Patience is essential. Don't try to do too much too soon and don't quit before you have a chance to experience the rewards of improved fitness. You can't regain in a few days or weeks what you have lost in years of sedentary living, but you can get it back if you persevere. And the prize is worth the price. . . .

CHECKING YOUR HEALTH

If you are under 35 and in good health, you don't need to see a doctor before beginning an exercise program. But if you are over 35 and have been inactive for several years, you should consult your physician, who may or may not recommend a graded exercise test. Other conditions that indicate a need for medical clearance are:

- High blood pressure.
- Heart trouble.
- Family history of early stroke or heart attack deaths.
- Frequent dizzy spells.
- Extreme breathlessness after mild exertion.
- Arthritis or other bone problems.
- Severe muscular, ligament or tendon problems.
- Other known or suspected disease.

Vigorous exercise involves minimal health risks for persons in good health or those following a doctor's advice. Far greater risks are presented by habitual inactivity and obesity.

DEFINING FITNESS

Physical fitness is to the human body what fine tuning is to an engine. It enables us to perform up to our potential. Fitness can be described as a condition that helps us look, feel and do our best. More specifically, it is:

"The ability to perform daily tasks vigorously and alertly, with energy left over for enjoying leisure-time activities and meeting emergency demands. It is the ability to endure, to bear up, to withstand stress, to carry on in circumstances where an unfit person could not continue, and is a major basis for good health and well-being."

Physical fitness involves the performance of the heart and lungs, and the muscles of the body. And, since what we do with our bodies also affects what we can do with our minds, fitness influences to some degree qualities such as mental alertness and emotional stability.

As you undertake your fitness program, it's important to remember that fitness is an individual quality that varies from person to person. It is influenced by age, sex, heredity, personal habits, exercise and eating practices. You can't do anything about the first three factors. However, it is within your power to change and improve the others where needed.

KNOWING THE BASICS

Physical fitness is most easily understood by examining its components, or "parts." There is widespread agreement that these four components are basic:

Cardiorespiratory endurance—the ability to deliver oxygen and nutrients to tissues, and to remove wastes, over sustained periods of time. Long runs and swims are among the methods employed in measuring this component.

Muscular strength—the ability of a muscle to exert force for a brief period of time. Upper-body strength, for example, can be measured by various weight-lifting exercises.

Muscular endurance—the ability of a muscle, or a group of muscles, to sustain repeated contractions or to continue applying force against a fixed object. Pushups are often used to test endurance of arm and shoulder muscles.

Flexibility—the ability to move joints and use muscles through their full range of motion. The sit-and-reach test is a good measure of flexibility of the lower back and backs of the upper legs.

Body composition is often considered a component of fitness. It refers to the makeup of the body in terms of lean mass (muscle, bone, vital tissue and organs) and fat mass. An optimal ratio of fat to lean mass is an indication of fitness, and the right types of exercises will help you decrease body fat and increase or maintain muscle mass.

A WORKOUT SCHEDULE

How often, how long and how hard you exercise, and what kinds of exercises you do should be determined by what you are trying to accomplish. Your goals, your present fitness level, age, health, skills, interest and convenience are among the factors you should consider. For example, an athlete training for high-level competition would follow a different program than a person whose goals are good health and the ability to meet work and recreational needs.

Your exercise program should include something from each of the four basic fitness components described previously. Each workout should begin with a warmup and end with a cooldown. As a general rule, space your workouts throughout the week and avoid consecutive days of hard exercise.

SOURCE:
President's Council on Physical Fitness and Sports. *Fitness Fundamentals: Guidelines for Personal Exercise Programs.* 1985. pp. 1-4.

EXERCISE—AND HEART DISEASE

Ask almost anyone about exercise, and they'll say "It's good for you." Ask most doctors, and they'll say "It's particularly good for your heart."

Of course it's unlikely that exercise alone will prevent or cure heart disease. But it is true that a sedentary lifestyle may increase the risk of heart attack. Regular exercise is one important way to help reduce heart attack risk.

Regular exercise brings gains in many ways:

- It improves blood circulation throughout the body. The lungs, heart and other organs and muscles work together more effectively.
- It improves your body's ability to use oxygen and provide the energy needed for physical activity.
- It helps people handle stress, so they can do more and not tire so easily. It bolsters enthusiasm and optimism.
- It's good for psychological well-being, because it releases tension and helps relaxation and sleep.
- Along with proper diet, it can help people control their weight.

Exercise isn't a remedy for all physical ills, though. In some cases, without proper guidance, it can be damaging. An exercise program appropriate for a person's individual capacity and suited to his or her needs can improve personal outlook and well-being, however.

Remember: Lack of exercise may be a risk factor leading to heart disease. But if the major controllable risk factors—high blood pressure, a high cholesterol level and cigarette smoking—are ignored, exercise alone probably won't help much. It's only one factor in a total program of cardiovascular health.

Check with your doctor if you plan to start a regular exercise program—particularly if you have been sedentary. Your doctor will help you find a program suited to your needs and physical condition. You may be given an exercise tolerance test to determine your present capabilities and identify potential hazards.

Chances are, if you're in good health, your doctor will recommend a program of frequent, ongoing physical activity that

- is rhythmic,
- is repetitive,
- involves motion and using large muscles, and
- challenges the circulatory system.

Such exercises are called isotonic, dynamic or aerobic.

Only those exercises that significantly increase the blood flow to the working muscles for an extended time promote "cardiovascular fitness." When a person's cardiovascular system is fit, he or she can exercise vigorously for long periods without undue fatigue. The person is able to respond to sudden physical or emotional demands more readily and with less strain. Activities often recommended for improving cardiovascular fitness include walking or hiking, jogging, bicycling, swimming, roller skating, jumping rope and active sports or games.

Exercises such as weight lifting or isometrics may build muscle strength, but they do little to promote cardiovascular fitness. They may be a part of your regular exercise program—that's for you and your doctor to decide. But don't depend on them to build cardiovascular endurance.

SOURCE:
American Heart Association. *"E" Is for Exercise*. 1989. pp. 1-2.

* * *

Epidemiologic studies published in the 1950s began to link physical activity to decreased incidence of myocardial infarction and sudden death. London bus conductors (on their feet all day collecting fares), postmen, physically active railroad workers, and longshoremen doing heavy physical labor have all been found to have fewer heart attacks than more sedentary fellow workers. While all of these studies have been criticized for certain shortcomings, they provided a stimulus for further inquiry into the potential links between physical activity and improved cardiovascular health. In the past 25 years, more than 40 major studies have continued to explore this association.

Perhaps the most convincing evidence linking physical activity to improved cardiovascular health has come from three recent studies. In the College Alumni Study, in which more than 16,000 men who entered college between 1916 and 1950 have been tracked for more than 25 years, individuals who regularly expended between 2,100 and 14,600 kJ (500 and 3,500 kcal) in physical activity each week showed reductions in myocardial infarction and sudden death when compared with more sedentary counterparts. A recent report from the Multiple Risk Factor Intervention Trial showed that even low-intensity activity (such as gardening) results in significant reduction in the manifestations of CHD [coronary heart disease]. The Centers for Disease Control analysis of 43 previous exercise trials showed a significant decrease in the incidence of CHD when comparing the most active with the least active groups of people.

SOURCE:
Rippe, James M., and others. "Walking for Health and Fitness." *JAMA* 259, no. 18 (May 13, 1988): 2720-2724. Copyright 1988, American Medical Association.

EXERCISE—DURING PREGNANCY

The general benefits of aerobic exercise for most nonpregnant individuals are familiar to most clinicians. Some benefits that might also help pregnant women include (1) reducing blood pressure, (2) decreasing other cardiovascular risks such as clot formation, (3) helping to maintain an ideal body weight, and (4) managing stable diabetes. In addition, some beneficial effects of exercise on labor and delivery have been documented.

Pregnant women who exercise have generally shorter labors, and faster, easier deliveries. A study of conditioned female athletes showed that the second stage of labor was shorter, presumably owing to strengthened abdominal muscles. The first stage, however, was prolonged because of the rigidity of the uterus and strong muscle tone. . . .

Exercise prescriptions should be individualized, taking into account the woman's total medical status along with her home situation. A patient education plan should encourage those physical activities that promote the potential benefits of exercise during pregnancy. Pregnant women should be instructed to monitor their own heart rates accurately and to avoid overexertion. An easy way to monitor exertional stress is to use the exercise-talk test. If a woman cannot exercise and talk simultaneously, she is approaching a compromising respiratory or heart rate. The heart rate should increase no more than 60% to 70% of the predicted maximum (220 beats per minute minus age in years), and the heart and respiratory rates should return to their resting rates within 15 minutes after exercising. Even moderate exercise should not continue to exhaustion; frequent rest periods should be recommended.

SOURCE:
Jarski, Robert W., and Diane L. Trippett. "The Risks and Benefits of Exercise during Pregnancy." *The Journal of Family Practice* 30, no. 2 (February 1990): 187–188.

EXERCISE—AND OLDER ADULTS

We are in the exercise era—the age of aerobic workouts, marathons and triathalons. Unfortunately, adults over age 60 have been wary of joining the race to become physically fit. Young people are not the only ones who benefit from a regular fitness program; exercise is equally important and beneficial for older adults.

It is common for people to become less active as they grow older. Inactivity in older adults can lead to weakened and shortened muscles that in turn lead to stiffness and further immobility. Prolonged inactivity can also lead to other problems such as obesity, constipation, back pain and osteoporosis. All too often, these problems are accepted as a natural part of aging. In fact, exercise can do much to prevent them. Adults 60 or older who follow a safe exercise program that is designed for their needs and capabilities can improve their muscle strength, cardio-respiratory fitness, physical endurance and mobility. In addition, regular exercise may help lower blood pressure and prevent the bone loss that leads to osteoporosis. Exercise may lower the concentration of fatty substances in the blood and help prevent weight gain by encouraging better eating habits, burning off excess calories and regulating metabolism.

Exercise can also provide important psychological benefits. Older adults who exercise regularly appear to be more self-confident and self-sufficient than their sedentary peers. Participating in a physical fitness program can help offset the depression often associated with the inactivity of retirement and teach people to relax and better cope with stress.

If you have never maintained a regular exercise program, don't be afraid to start one now. It is important, however, for you to consult your physician before starting. He or she may perform a stress test which will help determine your target heart rate for exercise and the types of exercise that are appropriate. It may be necessary to try many different activities or programs in order to find one that feels good and is enjoyable. Exercise can be performed dally, but should be done at least three to five times per week. Remember that for young and old alike, exercise training should begin slowly and build gradually. Do not expect immediate results—you will build strength and endurance over time. Listen to your body and know your limitations. If you experience pain other than the temporary stretching or soreness sensation, try to modify the way in which you did the exercise. Never exercise in spite of pain and don't try to compete with your peers. Be sure to warm up for five to ten minutes before exercising, rest between movements and stretch with a slow cool-down until your pulse rate is less than 100. It is important to set realistic goals; age is less of a factor in exercising than your previous levels of fitness and activity. The best types of exercise for older adults are those designed to improve flexibility and cardiovascular fitness. Walking is perhaps the most convenient exercise for older adults and is extremely beneficial since it places little stress on the heart and joints while improving musculoskeletal function and benefitting the cardiovascular system. Good quality, shock-absorbing shoes with traction soles are a must; they provide stability and absorb impact. Dancing (using sliding steps), cycling (stationary), gardening and swimming are also ideal exercises for older adults. Those that are fit may enjoy low impact aerobics, tennis, racquetball, cross-country skiing and running. Less mobile individuals, or those who use wheelchairs, can develop a routine of sitting exercises using the upper body, arms, neck, shoulder and stomach. These kinds of workouts can be particularly beneficial when followed by deep breathing and a relaxation period.

Some individuals may find they dislike exercising alone and need the motivation of a group program. You may wish to contact physical education specialists at your local "Y," senior citizen center, hospital, school or college. They will probably be able to help you find a fitness program suited to your needs. Another excellent source for information on exercise and older adults is the National Association for Human Development (NAHD). . . . There may be a variety of programs to choose from in your area. Look for those programs which improve cardiovascular fitness and maintain joint flexibility without stressing the joints.

Keep certain precautions in mind. When you exercise, your heart rate should increase but there should be no chest pain. Avoid holding your breath during exercise, and beware of exercises that stress the lower back, such as leg lifts or side stretches. Dehydration is more common among older adults, so drink water before, during and after exercising. It is not wise for some people to do isometric exercises which tense one set of muscles against another or against weights. These may substantially increase blood pressure and strain the heart. Some people with degenerative arthritis of the elbow or shoulder may find that isometric exercises help control joint pain and prevent further joint damage. However, such individuals should check with their physician before doing isometric exercises. Stop any activity that causes discomfort, and contact a physician if you have persistent joint and muscle pain. Also seek help if you have chest pain, headache, dizziness, breathlessness or unusual fatigue on the day of or day after exercising.

Exercise—even when begun at a late age—can significantly improve your quality of life. Not only can older individuals who participate in a regular fitness program slow the onset of health problems, they can also reap important psychological benefits.

SOURCE:
California Medical Association. "Exercise and Older Adults." *HealthTips* no. 461 (May 1990): 1–2.

RESOURCES

ORGANIZATIONS

American Heart Association. 7320 Greenville Ave., Dallas, TX 75231.

President's Council on Physical Fitness and Health. 450 Fifth St. NW, Washington, DC 20001.

PAMPHLETS

California Medical Association:

"Exercise and Heart Disease." *HealthTips* index 4 (April 1989): 2 pp.

"Exercise During Pregnancy." *HealthTips* index WH-6 (June 1990): 2 pp.

BOOKS

Pleas, John. *Walking.* New York: Norton, 1987. 158 pp.

Simon, Harvey B., and Steven R. Levisohn. *The Athlete Within: A Personal Guide to Total Fitness.* Boston: Little, Brown, 1987. 314 pp.

RELATED ARTICLES

Gillis, Angela, and Anne Perry. "The Relationships Between Physical Activity and Health-Promoting Behaviours in Mid-Life Women." *Journal of Advanced Nursing* 16 (1991): 299-310.

Harris, Sally S., and others. "Physical Activity Counseling for Healthy Adults as a Primary Preventive Intervention in the Clinical Setting. Report for the US Preventive Services Task Force." *JAMA* 261, no. 24 (June 23/30, 1989): 3590-3598.

"Surgeon General's Workshop on Health Promotion and Aging: Summary Recommendations of Physical Fitness and Exercise Working Group." *JAMA* 262 (November 10, 1989): 2507-2508.

"Tips for Sensible Winter Exercise." *University of Toronto Faculty of Medicine Health News* 8, no. 6 (December 1990): 1-3.

FIBROCYSTIC BREAST DISEASE

(*See also:* MAMMOGRAMS AND BREAST BIOPSY)

OVERVIEW

Fibrocystic breast disease is a noncancerous condition. It is usually marked by the presence of nodules or cysts (sacs filled with fluid), which may or may not be accompanied by pain and tenderness. Its symptoms fluctuate in response to hormonal changes, especially those associated with menstruation.

Fibrocystic breast disease can occur in one or both breasts. The nodules or cysts can be spread throughout the breast, be located in one general area, or simply appear as one or more large cysts.

It is the most common noncancerous disease of the breast. In fact, at some point in her life, one woman out of four in the United States requires medical attention for a breast problem, which will often be diagnosed as fibrocystic breast disease.

Fibrocystic breast disease can occur at any age after menstruation begins, but it is more likely to appear between the age of 30 and menopause. After that, it rarely occurs.

The cause or causes are unknown, but the condition is believed to result from an imbalance of the female sex hormones. It does not appear before the onset of menstruation, when the production of these female sex hormones begins, and it rarely appears after menopause, when their production ceases.

Fibrocystic breast disease is usually diagnosed when a patient goes to her doctor for a checkup or seeks help for pain, tenderness, or a lump that was probably discovered during breast self-examination.

At times, the doctor may wish to further confirm the diagnosis, in which case he or she will probably recommend additional routine tests. These tests may help the doctor get a more complete picture of your breasts than can be obtained simply from a manual examination.

In the past, there were no specific treatments for fibrocystic breast disease other than those to minimize discomfort. Today, the primary goal of treatment is the relief of pain and the tenderness as well as the reduction and/or elimination of cysts.

Fibrocystic breast disease by its very nature is cyclical, so symptoms that may be mild at one point in your life can become progressively more severe later. The condition usually disappears during pregnancy and nursing. Sometimes it will disappear permanently, or it may return in the future. Therapy might be different each time.

Hormonal drug therapy can provide relief of the symptoms of pain, tenderness, and nodularity by helping to correct the underlying hormonal imbalance. In this way, the breasts are less stimulated and are, in effect, "given a rest."

SOURCE:

Winthrop Pharmaceuticals. *Fibrocystic Breast Disease: What Should I Know about It?* 1987, pp. 2-5.

FIBROCYSTIC BREAST DISEASE—A USELESS DIAGNOSIS?

"Fibrocystic disease" is a meaningless umbrella term—a wastebasket into which doctors throw every breast problem that isn't cancerous. The symptoms that it encompasses are so varied and so unrelated to each other that the term is wholly without meaning. Some doctors recognize this and have stopped using the term. Others, unfortunately, have not. Still others will use equally bad terms such as "chronic cystic mastitis" or just "cystic mastitis."

What are doctors talking about when they use the term "fibrocystic disease?" Well, to begin with, it depends on what kind of a doctor is using the term. First, there's the doctor who examines you. This doctor can be addressing one or more symptoms. His (or her) "fibrocystic disease" can be swelling, pain, tenderness, lumpy breasts (a condition that should not be confused with breast lumps), nipple discharge—any noncancerous thing that can happen in or on the breast. That's the clinical version of our mythical disease.

If the doctor is concerned that your problem might be a symptom of cancer, your breast will be biopsied, and the tissue examined under a microscope by another doctor called a pathologist. And what does the pathologist find? You've got "fibrocystic disease." But the trick is, it's not the same fibrocystic disease the examining doctor discovered. The pathologist's report has to do not with your original symptom, but with any one of about 15 microscopic findings that exist in virtually every woman's breasts, and which never reveal themselves except through a microscope. They cause no trouble, and they have no relation to cancer—or to anything else, except the body's natural aging process. They are the result of natural wear and tear, no more a disease than gray hair or age lines. And the only reason they showed up in the particular breast tissue that was biopsied was because it was biopsied. If you'd had another area of your breast biopsied, they'd find them there, too: those harmless little changes that take place throughout your breasts. (Only one of these—a fairly rare one—is a danger sign: it's called atypical hyperplasia, and, combined with a family history of breast cancer, it can suggest an increased breast cancer risk.) But your doctor won't make this distinction. . . The doctor will just tell you what you already know: you've got "fibrocystic disease." Again, you're grateful not to have cancer, but upset that you're diseased.

If this isn't confusing enough, there's a third kind of fibrocystic disease, discovered by the radiologists who read your mammogram. Mammography is the new kid on the block—it's only been around 10 or 15 years—and the radiologists want to get in on the game. So when the radiologists began reading mammograms, they discovered that younger women tended to have very dense breast tissue, while older women tended to have less dense breast tissue. "Why?" they asked the surgeons. And the surgeons answered—what else?—"fibrocystic disease." And now the radiologists have their very own fibrocystic disease to diagnose—completely different from the clinical or pathological versions.

What really causes the radiologists' fibrocystic disease? Interestingly enough, it's exactly the opposite of what causes the pathologists' version: it's simply youth. You know those firm, unsagging breasts that women in their teens and early 20s so often have—the breasts the rest of us are supposed to envy? Well, they're firm because they've got comparatively little fat and comparatively more breast tissue, and the more breast tissue you've got, the denser the tissue is. . . Dense breast tissue is in fact very normal, especially in young women. There's nothing diseased about it, except in the imaginations of some doctors.

If you're beginning to feel a little like Alice after she fell through the looking glass, you should. "Fibrocystic disease" is as fanciful as anything Lewis Carroll ever invented. It's not only fanciful, however; it's dangerous. It causes a number of problems for those women who, as we say in the medical world, "carry the diagnosis." The dangers fall into three categories.

The first danger isn't a medical one; it's economic. Many insurance companies won't insure a woman who's been diagnosed as having fibrocystic disease—as they won't insure people diagnosed as having any chronic disease. If they'll insure you at all, they may exclude breast problems—with the result that you won't have insurance coverage should you ever get a real breast disease.

At the same time, if you're already insured when you're diagnosed as having fibrocystic disease, your company may pay for your mammograms. Because of this, a well-meaning doctor is often tempted to diagnose fibrocystic disease so your mammogram will be paid for. But your advantage then lasts only as long as you remain with the same insurance company: should you ever want to sign up with another company, your "disease" will work against you, and you'll be stuck with the label for the rest of your life.

Medically, the dangers range from minor to very serious indeed. First of all, your mental health isn't going to be improved by your conviction that you're especially prone to breast cancer. Second, the medical "treatments" can be anything from ineffective (like eliminating caffeine from your diet) to devastating; some doctors even recommend a form of mastectomy to prevent the cancer you're supposedly likely to get.

SOURCE:

Love, Susan. *Dr. Susan Love's Breast Book.* Addison-Wesley, 1990. pp. 76–78.

SYMPTOMS

Fibrocystic disease takes many forms. Approximately half of all premenopausal women report discomfort, ranging from tenderness and mild swelling to insistent pain. They may also experience changes in the texture of the breast tissue, lumps, nipple discharge, or inflammation. Regardless of the symptoms and physical findings, benign breast disorders stem from the same underlying cause: the normal hormonal fluctuations that occur throughout a woman's reproductive years.

Each month, the breasts respond to the cyclic peaks and troughs of estrogen and progesterone. As hormone levels rise just before and during menstruation, mammary blood vessels swell, ducts and alveoli expand, and cell growth proliferates. Breast tissue retains fluid and grows larger. After menstruation, these processes reverse.

Years of such fluctuations eventually produce areas of dense or fibrotic tissue. Multiple small cysts and an increasing level of breast pain commonly develop when a woman hits her 30s. Larger cysts usually don't occur until after age 35. . . .

There are good data showing that breast pain and lumpiness, for example, do not necessarily occur together, and that women with nodularity do not experience the same hormonal changes as women with cyclic breast pain. To account for these differences, a new classification system, based on clinical symptoms and physical findings, divides fibrocystic disease into six diagnostic categories:

- Swelling and tenderness (cyclic discomfort)
- Mastalgia (severe pain, both cyclic and non-cyclic)
- Nodularity (lumpiness, both cyclic and non-cyclic)
- Dominant lumps (including cysts and fibroadenomas)
- Nipple discharge (including intraductal papilloma and duct ectasia)
- Infections and inflammations (including subareolar abscess, lactational mastitis, breast abscess, and Mondor's disease).

SOURCE:
Mack, Ellie. "Most Breast Lumps Aren't Cancer!" *RN* 53 (December 1990): 20–23.

TREATMENT

Perhaps the best known—and most controversial—treatment for benign breast symptoms is to reduce intake of foods and substances containing caffeine to relieve pain, tenderness and swelling and eliminate lumps. A plethora of studies shows little consensus on whether or not caffeine is linked to breast symptoms. "There's not a solid body of scientific knowledge that says yes or no," says Bruce H. Drukker, M.D., chairman of obstetrics and gynecology and reproductive biology at the College of Human Medicine, Michigan State University in East Lansing. Based on clinical observation, he believes that about two thirds of women with benign breast symptoms are helped by giving up all caffeine. Other experts, however, aren't convinced that caffeine is a culprit. . . .

Advice abounds on the use of vitamins to relieve various symptoms, from rubbing vitamin E oil on the breasts to taking vitamin B1 to help the liver process estrogen. At the moment there is no firm scientific evidence to support these or any other vitamin-related suggestions. The best strategy, say many doctors, is to use analgesics such as aspirin for combatting pain and to reduce salt intake—especially during the two weeks before the menstrual period. This will limit water retention, which contributes to swelling. Taking a diuretic under a doctor's supervision for about 10 days before menstruation may also cut down on fluid retention.

For severe symptoms, doctors may prescribe hormonal therapies. Some women find relief by going on birth control pills, which help regulate estrogen and progesterone levels. If this doesn't work, stronger therapies are available; unfortunately, these may bring debilitating side effects. For example, Danocrine, a synthetic version of the male hormone testosterone, works by shutting down the menstrual cycle. But it can also cause weight gain, growth of facial and bodily hair, acne, deepening of the voice and other undesirable side effects. Bromocriptine suppresses the hormone prolactin (which is elevated in about two thirds of women with benign breast changes) but may also lower blood pressure and cause headache and fatigue. Some doctors try tamoxifen, an anti-estrogen drug, but it can lead to loss of appetite, depression, blood clots and nerve problems.

Many women can make themselves more comfortable through nondrug means. For example, switching to a larger bra cup size in the days before the period may make swelling and tenderness more bearable. Wearing loose clothing, sleeping on your back and avoiding jarring activities such as jogging and high-impact aerobics also may help.

SOURCE:
McCarthy, Laura Flynn. "The Benign Breast Syndrome." *Health* (March 1991): 56–57.

RESOURCES

RELATED ARTICLES

Boyd, N. F., P. Shannon, and others. Effect of Low-Fat High-Carbohydrate Diet on Symptoms of Cyclical Mastopathy. *The Lancet* 2 (July 16, 1989): 128–142.

"Fibrocystic Breast Conditions. *University of Texas Lifetime Health Letter* 1, no. 7 (August 1989): 6–7.

Love, Susan M. "Fibrocystic Disease: What's in a Name?" *Patient Care* 24 (July 15, 1990): 65–75.

Love, Susan M., and Karen Lindsey. "Fighting Back against Breast Pain." *Prevention* 7 (August 1990): 56–62.

Vorherr, H. "Fibrocystic Breast Disease: Pathophysiology, Pathomorphology, Clinical Picture, and Management." *American Journal of Obstetrics and Gynecology* 154 (1986): 161–179.

FLU

(*See also:* VACCINES)

OVERVIEW

Most flu cases result from the influenza A and B viruses. Both cause fever, coughs, and muscle aches and headaches, but B often evokes a milder form of influenza and fewer deaths than A, says Dr. Roland Levandowski, a virologist and internist with FDA's Center for Biologics Evaluation and Research.

Influenza A has been the virus responsible for most widespread flu epidemics, according to CDC's [Nancy] Arden [epidemiologist with the Centers for Disease Control in Atlanta], including the 1918–19 "Spanish" flu that killed an estimated 500,000 Americans and 20 million people elsewhere. The nickname "Spanish" and others, like "Hong Kong," refer to the place where outbreaks first appeared, Levandowski says.

There are three different strains of the influenza A virus. The one scientists call H1N1 dominated flu cases from 1918 to 1957. Then it disappeared, only to mysteriously reappear in 1977. "It was like someone put it in a freezer for 20 years and then took it out again," Arden says.

The second type, H2N2, first emerged in 1957 as the cause of that year's "Asian" flu, an outbreak that killed 70,000 Americans. Like H1N1, the H2N2 strain disappeared in 1968 as suddenly as it had come. In its place came the third strain, H3N2. It has reappeared yearly since 1968. Thus, two strains of influenza A—H1N1 and H3N2—have circulated together since 1977, a first in known medical history, Arden says.

Which virus (A or B) or which strain will strike in any given year is hard to say. Sometimes all types and strains will cause influenza cases; other times one virus or strain will dominate. Yet, in other years (as in 1957 or 1968), a wholly new or a mutated version of an older strain will appear.

"It is almost impossible to predict which one will dominate," says FDA's Levandowski, a sentiment with which CDC's Arden agrees. "One thing you can be sure of," Levandowski adds, "whatever you predict will be wrong. That's what makes us go gray and pull our hair out."

SOURCE:

Cohn, Jeffrey P. "Here Come the Bugs: Cold and Flu Season's Back." *FDA Consumer* 22 (November 1988): 6–9.

* * *

The spread of viruses that cause flu is primarily through direct person-to-person routes, especially coughing and sneezing (via the airborne droplets of respiratory fluids). Because these viruses can survive on objects for brief periods, a person can also acquire the flu by touching a contaminated object and then touching the mucous membranes of the eye, nose, or mouth.

The greatest risk of infection is found in highly populated areas, where people live in crowded conditions, and in schools. Isolating people with flu symptoms, as a means of disease control, is not considered useful since an infection may be spread by someone whose symptoms are not immediately obvious.

After a person has been infected with the virus, the symptoms usually become apparent in 2 to 4 days. From this stage in the disease, the infection is considered contagious for another 3 to 4 days.

Flu is usually signaled by headache, chills, and dry cough, which are rapidly followed by aches, fever, and sore muscles. Typically, the fever starts declining on the second or third day of the illness. It is then that the upper respiratory symptoms become noticeable, and nasal congestion and sore throat develop. Flu almost never causes gastrointestinal symptoms; the illness that people often call "stomach flu" is not influenza.

Usually, a diagnosis of flu is based simply on whether there is a flu outbreak in the community and whether the patient's complaints fit the current pattern of symptoms. Laboratory testing to identify the virus is rarely necessary, but it is sometimes done by health officials to determine which type of flu virus, A or B, is responsible for the epidemic.

SOURCE:
National Institute of Allergy and Infectious Diseases, Office of Communications. *Flu.* NIH Pub. No. 87-187. September 1987. p. 5.

SYMPTOMS

A bout of influenza generally lasts from a few days to a couple of weeks, depending on the strain, individual susceptibility, age and personal state of health. The illness usually starts with a sore throat, fever, chills, headache, muscle and joint pains, dry cough and sometimes a runny nose. The nasal involvement is usually far less pronounced than with a common cold. And, unlike a typical cold, with flu the fever may be quite high, depending on the influenza strain. The cough often becomes irritating, with consequent chest soreness and interrupted sleep. The complications of influenza, such as pneumonia, can be serious. Secondary infection of the lungs with pneumococci, the bacteria responsible for pneumonia, may follow influenza, and requires prompt medical attention. But for a mild bout of influenza, treatment with bedrest, fluids, and antipyretics (fever reducers) usually suffices. However, ASA/aspirin [acetylsalicylic acid] should not be used in children (because of possible danger of Reye's syndrome linked to ASA-treated influenza B). Antibiotics do not help influenza since they're ineffective against viral illnesses, but they may be required for a secondary bacterial lung infection, such as pneumonia.

SOURCE:
"Flu Shots: Yes or No?" *Health News* (October 1988): 6-7.

TREATMENT

Once a person has the flu, treatment usually consists of resting in bed, drinking plenty of fluids, and taking medication such as acetaminophen to relieve fever and discomfort.

At present, there is only one drug, amantadine, that has been licensed for the treatment of influenza A (amantadine is not effective against influenza B). When amantadine is given within 24 to 48 hours after the onset of illness, it reduces the duration of fever and other symptoms and allows flu sufferers to return to their daily routines more quickly.

Amantadine can also prevent infection; to be effective, however, it must be taken during the entire 4- to 6-week course of an epidemic. The drug has been shown to be 70 to 90 percent effective when used in this way. After people stop taking the preventative amantadine therapy, they again become susceptible to the virus.

About 7 to 10 percent of the people taking amantadine experience some side effects (nausea, dizziness, sleep disturbances, and depression). These symptoms are more pronounced among older persons, especially those with impaired kidney function.

SOURCE:
National Institute of Allergy and Infectious Diseases, Office of Communications. *Flu.* NIH Pub. No. 87-187. September 1987. p. 5.

PREVENTION

All current influenza vaccines are inactivated (i.e., killed) and cannot cause influenza. Influenza vaccine is reformulated annually each spring to contain antigens of influenza A and B viruses expected to circulate in the population during the next influenza season. Because influenza viruses tend to change each year and because immunity in the elderly may wane rapidly, it is recommended that high-risk persons receive an influenza vaccine annually. . . .

Influenza vaccine should be administered annually to all high-risk patients with chronic lung or cardiovascular disease, diabetes, renal disease, hemoglobinopathy, or immunosuppression (including those infected with human immunodeficiency virus). Pregnant women with high-risk medical conditions should be vaccinated because the vaccine is considered safe during pregnancy. When feasible, the vaccine should be administered after the first trimester, unless the influenza season begins during that time. In addition, all persons who are older than 65 years of age should receive an influenza vaccine annually. Physicians, other health care workers, care providers, and household associates of high-risk patients should be strongly encouraged to receive annual influenza vaccinations to reduce the likelihood of transmitting the virus. The same patient groups, especially those with chronic lung disease, are also candidates for the pneumococcal vaccine (given only once.) Other persons who are candidates for the pneumococcal vaccine are those older than two years of age with sickle-cell disease or splenic dysfunction of other causes. Children younger than two years of age are not included because their immunologic responses to pneumococcal vaccine are generally poor.

Influenza vaccine should usually be administered during the fall months, optimally in November so that antibody titers will be at their peak when the outbreaks start, usually in December or January, but it may be offered up to and after influenza virus activity is documented in the community. Pneumococcal vaccine can be administered at any time during the year. Influenza and pneumococcal vaccines can safely be given at the same time in different sites with efficacy similar to that when they are given at different times. Vaccinations should be intramuscular in the deltoid muscle or, for infants and young children, in the anterolateral aspect of the thigh.

SOURCE:
Mastow, S. R., T. R. Cate, and F. L. Ruben. "Prevention of Influenza and Pneumonia." *American Review of Respiratory Diseases* 142, no. 2 (August 1990): 487-488.

* * *

For most people, the flu vaccine is the easiest, most effective way to avoid influenza and its complications, or at least to decrease their severity. But for those who can't tolerate a flu shot, the prescription drug amantadine (Symadine, Symmetrel) can help prevent influenza. Amantadine can also provide additional protection for people who are not adequately protected by the vaccine. And when taken as treatment for flu, the drug can reduce the severity of symptoms and shorten their duration. . . .

Despite some disadvantages, amantadine is clearly beneficial for many people who can't take a flu shot, such as those who are allergic to eggs (used to manufacture the flu vaccine) and those who have had severe allergic reactions to the shot.

Certain people should consider using the drug as well as the vaccine to prevent influenza:

- Those who get the shot after flu season starts. Daily doses of amantadine will protect them during the two or three weeks it takes to build immunity.
- Those exposed to strains of influenza A virus not included in the vaccine.
- Those who live in nursing homes or similar institutions during flu outbreaks there.
- Those with AIDS or any other condition that weakens the immune system.

To prevent flu, amantadine must be taken daily while flu is in the community. A six-week supply of the generic drug costs $15 to $30; brand-name versions cost twice as much.

SOURCE:
"Drugs to Prevent and Treat Influenza: Are They for You?" *Consumer Reports Health Letter* (October 1990): 76-77.

RESOURCES

ORGANIZATIONS
American Lung Association. 2250 Palm Avenue, San Mateo, CA 94403.

National Institute of Allergy and Infectious Diseases. 9000 Rockville Pike, Bethesda, MD 20205.

PAMPHLETS
American Academy of Allergy and Immunology:

Should You Get the "Flu Shot" and How About the Pneumococcal Vaccine. November 1990.

American Lung Association:

Flu. September 1988.

RELATED ARTICLES
Douglas, R. Gordon. "Prophylaxis and Treatment of Influenza." *The New England Journal of Medicine* 322, no. 7 (February 15, 1990): 443-450.

"Flu Inoculation Innocuous." *Consumer Reports Health Letter* (December 1990): 44.

"Flu Shot: If You Need One, Now Is the Time to Get It." *Mayo Clinic Health Letter* (October 1990): 6.

"Influenza Prevention, 1989-1990." *Medical Letter on Drugs and Therapeutics* 31 (October 20, 1989): 95-96.

la Montagne, J. R. "Influenza: Status and Prospects for its Prevention, Therapy, and Control." *Pediatric Clinics of North America* 37, no. 3 (June 1990): 669-688.

Nicholson, K. G. "Influenza Vaccine and the Elderly." (Editorial). *British Medical Journal* (September 29, 1990): 617-618.

Shann, F. "Modern Vaccines: Pneumococcus and Influenza" (Review). *The Lancet* 335, no. 8694 (April 14, 1990): 898-901.

FLUORIDATION

OVERVIEW

Fluorine is an essential trace element and as fluoride it is a natural constituent of all water and some foods. However, the amounts found from "natural" sources are often not sufficient to help develop decay-resistant teeth and strong bones. Fluoridation is an adjustment of fluoride levels in our water supply to a level of 0.7 to 1.2 parts of fluoride per million parts of water (ppm).

Fluoride ingested in water that has been fluoridated is completely safe. Fluoridation reduces tooth decay by 50–70%, depending on how soon after birth one uses fluoridated water on a daily basis. Fluoride's effectiveness is ongoing as long as an individual continues to receive fluoridated water. There are substitutes for fluoridation in the form of fluoride drops, and fluoride tablets. Toothpastes and mouthrinses containing fluoride and dental treatments with topical fluoride solutions help to potentiate the benefits of fluoridation. But none of the substitutes are as effective as fluoridation and all are more expensive.

In addition to greatly reducing tooth decay, fluoridated water helps decrease the prevalence and severity of osteoporosis, a common disease of ageing. Some evidence suggests that fluoride may help reduce the development of arteriosclerosis and thus of coronary heart disease and cerebral hemorrhage (stroke). . . .

Fluoridation is simply the adjustment of the naturally occurring amount in fluoride in drinking water to a level known to promote the development of decay-resistant teeth and strong bones. Water levels are adjusted to 1 part of fluoride per million parts of water (ppm). This amounts to 1 mg fluoride per 1,000 ml of water (1 liter). This level applies to Temperate Zones. In warmer areas where more water is consumed, the water is adjusted to 0.7 ppm fluoride. In cooler areas where less water is consumed, a level of 1.2 ppm is used.

SOURCE:

American Council on Science and Health. *Fluoridation*. September 1990. pp. 1, 3.

POTENTIAL BENEFITS

The American Dental Association has endorsed fluoridation for the last forty years as the safest, most economical method to provide public access to fluoride.

Fluoride protects against cavities in two ways. First, if fluoride is present while a child's teeth are forming, it is incorporated into the crystalline substance that forms the hard surfaces of the teeth, hydroxyapatite (HAP). HAP that forms with fluoride becomes fluoridated hydroxyapatite (FAP), which is more resistant to erosion by acid in the mouth.

Fluoride also benefits adult teeth. As we age, the gums recede or pull away from the base of the teeth, exposing more of the tooth to the acids in the mouth. Fluoride helps prevent root cavities in these exposed sections, which are prone to decay.

When fluoride is present in saliva, the natural healing properties of the saliva are enhanced. Both calcium and phosphate, the two predominant minerals in teeth, are present in saliva. These minerals move from the saliva into the surfaces of teeth when teeth have been eroded by acids. Fluoride enhances this movement of minerals in response to tooth erosion.

Only ingested fluoride, is secreted in the saliva. Topical fluoride is considered an additional therapy.

Fluoride is one of only two known substances that can actually increase bone mass. Other osteoporosis treatments only prevent further bone loss. A recent study completed at the Mayo Clinic, however, found that although fluoride supplementation increases bone mass up to 35%, the bones are of inferior quality. The bones are thicker, but not stronger and there was no reduction in the number of bone fractures in people taking fluoride supplements. Whether or not other dosages or other methods of administration might be helpful in treating osteoporosis are questions to be answered by further research.

SOURCE:
Weinberg, Linda. "Does Fluoride Cause Cancer or Doesn't It." *Environmental Nutrition* 13 (August 1990): 1-2.

GENERAL SAFETY

Is fluoridated water safe to drink? Experts say it's the most effective dental public health measure available. Yet some 40 percent of Americans are still drinking water not yet treated with fluoride, a mineral that helps strengthen tooth enamel and thereby fights cavities. One reason for the lapse is the publicity generated by antifluoridation groups who allege that the mineral promotes chronic diseases such as AIDS, cancer, and sickle cell anemia. But that publicity is ill-founded. Concurrent with the antifluoridationists' efforts to stir controversy, the American Dental Association reports that fluoridation has never been shown to increase the incidence or mortality of any chronic disease. Taking that reassurance one step further, the Surgeon General's recent Report on Nutrition and Health says the evidence is "conclusive" that the levels of fluoride recommended for drinking water "are safe." Perhaps more to the point, the prevalence of cavities has been shown to drop as much as 60 percent among people who drink fluoridated water from birth to adolescence, saving families thousands of dollars in dental bills, not to mention eliminating the discomfort of sitting under the drill. It's true that a condition known as dental fluorosis, a harmless mottling of the teeth, does afflict some people who live in communities where the naturally occurring fluoride levels run exceedingly high. But the amount of fluoride that is added to fluoride-less or low-fluoride water supplies is relatively low—definitely not enough to discolor teeth. If you are unsure about whether your tap water contains adequate fluoride to prevent tooth decay, check with your dentist.

SOURCE:
"Is Fluoridated Water Safe to Drink?" *Tufts University Diet and Nutrition Letter* 7 (October 1989): 1.

NEGLIGIBLE CANCER RISKS

James Mason, Assistant U.S. Secretary for Health, says tests in animals have shown that fluoride carries a negligible cancer risk.

"There is no information available at this time that would indicate a need for any changes in the Public Health Service policy of continued support for the use of fluorides for the prevention of tooth decay," Mason says.

A National Toxicology Program review panel studied the effects of large doses of sodium fluoride in 520 rats and 520 mice given concentrations up to 79 parts per million and found no increased cancer rates in male or female mice or among female rats. The recommended limit for fluoride in drinking water is 4 ppm.

However, the study found osteosarcomas in bones in one of 50 male rats receiving 45 ppm and three of 80 rats receiving 79 ppm. Another male rat receiving the higher dose had evidence of osteosarcoma of the subcutaneous tissue.

The Academy of General Dentistry says a person would have to drink 360 glasses of heavily fluoridated water per day to be exposed to as much chemical as the rats receiving the 45 ppm dose.

"The benefits of water fluoridation are undeniable," says Henry Finger, president of the academy. He says its effectiveness has been "documented in approximately 140 studies from 20 countries over several decades. Since 1945, community water fluoridation has helped create two generations of children who are 50 percent cavity-free."

SOURCE:
Cooper, Mike. "Cancer Risk of Fluoride Downplayed." *NCI Cancer Weekly* (June 11, 1990): 3-4.

RESOURCES

RELATED ARTICLES

Begley, Sharon. "Don't Drink the Water?: Brush Your Teeth, but the Fluoride from Your Tap May Not Do Much Good—and May Cause Cancer." *Newsweek* (February 5, 1990): 60-61.

Corbin, Stephen B. "Fluoridation Then and Now." *American Journal of Public Health* 79, no. 5 (May 1989): 561-564.

Jarvis, William T. "Fluoridation and the EPA." *Priorities* (Summer 1990): 24-27.

Sears, Cathy. "Fluoridation: Friends and Foes." *American Health: Fitness of Body and Mind* 8 (October 1989): 36-37.

FOOD/NUTRITION GUIDELINES

(*See also:* CHOLESTEROL; DIETARY FATS; DIETARY FIBER)

1990 DIETARY GUIDELINES FOR AMERICANS

What should Americans eat to stay healthy?

These guidelines help answer this question. They are advice for healthy Americans ages 2 years and over—not for younger children and infants, whose dietary needs differ. The guidelines reflect recommendations of nutrition authorities who agree that enough is known about diet's effect on health to encourage certain dietary practices by Americans.

Many American diets have too many calories and too much fat (especially saturated fat), cholesterol, and sodium. They also have too little complex carbohydrates and fiber. Such diets are one cause of America's high rates of obesity and of certain diseases—heart disease, high blood pressure, stroke, diabetes, and some forms of cancer. The exact role of diet in some of these is still being studied.

Diseases caused by vitamin and mineral deficiencies are rare in this country. But some people do not get recommended amounts of a few nutrients, especially calcium and iron.

Food alone cannot make you healthy. Health also depends on your heredity, your environment, and the health care you get. Your lifestyle is also important to your health—how much you exercise and whether you smoke, drink alcoholic beverages to excess, or abuse drugs, for example. But a diet based on these guidelines can help you keep healthy and may improve your health.

The first two guidelines form the framework for the diet: "Eat a variety of foods" for the nutrients you need and for energy (calories) to "Maintain healthy weight." The next two guidelines stress the need for many Americans to change their diets to be lower in fat, especially saturated fat, and higher in complex carbohydrates and fiber. Other guidelines suggest only moderate use of sugars, salt, and, if used at all, alcoholic beverages.

These guidelines call for moderation—avoiding extremes in diet. Both eating too much and eating too little can be harmful. Also, be cautious of diets based on the belief that a food or supplement alone can cure or prevent disease.

Your good health may depend on your learning more about yourself. Are you at your healthy weight? Are your blood pressure and your blood cholesterol levels too high? If so, diet or medicine your doctor prescribes may help reduce them. Generally, the sooner a problem is found, the easier it is to treat.

The foods Americans have to choose from are varied, plentiful, and safe to eat. These guidelines can help you choose a diet that is both healthful and enjoyable. . . .

Dietary Guidelines for Americans

- Eat a variety of foods
- Maintain a healthy weight
- Choose a diet low in fat, saturated fat, and cholesterol
- Choose a diet with plenty of vegetables, fruits, and grain products
- Use sugars only in moderation
- Use salt and sodium only in moderation
- If you drink alcoholic beverages, do so in moderation

SOURCE:
U.S. Department of Agriculture, and U.S. Department of Health and Human Services. "Nutrition and Your Health: Dietary Guidelines for Americans." *Home and Garden Bulletin* no. 232. November 1990. pp. 3–4.

NATIONAL ACADEMY OF SCIENCES REPORT ON DIET AND HEALTH

In summary, the diet recommended by the committee should contain moderately low levels of fat, with special emphasis on restriction of saturated fatty acids and cholesterol; high levels of complex carbohydrates; only moderate levels of protein, especially animal protein; and only low levels of added sugars. Caloric intake and physical activity should be balanced to maintain appropriate body weight. The recommendation to maintain total fat intake at or below 30% of total caloric intake and saturated fatty acid as less than 10%, combined with the recommendation to maintain protein intake only at moderate levels, means that for most North Americans it will be necessary to select leaner cuts of meat, trim off excess fat, remove skin from poultry, and consume fewer and smaller portions of meat and poultry. Fish and many shellfish are excellent sources of low-fat protein. By using plant products (e.g., cereals and legumes) instead of animal products as sources of protein, one can also reduce the amount of saturated fatty acids and cholesterol in the diet.

Dairy products are an important source of calcium and protein, but whole milk, whole-milk cheeses, yogurt, ice cream, and other milk products are also high in saturated fatty acids. Therefore, low-fat or skim milk should be substituted. Furthermore, it is desirable to change from butter to margarine with a low saturated fatty acid content, to use less oils and fats in cooking and in salad dressings, and to avoid fried foods.

For most people, the recommended restriction of fat intake, coupled with the recommendation for moderation in protein intake, implies an increase in calories from carbohydrates. These calories should come from an increased intake of whole-grain cereals and breads rather than from foods or drinks containing added sugars. For example, baked goods, such as pies, pastries, and cookies, although they provide complex carbohydrates also tend to contain high levels of total fat, saturated fatty acids, and added sugars, all of which need to be curtailed to meet the committee's recommendations.

In general, vegetables and fruits are unlikely to contribute substantially to caloric intake but are major sources of vitamins, minerals, and dietary fiber. The committee places special emphasis on increasing consumption of green and yellow vegetables as well as citrus fruits, particularly since their consumption in North America is relatively low. The committee's recommendations would lead to a substantial increase in consumption frequency and portion sizes, especially of vegetables, for the average person. Thorough washing of fresh vegetables (especially leafy ones) and fruits will minimize the consumption of pesticide residues in the diet.

The need for restriction of certain dietary components—such as egg yolks; salt; salty, smoked, and preserved foods; and alcoholic beverages—is clearly explained in the recommendations. Further considerations include methods of preparation, cooking, and processing, which can have important effects on the composition of foods. The committee emphasizes the need to read the labels on prepared, formulated, and other processed foods to identify their contribution of nutrients in general and of salt, fats and cholesterol, and sugars in particular. With regard to the risk of chronic diseases, maximum benefit can be attained and any unknown, potentially harmful effects of dietary constituents minimized by selecting a variety of foods from each food group, avoiding excessive caloric intake (especially excessive intake of any one item or food group), and engaging regularly in moderate physical exercise.

SOURCE:

Interdisciplinary Committee on Diet and Health. "National Academy of Sciences Report on Diet and Health." *Nutrition Reviews* 47, no. 5 (May 1989): 149.

DEFINITION OF A GOOD DIET

A good diet includes variety and avoids both excesses and deficiencies of nutrients. A diet that fulfills these requirements is one that is likely to contain all essential nutrients in appropriate proportions. A well-balanced diet provides enough calories to maintain your optimal body weight. It provides sufficient protein for growth and replacement of lost tissue; adequate carbohydrates and fats for your energy needs; enough fat to help you absorb fat-soluble vitamins; sufficient essential fatty acids; and sufficient vitamins and minerals to allow your enzymes to do their best job in breaking down food and producing new tissue and energy. Adequate intake of these nutrients helps all tissues (liver, lungs, kidney, brain, etc.) do their assigned duties to the best of their ability. For your body to function at its best, it has to have everything it needs when it needs it—not more and not less.

The four basic food groups have been developed by the U.S. Department of Agriculture to aid the consumer in selecting a balanced diet. Each of the four basic food groups is specialized in providing generous amounts of a certain group of nutrients. Recommended daily servings for adults are given below:

The Fruit and Vegetable Group

Includes: fruits, vegetables, greens.

It supplies: vitamin A (in form of beta carotene), folic acid, vitamin C, and smaller amounts of many other vital nutrients. Four of five servings. (Typical serving size: ½ cup fruit or cooked vegetables or 1 cup raw, 1 medium apple)

The Grain Group

Includes: cereals, bread, pasta, rice.

It supplies: carbohydrates, B vitamins, and some minerals and smaller amounts of many other vital nutrients. Four servings. (Typical serving size: 1 slice bread, 1 small roll, 1 cup cereal, ½ cup cooked rice, oatmeal, pasta.)

The Dairy Group

Includes: milk, cheese, yogurt and ice cream.

It supplies: calcium, protein, and vitamin B2, and smaller amounts of many other vital nutrients. Two servings. (Typical serving size: 1 cup milk or yogurt, 1–2 oz cheese.)

The Meat Group

Includes: meat, fish, fowl, eggs, nuts and legumes.

It supplies: protein, iron, Vitamin B1, niacin, and trace elements and smaller amounts of many other vital nutrients. Two servings. (Typical serving size: 3–4 oz raw meat, 2 eggs, 1 cup cooked legumes.)

NOTE: The U.S. Department of Agriculture recognizes 5 food groups (the fifth being the sugar, fats and oils, and alcohol group). In order to avoid promoting alcohol, the existence of 5 food groups is acknowledged but not promoted. Our body is designed to maintain an inner chemical balance, called homeostasis, in spite of varying intake of nutrients. We therefore can afford occasional excesses or deficiencies.

SOURCE:
American Council on Science and Health. *Food and Life: A Nutrition Primer.* July 1990. pp. 34–35.

NUTRITIONAL VALUE OF FAST FOOD

Contrary to common belief, fast food has substantial nutritional value. In fact, its potential nutritional contribution to the diet is limited only by the variety of menu items available and the choices made by individual consumers. Individuals who want to eat healthfully can incorporate fast food into a balanced diet by varying their fast food selections, choosing menu items that contribute to nutrient needs, and choosing meals of appropriate calorie content. . . .

The popularity of fast foods is well documented. A 1978 consumer survey showed that in one six month period, 90 percent of Americans ate in a fast food restaurant at least once. On any given day, about 7 percent of the American population eats a meal at McDonald's—and while McDonald's is by far the largest of the fast food chains, in terms of sales it comprises only 18 percent of the total fast food industry. Most fast food consumers eat from one to three fast food meals a week. Ten percent eat fast food more than five times weekly. Young families with three or more members patronize fast food restaurants most frequently. As family income increases, fast food consumption increases also, through the upper-middle-class level. . . .

It is possible to eat healthfully at fast food restaurants, just as it is possible to do so at home. In either case, the consumer must know some basic nutrition rules and apply them.

However, it would be best for consumers to make fast food only a part of their total daily diets, rather than choosing all their meals and snacks from the relatively limited selection of foods available at fast food restaurants. The limited number of items on many fast food restaurant menus is a nutrition drawback, particularly for frequent consumers, because variety is important for good nutrition. Meals eaten at fast-service restaurants should be incorporated into a varied diet that includes many other food choices.

SOURCE:
American Council on Science and Health. *Fast Food and the American Diet.* 1985. pp. 3, 5, 6–7.

PRACTICAL ADVICE ON NUTRITION

- Replace the outdated concept of "good" versus "bad" foods with the principle of balance and moderation.
- Ignore trendy nutritional news unless it's based on scientific fact. Never shun or favour a food because of unvalidated rumours about its possible dangers or benefits.
- Shop for nutritional value and pleasure rather than fads and fashions.
- Demand clear nutrition information on foods and learn how to assess it.
- Become a conscientious label reader, evaluating what you read, comparing the nutrient values of foods chosen. (Take a pocket calculator if inclined to work out fat percentages!) Remember that fat has nine calories per gram, while protein, sugars and other carbohydrates each have four calories per gram. To work out the percentage of fat in a serving, multiply the fat grams by nine and calculate its percentage of the total calorie value listed on the label.
- Eat a great variety of foods, especially those from plant sources. Consume an array of differently coloured fruits and vegetables (to get the required vitamins and minerals).
- Consume more starchy foods and abandon the mistaken idea that starch is fattening. The latest research suggest that starch (a complex carbohydrate) as well as the fibre in plant foods may confer health benefits and reduce the risk of colon and other cancers. While it's hard to separate the benefits of starch from those of fibre, since they're often present in the same foods, enjoying more pastas, cereals, grains, bananas, yams, rice, potatoes and legumes may promote health.
- Note that carbohydrate-rich diets make weight control easier because any calories from starch, sugar and other carbohydrates are less efficiently stored than those from fat.
- Choose a sensible fat mix, reduced in saturated (solid or animal) fats, but don't eliminate dietary fat altogether—it's a nutrient essential for energy, especially in young children, and crucial for the absorption of fat-soluble vitamins.
- Favour olive oil, a monounsaturated fat, which has unique antioxidant and health-promoting proper-

ties. Among the cooking oils, olive oil is the only one that contains natural antioxidants which keep it stable and stop it from going rancid for many years. (The health benefits of olive oil may stem more from its antioxidant levels than, as previously assumed, from its fatty acid composition.)

- To reduce fat to the recommended "30 per cent of calories," steam, bake or poach foods. (Deep-fat frying or flaming of foods produces oxidized components, known to be toxic at very low concentrations.)
- Make sauces with skim, not whole milk, use low-fat yogurt instead of cream.
- Become a "hidden fat" detective. Watch for fat in crackers, cookies, desserts, dressings and sauces.
- Choose leaner cuts of meat and trim off the fat; eat smaller portions, boil or bake rather than broiling or frying. No need to shun meat—besides high quality protein, it provides many other vital nutrients, such as iron, zinc, vitamins B6 and B12 (to name a few).
- Eat fish two to three times weekly. Cold-water, deep sea fish are rich in long-chain omega-3 fatty acids. Eaten two or three times a week they may protect the heart and cardiovascular system. Eating deep sea fish is known to lower heart attack risks in some populations (by reducing the blood's clotting action). Even the higher-fat fish (such as salmon, swordfish, herring and mackerel) are healthy choices. Low in saturated fats, fish also provide high quality protein. Finfish are generally low in cholesterol, shellfish somewhat higher. Canned fish is equally healthy.
- Skip supplemental vitamins unless medically advised to take them. Intakes of vitamins and minerals in excess of the RNIs aren't recommended, except for specific situations such as pregnancy (folic acid) and vitamin D for infants and perhaps older people—when there's too little sun-exposure.
- A little of what you fancy does you good. There's nothing wrong with occasional "junk" food such as chips, candy, donuts, cream cake or chocolates, provided they're not invariably the major part of your diet.
- Relax, and enjoy food!

SOURCE:
"So, What Should We Eat? (Practical Tips for Healthier Eating in the '90s)." *University of Toronto Faculty of Medicine Health News* 9, no. 2 (April 1991): 7.

FOOD LABELING

Regulators have targeted three major areas of label abuse: deceptive definitions, hazy health claims, and slippery serving sizes. Phase I of their program, already under way, covers fresh fruit, vegetables, seafood and other edibles that have never before been subject to nutritional labeling requirements. Grocers will not be asked to plaster ingredients labels on an apple or haddock; instead, they will post nutritional information at their produce bins and fish counters. In addition, the FDA is under congressional orders to standardize the requirements for such terms as juice and juice drink.

Scheduled for completion this fall [1991], Phase II will focus on making labels mean exactly what they say. Among the worst culprits are products that claim to be 80%, 90% or even 99% fat free. Although technically correct, the labels are misleading because virtually all manufacturers base their calculations not on the composition of calories, but on weight, including water, which occurs naturally in most food. For example, Louis Rich Turkey Bologna accurately claims to be "82% fat free, 18% fat." It sounds perfect for people who are trying to keep their fat consumption below 30% a day. Yet each 60-calorie slice, which weighs 28 g (or 1 oz.), contains 5 g of fat. Since each gram of fat accounts for nine calories, 75%—not 18%—of the calories in a slice of Louis Rich Turkey Bologna come from fat.

SOURCE:
Gorman, Christine. "The Fight over Food Labels." *Time* (July 15, 1991): 55.

RESOURCES

ORGANIZATIONS

American Dietetic Association. 208 S. LaSalle St., Suite 1100, Chicago, IL 60604.

American Nutritionists Association. P.O. Box 34030, Bethesda, MD 20817.

American Society for Clinical Nutrition. 9650 Rockville Pike, Bethesda, MD 20814.

Food and Nutrition Information Center. National Agricultural Library, Beltsville, MD 20705.

PAMPHLETS

National Research Council, National Academy of Sciences:

Diet and Health: Implications for Reducing Chronic Disease Risk. 1989.

Recommended Dietary Allowances. 10th ed. 1989.

Public Health Service:

The Surgeon General's Report on Nutrition and Health. 1988.

BOOKS

Brody, Jane. *The Good Food Book*. New York: Bantam, 1990.

Gershoff, Stanley, and others. *The Tufts University Guide to Total Nutrition*. New York: Harper, 1990.

Hamilton, Michael, and others. *The Duke University Medical Center Book of Diet and Fitness*. New York: Ballantine, 1990.

Herbert, Victor, and Genell J. Subak-Sharpe. *Mount Sinai School of Medicine Complete Book of Nutrition*. New York: St. Martin's, 1990.

Kaufman, Phyllis. *The Good Eating: Good Health Cookbook*. Fairfield, OH: Consumer Reports Books, 1991.

RELATED ARTICLE

"Feeding Frenzy." *Newsweek* (May 27, 1991): 46–52.

FOOD POISONING

OVERVIEW

Each year food poisoning causes gastrointestinal disease in some 33 million Americans, *The New York Times* reported recently. *Salmonella enteritidis* alone, CDC officials estimate, is responsible for approximately 2.5 million cases, and statistics indicate that the problem is growing. From 1960 to 1987, the number of cases of salmonellosis per 100,000 population that were reported to state health departments, for instance, had climbed from 3.85 to 20.92.

Why do foodborne diseases continue to plague a nation where refrigerators are rampant and food processing is a way of life? One survey suggests that the public doesn't know enough about food hygiene. Others point to the unsanitary conditions in processing plants and inadequate government inspection. Whatever the cause, clinicians must still cope with these infections.

A nearly endless array of microorganisms can contaminate food, but four infections are most common among patients who complain of diarrhea or related GI symptoms.

Staphylococcus aureus infection is brought on by the enterotoxin of *S. aureus*. Since the pathogen's byproduct is the culprit, there's often no trace of the bacteria itself in the stool culture. The diagnosis must therefore depend on the clinical picture.

Look for severe nausea and vomiting, along with abdominal cramps, diarrhea, and occasionally headache and fever. The infection seldom lasts for more than 24 hours and is rarely life-threatening. In elderly and seriously ill patients, however, fluid and electrolyte imbalances can be dangerous.

A diet history may turn up important clues. Ask about intake of cream- or custard-filled pastries, 30 minutes to eight hours before symptoms appeared. Keeping such foods at room temperature allows bacteria to grow quickly, and release toxin.

Also find out if the patient has been to a picnic or barbecue, where food often lies around for hours, or has made a stop at a roadside food truck or street vendor—*S. aureus* can be passed on by food handlers who don't wash their hands properly.

Salmonellosis is caused by *Salmonella enteritidis*. Unlike *S. aureus* infection, in which nausea and vomiting are most prominent, many dinner partners will more likely develop sudden abdominal pains and loose, watery diarrhea. A fever around 102° F (38.8° C) is also common. Diagnosis can be confirmed by stool culture, and symptoms subside in two to five days.

A food history may reveal consumption of contaminated milk and water, or undercooked pork, poultry, or fish, within the last 12 to 72 hours. A recent *JAMA* study found widespread *S. enteritidis* infestation in Grade A raw eggs. The CDC recently reported outbreaks linked to omelets and scrambled eggs, and homemade ice cream.

Ask the patient what medication he's been taking, since some drugs can increase the risk of salmonellosis. Antacids reduce gastric acidity, one of the protective defenses that destroy the pathogen. So too, antibiotics kill the intestinal flora that inhibit its growth.

Salmonellosis usually clears up within three days, although severe cases can cause complications, including septicemia.

Campylobacter infection, which is caused by *C. jejuni* and *C. fetus*, among other species, can be passed on through the consumption of unpasteurized milk, raw clams, and contaminated infant formula or water. Experts suspect that approximately two million infections occur annually in the United States, and a recent National Research Council study concluded that 48% of all infections can be traced to chicken.

You can often distinguish the disease from staph and salmonella poisoning by its long incubation period: Watery diarrhea, the first symptom, may not appear until 10 days after infection, and two days is a minimum. As the disease progresses, stool becomes more bloody and mucus-filled, and the patient is sometimes mistakenly diagnosed as having ulcerative colitis. Sometimes, abdominal pain—especially in the right lower quadrant—is more prominent than diarrhea.

The condition may last a week or so, and require a course of antibiotics. In debilitated patients, *C. fetus* can cause life-threatening sepsis.

Because the sources and symptoms of campylobacter infection and salmonellosis are similar, a stool culture is usually required to tell them apart.

Clostridium perfringens infection often develops when meat is partially cooked, allowed to cool slowly, and then recooked the following day. During cooling, remaining bacteria multiply quickly, and reheating causes any spores that survived the first cooking to germinate.

In a typical case, the patient develops severe, mid-epigastric cramps and watery diarrhea eight to 12 hours after eating. Fever and vomiting seldom occur, although nausea does. Definitive diagnosis can be made from food and fecal cultures.

The clinical course of the condition is generally mild and has seldom been known to last much longer than 24 hours. The treatment of all four infections have much in common: The patient often needs fluid and electrolytes to replace what's lost in vomiting and diarrhea. One study found that 20% of patients with staph poisoning needed IV fluids.

If nausea and vomiting are mild or have already ceased, give warm, sweetened tea, strained broth, or bouillon with salt. Bland solid foods can follow in time, including gelatin, cereal, and jellied consomme.

The physician may order tetracycline or erythromycin for campylobacter infection and may give antibiotics or infants and elderly patients with salmonellosis. Those with *C. perfringens* may receive codeine for abdominal cramps.

SOURCE:
Cerrato, Paul L. "Food Poisoning Makes a Dangerous Comeback." *RN* 52 (October 1989): 73–76.

SALMONELLA

Salmonellosis, a disease that strikes at least 40,000 and up to 2 million Americans each year and kills from 500 to 2,000, is almost entirely preventable. Food poisoning caused by Salmonella bacteria, which gives victims flu-like symptoms for as long as a week, usually can be traced to careless food handling, improper cooking and incorrect cooling. The spread of the Salmonella bacteria can best be prevented by monitoring the temperature at every stage of food processing. Fortunately, Salmonella does not spread easily, although victims can transmit it for a few weeks after they have been sick. It can be carried by any food of animal origin. For instance, milk was the culprit in a major Chicago-area outbreak, and chicken is frequently suspect because the large-scale processing can cause sanitation problems. Because it is unlikely that Salmonella bacteria can be eliminated, consumer education is the main weapon against further outbreaks. Prompt refrigeration for all perishable foods, especially in warm weather, cooking poultry to an internal temperature of 140 [degrees] F and refrigerating all leftovers at once to discourage the multiplication of bacteria are important precautions. While food is the main carrier of Salmonella bacteria, kitchen surfaces, utensils and dishes are easily contaminated. For instance, if you put cooked meat on the same plate you used for raw meat, the cooked meat can be contaminated. Clean-up is crucial, too. Using a dishwasher reduces risk, and hand-washed dishes left to air dry are safer than those that are wiped dry. Even sponges and dishtowels can carry bacteria . . . Because Salmonella symptoms are uncomfortable and frightening, but usually not severe, it is often underreported.

Public awareness is the only way to reduce Salmonella infection.

SOURCE:
"Salmonella Spread Can Be Controlled." *Nutrition Today* 24 (February 1989): 5.

SALMONELLA—IN EGGS

From 1976 to 1986, reported *Salmonella enteritidis* infections increased more than sixfold in the northeastern United States. From January 1985 to May 1987, sixty-five foodborne outbreaks of *S enteritidis* were reported in the Northeast that were associated with 2119 cases and 11 deaths. Twenty-seven (77%) of the 35 outbreaks with identified food vehicles were caused by Grade A shell eggs or foods that contained such eggs. . . .

Limited public awareness that raw eggs, like other foods of animal origin, constitute a potential source of *Salmonella* is suggested by the widespread use of raw or near raw eggs in Caesar salad dressing, hollandaise sauce, eggnog, homemade ice cream, and many other foods. In the short-term prevention of *S enteritidis* and other *Salmonella* infections associated with eggs will depend on not eating raw or undercooked eggs. In addition, some standard egg cooking practices may be inadequate to kill *Salmonella* in eggs. In one set of experiments, cooking eggs longer than usual—boiling for seven minutes, poaching for five minutes, and frying on each side for three minutes—was necessary to destroy *Salmonella* that was artificially inoculated into yolks; no duration of frying "sunnyside" (not turned) eggs was sufficient to kill all the *Salmonella.*

SOURCE:
St. Louis, Michael E., and others. "The Emergence of Grade A Eggs as a Major Source of *Salmonella enteritidis* Infections: New Implications for the Control of Salmonellosis." *JAMA* 259, no. 14 (April 8, 1988): 2103-2106. Copyright 1988, American Medical Association.

BOTULISM

Botulism is a serious form of food poisoning, usually caused by eating improperly canned foods which are contaminated with *Clostridium botulinum.* Eating, or even tasting, the poisoned food can be fatal.

Unless strict precautions are followed, home-canned non-acid foods may be contaminated with the bacteria *Clostridium botulinum.* Non-acid foods include vegetables, meat, poultry and fish; acid foods include fruits, tomatoes and pickles. These acid foods are usually safe. The poison comes from tiny spores (seed-like structures with hard, heat resistant coverings) produced by the bacteria. The danger does not come directly from eating the bacteria; in fact, a lot of fresh food contains the bacteria and it passes harmlessly through the digestive tract when it is eaten. However, in the absence of air (as in cans), *Clostridium botulinum* produces a toxin—a substance which may be the most lethal human poison in existence. Non-acid food canning, if improperly carried out, can provide perfect conditions for the production of this poison.

The first symptoms appear abruptly, usually 18 to 48 hours after the food was eaten. These symptoms include nausea, dry mouth, vomiting, abdominal pain and blurring of vision. The toxin has a paralyzing effect on the nervous system; it prevents the nerves from conducting messages from the brain. Control of the muscles is lost, beginning with those around the face and neck. Loss of the ability to swallow makes it impossible to eat. It leads to choking and may introduce foreign materials into the lungs. The victim usually dies within several days. If medical aid is quickly obtained and the correct diagnosis rapidly made, it may be possible to save the patient. A serum may be injected which is sometimes able to neutralize a portion of the toxin and limit further paralysis. This serum cannot help the nerves that are already damaged. The speed with which symptoms appear depends largely on the amount of toxin-containing food that is eaten. . . .

If you have a supply of non-acid home-canned food, you can make sure it is safe by following one simple precaution—boil before eating!

SOURCE:
"Home-Canned Foods Can Be Dangerous." *HealthTips* no. 130 (September 1989): 7-8.

RESOURCES

PAMPHLET
U.S. Department of Agriculture, Food Safety and Inspection Service:

"A Quick Consumer Guide to Safe Food Handling." *Home and Garden Bulletin* No. 248, September 1990. 8 pp.

RELATED ARTICLES

"Botulism Outbreaks May Escape Diagnosis." *Patient Care* 22 (August 15, 1988): 31–32.

Eastaugh, Janet, and Suzanne Shepherd. "Infections and Toxic Syndromes from Fish and Shellfish Consumption." *Archives of Internal Medicine* 149 (August 1989): 1735–1740.

"Food-Borne Illness: How to Prevent Foods from Making You Sick." *Mayo Clinic Nutrition Letter* 3, no. 4 (April 1990): 1–2.

Heinz, Agnes. "Salmonella Poisoning." *Priorities* (Fall 1989): 10–12.

Young, Frank A. "Seafood Safety: Current Issues." *Nutrition Today* 25 (June 1990): 25–26.

GALLSTONE DISEASE

OVERVIEW

An estimated 25 million Americans—over 10 percent of the population—have gallstones. In the next year, 1 million more people will discover that they have them. Even though gallbladder disease is not usually fatal, approximately 6,000 people will die from complications this year.

Gallstones are lumps of solid material that form in the gallbladder. Though in many patients these stones remain "silent" and cause no problems, in many other patients they do. Indeed, each year 500,000 people have their gallbladders removed in order to treat or prevent serious or even life-threatening complications. This makes cholecystectomy—the surgical removal of the gallbladder—the fifth most common operation performed in the United States. . . .

The gallbladder is a sac located beneath the liver on the right-hand side of the abdominal cavity. Its primary job is to store the bile secreted by the liver until it is needed in the small intestine for digestion. When digestion begins, the gallbladder contracts and sends the bile into the intestine through a series of ducts. When digestion is completed, the bile is routed to the gallbladder for storage.

Bile helps break up fat so that it can be further digested by the pancreatic enzymes and absorbed by the intestines. Bile contains bile salts, cholesterol, bilirubin, and lecithin. In one day, the liver may produce as much as 700 milliliters (almost 3 cups) of bile to aid in digestion.

Gallstones form when there is a precipitation of chemicals in the bile. Two types of gallstones can occur: cholesterol gallstones or pigment gallstones. Cholesterol gallstones are composed chiefly of cholesterol and pigment gallstones are composed of bilirubin and other compounds. About 80 percent of the patients with gallbladder disease in the United States have cholesterol gallstones.

Cholesterol and other components of bile are collected in the gallbladder during periods of fasting—for instance, during sleep or between meals. For some reason that is not yet understood, in those patients who develop gallstones, the cholesterol comes out of solution and forms crystals. These crystals provide the cores around which the stones develop.

Researchers are uncertain about the relative importance of the liver and the gallbladder in the formation of gallstones. (But removing the gallbladder does prevent the formation of additional gallstones in the great majority of patients in the United States.) It is possible that the mixture of chemicals secreted by the liver of a patient with gallstones is not able to hold cholesterol in solution. On the other hand, some chemical may be present in the gallbladder of a patient with gallstones that disturbs the mixture and leads to the formation of crystals. . . .

The people most likely to develop gallstones are women who have been pregnant; overweight people who eat a lot of dairy products and animal fats; and people over 60. In the 20 to 60 age group, women are three times more likely to develop gallstones than men. By the age of 60, however, almost 30 percent of all men and women have gallstones. . . .

A great many people have gallstones but do not have symptoms. These people have silent gallstones and their stones may remain silent for the rest of their lives.

When symptoms are evident, a person with gallstones may have severe, steady pain in the upper abdomen. It lasts at least 20 minutes and usually up to 2 to 4 hours. There may be pain between the shoulder blades or in the right shoulder. There may be nausea or vomiting.

Gallstones cause more severe problems when they make their way out of the gallbladder. Gallstones can lodge in the channel that allows the bile to enter and leave the gallbladder. This channel is called the cystic duct. If gallstones block the channel for a prolonged period, the gallbladder may become inflamed. This condition is called cholecystitis. Obstruction of the cystic duct is a relatively common complication of gallbladder disease.

Other complications are less common. For example, gallstones can enter and block the channel that drains the liver. This is called common bile duct obstruction. Gallstones can lodge in the main channel that drains the pancreas, called the pancreatic duct, and cause pancreatitis.

The major symptom of all the complications of gallstone disease is abdominal pain. The pain is usually sudden, often severe, and located in the middle or right portions of the abdomen. The pain may spread out and it may be felt on both sides, in the back, or throughout the abdomen. It may shift from side to side or it may lodge in the right shoulder. This pain is often so intense that the sufferer may perspire heavily or vomit. The patient will have a chill with a high fever. An attack of this kind may be over in a few minutes, but usually lasts several hours. If this occurs, the patient should check with a physician as soon as possible.

Many silent gallstones are identified when X-ray or ultrasound examinations are performed as part of a routine medical checkup or because some other illness is suspected. In patients who develop the typical symptoms of complications associated with gallbladder disease noted in the previous section, the physician will begin by taking a medical history and performing appropriate laboratory tests to help rule out other possible illnesses.

The diagnosis of patients with silent gallstones and those who have had complications that have subsided can be made with at least 95 percent accuracy. There are several methods available to do this. Oral cholecystography is a procedure in which X-rays of the gallbladder are taken after the patient has swallowed pills containing a dye that is absorbed and later appears in the bile outlining the gallbladder.

Ultrasonography is as sensitive as any method available to detect gallstones. It provides the physician with an immediate set of rules from which to make a diagnosis. Additionally, ultrasound pictures allow the physician to detect other disorders that may be present.

To get a picture of the extensive network of ducts and any stones that may be lodged in them, the doctor may perform a PTC—percutaneous transhepatic cholangiography. In this procedure, dye is injected into the small bile ducts in the liver. Once the dye had spread through the system into the common bile duct, an X-ray is taken.

Another method, ERCP (endoscopic retrograde cholangiopancreatography), uses a flexible tube in the intestine to deliver the dye through another, smaller tube into the common bile duct. While both of these procedures provide a good look at the ducts, they carry a slight risk of complications. For this reason they are used only with certain patients.

The surgical removal of the gallbladder—cholecystectomy—is by far the most common course of treatment for patients who develop complications of gallbladder disease. This is because, until recently, removal of the gallbladder was the only way to get rid of gallstones. Even with the introduction of new drugs, many patients with gallstones will require surgery when life-threatening complications occur. Removal of the gallbladder does not seem to interfere with the normal digestive process. After the gallbladder is removed, the bile produced by the liver flows directly to the intestine.

SOURCE:
Tyor, M. P. "Gallstone Disease." National Digestive Diseases Education and Information Clearinghouse. n.d.

GALLSTONES—REMOVAL

Almost 25 percent of women and 10 percent of men in the United States develop gallstones.

Here are the main ways to remove gallstones:

- **Traditional surgery**—Removes the gallbladder, preventing a recurrence of stones. Leaves a three- to six-inch scar across the abdomen. Five to eight days in the hospital. Up to six weeks of recovery time.
- **Laparoscopic cholecystectomy**—New form of surgery. A few small incisions. One day in the hospital. About a week of recovery time.
- **Percutaneous cholecystolithotomy**—Procedure in which a radiologist and general surgeon insert an instrument into the gallbladder. Gallstones are fragmented and removed; gallbladder remains intact. Requires general anesthesia.
- **Lithotripsy**—Ultrasound waves break up gallstones. Less cost and faster recovery than conventional surgery. General anesthesia isn't necessary. Stones can recur in up to 50 percent of people within five years. Technique works best on a single small stone.
- **MTBE**—Chemical called methyl tert-butyl ether dissolves gallstones. Leaves a residue that can be removed with suction.

SOURCE:
"Gallbladder Removal." *Mayo Clinic Health Letter* 8, no. 11 (November 1990): 2.

RISKS OF DIETING

Several recent medical studies have linked rapid weight loss to the formation of cholesterol gallstones, according to [Daniel R.] Ganger, [M.D. of Northwestern University in Chicago]. "The gallbladder is connected to the liver by bile ducts and is sued to store bile—a greenish-brown fluid used to digest fatty foods. Cholesterol gallstones are generally composed of the cholesterol made by our own systems and are not necessarily related to high-cholesterol diets," says Ganger.

"They may form in dieters because when people don't eat enough, their gallbladders don't empty properly, and the cholesterol in their gallbladders remains inside and has time to solidify." . . .

Doctors who treat digestive disorders urge dieters to learn the signs and symptoms of gallstones. "Early signs of the disease include gas, nausea, bloating, and belching," says Ganger. "Anyone experiencing gas and bloating that lasts several weeks and is not alleviated by changes in diet, such as reducing fiber intake, should see a physician." . . .

Dieters who "yo-yo" back and forth, gaining and losing five to 10 pounds once or twice each year, may be at an even greater risk for gallstone development, says Ganger. "Gallstone disease can be asymptomatic in the early stages. A dieter may develop gallstones without knowing it during one diet, gain a few pounds and go on a second diet which triggers very painful symptoms of gallstone disease."

SOURCE:
"Warning: Rapid Weight Loss May Cause Gallstones." *Employee Health & Fitness* 12, no. 6 (June 1990): 106.

SURGICAL TREATMENT

As lithotripsy's stock plummets under the weight of unfavorable data, laparoscopic cholecystectomy is rapidly assuming the role of gallstone therapy's rising star.

Though the laparoscopic procedure has been in clinical use less than two years, some physicians think that it will render other gallstone therapies obsolete. They're making that prediction despite disturbing reports of injuries to patients, and amid extensive media hype and provider advertising.

Even physicians taking a wait-and-see stance understand the advocates' enthusiasm. When all goes well, the gallbladder can be removed laparoscopically in about 45 minutes. The patient usually goes home in less than a day and returns to work within a week. Costs of inpatient care and lost time from work are much less than those for open cholecystectomy, and patients don't have to worry about stone recurrence, a problem with nonsurgical therapy.

Mayo surgeon Jon van Heerden, who has been working with endoscopic laser destruction of gallstones, is among those who expect laparoscopic cholecystectomy to make other therapies obsolete. But, like lithotripsy and dissolution therapy, the laparoscopic procedure will likely be limited to carefully selected patients who aren't surgical candidates.

SOURCE:
Bankhead, C. D. "One-Day Cholecystectomy Popular." *Medical World News* 31 (July 1990): 48.

NONSURGICAL TREATMENT

During the past 18 years, three approaches have been introduced as alternatives to surgical treatment of gallbladder stones, a condition known since antiquity. All have as their objective the dissolution of the stones, leaving the gallbladder intact and stone-free. Elimination of the stones should be accompanied by relief of symptoms and should prevent the development of more serious complications—e.g., cholecystitis, pancreatitis, cholangitis, or obstructive jaundice.

In contrast to cholecystectomy, for which prior knowledge of the composition of the stones is unnecessary, dissolution therapy is effective only for cholesterol stones. Gallstones composed predominantly of pigment (bilirubin polymers) or calcium salts cannot be dissolved by the litholytic therapy now available. However, since about 80 percent of gallbladder stones contain mostly cholesterol, the majority of patients with symptomatic gallstones can be considered for alternative therapy.

The first of the new litholytic treatments involves the oral administration of bile acids. The treatment is most effective in patients with a few small stones. Unfortunately, gallstones may re-form after bile acid therapy has been discontinued.

Thistle and colleagues report from the Mayo clinic on a second method of nonsurgical treatment: the rapid dissolution of cholesterol gallbladder stones with methyl tert-butyl ether (MTBE). The results are impressive: almost complete dissolution of stones in 96 percent of the carefully selected patients. However, several features of this study need emphasis. MTBE is a volatile, highly flammable solvent. It must be instilled directly into the gallbladder to come into contact with the stones, since it tends to float on bile. Unlike litholytic bile acids, which are taken orally and are secreted by the liver into bile, MTBE treatment requires careful placement of a catheter by percutaneous puncture and passage through the liver to the narrow infundibular portion of the gallbladder in order to minimize leakage of bile.

The third nonsurgical treatment for gallstones is extracorporeal shock-wave biliary lithotripsy. Shock waves may be generated by spark-gap, electromagnetic, or piezoelectric sources and are focused on the gallstones with the aid of ultrasound imaging. These devices fragment large stones, producing many small ones. However, the fragments need to be dissolved to prevent their passage into the bile duct, where they may cause pain or serve as a nidus for new stone formation.

At present, lithotripsy seems most useful for fragmenting stones in the 25 to 30 percent of patients with one to three moderate-to-large stones. The side effects of lithotripsy have not been serious.

Thus, the three litholytic treatments are not mutually exclusive but can be used together to overcome disadvantages inherent in the individual therapies. Large stones can be fragmented into small stones, which can be dissolved more rapidly with either ursodiol or MTBE. Stone re-formation may be retarded by ursodiol, which normalizes hepatic cholesterol secretion. Impending cholecystitis may be prevented by rapid dissolution of stones with MTBE. For the present, cholecystectomy remains the standard treatment for gallstones, but the considerable progress in nonsurgical therapies now gives patients and their physicians alternative choices. More experience will be needed to put these choices into proper perspective.

SOURCE:

Salen, G., and G. S. Tint. "Nonsurgical Treatment of Gallstones." *New England Journal of Medicine* 320, no. 10 (March 9, 1989): 665–666.

DRUG TREATMENT

Drug treatment to dissolve gallstones began about 20 years ago, when researchers found that a deficiency of bile salts enabled cholesterol to crystallize out of solution and form stones. Today, drugs are typically given for small stones or if a person cannot tolerate surgery.

The two approved cholesterol gallstone dissolution drugs are the natural bile constituents chenodeoxycholic acid (Chenix) and its chemical non-identical twin ursodeoxycholic acid (Actigall).

"These drugs can change the cholesterol saturation in the gallbladder and permit cholesterol in the stone to go into solution, so that it dissolves," says Stepen Fredd, M.D., director of FDA's division of gastrointestinal and coagulation drug products at FDA. "Ursodeoxycholic acid is less likely to be toxic to the liver, but is more expensive."

But the drugs have major drawbacks. "In 50 percent of patients, stones recur within five years of drug treatment," explains Fredd. "A common side effect of these drugs is diarrhea. The drugs work slowly and must be taken daily for a long time and, even then, are not always effective." About 12 percent of patients improve after six months, and up to 50 percent show improvement by a year. The cost of drug treatment is about $1,200 a year.

A new investigational drug is methyl-tert-butyl-ether. It works fast on cholesterol stones, dissolving them in 24 to 48 hours, but administering the drug is an invasive procedure.

"It is not taken orally," explains Fredd. "It is put in the gallbladder by a catheter through the liver to the gallbladder. This is not minor stuff, but in expert hands, it can be done safely. But it has dangerous propensities. It is an ether, and can put you to sleep. It can irritate the intestines."

Another new drug is mono-octanoin (Moctanin), which is approved only to treat stones lodged in the bile duct. This sometimes happens after the gallbladder is removed and small stones migrate into the duct.

SOURCE:

Lewis, Ricki. "The Gallbladder: An Organ You Can Live Without." *FDA Consumer* (May 1991): 14-15.

RESOURCES

ORGANIZATIONS

American Liver Foundation. 998 Pompton Avenue, Cedar Grove, NJ 07009.

National Digestive Diseases Information Clearinghouse. Box NDDIC, Bethesda, MD 20892. (301) 468-6344.

PAMPHLETS

American Liver Foundation:

Gallstones and Other Gallbladder Disorders: A National Health Problem. n.d. 7 pp.

National Institutes of Diabetes and Digestive and Kidney Diseases:

Gallstones. NIH Pub. No. 87-2897. May 1987. 15 pp.

RELATED ARTICLES

Cuschieri, A., G. Gerci, and others. "Laparoscopic Cholecystectomy." *American Journal of Surgery* 159 (March 1990): 273.

Gilliland, T. M. and L. W. Traverso. "Modern Standards for Comparison of Cholecystectomy with Alternative Treatments for Symptomatic Cholelithiasis with Emphasis on Long Term Relief of Symptoms." *Surgery, Gynecology & Obstetrics* 170 (January 1990): 39–44.

Lu, Shelly C. "Frontiers of Gallstone Therapy: How Far Have We Come with Nonsurgical Methods?" *Postgraduate Medicine* 85, no. 3 (February 15, 1989): 90–104.

McSherry, C. K. "Cholecystectomy: The Gold Standard." *American Journal of Surgery* 158 (September 1989): 174–178.

"Shock Waves for Gallstones." *Harvard Medical School Health Letter* (July 1988): 3–4.

Taylor, M. C., J. C. Marshall, and others. "Extracorporeal Shock Wave Lithotripsy (ESWL) in the Management of Complex Biliary Tract Stone Disease." *Annals of Surgery* 208 (November 1988): 586–592.

GENERIC DRUGS

OVERVIEW

Generics are here to stay. The government, for one, has a major stake in them. The Veterans Administration, which runs the largest drug program in the country, and state Medicaid programs, which are subsidized by the federal government, either mandate generics or provide financial incentives to use them. Insurance companies, HMO's and hospitals also have a vested interest in containing the soaring cost of health care.

Any way you cut it, you're likely to be touched by generic drugs—whether or not you particularly care about saving money. Of course, if you do, generics can save you anywhere from 30% to 70% of what you'd pay for the branded version—sometimes even more. That's no small potatoes, especially for people over 65, who buy 30% of all prescription drugs.

Then there's this economic fact of life: Where there's money to be made, people will try to make it. The generic drug industry brought in some $1.9 billion in 1989; about 500 million prescriptions—one-third of all those dispensed in the U.S.—were filled with clones, according to Hemant Shah, a health care analyst with HKS and Company of Warren, NJ. If that's not enough to keep generic pills popping, consider that $10 billion worth of brand-name products will be going off patent between 1991 and 1995.

There's never exactly been a love affair between generics manufacturers and the brand-name ("innovator") drug companies. After spending millions of dollars and perhaps years of testing on developing new drugs, major firms hate it when their "babies" lose patent protection and become open to competition from the 300 or so smaller companies that make knock-offs. For example, why should Hoffmann-LaRoche, originator of Valium, be happy about sharing the pie with some dozen other firms who now make generic diazepam?

For years, says Jay Molishever, director of public affairs for the Generic Pharmaceutical Industry Association, the big-name companies have waged a smear campaigns generics, underwriting "scientific" studies that knock their safety, paying physicians and publicists to talk up instances where generics caused harm—even though the cases are always anecdotal and can't be substantiated. Congressman Henry Waxman (D.-Calif.), a sponsor of the 1984 law that simplified the generic drug approval process, recently called such disinformation campaigns "blatantly dishonest." And the FDA labeled some "false and misleading."

Says Molishever: "Consumers should be aware that the brand-name companies put out a great deal of disinformation about generics to try to scare consumers. Why should someone continue paying $70 for a medication when he can get if for $7? Because he's scared, that's why."

SOURCE:
Avery, Caryl S. "Can You Trust Generic Drugs? In the Wake of Scandal, Here's What You Need To Know." *American Health* (April 1990): 82.

COST SAVINGS

Rising costs of brand-name drugs are also contibuting to generic drugs' popularity. According to a Federal Trade Commission report, generic drugs saved consumers approximately $236 million in 1984. Some examples: A major national pharmacy chain charges $31.54 for 100 tablets of the leading, branded oral insulin. By contrast, the same chain charges $7.59 for 100 tablets of the generic version of the drug. If you were taking one tablet per day, the cost would be $115 a year for the branded product versus $28 for the generic product. The FDA estimates that generic drugs generally cost 30 to 40 percent less, and sometimes as much as 80 percent less than their brand-name equivalents. The elderly, who must often take drugs regularly, play a major role in growing generic sales. Although people over 65 constitute only 12 percent of the population, they consume 30 percent of all prescription drugs. According to a 1987 General Accounting Office report to the U.S. Senate, 15.5 percent of elderly patients who require prescriptions say they are unable to pay for their drugs.

Besides cost-conscious consumers, hospital pharmacies are increasingly using generic drugs to contain costs. Group purchases of generic drugs are leading to price discounts, further enhancing the attractiveness of brand substitutions. One example is the 256-bed University of Nebraska Medical Center. In 1986, the hospital reported saving $280,000 on $1.5 million in generic drug purchases through the University Hospital Consortium.

SOURCE:
Sweet, Cheryl. "The Real Cost of Generic Drugs." *Priorities* (Summer 1989): 37.

SAFETY

Some pharmacists and doctors warn that substitution of brand-name drugs by generics—especially when doctors and patients are not told that it is happening—can be dangerous. Generics are not exact copies of brand-name drugs. While the amount of active ingredients in generics and their brand-name counterpart may be the same, the inert ingredients that bind, color, and fill the dosage form may differ. These inactive ingredients can affect the way the drug dissolves in your stomach and, therefore, how thoroughly and rapidly it is absorbed into the body. For many drugs and medical conditions, this makes little or no difference. Some conditions, however, require maintaining a constant and precise blood level of medication over long periods. There are four categories of drugs in which generic substitutes may not always be safe: antiepileptic drugs, antipsychotic drugs, antiarrhythmic drugs, and warfarin, a blood thinner. For people with conditions that are treated with these drugs, such as epilepsy, asthma, diabetes, heart ailments, mental disorders, and thyroid problems, substituting drugs may upset a delicate balancing act. The age and health of the patient is another factor that can cause problems since the absorption of generic drugs in the sick and elderly may not be equivalent to that in the healthy, young men in whom generic drugs are tested.

If you opt for generics, make an effort to know what you are purchasing. If your physician wants you only to take a brand-name drug, be sure your physician notifies your pharmacist. In some states physicians must write "dispense as written" or check a box on the prescription form to prevent automatic switching to a generic.

SOURCE:
Sweet, Cheryl. "The Real Cost of Generic Drugs." *Priorities* (Summer 1989): 39.

EFFICACY

There is evidence that brand-name companies have supplied information to federal investigators probing generics firms, according to *The Wall Street Journal.* But even without a scandal, brand-name makers have managed for years to raise serious doubts in the minds of health care professionals and consumers, says the FDA. Their arguments center on two issues: "bioequivalence" vs. "therapeutic" equivalence, and the "plus-or-minus 20% rule."

Brand-name makers claim that just because a generic is bioequivalent (which means it reaches the target tissue with the same payload about as quickly as the brand-name product) doesn't mean it has therapeutic equivalence (the same medicinal effect). Brand-name companies argue that different inert ingredients—such as binders and coloring agents—can alter the drugs' overall effect.

In response to such concerns, the FDA convened a hearing on the subject in 1986, attended by over 800 representatives of academia, industry, medicine and the government. A task force was appointed to review the issues. In effect, its 1988 report held fast that bioequivalence does equal therapeutic equivalence.

Still, many doctors remain unconvinced. The American Academy of Family Physicians (AAFP), representing some 60,000 family practitioners, recently reviewed the medical literature and concluded that so many generics are not chemically the same drug entitity in the same dosage form, because of different additives and inert compounds, that the drugs should not be considered bioequivalent.

Says Dr. Jerry Mann, former chairman of the AAFP committee on drugs and devices: "I kind of regret having to admit that for years I—and I think most doctors—felt that if the FDA said something's true, it must be true. Now our study says that's not necessarily so."

The generics industry's [Jay] Molishever says such statements show a lack of awareness about basic pharmacological concepts. "Unfortunately, physicians get most of their information about pharmaceuticals from brand-name companies—drug salespersons," he says. "Brand-name firms spend $9,000 per year per physician on promotion."

SOURCE:
Avery, Caryl S. "Can You Trust Generic Drugs? In the Wake of Scandal, Here's What You Need To Know." *American Health* (April 1990): 82–83.

GENERIC DRUGS—FDA RECOMMENDATION

MYTH: Generic drugs just won't do the same job as well as brand-name drugs.

FACT: Under the new law, generic drugs must be bioequivalent to their brand-name counterparts to gain FDA approval. That means that the generics must contain the same active ingredients and must be identical in strength, dosage form (tablet, solution, etc.), and rout of administration (for example, taken by mouth or through injection). Further, they must release the same amount of drugs into the body as the brand-name drug.

MYTH: Generic drugs are not as potent as brand-name drugs

FACT: Generic drug manufacturers have to ensure that their products are of the same quality, strength, purity, and stability as the brand-name products.

MYTH: Generics take longer to act in the body.

FACT: In seeking FDA approval for their products, generic makers must submit evidence that their drugs will have the same therapeutic effect as the brand-name counterparts. This means that a generic product can be expected to deliver to the bloodstream, or other site where the drug does its work, the same amount of active ingredient as the original product.

MYTH: Generics are not as safe as brand-name drugs.

FACT: FDA requires that all drugs products be safe and effective. Since generics use the same active ingredients as their brand-name counterparts and work the same way in the body, generics are as safe and effective as their brand-name equivalents.

SOURCE:
Food and Drug Administration. *Myths and Facts of Generic Drugs*. DHHS Pub. No. (FDA) 89-3167. September 1987. pp. 1-2.

SELECTION GUIDELINES FOR CONSUMERS

With all that in mind it's clear that consumers today need to pay a lot more attention to their prescriptions than in the past. If your doctor is prescribing medication, ask if it matters in your particular circumstance whether you get a brand name. Some states require doctors to tell you whether they are prescribing brand or generic. Still, they seldom do. So talk to your doctor before you leave the office.

Some states actually mandate pharmacists to substitute a less expensive generic for the brand. All other states merely permit it. In a mandatory-substitution state the pharmacist must fill a prescription with a lower-priced generic unless the physician has checked the "dispense as written" box on the scrip. After the prescription is handed over, neither the patient nor the pharmacist has any choice in the matter.

If you are taking medication for a chronic condition, ask your doctor whether switching—from brand to generic, vice versa or one generic to another—could have any adverse effect on your medical condition. If so, the doctor may restrict you to a brand-name drug. No problem. But if you've been doing well on a generic, getting the same one each time you refill your prescription may be difficult; most pharmacies—at least until now—have tended to take whatever generics their wholesaler happens to stock.

What can you do? First, ask your pharmacist for the kind you were taking. If it's unavailable, ask that the label note the new manufacturer. Some states require this. Notify your physician that you will be taking a different maker's generic in case he or she thinks it's necessary to monitor the level of the drug in your blood. If you don't tell your doctor you've switched and your symptoms get worse, the physician may assume it's you when it could be the drug.

Finally, find and stick with a pharmacist you trust. "Going to different pharmacies to have prescriptions filled is one of the worst mistakes people can make," says Dr. Arthur Kibbe, director of scientific affairs for the American Pharmaceutical Association, which represents independent pharmacists. "Having one pharmacist who knows you—knows your allergies and has your records—provides a certain continuity in health care."

SOURCE:
Avery, Caryl S. "Can You Trust Generic Drugs?" *American Health* (April 1990): 86.

RESOURCES

ORGANIZATIONS

Food and Drug Administration. 5600 Fishers Lane, Rockville, MD 20857.

Generic Pharmaceutical Industry Association. 12 Stoneleigh Ave., P.O. Box 990, Carmel, NY 10512.

PAMPHLET

GPIA (Generic Pharmaceutical Industry Association):

Guide to Interchangeable Drugs. 1988. 32 pp.

RELATED ARTICLES

"AAFP Approves Policy against Mandatory Generic Substitution." (American Academy of Family Physicians). *American Family Physician* (November 1989): 297–298.

"FDA Says Tests of Generic Drugs Find Only 1.1% Deficient in Safety, Quality." *Heart Care* 2 (June 1990): 10.

"The Generic Drug Scandals: What Do They Mean for Consumers?" *HealthFacts* (November 1989): 2.

Schneider, Michael. "Generic Drugs: The Hidden Problems." *Mature Health* (February 1990): 5–6.

GLAUCOMA

OVERVIEW

Glaucoma occurs when there is too much fluid pressure in the eye, usually because the eye's plumbing system is not working correctly. The drainage canals may become clogged or covered over, but the ciliary tissues continue to produce fluid. In other words, the faucet is still turned on, but the sink's drain is blocked or its drainage pipes are clogged.

The extra fluid that builds up in the eye presses against its weakest point: the optic nerve at the back of the eye. The increased fluid pressure actually pushes the optic nerve back into a "cupped" or concave shape. If the intraocular pressure remains too high for too long, the extra pressure damages parts of the optic nerve. This damage appears as gradual visual changes and then loss of vision. The early visual changes are very slight and do not affect the central vision—the center portion of what is seen when looking straight ahead or reading. Certain parts of the peripheral vision—the top, sides, and bottom areas of vision—are affected first. Glaucoma usually occurs in both eyes, but extra fluid pressure often begins to build up first in only one eye.

In the most common form of glaucoma, this build-up of fluid pressure happens very gradually, usually without any uncomfortable or painful symptoms. The symptoms of less-common kinds of glaucoma are severe, such as: hazy vision, eye and head pain, nausea or vomiting, the appearance of rainbow-colored halos around bright lights, and rapid loss of vision.

Glaucoma occurs in people of all ages, from children to older adults, but it is more likely to develop in people who are over 35 years old, very nearsighted, or diabetic. The tendency to develop glaucoma may be inherited, since relatives of glaucoma patients are more likely to develop glaucoma themselves. Glaucoma also seems to occur more frequently in Blacks.

Ophthalmologists recommend a glaucoma check as part of regular eye examinations for children, teenagers, and adults. Most people should have an especially thorough glaucoma check around the age of 35. Another check-up is recommended at age 40 and then every two or three years after age 40. People over 35 who are more likely to develop glaucoma should continue to have an ophthalmologist check their intraocular pressures and optic nerves every year or two after age 35.

Doctors are not sure why the eye's drainage canals stop functioning correctly. Doctors do know, however, that glaucoma is not contagious, is not life-threatening, and seldom leads to blindness if diagnosed early and treated carefully. Doctors also know that glaucoma is generally not caused by too much reading, reading in poor light, improper diet, wearing contact lenses, or other activities in normal lifestyles.

Vision lost as a result of glaucoma usually cannot be recovered, but early diagnosis and careful, lifelong treatment can help prevent further visual damage. Most cases of glaucoma can be controlled with medication or surgery. Ophthalmologists in research centers all over the world are searching for the causes of glaucoma and for more effective treatments.

SOURCE:
Foundation for Glaucoma Research. *Understanding and Living with Glaucoma: A Reference Guide for Patients and Their Families.* 1990, pp. 6-8.

MAJOR TYPES OF GLAUCOMA

- Primary open or wide angle glaucoma, accounting for 75–80 percent of all cases, progresses slowly and painlessly over many years. It usually involves a build-up of eye pressure related to blocked fluid outflow. This type of glaucoma tends to be more severe in blacks than whites. People with first degree relatives who have glaucoma are at above average risk of this disorder. Those with diabetes, hypertension (high blood pressure) and strong myopia or shortsightedness are also at elevated risk. The gradual vision loss in open angle glaucoma occurs in a typical fashion. Peripheral or side vision goes first. Tiny blind spots appear at the edges of the visual field, slowly getting larger and spreading until, in serious cases, peripheral vision is altogether wiped out, leaving only central or "tunnel vision"—rather like looking through a telescope. When central or tunnel vision also disappears, the result is total blindness.

- Acute, closed or narrow angle glaucoma accounts for six to 10 percent of glaucoma cases. The angle between the iris and the cornea becomes too narrow or closes up, blocking the eye's fluid drainage. This type of glaucoma may hit suddenly with blurred vision, eye pain, headaches, coloured haloes around lights, nausea and vomiting—symptoms sometimes mistaken for migraine, a digestive attack, stroke or uveitis (eye inflammation). Acute glaucoma is an emergency and must be treated quickly to reduce the elevated eye pressure, which can lead to sight loss.
- Various types of "secondary" glaucoma may arise from several causes—for instance, congenital glaucoma, which occurs in about one per 10,000 births (where the eye's draining system doesn't develop properly). In some cases glaucoma stems from eye trauma (injury), diabetes and various vascular diseases. It may also arise from the use of certain drugs which damage the eye's draining meshwork such as topical steroids (prednisone or cortisone) sometimes dispensed for trivial eye complaints and over-lavishly applied.

SOURCE:

"Glaucoma Update." *Health News* (University of Toronto) (April 1991): 9.

TREATMENT

Drugs for open-angle glaucoma are the most widely used method of treating this disease. These medications are taken as eyedrops or pills. Some improve fluid drainage, while others lower pressure by inhibiting fluid formation. Most cases of glaucoma can be controlled with one or more medications, and a majority of patients tolerate these drugs well.

However, in a few patients intraocular pressure is not adequately controlled by medications. Also, some people find that the drug's side effects—such as stinging in the eye, blurred vision, or headaches—do not go away after the first few weeks of use but continue to be a problem. The patient may have trouble adhering to the prescribed dosage schedule and may be tempted to stop taking the medication or cut back on the dosage. In this situation, the patient should contact his or her eye doctor to discuss the problem and the best means of dealing with it. Changing the treatment plan without proper medical advice may allow intraocular pressure to rise again, and the patient may suffer needless visual loss as a result.

So, in spite of the fact that glaucoma can by controlled by medications in a majority of patients, other forms of treatment also play an important role in glaucoma therapy.

SOURCE:

National Eye Institute. *Glaucoma.* NIH Pub. No. 89-651. n.d.

* * *

Surgery is another way to treat glaucoma. Surgery of any kind always carries some risk of complications, so doctors try to avoid or delay surgery. However, modern glaucoma surgery is remarkably successful for most patients.

Surgery is the primary treatment method for acute and congenital glaucoma because it is generally the only way that the blocked or incorrectly formed drainage canals can be opened up. In cases of open-angle glaucoma, surgery is considered only when the maximum dosage of medications does not control the intraocular pressures, or when a patient cannot tolerate the medications needed to control eye pressures. Surgery is usually scheduled for only one eye at a time, as a safety measure and because one eye will often need surgery before the other.

There are two different ways of doing surgery now: laser treatment and microsurgery.

- Laser treatment is a technique that is used in cases of acute and chronic glaucoma. A laser is a tiny, powerful beam of light that can make a small burn or opening in tissue, depending on the strength of the light beam. Laser treatments are performed in a doctor's office or in a hospital clinic. Drops are used to anesthetize the eye. Then the doctor, with the help of a microscope, focuses the light beam on exactly the right place in the eye. The laser can be used to make an opening in the iris. This has become the treatment of choice for acute glaucoma. The laser also can be used to open some of the eye's drainage canals. The light beam passes harmlessly through the outer covering of the eye and makes an opening only where it is focused on the iris or drainage canals. During laser treatments, patients see a bright light—like a camera flash—and may feel a faint tingling sensation. The eye may be slightly irritated, and patients are advised to take it easy for a day or so. Eye pressure must be checked frequently right after laser treatment, and the pressure may not go down to a safe level for several weeks. Although laser treatments may not permanently control eye pressure, they can often delay the need for microsurgery. Ophthalmologists are still evaluating the long-term effects of laser treatments for glaucoma.

- Microsurgery is a technique that is successful in cases of acute, chronic, congenital, and secondary glaucoma. Same-day surgery is usually possible and can reduce hospitalization expenses. Microsurgery is usually done with a local anesthetic, often combined with relaxing medications. Patients sleep or feel drowsy and do not experience any discomfort during surgery. General anesthesia is not routinely used in glaucoma microsurgery for adults because there is some risk of heart or breathing complications, but general anesthesia is always used for infants and young children.

SOURCE:
Foundation for Glaucoma Research. *Understanding and Living with Glaucoma: A Reference Guide for Patients and Their Families.* 1990, pp. 19-21.

RESOURCES

ORGANIZATIONS

American Academy of Ophthalmology. 655 Beach Street, P.O. Box 7424, San Francisco, CA 94120–7424.

American Optometric Association. 243 Lindbergh Boulevard, St. Louis, MO 63141.

American Foundation for the Blind. 15 West 16th St., New York, NY 10011.

Foundation for Glaucoma Research. 490 Post Street, Suite 830, San Francisco, CA 94102.

PAMPHLETS

American Academy of Ophthalmology:

Glaucoma: It Can Take Your Sight Away. April 1987, 8 pp.

Foundation for Glaucoma Research, Fact Sheets:

Developmental Glaucoma.

Glaucoma in Blacks.

Lasers Used in Ophthalmology: An Overview.

Medications Used in Glaucoma.

What Is Glaucoma.

National Eye Institute:

Glaucoma. November 1990, 10 pp.

BOOKS

Epstein, D. L. (ed.). *Chandler's and Grant's Glaucoma.* 3d ed. Philadelphia: Lea and Febiger, 1986.

Ritch, R., M. B. Shields, and T. Krepin. *The Glaucomas.* St. Louis: Mosby, 1989.

ADDITIONAL ARTICLES

Anderson, Douglas R. "Glaucoma: The Damage Caused by Pressure." *American Journal of Ophthalmology* 108, no. 5 (November 15, 1989): 485–495.

Capino, Diosdada G., and Howard M. Leibowitz. "Glaucoma: Screening, Diagnosis, and Therapy." *Hospital Practice* 25, no. 5A (May 30, 1990): 73–91.

Elkington, A. R., and P. T. Khaw. "The Glaucomas." *British Medical Journal* 297, no. 6649 (September 10, 1988): 677–680.

Everitt, Daniel E., and Jerry Avorn. "Systemic Effects of Medications Used To Treat Glaucoma." *Annals of Internal Medicine* 112, no. 2 (January 15, 1990): 120–125.

"The First Line of Treatment for Glaucoma." *Health After 50* (April 1991): 6.

"Glaucoma: A Brighter Future in Sight." *Weight Watchers Women's Health and Fitness News* (March 1991): 5.

Patlack, Margie. "Lights for Lasers: Lasers Beginning to Solve Vision Problems." *FDA Consumer* 24 (July-August 1990): 14–17.

Spaeth, George L., and Lawrence F. Jindra. "Glaucoma Can Impair Your Vision." *Executive Health Report* (January 1989): 1–4.

GONORRHEA

(*See also:* CHLAMYDIA; PELVIC INFLAMMATORY DISEASE; SEXUALLY TRANSMITTED DISEASES; SYPHILIS)

OVERVIEW

Nearly 1 million cases of gonorrhea are reported annually in the United States. Another million unreported cases, mostly among teenagers and young adults, are believed to occur each year. Gonorrhea is caused by the gonococcus, a bacterium that grows and multiplies quickly in moist, warm areas of the body such as the cervix, urinary tract, mouth, or rectum. In women, the cervix is the most common site of infection. However, the disease can spread to the ovaries and fallopian tubes, resulting in pelvic inflammatory disease (PID); this can cause infertility and other serious problems.

Gonorrhea can also be spread from a man's penis to the throat of his sex partner during oral sex (pharyngeal gonorrhea). People can transfer the bacteria from the genital area to the mouth with their fingers. Gonorrhea of the rectum may develop in women due to spread of the infection from the vaginal area, and it can also occur in homosexual men who practice receptive anal intercourse.

Gonorrhea can be passed from an infected woman to her newborn infant during delivery. The infection also occurs in children, most commonly in young victims of sexual abuse.

The early symptoms of gonorrhea often are mild, and some who are infected have no symptoms of the disease; this is one reason why it is so readily transmitted. If symptoms of gonorrhea develop, they usually appear within 2 to 10 days of sexual contact with an infected partner, although a small percentage of patients may be infected for several months without showing symptoms. The initial symptoms in women include a painful or burning sensation when urinating or a yellowish vaginal discharge. More advanced symptoms include abdominal pain, bleeding between menstrual periods, vomiting, or fever. Men usually have a discharge from the penis and a burning sensation during urination that may be severe. Symptoms of rectal infection include anal itching, and sometimes painful bowel movements.

Two techniques, Gram stain and culture, are generally used to diagnose gonorrhea. Many doctors prefer to use both tests to increase the chance of an accurate diagnosis. The Gram stain is quite accurate for men but less so for women. The test involves placing a smear of the discharge on a slide that has been stained with a dye and then examining it under a microscope for the presence of the gonococcus. A Gram stain of the discharge from a man's penis or a woman's cervix is correct in diagnosing gonorrhea more than 90 percent of the time. Test results usually can be given to the patient at the time of an office or clinic visit.

The culture test involves placing a sample of the discharge onto a culture plate and incubating it for up to 2 days in order to allow the bacteria time to multiply. The accuracy of this test depends on the site from which the sample is taken. Cervical samples are accurate, for example, approximately 90 percent of the time. Throat cultures can also be done to detect pharyngeal gonorrhea.

SOURCE:

National Institute of Allergy and Infectious Diseases. *Gonorrhea.* NIH Pub. No. 87-909E. August, 1987.

TREATMENT

Because one in four men and two in five women who have gonorrhea also have chlamydia, your treatment should be designed to cure both infections. Your partner(s) must be treated at the same time you are.

Gonorrhea is quickly eradicated in about 95% of cases by a single (large) dose of ampicillin, amoxicillin, or penicillin. Probenecid is used along with these drugs to increase their effectiveness. Probenecid temporarily slows down kidney excretion of penicillin-type antibiotics so that a high bloodstream antibiotic level can be quickly achieved and sustained. After an initial single-dose treatment for gonorrhea you should take tetracycline or doxycycline faithfully for seven days to cure chlamydia as well. Erythromycin will be substituted if you are pregnant. Tetracycline and doxycycline are also effective against gonorrhea, but are not preferred treatments because cure depends on precise and faithful doses over the entire seven days. Anyone (woman or man) exposed to a partner with gonorrhea should be treated. An exam and cultures should also be done, but treatment should be started immediately even if no symptoms are present.

Treatment options recommended by the Centers for Disease Control for uncomplicated gonorrhea infection, with no evidence of infection spread to uterus or tubes, are:

An initial antibiotic single dose of:

- Amoxicillin, 3 grams (six capsules) taken all at once, plus Probenecid, 1 gram (two capsules) taken at the same time
- or Ampicillin, 3.5 grams (seven capsules) taken all at once, plus Probenecid, 1 gram (two capsules) taken at the same time
- or Penicillin injection (procaine penicillin, 4.8 million units total given by injection into muscle in two different sites), plus Probenecid, 1 gram (two capsules) taken at the same time

Followed by:

- Tetracycline, 500-mg capsules taken four times a day for seven days
- or Doxycycline, 100-mg capsules taken two times a day for seven days
- or (if you are allergic to tetracycline or pregnant) Erythromycin base or stearate, 500-mg capsules taken four times a day for seven days or Erythromycin ethylsuccinate, 800-mg capsules taken four times a day for seven days

SOURCE:

Stewart, Felicia H., and others. *Understanding Your Body: Every Woman's Guide to a Lifetime of Health.* New York: Bantam Books. 1987. pp. 487–488.

COMPLICATIONS

If the bacteria spread to the bloodstream, they can infect the joints, heart valves, or the brain. The most common consequence of gonorrhea, however, is pelvic inflammatory disease (PID), a potentially serious infection of the female pelvic organs, which occurs in an estimated 1 million American women each year. PID can cause scarring of the fallopian tubes, resulting in infertility in as many as 10 percent of women affected. In others, the scarring blocks the proper passage of the fertilized egg into the uterus. If this happens, the egg may implant itself in the tube; this is called an ectopic pregnancy and is life-threatening to the mother if not detected early.

An infected woman who is pregnant may pass the infection to her infant as the baby passes through the birth canal during delivery. Most states require that the eyes of newborns be treated with silver nitrate or other medication immediately after birth to prevent gonococcal infection to the eyes, which can lead to blindness. Because of the risk of gonococcal infection to both mother and child, most doctors now recommend that a pregnant woman have at least one test for gonorrhea during her pregnancy.

SOURCE:

National Institute of Allergy and Infectious Diseases. *Gonorrhea.* NIH Pub. No. 87-909E. August 1987.

PREVENTION

Prevention is based on education, mechanical or chemical prophylaxis, and early diagnosis and treatment. The condom, if properly used, can reduce the risk of infection. Effective drugs taken in therapeutic doses within 24 hours of exposure can abort an infection, but prophylaxis with penicillin is ineffective and contributes to the selection of penicillinase-producing gonococci.

Ophthalmic infection of the newborn is prevented by the installation of 0.5% erythromycin ointment, 1% tetracycline ointment, or 1% silver nitrate solution into each conjunctival sac immediately after birth. Ceftriaxone, 125 mg intramuscularly once, is effective against both eye and systemic infections.

SOURCE

Schroeder, Steven A., and others (eds.). *Current Medical Diagnosis & Treatment 1992.* Norwalk, Connecticut: Appleton. 1992. p. 996.

RESOURCES

ORGANIZATION

National Institute of Allergy and Infectious Diseases. 9000 Rockville Pike, Bethesda, MD 20205.

RELATED ARTICLES

Goldstein, A. M. B., and J. H. Clark. "Treatment of Uncomplicated Gonococcal Urethritis With Single-Dose Ceftizoxime." *Sexually Transmitted Diseases* (October-December 1990): 181–183.

"Gonorrhea and Syphilis Pose Renewed Threats." *Patient Care* 22 (April 30, 1988): 23–24.

"Screening for Sexually Transmitted Diseases: Gonorrhea." *American Family Physician* 42 (September 1990): 694–696.

GUM DISEASE

OVERVIEW

In the broadest sense, periodontal disease can be considered any form of ill health affecting the periodontium—the tissues that surround and support the teeth. These include the gums (or gingiva), the bone of the tooth socket, and the periodontal ligament, a thin layer of connective tissue that holds the tooth in its socket and acts as a cushion between tooth and bone.

Inflammation or infection of the gums is called gingivitis; that of the bone, periodontitis. These conditions can arise for a variety of reasons. A severe deficiency of vitamin C can lead to scurvy and result in bleeding, spongy gums, and eventual tooth loss. And at least one periodontal disease—the uncommon but highly destructive juvenile periodontitis—is thought to have a strong genetic basis. But as the terms periodontal disease, gingivitis, and periodontitis are most commonly used, they refer to disease that is caused by the buildup of dental plaque.

Plaque is a combination of bacteria and sticky bacterial products that forms on the teeth within hours of cleaning. Its source is the natural bacteria in the mouth, of which more than 300 different species have been identified. In small amounts and when newly formed, plaque is invisible and relatively harmless. But when left to accumulate, it increases in volume (in large amounts, plaque can be seen as a soft whitish deposit), and the proportion of harmful species in the plaque grows.

The role played by plaque in the development of gingivitis was demonstrated in the early 1960s. Dental researchers had people stop brushing their teeth and let the plaque in their mouths build up. Within two to three weeks, signs of inflammation appeared—redness, swelling, and an increased tendency to bleed—and when brushing resumed, the inflammation went away.

Gingivitis is fairly common. Just about everybody, says [Brian] Burt [dental epidemiologist, School of Public Health, University of Michigan], has it in some degree. A recent nationwide survey by the National Institute of Dental Research, for example, found that 40 to 50 percent of the adults studied had at least one spot on their gums with inflammation that was prone to bleeding.

At one time gingivitis and periodontitis were thought to be different phases of the same disease, meaning that the sort of inflammation detected in this study would lead inevitably to periodontitis if left untreated. Yet, dental researchers no longer believe this to be true. In the April 1988 *Dental Clinics of North America*, National Institute of Dental Research director Harald Loe, D.D.S., describes an ongoing study, then in its 15th year, of Sri Lankan tea workers who practice no oral hygiene. All have gingivitis—but not all have periodontitis.

This and other studies with similar results have led dental researchers to two conclusions. One, says dental epidemiologist Ronald J. Hunt, of the College of Dentistry at the University of Iowa, is that "gingivitis is not a particularly serious disease." The other is that "gingivitis and periodontitis are different disease entities."

Some people with gingivitis do, nonetheless, develop periodontitis. The plaque that causes gingivitis is located at or above the gum line and is referred to as supragingival plaque. With time, areas of supragingival plaque can become covered by swollen gum tissue or otherwise spread below the gum line (where it is called subgingival plaque), and in this airless environment the harmful bacteria within the plaque proliferate. These bacteria can injure tissues through the direct secretion of toxins. But they cause the greatest damage by stimulating a chronic inflammatory response in which the body in essence turns on itself, and the periodontal ligament and bone of the tooth socket are broken down and destroyed. This is similar to what happens in rheumatoid arthritis and, like rheumatoid arthritis, periodontitis is now considered primarily an inflammatory disease.

The bone destruction from periodontitis can be fairly even, resulting in receding gum lines. But more often it causes deep crevices between an individual tooth and its socket. These crevices are called periodontal pockets, and just as it once was thought that gingivitis inexorably progressed to periodontitis, so it was once believed that shallow periodontal pockets inevitably deepened, eventually becoming deep enough to jeopardize the socket's support of the adjacent tooth.

SOURCE:
Shepherd, Steven. "Brushing Up on Gum Disease." *FDA Consumer* 24 (May 1990): 9–10.

DIAGNOSIS

How can I be tested for gum disease?

By visiting your dentist. The dentist or dental hygienist will inspect the color and firmness of the gums and test the teeth for looseness. They will also check the way your teeth fit together when you bite. X-rays may be taken to evaluate the bone supporting the teeth.

A technique called periodontal probing is the cornerstone of testing for gum disease. In this procedure, a small measuring instrument is gently inserted between the tooth and gum to measure the depth of the pocket.

Can I test myself for gum disease?

You can—and should—check yourself for the warning signs of gum disease. However you may have gum disease that has spread into the bone and not have any of the symptoms. Most people do not experience any pain due to gum disease and therefore it often goes unnoticed. Many times gum disease is a silent epidemic.

Only a dentist can diagnose gum disease. That is why it is important to have regular dental checkups, including a periodontal examination.

The warning signs of gum disease are:

- bleeding gums during tooth brushing
- red, swollen or tender gums
- gums that have pulled away from the teeth
- persistent bad breath
- pus between the teeth and gums
- loose or separating teeth
- a change in the way your teeth fit together when you bite
- a change in the fit of partial dentures

You should contact your dentist if you notice any of these symptoms.

SOURCE:
American Academy of Periodontology. *Gum Disease: Be Tested to See If You Have It.* September 1989. pp. 2–4.

PREVENTION OF PLAQUE—USE OF MOUTHWASH

A prescription product (trade name Peridex) containing the antimicrobial chlorhexidine was approved by FDA in 1986 based on studies showing that it reduced gingivitis by up to 41 percent. Chlorhexidine mouthwashes have long been used in Europe, and an article that year in *The Journal of Periodontal Research* called chlorhexidine "the most effective and most thoroughly tested anti-plaque and anti-gingivitis agent known today."

Shortly after Peridex was approved for marketing, the American Dental Association awarded its "Seal of Acceptance"—the first ever granted a mouthwash by the ADA. This seal (which can have considerable marketing value and is probably most familiar as a result of its being displayed on many brands of toothpaste) indicated that Peridex had met a series of guidelines established by the ADA for evaluating products making anti-plaque, anti-gingivitis claims.

In 1987, the ADA awarded its second (and so far only other) Seal of Acceptance to a mouthwash for use in the reduction of plaque and gingivitis. This seal went to Listerine, and its manufacturer has since used the ADA seal in promoting the product as a plaque-fighter. FDA, however, has not yet approved Listerine for this use. In fact, FDA has sent letters to the makers of Listerine and several other over-the-counter (OTC) products making anti-plaque claims stating that in its opinion the products are being marketed in violation of the Federal Food, Drug, and Cosmetic Act and are "at risk of regulatory action."

SOURCE:
Shepherd, Steven. "Anti-Plaque Mouthwashes." *FDA Consumer* 24 (May 1990): 14.

PREVENTION OF PLAQUE—BY BRUSHING

The most effective nonprescription tool available for this job is the toothbrush. Because a toothbrush's ability to remove plaque is markedly reduced by splayed or matted bristles, toothbrushes need to be replaced at the first sign of wear. Soft bristles are superior to hard for removing plaque, but with this exception the kind of brush you buy is less important than how well you use it. Several techniques have been developed for effective toothbrushing and it is advisable to be instructed in at least one by a dentist. Estimates are that less than a third of the population cleans its teeth adequately when brushing; according to one textbook, "periodontists generally find that uninstructed patients usually miss entirely or only partially clean several areas of their mouths in toothbrushing."

Electric toothbrushes have not been shown any more effective at removing plaque than manual toothbrushes when properly used. Water-jet devices may be useful in dislodging food particles but they are only minimally effective at removing plaque and some experts worry that they may actually drive harmful bacteria deeper into the periodontal tissues if misused; the advisability of using such a device is best determined by consulting your dentist. There is no question about the usefulness of floss. Floss is the best available aid for removing plaque from between the teeth—an area where the toothbrush is typically ineffective.

Fluoride toothpastes can help prevent cavities and should be used for this reason. So far, though, no toothpaste has been recognized by the American Dental Association as having effective plaque-fighting capabilities. Many products, toothpastes among them, are now being marketed as plaque-fighters. However, a product may have some effect against plaque but not enough to make a difference in a person's oral health. Such products are not considered by the ADA to be effective and for this reason it is worth looking for the ADA seal of acceptance when trying to determine if a product is an effective anti-plaque agent.

SOURCE:

Shepherd, Steven. "New Progress on the Periodontal Diseases." *Executive Health Report* 25 (June 1989): 3–4.

RESOURCES

ORGANIZATIONS

American Academy of Periodontology. 211 East Chicago Avenue, Room 924, Chicago, IL 60611.

National Institute of Dental Research. 9000 Rockville Pike, Building 21, Room 8A-06, Bethesda, MD 20205.

PAMPHLET

National Institute of Dental Research:

Periodontal (Gum) Disease. n.d. 8 pp.

RELATED ARTICLES

"Combatting Periodontal (Gum) Disease." *Health News* 7 (June 1989): 3–7.

McVeigh, Gloria. "High-Tech Tooth Savers from the American Academy of Periodontology." *Prevention* (May 1990): 86–92.

Suzuki, Jon B. "Diagnosis and Classification of the Periodontal Diseases." *Dental Clinics of North America* 32, no. 2 (April 1988): 195–216.

Williams, Ray C. "Periodontal Disease." *The New England Journal of Medicine* 322, no. 6 (February 8, 1990): 373–382.

HEAD LICE (PEDICULOSIS)

OVERVIEW

The head louse, technically known as *Pediculus capitis humanus*, is by no means a new nuisance. The insect has been an unwelcome companion to humans probably from the beginning, as have its close relatives, the body louse and the pubic or crab louse. But head lice infestations seem to be on the rise in recent years—as almost any parent of an elementary school-aged child can tell you.

A parent's first reaction to head lice is often revulsion, sometimes accompanied by a sense of shame due to the misperception that head lice only live on "dirty" people. In truth, the only thing that the presence of head lice tells about children is that they've been around other kids with head lice.

Head lice are parasites about the size of a small ant. They get their nourishment by sucking small amounts of blood from humans. Their favorite feeding area is the scalp behind the ears and at the nape of the neck. Their feeding and sucking activity is responsible for the itching that is so frequently the first hint of infestation. Left untreated, rash and infection can occur. In severe cases, the lymph glands in the neck may swell. Although usually confined to the head, head lice sometimes also set up shop in beards, eyebrows and, rarely, eyelashes.

Though they don't fly, lice are quite adept at getting from head to head, especially when those heads are close together. Good hygiene is always an admirable goal, but a clean head of hair is no guarantee that they won't invade. Because children play so closely together, often in large groups, lice have an easy time traveling from child to child. Cases of lice seem to increase in the winter, possibly because kids are inside and close together, sometimes sharing hats, combs and, consequently, "cooties," as kids sometimes call them. The creepy critters can live up to two to three days apart from the body and, in closets where clothes hang close together, may hop from hat to scarf. They also may be lurking on the headrest of a school bus seat, just waiting to get aboard an attractive head. (The stitchings of those upholstered headrests can hide the tiny gray-white lice eggs called nits.)

It's easier to spot the nits than the lice themselves. And, because nits are dandruffy in appearance, they are easier to see on brunettes than on blonds. To distinguish them from dandruff or hair spray, pick up a strand of hair close to the scalp and pull your fingernail across the area where the whitish substance appears. Dandruff (or hairspray) will come off easily, but nits will stay firmly attached to the hair. If you look real hard, you may be able to see the bugs themselves on the back of the head and around the ears.

Once you have discovered head lice on one family member, all other members of the family, as well as close friends, should be checked. Also, look for lice or their nits in fabrics of stuffed toys, upholstered furniture, and bedding.

SOURCE:

Young, Theresa A., and Judith Levine Willis. "Of Lice and Children: Going to the Head of Class." *FDA Consumer* 23 (November 1989): 28–29.

TREATMENT

For all types of pediculosis, lindane lotion (Kwell, Scabene) is used extensively. A thin layer is applied to the infested and adjacent hairy areas. It is removed after 12 hours by thorough washing. Remaining nits may be removed with a fine-toothed comb or forceps. Sexual contacts should be treated. Permethrin (Nix), 1% cream rinse, is a topical pediculocide and ovicide for the treatment of head lice and eggs. It is applied to the scalp and hair and left on for 10 minutes before being rinsed off with water. Synergized pyrethrins (A-200 Pyrinate, Pyrinyl, Rid) are over-the-counter products that are applied undiluted until the infested areas are entirely wet. After 10 minutes, the areas are washed thoroughly with warm water and soap and then dried. Nits may be treated as indicated above. For involvement of eyelashes, petrolatum is applied thickly twice daily for 8 days, and the remaining nits are then plucked off. There is controversy about whether lice and the acarus of scabies can develop resistance to lindane.

Malathion lotion, 0.5% (Ovide), compared with A-200 shampoo, R&C shampoo, RID, lindane shampoo, and A-200 Pyrinate gel, is the only product for pediculosis capitis that shows excellent ovicidal activity. Hatching of eggs following treatment with the other agents leads to recurrence of the infestation.

SOURCE:
Schroeder, Steven A., and others (eds.). *Current Medical Diagnosis & Treatment 1992.* Norwalk, CT: Appleton & Lange, 1992. p. 110.

"NIT PICKING"

While parents hate to be "nit-pickers," nit-picking is usually the worst problem associated with head lice. To get rid of all the nits left after a de-lousing shampoo, either a special fine-toothed metal nit comb is used to dislodge the eggs or they are picked off with fingernails or tweezers—a tedious procedure! Nit combs (fine-toothed metal combs, sometimes with tiny blades at the base) may cut the individual hairs to which a louse egg is attached. But nit combing can take hours per head, depending on the length of hair and the number of nits. Although effective for thick hair, nit combs are useless for the very fine hair of a young child. Each egg-bearing hair can be cut out with scissors or one might end up using the fingernails! Some experts recommend soaking the hair in warm, diluted vinegar to make nit-picking easier—a strategy of unproven usefulness. A haircut may make nit removal less time-consuming, but stigmatizes children. For lice of the pubic variety on the eyelashes or eyebrows, petrolatum or Vaseline may be used to suffocate them (cuts off their oxygen supply.)

SOURCE:
"A Lousy Problem: Nit-Picking." *Health News* (University of Toronto) 8 (August 1990): 9.

PREVENTING RE-INFESTATION

To prevent reinfestation, the following may be helpful:

- Make sure all family members and friends of the infested person have been closely scrutinized for signs of lice. If any of them appear to have lice, make sure they are treated.
- Wash all clothing and bed linens used by the infested members of your family in hot water and place in a hot dryer for at least 20 minutes. If this cannot be done, place the linens and clothing into an air-tight bag for two weeks. Dry cleaning also kills lice and nits.
- Vacuum backs of chairs, pillows in living and bedroom areas, mattresses, car seats and headrests, and rugs that might be in contact with infested hair. Empty the vacuum bag (if it is the paper disposable sort, discard the bag). There are some OTC sprays for disinfecting furniture and bedding. They contain insecticides that are not suitable for humans or animals, so be careful not to confuse them with the products that are for human use.
- Disinfect combs, brushes, sports helmets, and other objects that come in contact with the head by soaking in medicated shampoo or very hot soapy water.
- Recheck all family members and friends 7 to 14 days and 21 to 28 days after initial treatment to be sure lice have not reappeared (eggs that remain after treatment will hatch in 7 to 14 days).

Though discovering that your child has head lice is no picnic, neither is it cause for panic or shame. The problem is shared by a good portion of the American school population and can be controlled by vigilance and appropriate treatment.

SOURCE:
Young, Theresa A., and Judith Levine Willis. "Going to the Head of the Class." *Pediatrics for Parents* 11 (October 1990): 2-3.

RESOURCES

ORGANIZATION
National Pediculosis Association. P.O. Box 149, Newton, MA 02161.

RELATED ARTICLES
DiNapoli, Joan B., and others. "Eradication of Head Lice with a Single Treatment." *American Journal of Public Health* 78, no. 8 (August 1988): 978-980.

"Malathion for Head Lice." *Medical Letter on Drugs and Therapeutics* 31 (December 15, 1989): 110-111.

HEADACHE

OVERVIEW

Except perhaps for head colds, headaches are the most common human ailment. Three out of four Americans had a headache during the past year, according to the National Headache Foundation. Usually headaches are merely passing annoyances that go away with aspirin or after a nap. But as many as 45 million people suffer from chronic and/or severe headaches that seriously interfere with their lives. All told, headaches account for 80 million doctors' office visits and more than $400 million spent on over-the-counter pain relievers each year.

Like colds, headaches are not completely understood by scientists. There appear to be various types of headache, but any hard and fast classification is open to debate, in part because the types often overlap—both in their symptoms and their response to medication. Moreover, triggering factors and modes of relief vary from person to person. Still, the great majority of primary headaches (that is, those not due to underlying disease) fall into three categories, according to the International Headache Society: tension, migraine, and cluster.

Tension headaches

Also called a muscle-contraction or stress headache, this is the type almost everyone gets occasionally. The dull, steady pain—mild compared to migraine or cluster headaches—may be felt in the forehead, temples, back of neck, or throughout the head. A feeling of tightness around the scalp is typical; muscles in the back of the upper neck may feel knotted and tender to the touch. It's not known whether it's the sustained muscle tension itself or the subsequent restricted blood flow that causes the pain. Tension headaches are associated with stress (often the pain actually comes after the stress has ended), fatigue, or too much or too little sleep. Assuming a posture that tenses your neck and head muscles for long periods, such as holding your chin down while reading, can trigger these headaches; so can gum chewing, grinding your teeth, or tensing head and neck muscles during sexual intercourse. Men and women are about equally likely to suffer tension headaches.

Tension headaches that occur daily may also be a sign of clinical depression. In some cases, the headaches may cause the depression; in others, treating the depression makes the headaches go away.

Migraines

The word migraine, derived from the Greek, means "half a skull"—an apt description of the pain, which usually occurs in only one side of the head. Migraines appear to involve the abnormal expansion and contraction of blood vessels in and around the brain. In some people, migraines start with distorted vision, called an "aura"—generally characterized by zigzag patterns of shooting lights, blind spots, and/or a temporary loss of peripheral vision. The throbbing, pulsating pain can be incapacitating. It can last anywhere from a few minutes to several days; if it lasts longer than that, it's probably not a migraine. Migraine sufferers may also experience nausea, vomiting, and sensitivity to both light and noise.

About 80% of migraine sufferers have a family history of the ailment; women are nearly four times more likely to be afflicted. The typical sufferer is young (under 35) and had her first attack during her teens or twenties. With age, attacks usually become less severe and less frequent. Hormonal changes can play a role: thus susceptible women may have more attacks if they take oral contraceptives, or around the time of menstruation; they may have fewer attacks during pregnancy and after menopause. Attacks can also be instigated by certain substances in foods, emotional factors, and environmental factors (such as glaring light, strong odors, and changes in weather).

Cluster headaches

These strike in a group or "cluster" for up to a few hours, and recur daily for days, weeks, or even months on end. There may be months of freedom between attacks. Some researchers consider cluster headaches a variant of migraines, largely because the excruciating pain is centered on one side of the head, as in a migraine. But unlike the throbbing of a migraine, this pain is steady and piercing. There are other notable differences: typically cluster headaches strike at night or early morning, and the pain is located around or behind one eye or in one temple. Cluster headaches are about six to nine times more likely to strike men than women; the first attack usually comes in a person's twenties or thirties. They are sometimes misdiagnosed as a sinus disorder (because stuffy nose or sinus congestion is a common symptom) or even an abscessed tooth. There's no clear cause, though heavy smoking and drinking are possible contributing or triggering factors.

SOURCE:
"Heading Off Headaches." *The University of California, Berkeley Wellness Letter* 7 (November 1990): 4–5. Excerpted from *The University of California, Berkeley Wellness Letter,* Copyright Health Letter Associates, 1990.

CHANGING MEDICAL VIEW OF HEADACHE

"The standard way to treat [chronic] headaches used to be this: the doctor would give the patient a drug like Fiorinal and if that didn't work, he'd send her to a psychiatrist," said Joel R. Saper, M.D., director of the Michigan Head Pain and Neurological Institute. . . . The idea that headaches, be they migraines or tension headaches, are due to disturbed emotions or a personality defect is slowly giving way—at least among the neurologists who dominate the hospital-based headache centers—to an emphasis on biochemical imbalances in the brain. Drawing a distinction between cause and provoking influences, Dr. Saper sees emotions as an important aggravating factor in people who have an inherited vulnerability to headaches. Other triggering factors include hormonal fluctuations (in women), weather changes, skipping a meal, and flying across time zones. The health care community's failure to comprehend headache as an illness, said Dr. Saper, has contributed to mistreatment with everything from hysterectomy to tooth extractions.

"I was taught in medical school that migraine is a disease of the blood vessels because it causes them to constrict, dilate, and become inflamed," said Dr. Lipton. "But over the last ten years, it has become clear that the blood vessels are sort of bystanders and migraine is really a disease of the brain." The blood vessel changes take place because of fundamental changes in the brain, he said, explaining that there has been a new understanding of chemical imbalances in the brain, particularly the contribution of serotonin. Elevating levels of this brain chemical which regulates the body's response to stress is an effect of some drugs (anti-depressants) commonly prescribed to prevent migraines.

Chronic migraine or tension headaches are not curable, but they can be controlled. The goal of treatment is to reduce the frequency with as little reliance upon drugs as possible.

SOURCE:
"Changing Medical View of Chronic Headache." *HealthFacts* (March 1991): 4.

TREATMENT

Most headaches are tension headaches, caused by muscle spasm in the back of the head and neck. In some people, those headaches are virtually continuous for years at a time. The spasm can be sparked by emotional stress or by holding the head in a fixed position (for example, while facing a computer screen or driving for hours). Sometimes the pain can be severe. You'd usually feel it in the back of your head, but it could encircle the head in a vise-like band.

Tension headaches are sometimes helped by measures to relax the tight muscles. These include massage, hot showers, and heating pads on the back of the neck (some people respond better to cold packs). Biofeedback and muscle-relaxation training may be helpful. And some people find relief with other nontraditional techniques such as acupuncture, hypnosis, or meditation.

Nonprescription pain relievers often help occasional tension headaches. If not, prescription analgesics may do the trick. These include aspirin with codeine (Empirin with Codeine); acetaminophen with codeine (Tylenol with Codeine); aspirin, caffeine, and butalbital (Fiorinal); and aspirin and oxycodone (Percodan).

But for chronic tension headaches, even prescription analgesics aren't always useful. They tend to lose their effectiveness, encourage dependency, and even cause "rebound" headaches when they wear off.

A less addictive, often more effective alternative is a tricyclic antidepressant such as amitriptyline (Elavil) or imipramine (Tofranil), which can affect the pain pathways in the brain. Tricyclics must be used for several weeks before they take effect. Since much lower doses of the antidepressant are needed for pain than for depression, there are generally few or no side effects.

Much less common than the tension headache is the vascular headache. This kind occurs when the blood vessels on the surface of the brain widen excessively. Your head then literally throbs with pain. A few possible causes include severe hypertension, excessive alcohol, certain medications (such as nitroglycerine, for angina), and caffeine withdrawal. Vascular headaches range from mild hangovers to migraines to savage "cluster" headaches.

Migraines are often accompanied by nausea and vomiting, and frequently affect only one side of the head. In the classic form, the pain follows certain warning signs (the aura), such as flashing lights, blind spots, or tingling or numbness on one side of the body. The aura is always the same for each individual. An "abortive" migraine features the aura without the headache.

Biofeedback and other nontraditional techniques occasionally help prevent, though not relieve, migraines; heat and other muscle-relaxing steps generally don't do either.

Since migraines may be sparked by specific factors, sufferers should keep a headache diary to pinpoint any possible triggers. People have blamed their migraines on alcohol, monosodium glutamate (MSG), nitrites, and a host of other foods and drinks. Birth-control pills, estrogen replacement therapy, menstruation, irregular eating and sleeping schedules, and bright lights or noises have also been linked to migraines.

The supposed migraine personality—compulsive, neat, and rigid—is probably a myth.

Drugs that constrict blood vessels, notably ergotamine (Ergostat), may relieve migraines if taken at the first sign of the headache. Once a migraine is established, the only recourse is to take a narcotic such as meperedine (Demerol) or codeine, head for a darkened room, and try to sleep it off. Recent studies show that nonsteroidal anti-inflammatory agents—such as ibuprofen (Motrin), indomethacin (Indameth), and others—can alleviate migraines, sometimes as effectively as ergotamine. An experimental drug, sumatriptan, appears to ease migraine about as well as ergotamine, with much milder side effects.

Preventing migraines requires different drugs than those used for relieving them. While neither aspirin nor acetaminophen will relieve migraines, recent research suggests that a regular aspirin regimen may help prevent them. Beta blockers taken daily are often effective—provided side effects, such as lowered pulse or blood pressure, don't develop. If you have asthma, don't take beta blockers. Propranolol (Inderal) is the only beta blocker approved for migraines, but others may also help forestall attacks.

Cluster headaches seldom last more than an hour or two, but those hours—usually in the middle of the night—can be miserable. The attacks can occur daily for weeks at a time, and then disappear for long stretches. These headaches don't usually last long enough to be treated effectively. Some sufferers need prescription narcotics.

SOURCE:

Lipman, Marvin M. "Headaches—What to Do and When to Worry." *Consumer Reports Health Letter* (July 1990): 54.

PREVENTION

Preventing a headache can take many routes. For most people, prevention centers around knowing themselves: that is, knowing what they do that sets them off.

It can be something as simple as sleeping in late on Saturday or Sunday, or not having your 9 A.M. fight with the boss, or eating dinner at 8 instead of 6, or drinking that wine at a susceptible time.

Principle of Sameness

The concept of chronobiology works with the idea that the body gets into routines which it then attempts to perpetuate. If you eat at the same time Monday through Friday, your body will start putting out digestive enzymes when it gets close to that time. If on Saturday you decide to eat two hours later, your body may have tried to start digestion a good two hours earlier. If this response plays out in the entire body, then it means your body expectantly prepares for anything and everything you routinely do. If you then disappoint that expectation, what's left is a response with no reaction, which may well provoke a headache.

The idea, then, is to go by the principle of sameness: try to keep each day as close to the others as you reasonably can. If you normally get up at 6 A.M., then do the same on your days off, too. Keep mealtimes relatively constant.

And, strange as it might sound, if your routine includes a certain amount of stress at a certain time, be aware that the lack of stress or having it occur earlier or later may result in a headache. It won't be caused by stress, per se, but rather by your body's inability to play out a situation for which it is prepared.

Avoidance

Another way to head off a headache is to avoid things you know bother you, like smoke, perfumes or polluted air.

Noise probably won't cause you trouble except when you're actually in the throes of a headache. Bright lights might, particularly fluorescents since many people find those more troublesome than incandescent lights.

The jury's still out on whether computer terminals can cause headaches. Certainly they combine some of the worst of the triggers—poor posture, bad lighting, a fixed focus, and perhaps harmful emissions. As of now there's no hard evidence implicating computer terminals alone in causing headaches.

If you have headaches every day you work at a computer, but you don't have them when you're doing something else, that might be a good place to start. But before you implicate the computer itself, be sure you've eliminated other potential problems.

As with everything having to do with headaches, diagnosis and treatment must be individualized.

SOURCE:

"Heading Off a Headache." *Executive Health's Good Health Report* 28, no. 5 (February 1992): 4-5.

RESOURCES

ORGANIZATIONS

National Headache Foundation. 5252 Western Avenue, Chicago, IL 60625.

PAMPHLETS

National Headache Foundation:

The Headache Handbook. 1990.

National Institute of Neurological and Communicative Disorders and Stroke:

Headache: Hope Through Research. NIH Pub. No. 84-158. 1984. 36 pp.

BOOKS

Falleta, Betty Ann. *Headaches*. Springhouse, PA: Springhouse Corporation, 1986.

Rapaport, Alan, and Fred Sheftell. *Headache Relief*. New York: Simon and Schuster, 1990.

Solomon, Seymour, and Steven Fraccaro. *The Headache Book*. Fairfield, OH: Consumer Reports Books, 1991. 208 pp.

RELATED ARTICLES

Diamond, Seymour. "Management of Headaches: Focus on New Strategies." *Postgraduate Medicine* 87, no. 4 (March 1990): 189–192, 195.

Drexler, Ellen D. "Severe Headaches: When to Worry, What to Do." *Postgraduate Medicine* 87, no. 4 (March 1990): 164–180.

Foster, R. Daniel. "Head Bangers." *Men's Health* 6 (February 1991): 24.

"Preventing Migraines." *Prevention* 42 (August 1990): 14–15.

HEALTH INSURANCE

(*See also:* HEALTH MAINTENANCE ORGANIZATIONS [HMOs]; MEDICARE)

OVERVIEW

There are three basic kinds of health-insurance coverage:

- **Major-medical policies.**

These are the most comprehensive, covering both hospital stays and physicians' services in and out of the hospital.

- **Hospital-surgical policies.**

These cover hospital services and surgical procedures only.

- **Hospital-indemnity and dread-disease policies.**

These policies are vastly inferior to the other two types and offer very limited benefits.

Major medical policies typically pay for most hospital services, including room and board; operating and recovery rooms; nursing care; and treatment in intensive-care units, emergency rooms, and outpatient facilities. They also pick up the tab for lab tests, X-rays, anesthesia, medical supplies, ambulance services, and physicians' office visits. Most pay for prescription drugs and cover confinements in skilled-nursing facilities, if necessary, following a hospital stay.

Some policies, however, don't pay for assistant surgeons or for stand-by surgeons. Others won't cover emergency treatment unless the policyholder is admitted directly to the hospital. (That's to discourage the use of emergency rooms for routine treatment.) Still others limit the number of times they'll pay for doctors' visits in the hospital. Even a comprehensive policy may pay for only one visit each day.

Hospital-surgical policies cover hospital room and board, often for a specified number of days; treatment in intensive-care and outpatient facilities; medical supplies; surgeon's fees; diagnostic tests relating to an operation; some radiation and chemotherapy; and sometimes second opinions. But they cover almost no expenses incurred outside a hospital. They won't pay for a doctor's office visit to check on a persistent cough, or to have your child's cast removed, or for any medical condition that does not require hospitalization. Most don't cover prescription drugs that you may need outside a hospital.

Generally, both major-medical and hospital-surgical policies pay for 30 days of inpatient treatment for mental illness and substance abuse. Some major-medical policies cover outpatient treatment as well. If they do, insurers limit the number of visits per year or even the dollar amount of their payments. . . .

The worst buys in health insurance are hospital-indemnity policies and dread-disease policies. Hospital-indemnity policies pay a fixed amount each day you're in the hospital. Dread-disease policies pay benefits only if you contract cancer or some other specified illness.

Such policies are a profitable staple for many well-known insurance companies and for the American Association of Retired Persons (AARP). They're sold to unsophisticated buyers through enticing but sometimes misleading advertising.

"Cash benefits of $2250 a month, $525 a week, $75 a day . . . You cannot be turned down . . . No salesman will call . . ." reads a flyer for a hospital-indemnity policy from Physician's Mutual. "Use these cash benefits any way you choose . . . Get extra benefits when you may need them the most," promises an ad for a policy sold by the AARP.

The deal is simple and understandable. You get a fixed dollar amount for each day you spend in the hospital.

No complicated deductibles or coinsurance. Trouble is, the fixed benefit is skimpy to start with and grows less valuable with each passing year. . . .

Dread-disease policies offer similarly inadequate benefits. We measured two cancer policies against a $19,774 claim for colon-cancer surgery and follow-up chemotherapy that we also used to rate the policies in out survey. A policy from American Family Life, a large seller of this type of insurance, would pay a maximum of $4100; a policy from American Fidelity Assurance would cover as much as $6210—but only if the policyholder had purchased some optional coverage. (These policies may also pay an additional benefit based on the number of months you own the policy before you contract cancer.)

Companies also sell riders to cover such dread diseases as smallpox, polio, rabies, diphtheria, and typhoid fever. We don't know why anyone would buy them, since these diseases are now extremely rare.

SOURCE:
"The Crisis in Health Insurance." *Consumer Reports* (August 1990): 538, 539.

LEAVING A GROUP PLAN (COBRA)

If you leave a job, you may have two options for continuing your health insurance short of shopping for an individual policy on your own. Depending on the size of the firm you worked for and on your state's insurance regulations, you may be able to continue your group coverage for a short time as provided under the Consolidated Omnibus Budget Reconciliation Act of 1985 (COBRA). Or you may be able to obtain an individual policy through a process known as conversion. Both options, though, will usually cost a lot more than you would spend for group coverage.

Because it is less expensive and generally offers better coverage than a conversion policy, your first line of defense should be COBRA.

If you worked for a business with 20 or more employees, COBRA entitles you and your dependents to continued coverage for at least 18 months under your former employer's plan. If you are disabled and eligible for Social Security disability benefits when your employment ends, you can obtain an additional 11 months of coverage, for a total of 29 months.

If you are insured through your spouse's plan at work and your spouse dies, you become divorced or separated, or your spouse becomes eligible for Medicare, COBRA provides for coverage of up to 36 months.

COBRA requires that you pay 102 percent of your group insurance premium. If your employer has been paying a portion, you will have to assume that cost in addition to what you were already paying, plus an extra 2 percent for administrative costs. Disabled people who take COBRA coverage must pay as much as 150 percent of the premium for the extra 11 months.

You can lose coverage if you don't pay the premiums, if you become eligible for Medicare, if your employer discontinues health insurance for employees still working there, or if you join another plan.

However, if you join another plan and have an existing medical condition for which that plan imposes a waiting period, you can still keep your COBRA benefits until they would normally run out. By that time, your preexisting condition may be covered under the new plan. But you could be without coverage for that condition if your COBRA benefits stop before the waiting period on the new policy is over.

SOURCE:
"The Crisis in Health Insurance." *Consumer Reports* (August 1990): 545.

RIGHT TO APPEAL A REJECTED CLAIM

When an insurance company refuses to pay for a medical expense or denies part of a claim you believe should be paid in full, one expert offers this advice: "The insurance company owes the claim unless it can affirmatively demonstrate why it should not be paid."

That is the word from Earl Pomeroy, the Insurance Commissioner of North Dakota, who is also president of the National Association of Insurance Commissioners. He adds, "Millions of dollars are recovered for consumers every year."

Insurers are not always wrong, of course, and if a claim has been rejected the first thing to do is make certain you or your doctor or dentist filled out the required form correctly. Another bit of advice is to have copies of documents at hand that prove your case.

Here, in summary, are the basic steps to take when you believe an insurance company has erred:

- Appeal to a high official at the insurance company and, if you can, include additional documentation for your claim.
- If that is unsuccessful, write to your state insurance commissioner, enclosing copies of all correspondence between you and the insurer.
- If the response is still not satisfactory, decide whether the amount you feel you are owed is worth suing.

Why are most insurance claims turned down, fully or partly? These are among the reasons given most frequently by insurers:

- The medical service or treatment is not covered by the contract.
- The charge is incurred before the effective date of coverage.
- The doctor's fee is considered to be in excess of the usual, prevailing and customary fees in the area.
- The doctor entered the wrong code number for the procedure on the insurance form.

"You should become more aware of what is and what is not compensable under the plan by reading the booklet," said Gary Cain, vice president of the Principal Financial Group, a major insurer based in Des Moines. "When there is a question in your mind whether a service is covered, ask the company in advance."

Denials or partial denials of medical insurance claims are made on an explanation of benefits form, on which the company explains its decision. The Employment Retirement Income Security Act says this E.O.B. form must specifically state that consumers have the right of appeal within 60 days of receiving the notice.

That means you should initiate any appeal in writing as soon as you receive an unsatisfactory explanation form. Some consumer advocates believe that a letter to the president of the insuring company is the best approach, even though it may be bucked down to a lower level for response. The letter should summarize the elements of the dispute and contain the insured's and the patient's names, the policy number and the claim number.

Any additional documents—copies, not originals—that might have a bearing on the case should be included, too. Sometimes simply resubmitting the information will result in a claims payment.

"If they see that you are serious and have the facts, good records increase your chance of settlement significantly," said J. Robert Hunter, president of the National Insurance Consumer Organization, a nonprofit public-interest group.

If you decide to take the next step, writing to your state insurance department, you should know that every state has such a department and that it has a consumer-complaint section to intercede on your behalf. And while an insurance department cannot order an insurance company to pay a claim, it at least has the leverage to make sure that requests for information or further explanations are reviewed and answered promptly. . . .

If all else fails, you have the option of bringing legal action against the insurer. Depending on the amount in question, you can go to small claims court on your own or consult a lawyer about a full-scale suit for larger amounts.

SOURCE:

Sloane, Leonard. "Coping with Medical Insurance Claims: When You Feel a Payment Was Unfairly Rejected, Don't Be Afraid to Go the Top." *The New York Times* (October 13, 1990): 16.

UNIVERSAL HEALTH INSURANCE

America's health care economy is a paradox of excess and deprivation. We spend more than 11 percent of the gross national product on health care, yet roughly 35 million Americans have no financial protection from medical expenses. To an increasing degree, the present financing system is inflationary, unfair, and wasteful. In its place we need a strategy that addresses the whole system, offers financial protection from health care expenses to all, and promotes the development of economical financing and delivery arrangements. Such a strategy must be designed to be broadly acceptable in our society.

To remedy the deprivation, we propose that everyone not covered by Medicare, Medicaid, or some other public program be enabled to buy affordable coverage, either through their employers or through a "public sponsor." To attack the excess, we propose a strategy of managed competition in which collective agents, called sponsors, such as the Health Care Financing Administration and large employers, contract with competing health plans and manage a process of informed cost-conscious consumer choice that rewards providers who deliver high-quality care economically.

SOURCE:

Enthoven, Alain, and Richard Kronick. "A Consumer Choice Health Plan for the 1990s: Universal Health Insurance in a System Designed to Promote Quality and Economy. First of Two Parts." *The New England Journal of Medicine* 320, no. 1 (January 5, 1989): 29.

RESOURCES

ORGANIZATIONS

Health Insurance Association of America. Public Relations Division, 1025 Connecticut Avenue NW, Suite 1200, Washington, DC 20036.

Health Insurance Institute. 110 William Street, New York, NY 10038.

National Insurance Consumer Organization. 344 Commerce Street, Alexandria, VA 22314.

BOOK

Berman, Henry, and Louisa Rose. *Choosing the Right Health Care Plan*. Fairfield, OH: Consumer Reports Books, 1990. 272 pp.

RELATED ARTICLES

Carpenter, E. Karen. "What to Do When They Won't Pay." *American Health* (October 1990): 66–68.

Fox, Harriette B., and Paul W. Newacheck. "Private Health Insurance of Chronically Ill Children." *Pediatrics* 85, no. 1 (January 1990): 50–57.

Johnson, Kirk. "Winning the Health Insurance Hustle." *East West* (April 1990): 64–67, 92–94.

HEALTH MAINTENANCE ORGANIZATIONS (HMOs)

(*See also:* HEALTH INSURANCE; MEDICARE)

OVERVIEW

An HMO is a closed system of care operating in a defined geographic area. All services are paid for in advance usually by a stated fixed monthly fee which has nothing to do with how many times you or your family use the HMO services during the month. Many HMOs will also require payment of a small office visit fee, usually $10 at the most. Once you join that system, you can't leave it without incurring additional expense during the period of your membership—normally one year. That is, if you seek medical care "outside" the HMO system, you must pay for it yourself.

The HMO system also restricts your freedom to choose whichever hospital or clinic you might want to use. Certain facilities which render care at lower costs than others in the area become part of the HMO network, and you must use these even if they are inconveniently located.

Also, since most HMOs have limited service areas, if you should leave one locale and move to another, your HMO membership will not go with you. Nor are you likely to have coverage when you travel. A few HMOs have entered into cooperative network arrangements to alleviate this problem but the network may not cover the entire nation, and may not be available for emergencies that occur when you travel. Insurance (indemnity) plans on the other hand are generally portable and can be used nationwide, and in some cases worldwide.

When you and your family initially enroll in an HMO, you will be asked to select a "primary care" physician. That physician will provide all of your medical care and will also act as a "gatekeeper" in directing further treatments, use of specialists, selection of drugs and the like.

It's important that you understand that the primary care physician has full control over your treatment, the tests that are ordered and all procedures that are performed. If you are dissatisfied with your primary care physician, most HMOs will allow you to choose another one with little or no hassle, but there is no guarantee that will happen. Remember, HMOs may operate in a number of different ways, be sure you understand those differences before you choose any particular one.

When you are offered an HMO or any other health option by your employer, you are committed to that choice for one year. If, after the year, you decide to opt for a non-HMO plan, you can. That choice is again good for a year and you can change back to the HMO for the following year. If you join an HMO during an "open enrollment" period, you and all members of your family must be admitted to the HMO unless you or a family member have certain pre-existing medical conditions. Depending on the HMO, open enrollment periods last a few weeks or a month at most.

Normally, you won't find any fancy offices and a lot of hand holding by the physicians at an HMO. The goal of the HMO is to deliver health care to its patients in as efficient and cost-effective way as possible.

SOURCE:

American Council on Science and Health. *HMOs: Are They Right for You?* 1991. pp. 2–4.

MAJOR TYPES OF HMOs

There are two main types of HMOs:

- Group or staff HMOs have their own doctors in health-care centers, which also often have laboratories, X-ray departments, pharmacies, and even opticians on the premises. Group or staff HMOs offer the convenience of one-stop medical care. If you join, however, you may have to exchange your present doctor for one who works only for the HMO. Kaiser is the country's largest group HMO, but there are scores of others.

- IPAs (Individual Practice Associations) or network HMOs contract with individual doctors or small groups of doctors. These physicians see patients in their private offices for an agreed-upon fee paid by the IPA. Doctors often have contracts with several different IPAs or network HMOs. One advantage to this arrangement is that you may be able to keep the same physician who has been helping you manage your diabetes. United HealthCare is one of the largest IPAs.

To complicate matters further, the lines between the two are blurring. Staff HMOs are starting networks, IPAs are starting networks, and IPAs are starting small staff centers. While both IPAs and HMOs are trying new approaches, they share some common restrictions. In general, both group/staff HMOs and IPA/network HMOs usually require that patients use their contracted doctors, hospitals, and pharmacies in return for low and predictable out-of-pocket costs.

A third type of prepaid health plan is the PPO (Preferred Provider Organizations, sometimes called Preferred Provider Arrangements). These function much like traditional fee-for-service insurance plans. If you opt for a PPO, you can see almost any licensed doctor. However, if you use the PPO's "preferred providers"—contracted doctors, hospitals, pharmacies—you receive significant financial gains. For example, a preferred provider may have only a $100 deductible, or perhaps no deductible at all, while a nonpreferred provider may have a $500 deductible.

SOURCE:
Zuvekas, Ann. "HMOs: Are They Good for Your Health?" *Diabetes Forecast 42* (November 1989): 42-43. Reproduced with permission from *Diabetes Forecast,* November 1989. Copyright 1989 by American Diabetes Association, Inc.

FACTORS IN CHOOSING AN HMO

SERVICES AND COSTS

HMOs generally provide broad medical care at little or no cost beyond the monthly premium. PPO coverage is almost as comprehensive and, though you pay for each service, fees are cheaper than the usual rate, assuming you stick to the list of preferred doctors and facilities; since you'll sometimes stray from that list, you should analyze non-preferred services and costs just as you would for a traditional plan. Be aware of any plan's exclusions and restrictions. Some PPOs won't pay for expensive, cutting edge tests—certain allergy assays, for example, and chorionic villus sampling, a new procedure to check on the health of a developing fetus.

Generally HMOs stress preventive medicine, offering treatment and training in such areas as nutrition, back pain, quitting smoking, and drug abuse. Choose a plan with special programs that you'd most likely use.

ARE THE DOCTORS QUALIFIED?

When you choose a particular HMO or PPO, you automatically limit your choice of physicians, so make sure they're a capable bunch. Ask what percentage of the doctors are board certified, a credential that requires a certain level of training and practice for a given specialty. Nationally, 66 percent of practicing physicians are board certified. Try to find a plan with 75 percent or more. The same percentage of doctors ought to be graduates of U.S. or Canadian medical schools. The member services department of most HMOs and PPOs should be able to furnish at least one of these ratings.

HOW DO YOU CHOOSE YOUR DOCTOR?

Most plans let you select your primary physician, a crucial choice with HMOs because this is the doctor who decides whether you can see a specialist, whether you need to enter the hospital, whether a second opinion you're seeking will be paid for by the plan. Make sure the HMO or PPO you're considering can give you a list of doctors, describing education, experience, and other biographical details. HMOs should also allow you to switch primary doctors if you're unhappy with your first choice. At some, you can change only at designated times, which can make for a miserable year.

GETTING TO THE OBSTETRICIAN/ GYNECOLOGIST

If you cannot see an obstetrician/gynecologist at your HMO without first seeing a primary physician, find an obstetrician/gynecologist who will also serve as your primary doctor—or find another HMO.

CAN YOU GET TO ALL THE SPECIALISTS YOU NEED?

Check that a plan has a sizeable number of board-certified specialists in areas that concern you. Under a PPO plan, if you're forced to go to outside specialists you'll have to pay more. For HMOs, if you think you'll need a specialty that their staff doesn't cover, make sure before you join that they have a convenient arrangement with an outside person and that it won't cost extra. It may not be easy, but try to find out how plans compensate their doctors. At HMOs some primary physicians lose income when they send patients to specialists and hospitals, not an ideal system from the patient's viewpoint.

HOW ACCESSIBLE AND CONVENIENT IS IT?

You should not have to travel more than 20 to 25 minutes to get to a clinic or a doctor's office. For checkups and other routine matters, it should never take more than a month to get an appointment and you shouldn't have to wait in the office beyond a half hour, at least not more than once or twice a year. For an urgent but not life-threatening problem, you should be able to get an appointment in 24 hours. Current members and receptionists are the best sources to ask about schedules and waiting times.

HOW DO THEY HANDLE EMERGENCIES?

The managed plans insist that you use their doctors and facilities whenever possible. Get them to explain how they would treat a late-night attack of food poisoning or a weekend sports injury. They should have a network of doctors and hospitals on standby, none of which is more than 20 minutes away. There should be a 24-hour hot line that can answer questions and arrange for help quickly; a tape machine is not enough. If possible, your primary physician should be reachable by beeper.

SOURCE:

Cohen, Paul. "Health Plan Roulette: Would You Rather Choose Your Own Doctor or Pay Less and Skip the Paperwork?" *In Health* 4 (July/August 1990): 82.

HMOs—AND MEDICARE

Many older Americans don't realize that they can pay for most of the services of an HMO through Medicare. Presently, Medicare has contracts with about 200 HMOs throughout the nation, that is, approximately 40% of all HMOs.

If you are an HMO member at the time you become eligible for Medicare, the HMO may offer you a Medicare "wrap-around" which will provide you with all the services covered under both Part A and Part B of Medicare. It is a kind of Medicare supplement and it would be offered by those HMOs that are not already under contract with Medicare.

According to the American Association of Retired Persons, which has studied this issue extensively, Medicare recipients have absolutely nothing to lose by either enrolling in or retaining membership in an HMO. If you are entitled to a benefit under Medicare, you will get it through the HMO. To take full advantage of your Medicare benefits, most of your health care will have to be provided through the HMO.

You must, however, meet certain eligibility requirements before you can join an HMO that contracts with Medicare.

As a Medicare beneficiary:

- You must participate in both Parts A and B of Medicare.
- At the time of your enrollment in the HMO, you do not have end-stage renal (kidney) disease. If, however, you should develop end-stage renal disease while a member of the HMO, the HMO cannot, under the present rules and regulations, ask you to leave.
- You have not elected hospice care through Medicare prior to your enrollment in the HMO.
- You must, of course, live within the geographic confines of the particular HMO's service area.
- Finally, to join the HMO, it must be currently accepting new members.

Eligibility requirements for "wrap-around" packages are determined by the state in which the HMO is doing business. Many states require that you first become an HMO member before you become a Medicare beneficiary.

SOURCE:

American Council on Science and Health. *HMOs: Are They Right for You?* 1991. pp. 15–16.

RESOURCES

ORGANIZATION

Health Care Financing Administration. 200 Independence Ave SW, Washington, DC 20201.

BOOK

Bloom, Jill. *HMOs: What They Are, How They Work, and Which One Is Best for You.* Tucson, AZ: The Body Press, 1987. 277 pp.

RELATED ARTICLES

Asnes, Marion. "Compromising Physicians? As HMOs Try to Solve Their Financial Crisis, Doctors May Be Cutting Corners on Your Medical Care." *Health* (January 1991): 58–63.

Cahn, Victor. "Making Your Health Care Plan Work for You." *Health Letter* (January 1990): 4–6.

Newcomer, Robert, Charlene Harrington, and Alan Friedlob. "Awareness and Enrollment in the Social/HMO." *The Gerontologist* 30 (February 1990): 86–93.

HEARING LOSS

OVERVIEW

The American Speech and Hearing Association estimates that three out of 100 school-age children, and 30 out of 100 persons 65 or older, are affected by hearing loss. More than 2.1 million cases of hearing impairment are reported in the US annually.

Although hearing impairment is one of the most prevalent disabilities, many persons who are affected do not fully understand the problem and often are unwilling to seek treatment. Those who have adjusted to a gradual loss of hearing through the years often do not realize that the sounds reaching them are greatly diminished. They have almost forgotten the sound of ocean waves, the chirping of birds, a loved one's whisper. Any suggestion that use of a hearing aid might be indicated is denied, and medical advice is strenuously avoided.

Since hearing impairment is an invisible condition, many people try to "pass" without it being detected, preferring lost sound to the perceived stigma of using a hearing aid. Despite wishful thinking, a hearing loss can never be successfully concealed. In the attempt, the significant benefits available through medical and scientific technology are missed, friendships may be severed, and the person may gradually retreat to a life of isolation.

There are three basic types of hearing impairments. With a conductive loss, sound waves are blocked as they travel through the auditory canal or middle ear and cannot reach the inner ear. Sounds seem muffled and an earache may be present. Children are often affected. Common causes of a conductive loss include wax blocking the ear canal, infection, or a punctured eardrum. Many conductive hearing problems can be treated successfully.

Another cause of conductive-type loss is otosclerosis. In this disorder, the bones of the middle ear soften, do not vibrate well, and then calcify. This problem can be corrected surgically.

A sensorineural hearing loss, commonly termed "nerve deafness," involves the inner ear and is the result of damage to the hair cells, nerve fibers, or both. Sounds are distorted, high tones are usually inaudible, and ringing or buzzing sounds (tinnitus) may be present. Speech can be heard, but is not easily understood. This type of loss is permanent and irreversible. Causes include high fevers, excess noise, heredity, adverse reaction to drugs, diseases such as meningitis, head injuries, and the aging process.

The third major type of hearing problem is the mixed loss. In this instance a person has both conductive and sensorineural losses.

As with any medical condition, early intervention is critical. When the telltale signs of hearing loss are noted—ringing in the ears, the need to have spoken material repeated frequently, high volume on TV or radio, or inattentiveness—an ear specialist (otologist) should be consulted. The problem may be a simple wax buildup, which can be remedied with one office visit. If the impairment cannot be treated medically, referral to an audiologist is in order.

SOURCE:

Kasper, Rosemarie. "Hearing Loss and You: Hearing Impairment Is One of the Most Prevalant Disabilities in the Country." *Independent Living* 5 (August-September 1990): 59–60.

HEARING AIDS

Federal regulation prohibits any hearing aid sale unless the buyer has first received a medical evaluation from a licensed physician. However, if you are at least 18 years old, you can sign a form that says you are fully aware of your rights but choose not to have the medical evaluation. Then, you can buy the hearing aid without seeing a physician. For people under 18 years of age, waiver of the medical evaluation is not permitted.

All hearing aids will make speech over the telephone louder. Many hearing aids will also have special "T" (telecoil) switches that are specifically designed for use with the telephone. Telephone sounds are amplified more efficiently and background noises are better eliminated with this switch than without it.

People with hearing impairment may also need a telecoil to use some of the special sound systems that are now available in many auditoriums, theaters, and other public places. Discuss your need for "T" switch with your audiologist.

With a hearing aid, you will hear some sounds you have never heard before, or at least haven't heard in a long time. Your own voice will sound louder. You will need to learn how to "tune out" background noises. Sometimes speech sounds will sound different than the way you think they should. It may take you several weeks to become adjusted to your hearing aid.

A hearing aid should help you hear, but not necessarily in all situations. Despite technological advances and good follow-up care, hearing when background noise is loud may still be difficult. . . .

All hearing aids work similarly and have similar parts. These include:

- a microphone to pick up sound
- an amplifier to make the sound louder
- a miniature loudspeaker (receiver) to deliver the louder sound into the ear
- batteries to power the electronic parts.

Some hearing aids also have earmolds (earpieces) to control the flow of sound into the ear, enhance sound quality, and help hold the hearing aid in place. . . .

The basic styles of hearing aids [are:]

Canal aids—these aids are contained in a tiny case that fits into the ear canal. They are the smallest aids available.

All-in-the-ear aids—all parts of the aid are contained in the outer part of the ear. These aids are larger than canal aids.

Behind-the-ear aids—all parts are contained in a small plastic case that sits behind the ear; the case is connected to an earmold by a piece of clear tubing.

Eyeglass aids—these aids are a different kind of behind-the-ear aid with the parts contained in side the frames of the glasses; again, clear plastic tubing connects the hearing aid to the earmold.

Body aids—the microphone, amplifier, and batteries are combined into a rectangular case that can fit into a shirt pocket; a cord connecting the case to the receiver runs along the neck; the receiver then snaps into an earmold.

Today more than three-quarters of hearing aids sold are canal or all-in-the-ear models. Only a very small percentage of eyeglass and body aids are dispensed.

SOURCE:

American Speech Language Hearing Association. *How to Buy a Hearing Aid.* July 1, 1991. pp. 3-6.

CHOOSING A HEARING HEALTH CARE SPECIALIST

There are three kinds of hearing specialists: otolaryngologists/otologists, audiologists, and hearing aid dealers (also called hearing instrument specialists). While not every otolaryngologist and audiologist tests and sells hearing aids, many do.

An otolaryngologist (ear, nose and throat specialist) is a physician who provides medical/surgical treatment for hearing disorders. These physicians don't normally dispense hearing aids, but about 70 percent of them have audiologists on staff to test hearing and dispense hearing aids.

More commonly, audiologists and hearing aid dealers evaluate hearing and dispense hearing aids. Audiologists have a graduate degree in the measurement and treatment of hearing impairment. They are licensed in 38 states and many are certified by the American Speech-Language-Hearing Association (certified audiologists are designated by the letters CCC-A).

Hearing instrument specialists are licensed in 46 states and the District of Columbia (Colorado, Massachusetts, Minnesota and New York do not currently license dealers) to test hearing and sell hearing aids, accessories, and batteries. While these specialists have less formal education, many have considerable experience. Dealers probably test and fit over half of all hearing aids sold nationwide. In many areas, dealers are the only hearing specialists available.

In most states, there are no formal educational requirements, but all states licensing dealers require that applicants pass an exam (with the exception of Alaska). Some dealers are certified by the National Board for Certification of Hearing Instrument Sciences (certified dealers are designated by the letters BC-HIS). Also be aware that some dealers have inaccurately called themselves "certified hearing aid audiologists."

SOURCE:

American Association of Retired Persons. *Product Report: Hearing Aids* 1, no. 4 (December 1989): 3–4.

COCHLEAR IMPLANTS

Some children who've been deaf from birth may now learn to hear words—and speak them—for the first time, thanks to a tiny device implanted in their ears. It's called a 22-channel cochlear implant, and the FDA has now approved its use in children two years of age and older.

Doctors began using implants in adults in 1984. Since then, half the adults who have received an implant after losing their hearing late in life can now comprehend speech.

Results promise to be even more dramatic for very young children. The implants will actually allow them to speak, an ability that depends on hearing spoken language during childhood, preferably before age seven.

The implant works this way: Sounds picked up by a tiny microphone behind the ear are sent to a speech processor about the size of a deck of playing cards and usually worn in a pocket. The processor's 22 channels select the sounds most useful for understanding speech and convert them to electronic signals. These signals are then sent back along wires to the implant, which is placed in the cochlea, a part of the inner ear. The implant's 22 electrodes transmit the signals as electric currents through nerve cells and on to the brain.

After the cochlear implant is in place, the child undergoes extensive training, learning to translate sounds into words—and ultimately learning how to speak those words intelligibly.

The implant does not restore normal hearing: It picks up a much narrower range of frequencies than is available to people with normal hearing. And what the child hears sounds a lot like Donald Duck talking. But with training, the cochlear implant can enable a deaf child to communicate with the world.

SOURCE:

Weiss, Gillian. "New Hope for Deaf Children: Implant Gives Them Hearing and Speech." *American Health* 9 (November 1990): 17.

RESOURCES

ORGANIZATIONS

American Association of Retired Persons (AARP). 1909 K St. NW, Washington, DC 20049.

American Speech-Language-Hearing Association. 10801 Rockville Pike, Rockville, MD 20852.

National Association for Hearing and Speech Action. 10801 Rockville Pike, Rockville, MD 20852.

National Hearing Aid Society. 20361 Middlebelt, Livonia, MI 48152.

National Information Center on Deafness. Gallaudet University, 800 Florida Ave. NE, Washington, DC 20002.

Self-Help for Hard of Hearing People. 7800 Wisconsin Ave., Bethesda, MD 20814.

PAMPHLETS

American Association of Retired Persons (AARP):

Have You Heard? Hearing Loss and Aging. D12219.

American Speech-Language-Hearing Association:

Answers Questions about Noise and Hearing Loss. January 1991. 3 pp.

BOOK

Combs, Alec. *Hearing Loss Help.* Santa Maria, CA: Alpenglow Press, 1986. 176 pp.

RELATED ARTICLES

"Am I a Candidate for a Cochlear Implant?" *Patient Care* 23 (April 30, 1989): 114.

"Cochlear Implants." *National Institutes of Health Consensus Development Statement* 7, no. 2 (May 4, 1988): 1–9.

"Finding the Right Hearing Aid." *Modern Maturity* 33 (June/July 1990): 85.

Furncamp, C. T. "Conductive Hearing Loss and Speech Development." *Journal of Allergy and Clinical Immunology* 81, no. 5, pt. 2 (May 1988): 1015–1020.

"Hearing Loss: Boom and Doom." *Harvard Health Letter* 16, no. 2 (December 1990): 1–4.

Weinstein, Barbara E. "Geriatric Hearing Loss: Myths, Realities, Resources for Physicians." *Geriatrics* 44, no. 4 (April 1989): 42–48, 58, 60.

HEART ATTACK

(*See also:* ANGIOPLASTY; HEART BYPASS SURGERY)

OVERVIEW

What Is a Heart Attack?

The human heart basically is a muscle that pumps blood. It has its own blood vessels, the coronary arteries, that nourish it and keep it alive. In most cases when a heart attack occurs, fatty deposits (composed mostly of cholesterol) have lined the coronary arteries. As these deposits build up, they progressively narrow the arteries and decrease or stop the flow of blood to the heart. When there's a decreased flow of blood to the heart, the heart muscle may be damaged, but when there's a complete blockage of the flow of blood so that the heart can't get the oxygen and food it needs, a part of the heart may actually die. This is a heart attack.

A heart attack most often results when a blood clot forms in a narrowed artery and blocks the flow of blood to the part of the heart muscle supplied by that artery. Doctors call this form of heart attack a coronary thrombosis, coronary occlusion or myocardial infarction. When a heart attack occurs, the dying part of the heart may trigger electrical activity that causes ventricular fibrillation. Ventricular fibrillation is an uncoordinated twitching that replaces the smooth, measured contractions that cause blood to be pumped to the organs of the body. In many cases, if trained medical professionals are immediately available, they can get the heart beating again by using electrical shock and/or drugs.

If the heart can be kept beating, and not too much heart muscle is damaged, small blood vessels may gradually reroute blood around the blocked arteries. This is the heart's own way of compensating for the clogged artery, and it's called collateral circulation.

The key to surviving a heart attack is promptly recognizing the warning signals and getting immediate medical attention.

How to Recognize a Heart Attack

If you feel an uncomfortable pressure, fullness, squeezing or pain in the center of your chest (that may spread to your shoulders, neck or arms) and your discomfort lasts for two minutes or longer, you could be having a heart attack. Sweating, dizziness, fainting, nausea, a feeling of severe indigestion, or shortness of breath also may occur, although not all symptoms necessarily occur. Sharp, stabbing twinges, on the other hand, usually aren't signals of a heart attack.

When a person has these symptoms, it's natural for him or her to deny what's happening. No one wants to think that he might be having a heart attack. But before you shrug off the symptoms, it's important to know that more 300,000 heart attack victims died before reaching the hospital last year, many of them because they refused to take their symptoms seriously.

What should you do if you think you might be having a heart attack? If you're uncomfortable for two minutes or more, call your local emergency medical service (EMS) immediately. If the EMS isn't available, get to a hospital offering emergency cardiac care as soon as possible.

Know in advance which route from home or work will take you to the hospital the quickest. You might even discuss your possible choices with your doctor. Another option is to call your local American Heart Association and ask which recognized emergency medical service and hospitals cover your area. Keep emergency information where you can find it easily and develop a "buddy system" with someone you know.

SOURCE:

American Heart Association. *Fact Sheet on Heart Attack, Stroke and Risk Factors.* 1987. pp. 1–2.

THROMBOLYTIC THERAPY

Each year, approximately 1.5 million Americans suffer acute myocardial infarctions (heart attacks). While coronary care units, the development of improved therapy for life-threatening arrhythmias and greater attention to coronary risk factors have led to a reduction in the mortality rate, myocardial infarction remains a major cause of morbidity and mortality in the United States. Although the number of deaths from coronary disease declined by about 27 percent between 1968 and 1979, more than 500,000 people still die each year of myocardial infarctions. . . .

The objective of thrombolytic therapy in acute myocardial infarction is to lyse [dissolve] the occluding coronary thrombus and reperfuse oxygenated blood to the myocardium before transmural infarction is completed. It is hoped that such intervention early in the course of infarction will limit infarct size, preserve left ventricular function, prevent pump failure and decrease morbidity and mortality. Lysis of the clot is accomplished by the administration of a thrombolytic agent, which activates the patient's fibrinolytic system.

The three thrombolytic agents approved for clinical use are streptokinase (Kabikinase, Streptase), urokinase (Abbokinase) and alteplase (Activase), a tissue-type plasminogen activator. Each agent initiates thrombolysis by converting plasminogen to plasmin. Plasmin is a nonspecific proteolytic enzyme that degrades various proteins in the circulation as well as in thrombi.

SOURCE:
Smucker, D. R., M. W. Burket. "Thrombolytic Therapy in Acute Myocardial Infarction." *American Family Physician* 37, no. 5 (May 1988): 265–266.

THROMBOLYTIC THERAPY—T.P.A. OR STREPTOKINASE?

Two drugs for treating people with heart attacks are equally effective in saving lives, according to two important studies. One drug costs $2,200 a dose, and the other $76 to $300. Which should be used?

In most countries, doctors usually choose the less expensive drug, known as streptokinase. But American doctors mostly prefer the more expensive one, known as T.P.A. Although some doctors have switched to streptokinase in recent months, many say there are theoretical reasons to believe that T.P.A. is better despite the recent studies.

The battle of the two heart drugs, both of which dissolve deadly blood clots, is polarizing the American medical community. The contest vividly portrays the important role that marketing plays in determining which therapies doctors will use. . . .

In 1990, about two-thirds of the roughly 150,000 American patients who received clot-dissolving therapy after a heart attack received T.P.A., resulting in sales of $210 million for its manufacturer, Genentech Inc., a biotechnology company in South San Francisco, Calif. Most of the rest received streptokinase at a cost of about $5 million. Had all the patients been given streptokinase, about $200 million would have been saved.

T.P.A., approved for sale in 1987, received a huge amount of publicity as one of the first wonder drugs created by biotechnology. It was promoted in an aggressive, some say unsavory, manner by Genentech, now majority-owned by the Swiss drug company Hoffman-La Roche. . . .

Keeping cardiologists in the T.P.A. camp is the job of Genentech's 278 sales people, who form one of the five largest sales forces that call only on hospitals. Intensifying their impact, Genentech sales people, unlike those from larger companies that have dozens of products, have only two major drugs to promote: T.P.A. and human growth hormone, another costly, controversial drug. . . .

As the marketing battle rages, many doctors and hospitals are switching from T.P.A.

"There's been a clearcut move away from the expensive therapy," said James Wilentz, a cardiologist at Lenox Hill Hospital in New York. He said 80 to 85 percent of heart attack patients transferred to Lenox Hill from smaller hospitals were treated with T.P.A. Now the figure is 50 percent at most.

At St. Joseph Mercy Hospital in Ann Arbor, Mich., which had been one of the biggest T.P.A. users in its state, cardiologists recently voted to use streptokinase. Some small financially strapped hospitals in rural Alabama have jumped on the new data and "pretty much gone to streptokinase totally," said Ross Davis, director of critical care at East Alabama Medical Center in Opelika. . .

So far, doctors say, insurance companies have not begun to pressure hospitals to use streptokinase. As for Medicare, it pays a fixed amount for treatment of a heart attack, so it does not care which drug is used. The main pressure to use streptokinase is instead coming from hospital administrators and pharmacists. Since the Medicare reimbursement for a heart attack can be as low as $5000, a hospital is bound to lose money if it spends $2,200 before the patient even leaves the emergency room. But except in some institutions like health maintenance organizations, hospital administrators cannot usually force doctors to use a particular therapy.

SOURCE:
Pollack, Andrew. "Both Heart Drugs Are Effective; Doctors Prescribe the Costly One: Genentech Pushes Its Medicine with a Hard Sell." *The New York Times* 140, no. 48,647 (June 30, 1991): 1, 10.

RESOURCES

PAMPHLETS
American Heart Association:

Heart Attack. 1989. 9 pp.

National Institutes of Health:

Heart Attacks. 1986. 20 pp.

RELATED ARTICLES

Bates, E. R., and E. J. Topol. "Thrombolytic Therapy for Acute Myocardial Infarction." *Chest* 95, no. 5 (suppl.) (May 1989): 257S–264S.

Brody, Jane E. "Sedentary Living, Not Cholesterol, Is the Nation's Leading Culprit in Fatal Heart Attacks." *The New York Times* (October 11, 1990): B7.

Chesebro, J. H., and others. "New Approaches to Treatment of Myocardial Infarction." *The American Journal of Cardiology* 65, no. 6 (February 2, 1990): 12C–19C.

Grines, C. L., and A. N. DeMaria. "Optimal Utilization of Thrombolytic Therapy for Acute Myocardial Infarction: Concepts and Controversies." *Journal of the American College of Cardiology* 16, no. 1 (July 1990): 223–231.

Gunnar, R. M., and others. "Guidelines for the Early Management of Patients with Acute Myocardial Infarction: ACC/AHA Task Force Report." *Journal of the American College of Cardiology* 16, no. 2 (August 1990): 249–292.

Lavie, C. J., and B. J. Gersh. "Acute Myocardial Infarction: Initial Manifestations, Management, and Prognosis." *Mayo Clinic Proceedings* 65, no. 4 (April 1990): 531–548.

Naylor, C. David, and S. B. Jazlal. "Impact of Intravenous Thrombolysis on Short-Term Coronary Revascularization: A Meta-Analysis." *JAMA* 264 (August 8, 1990): 697–702.

Pitt, Bertrand. "Acute Myocardial Infarction: Treatment in the Coronary Care Unit." *Postgraduate Medicine* 85, no. 2 (February 1, 1989): 145–152, 154.

White, Harvey D. "Comparison of Tissue Plasminogen Activator and Streptokinase in the Management of Acute Myocardial Infarction." *Chest* 95, no. 5 (suppl.) (May 1989): 265S–269S.

HEART BYPASS SURGERY

(*See also:* ANGIOPLASTY; HEART ATTACK)

OVERVIEW

Over 200,000 coronary artery bypass operations are currently being performed in the United States each year. Coronary artery bypass surgery was first attempted in the late 1960s to relieve the symptoms caused by a blockage in a coronary blood vessel. When a blockage occurs, the flow of blood carrying oxygen and nutrients to heart muscles is limited, resulting in chest pain with exertion, that is, angina.

In a coronary artery bypass operation, a large vein, called the saphenous vein, is removed from the leg. Occasionally other large veins or arteries in the body, for instance, the internal mammary artery in the chest, are used. One end of the vein is then implanted in the aorta and the other connected to the coronary vessel beyond the place of obstruction. This then provides a "bypass" route around the area of narrowing, just as in road construction, where blood can flow and thereby supply the heart with enough blood to prevent chest pain with exertion or at rest.

During the surgery, the pumping action of the heart is stopped so that the surgeon can perform the delicate repair. A heart-lung machine takes over the function of oxygenating and pumping blood through the body. . . .

Although an extensive operation, technological improvements and medical experience have helped to make coronary bypass quite safe, with a mortality rate of about 1–3 percent. Around 1.7 million Americans have had coronary artery bypass operations. In fact, in the last few years surgeons have accepted older patients than once would have been though advisable. In the early 1970s, the average patient was about age 50 and today the average age is nearer 60. It should be remembered, however, that although overall patterns of mortality and benefit establish broad guidelines, the specific risks and benefits for each person must be considered individually.

SOURCE:

National Heart, Lung, and Blood Institute. *Facts About Coronary Artery Bypass Surgery*. NIH Publication No. 87-2891. 1987. p. 1.

GRAFTING PROCEDURE

The first heart bypass was performed in 1967. But the procedure has changed since then, says cardiologist Eugene Passamani, M.D., director of the division of heart and vascular diseases at the National Heart, Lung, and Blood Institute.

"Initially," says Passamani, "the surgeon removed the long vein running from the thigh to the ankle, cut it into pieces, and then fashioned grafts going from the aorta [the largest artery coming from the heart] to each of the three coronary arteries—sometimes including several lesser arteries. But by 10 years later, a third of the grafts had closed up again, probably due in part to the fact veins weren't designed to be arteries.

"More recently, the consensus is that if you use the internal mammary artery from inside the chest wall, the graft tends to stay open longer."

The bypass patient undergoes general anesthesia, hours on the operating table, support from a heart-lung machine, and, barring complications, 10 to 13 days' hospital recuperation and several months' recuperation at home.

Geoffrey Hartzler, M.D., consulting cardiologist at the Mid-American Heart Institute in Kansas City, Mo., says that "a patient's first bypass procedure is associated with the lowest risk." With repeated bypass surgery, he says, deaths and complications such as heart attack and stroke "increase by two- to three-fold."

SOURCE:
Farley, Dixie. "Balloons, Lasers and Scrapers: Help for Hearts and Blood Vessels." *FDA Consumer* (April 1991): 22.

RECOVERY

For people who have sedentary office jobs, four to six weeks is the average. People who must perform heavy work will have to wait longer. In some cases, a person may not be able to return to his or her former job. If that's your case, contact the State Vocational Rehabilitation Agency for information and help.

Patients should follow these guidelines:

1. Arise at a normal hour.

2. Bathe or shower if possible.

3. Always dress in street clothes and never stay in sleeping clothes during the day. (It's important for you to think of yourself as healthy and active, rather than sick.)

4. Take a mid-morning and mid-afternoon rest following periods of activity.

Rest periods are helpful following activity, so after taking a morning walk of a few blocks, come home and take a short nap. You'll be able to perform more activities as more time passes, so be patient. And walking is particularly good exercise and will speed your recovery.

Aside from walking, you should have no problem doing any of the following: helping with light work around the house; going to the theater, restaurant, store or church; visiting friends; going for a ride in the car; or climbing stairs. In some instances, your doctor may prescribe a more formal, graded activity schedule which is part of the physical rehabilitation process. By following such a program, you should be able to walk two or three miles a day a few weeks after your operation. Such distances usually require walking outside, but if it's either very hot or very cold, you might try walking in an enclosed shopping mall. Extremes of temperature force the body to work harder to perform the same activity. It's unwise to force yourself to walk long distances outdoors if it's very hot or cold.

You can resume having sexual relations when you feel like it. If you have questions, ask your doctor.

SOURCE:
American Heart Association. *Coronary Artery Bypass Graft Surgery*. pp. 24–26.

ANGIOPLASTY—THE BALLOON ALTERNATIVE

This year alone, more than 500,000 Americans will be given a new lease on life in the form of coronary artery bypass surgery or balloon angioplasty.

These two techniques are the primary medical weapons against coronary heart disease, an insidious process that chokes off the blood supply to the heart. Of course, the wisest approach is to prevent heart disease in the first place by following a low-fat diet, stopping smoking, controlling high blood pressure, losing weight if necessary and getting regular exercise.

But for hearts already damaged by inattention to these measures, bypass surgery and angioplasty can mean the difference between life and death. Bypass reroutes the blood past potentially deadly blockages, and angioplasty opens blocked arteries by stretching open obstructions in vessel walls. . . .

If a physician suspects heart disease, the patient usually undergoes an exercise test to evaluate heart activity and to see whether chest pain occurs. If the stress test indicates a potential problem, the patient will then undergo angiography, an x-ray procedure used to study blood vessels. In angiography, a small catheter is passed from an arm or leg to the heart. Dye is then injected into the arteries of the heart to detect the location and severity of any blockages.

If angiography reveals one or more severe blockages, the physician will recommend either bypass surgery, now an old standby in heart disease care, or the newer balloon angioplasty technique.

Beyond some general guidelines, the decision over which technique to use may be open to considerable discussion, says Richard Smalling, M.D., Ph.D., an associate professor of medicine at The University of Texas Medical School in Houston.

Use of angioplasty has grown by leaps and bounds since it was first performed in 1977. An estimated 200,000 heart patients will undergo the technique this year, in which small balloons are used to enlarge the opening in arterial plaque, the wax-like buildup that restricts blood flow to the heart.

Dr. Smalling describes the ideal angioplasty candidate as a patient with one obstruction in a vessel that doesn't have a lot of twists and turns. The ideal blockage, or lesion, doesn't occur near a significant branch of the artery, doesn't completely block the vessel and doesn't contain a lot of calcium.

When the disease affects more than one vessel, the balance tends to shift in favor of bypass surgery, says Dr. [Michael] Sweeney [associate professor of surgery at The University of Texas Medical School in Houston]. "One should not look at multiple-vessel angioplasty as one procedure," he says. "Each vessel represents a separate procedure with all the potential risks and benefits."

SOURCE:
"Mending Hearts: Bypass Surgery and Angioplasty Explained." *The University of Texas Lifetime Health Letter* 2, no. 5 (May 1990): 1.

* * *

If you need treatment for blocked coronary arteries and don't have the right information, you could end up in the middle of one of the biggest controversies today—whether to have bypass surgery, balloon angioplasty and/or receive clot-dissolving drugs.

Ask very specific questions about the extent of your heart disease—primarily how many arteries are blocked and what the blockages look like. If you meet these criteria for angioplasty, your chances of being successfully treated are excellent. Angioplasty is less successful when there are more than two blocked arteries and when the blockages curve around bends in the artery or branch into smaller vessels. The best angioplasty candidates have only a single or perhaps two diseased arteries, and the plaque in those arteries is straight rather than branching out. Patients also should have good function of the heart muscle and be under the age of 65. "Ask to see your arteriograms (the pictures taken of your arteries). In this situation, a picture is worth a thousand words," says [Dr.] Ellis [Jones, bypass surgeon at Emory University School of Medicine].

Patients are encouraged and advised to ask very specific questions and seek several professional opinions before agreeing to undergo any major medical procedure.

SOURCE:
"Balloon or Bypass or Clot-Buster: What'll It Be?" *Heartcorps: A Self-Help Journal for Heart Patients and Those Who Love Them* 1 (March/April 1989): 8.

SURVIVAL OUTCOME

To elucidate the factors associated with improved survival following coronary artery bypass surgery, we studied 5809 patients receiving medical or surgical therapy for coronary artery disease. Three factors were associated with a significant surgical survival benefit: more severe coronary disease, a worse prognosis with medical therapy, and a more recent operative date. Patients with more extensive coronary obstruction had the greatest improvement in survival. Patients with a poor prognosis because of factors such as older age, severe angina, or left ventricular dysfunction had a reduction in risk that was proportionate to their overall risk on medical therapy. Survival with surgery progressively improved over the study period and by 1984 surgery was significantly better than medical therapy for most patient subgroups. Thus, contemporary coronary revascularization is associated with improved longevity in many patients with ischemic heart disease, especially in those with adverse prognostic indicators.

SOURCE:
Califf, Robert M., and others. "The Evolution of Medical and Surgical Therapy for Coronary Artery Disease: A 15-Year Perspective." *JAMA* 261, no. 14 (April 14, 1989): 2077-2086. Copyright 1989, American Medical Association.

MORTALITY RATES

Empirical evidence suggests that mortality rates for coronary artery bypass graft (CABG) surgery are lower in hospitals that perform a higher volume of the procedure. In recent years, the criteria for CABG surgery have been expanded to include patients with a wide variety of co-morbidities. To address the question of whether the volume-outcome relationship continues to exist for this new group of patients, discharge abstracts for 18,966 CABG operations at 77 hospitals in California in 1983 were analyzed using multiple-regression techniques. Higher-volume hospitals had lower in-hospital mortality (adjusted for case mix); this effect was greatest in patients who might be characterized as having "non-scheduled" CABG surgery. Higher-volume hospitals also had shorter average postoperative lengths of stay and fewer patients with extremely long stays. The results of this study suggest that the greatest improvement in average outcomes for CABG surgery would result from the closure of low-volume surgery units. . . .

The data suggest strongly that average outcomes would be improved if patients who require CABG surgery, particularly nonscheduled surgery, have this procedure in higher-volume hospitals.

SOURCE:
Showstack, Jonathan A., Kenneth E. Rosenfeld, and others. "Association of Volume with Outcome of Coronary Artery Bypass Graft Surgery: Scheduled vs. Nonscheduled Operations." *JAMA* 257, no. 6 (February 13, 1987): 785-789. Copyright 1987, American Medical Association.

RESOURCES

ORGANIZATIONS

American Heart Association. National Center, 7320 Greenville Avenue, Dallas, TX 75231. Or, see local affiliate.

National Heart, Lung, and Blood Institute. National Institutes of Health, 9000 Rockville Pike, Bethesda, MD 20892.

BOOKS

Hoffman, Nancy J. *Change of Heart: The Bypass Experience.* New York: Harcourt Brace, 1985. 384 pp.

Kra, Sigfried. *Coronary Bypass Surgery: Who Needs It?* New York: Norton, 1986.

Richards, Norman V. *Heart to Heart: A Cleveland Clinic Guide to Understanding Heart Disease and Open Heart Surgery.* New York: Atheneum, 1987. 220 pp.

RELATED ARTICLES

Allen, Jerilyn K. "Physical and Psychosocial Outcomes after Coronary Artery Bypass Graft Surgery: Review of the Literature." *Heart & Lung* 19, no. 1 (January 1990): 49–55.

Chatterjee, Kanu. "Is There any Long-Term Benefit from Coronary Artery Bypass Surgery?" *Journal of the American College of Cardiology* 12, no. 4 (October 1988): 881–882.

"Coronary Artery Bypass Surgery." *Mayo Clinic Health Letter* 8, no. 9 (September 1990): 1–2.

Johnson, W. Dudley, Jerold B. Brenowitz, and others. "Factors Influencing Long-Term (10-Year to 15-year) Survival After a Successful Coronary Artery Bypass Operation." *Annals of Thoracic Surgery* 48 (1989): 19–25.

Killip, Thomas "Twenty Years of Coronary Bypass Surgery." *The New England Journal of Medicine* 319, no. 6 (August 11, 1988): 366–368.

Weintraub, William S., Ellis L. Jones, and others. "Changing Use of Coronary Angioplasty and Coronary Bypass Surgery in the Treatment of Chronic Coronary Artery Disease." *The American Journal of Cardiology* 65 (January 15, 1990): 183–188.

Winslow, Constance Monroe, Jacqueline B. Kosecoff, and others. "The Appropriateness of Performing Coronary Artery Bypass Surgery." *JAMA* 260, no. 4 (July 22/29, 1988): 505-509.

HEARTBURN (GASTROESOPHAGEAL REFLUX)

OVERVIEW

People experience heartburn in a variety of forms. Usually heartburn is a burning chest pain located behind the breastbone. Often there is a sensation of food coming back into the mouth, accompanied by an acid or bitter taste. Typically, heartburn occurs after meals and is a common source of complaints of indigestion. Fried or fatty foods, tomato products, citrus fruits and juices, chocolate, and coffee often cause heartburn. Usually the burning-type chest pain lasts for many minutes—sometimes as long as 2 hours—and often is worse when the sufferer is lying flat or bending over. Heartburn is usually described as a burning sensation, although it may not be considered painful by some people. In addition, heartburn is neither brought on by exercise nor relieved with rest; most people obtain relief by standing upright or by taking an antacid.

Approximately 10 percent of the U.S. population suffers daily from heartburn, and at least one-third of otherwise normal individuals have this symptom occasionally. It is a common complaint among pregnant women, of whom 25 percent experience daily heartburn and more than 50 percent have occasional distress. Recent studies indicate that similar problems in infancy are more common than was previously recognized and may produce recurrent vomiting, failure to thrive, or coughing and other lung symptoms.

Although heartburn is a common malady in our society, it is rarely life-threatening. It can, however, limit an individual's daily activities and productivity. With proper understanding of the causes of heartburn and a rational approach to treatment, most people will find relief.

The esophagus is the tube-like structure that connects the mouth to the stomach. At the point where the esophagus joins the stomach, the esophagus is kept closed by a specialized muscle called the lower esophageal sphincter (LES). This muscle is important because the pressure in the stomach is normally higher than that in the esophagus. The muscle of the LES relaxes after swallowing to allow passage of food into the stomach, but then it quickly closes once again.

Backwash of stomach contents into the esophagus, commonly called reflux, occurs when the LES muscle is very weak or, more commonly, when it inappropriately relaxes. The reflux tends to be worse after big meals and when one lies down at night. The refluxed fluid irritates the esophageal lining.

The occurrence and severity of heartburn depend on LES dysfunction, but they are also affected by the type and amount of fluid brought up from the stomach, by the clearing action of the esophagus, by the neutralizing action of saliva, and by other factors. Although heartburn is the most common manifestation of acid reflux, it is important to recognize that other, more serious problems can result from chronic reflux. Some of these complications such as esophageal bleeding, ulcers, or stricture may require more vigorous treatment.

SOURCE:
Castell, Donald O. " Heartburn." *National Digestive Diseases Information Clearinghouse*. NIH Pub. No. 86-882 (April 1986): 1-2.

USE OF ANTACIDS

Millions of us take antacid tablets and seltzer tablets for ailments we call heartburn or acid indigestion. Over-the-counter antacids are so popular because most are effective, fast-working, and easy to use—neutralizing stomach acid and inhibiting the action of pepsin, a potentially irritating digestive enzyme.

All antacids are safe when used occasionally by healthy people. But, as we've reported, no over-the-counter medication is without its risks. Daily use of antacids can mask a serious problem, such as a peptic ulcer. In extreme cases, the "heartburn" may actually be an incipient heart attack. Taken irregularly without a doctor's supervision, antacids may cause bowel irregularities (constipation or diarrhea), aggravate kidney disorders, and cause other problems. And prolonged use can actually cause an increase in the production of stomach acid if you suddenly stop taking the antacids—this is called acid rebound.

Nine tips for effective antacid use

- Try to eliminate the cause of frequent heartburn or upset stomach (excess fatty food, alcohol, stress) instead of making antacid use a part of your daily life.
- Use antacids only occasionally for indigestion or heartburn. If symptoms persist despite antacid use, see your doctor.
- Liquid types generally neutralize acid more effectively than tablets. Chew tablets thoroughly to help them dissolve quickly in the stomach—and drink some water after swallowing them.
- If one brand doesn't work well, try another. Some formulations are more potent than others.
- Antacids may interfere with the absorption of many drugs (such as antibiotics, digitalis, and anticoagulants). If you take prescription medication, consult your pharmacist or doctor before using antacids.
- If you are on a salt-restricted diet, avoid sodium bicarbonate antacids, which contain whopping doses of sodium.
- Seek medical help immediately if your "heartburn" is severe and accompanied by chest pain, nausea, vomiting, weakness, breathlessness, fainting, and/or sweating. It may be a heart attack.
- Pregnant women and people with ulcers or kidney problems should consult a physician before using any antacid.
- If you are using antacids only to increase your calcium consumption, take doses yielding no more than 1,000 to 1,500 milligrams of calcium a day—and avoid aluminum-based antacids, which can actually deplete calcium.

Comparing antacid types

Sodium bicarbonate (such as Alka-Seltzer, Bromo Seltzer, and Brioschi). Baking soda, usually in effervescent form. For short-term use only: frequent use may interfere with kidney or heart function, promote urinary tract infection, and disrupt the body's acid balance. Very high sodium content. Brands containing aspirin can upset stomach and aggravate ulcers.

Calcium carbonate (such as Tums, Alka-2, and Titralac). A tablet containing 500 milligrams of calcium carbonate provides 200 milligrams of calcium, which is 20% of the U.S. RDA. Limit dosage according to instructions. May cause constipation.

Aluminum compounds (such as Amphojel and Alternagel). Less potent and slower acting than other types. Some types may promote calcium (or phosphorus) depletion and are not recommended for those with high calcium needs, such as postmenopausal women. People with kidney problems should check with their doctors before using. May cause constipation.

Magnesium compounds (such a Philip's Milk of Magnesia). May cause diarrhea.

Aluminum-magnesium compounds (such as Maalox, Digel, Mylanta, Riopan, and Gaviscon). May have the same side effects as either aluminum or magnesium compounds in some people, but generally less likely to cause constipation or diarrhea. Some brands add simethicone, which is supposed to reduce gas (or at least reduce the size of gas bubbles), but which has never been proven to provide relief.

Antacids are also available as generic products.

SOURCE:
"Antacids: How Do You Spell Relief?" *The University of California, Berkeley Wellness Letter* 7 (May 1991): 3. Excerpted from *The University of California, Berkeley Wellness Letter,* Copyright Health Letter Associates, 1991.

RESOURCES

ORGANIZATION

National Digestive Diseases Information Clearinghouse. 1255 23rd St. NW, Suite 275, Washington, DC 20037.

RELATED ARTICLES

Ament, Marvin E., and others. "Reflux Therapy: A Plan of Attack." *Patient Care* 23 (September 30, 1989): 30–39.

"Antacids: Part 6 in a Series on Safe and Effective Ingredients." *Consumer Reports Health Letter* (February 1990): 12–13.

Marshall, John B. "Gastroesophageal Reflux Disease: Medical Aspects." *Postgraduate Medicine* 85, no. 7 (May 15, 1989): 92–100.

"Omeprazole." *The Medical Letter on Drugs and Therapeutics* 32, no. 813 (March 9, 1990): 19–21.

Shepherd, Steven. "Taking the Fire out of Heartburn." *Executive Health Report* 26 (March 1990): 2–3.

HEMORRHOIDS

OVERVIEW

Hemorrhoids involve the blood vessels that line the anus. Pressure on the walls of the rectum weakens the muscles that support the hemorrhoidal vessels. They then become enlarged and lose their support, in a manner similar to the way varicose veins can develop in your legs. Result: a sac-like protrusion into the anal canal.

The problem of hemorrhoids is unique to humans; no other species develops a similar condition. Between 50 percent and 75 percent of Americans develop hemorrhoids. The problems can occur at any time, but becomes more common as you age. Among younger people, pregnant women and women who have had children are most apt to develop hemorrhoidal problems. The condition seems to run in families, and no group is immune.

Your risk of hemorrhoids increases if you are overweight, sit or stand for long periods of time or regularly lift heavy weights. Intense straining during bowel movements weakens your anal and rectal muscles, causing hemorrhoids to protrude or bleed.

Although hemorrhoids can be uncomfortable, they are not a life-threatening condition. They never develop into cancer.

Remember, however, that the common symptoms of hemorrhoids—rectal discomfort, itching, swelling around the anus, change in bowel pattern and blood in the stool—can resemble the signs of more serious problems.

In the early stages, symptoms tend to subside of their own accord. If they don't or if the problem recurs, talk to your doctor. A physician can distinguish hemorrhoids from other conditions and identify the type of hemorrhoid that bothers you:

- Internal—Located inside the rectum, these hemorrhoids usually are painless. Because they tend to bleed, you might notice some bright red blood after passing a stool.
- Prolapsed—some internal hemorrhoids protrude outside the anus. You may notice a mucous discharge.

Thrombosis is the formation of a clot within the hemorrhoid, preventing it from receding. This can lead to extreme pain.

- External—"Piles" develop under the skin at the entrance to the anus. As a hemorrhoid swells or develops a thrombosis, the overlying skin stretches, causing pain. A firm, sensitive mass, usually blue or purple, often forms outside the anal opening.

SOURCE:
"Hemorrhoids: Effective Treatments and Self-Care Techniques Are Available for This Ailment." *Mayo Clinic Health Letter* (March 1990): 4.

TREATMENT METHODS

The first step—which may prevent the formation of future hemorrhoids as well as treat existing ones—is to increase intake of fiber and water. Insoluble dietary fiber is found in whole grains, bran, fresh fruits and vegetables. This fiber remains untouched as it passes through the digestive tract; at the same time, it absorbs many times its weight in water. When it reaches the colon, it helps make a large, soft stool that is easy to pass.

It is important to avoid constipation; if the fiber-rich diet is not enough to help, a physician can prescribe a special type of laxative called a stool softener. Other types of laxatives may tend to worsen the constipation problem and should be avoided.

More involved treatment may be required if hemorrhoids don't clear up on their own and if they bleed enough to cause anemia, intolerable pain or discomfort. In recent years, a number of new treatments have appeared that avoid costly and time-consuming hospital stays with attendant pain and complications.

Rubber banding. This widely-used office treatment is effective for internal hemorrhoids that protrude. The band cuts off blood supply to the hemorrhoid, causing it to shrivel up. Several treatments may be necessary to eliminate multiple hemorrhoids, and the procedure is a little bit uncomfortable.

Injection. This procedure involves injecting a chemical solution into the mucous membrane near the hemorrhoid. It works well for small bleeding hemorrhoids and certain other types. Repeat treatments may be necessary every few years.

Photocoagulation. One of the newest of the outpatient procedures, this involves directing an infrared light into a fine point at the end of a probe, which is then used to attach—"spot weld," if you will—the hemorrhoid back in place.

Electric current. This new procedure involves the application of an electric current to the hemorrhoids. According to Robert D. Kaplan, M.D., of the section on gastroenterology at the University of Pennsylvania Hospital in Philadelphia, the electric current, emitted by an electrode probe, triggers a chemical reaction that shuts down the blood supply in the hemorrhoid and causes the inflamed tissue to shrink up. The process is painless, safe and effective. Most patients need one or two sessions, each lasting about 15 minutes. And since no recovery time is anticipated, the patient is able to return home or to work directly after the procedure. "All but the most severe hemorrhoids can be adequately treated by this new method," says Dr. Kaplan.

More recalcitrant hemorrhoids may require surgery. In the past, surgery usually required general anesthesia, a week in the hospital, and endurance of excruciating pain. Today, doctors use cryosurgery to freeze the offending hemorrhoid. Patients typically stay overnight in a hospital and return to work in a few days.

Recently, laser hemorrhoidectomy has been touted to replace conventional surgical procedures. Although this procedure can be faster and cheaper, it is not appropriate for more serious cases.

SOURCE:

Berkman, Sue. "Help for Hemorrhoids." *Weight Watchers Women's Health and Fitness News* (October 1990): 6.

TREATMENT BY ELECTRICITY

More and more doctors are using a quick, painless way to eradicate hemorrhoids using mild electrical currents. The procedure is carried out in a doctor's office and patients go back to work immediately after treatment. . . .

The new method for treating hemorrhoids joins an arsenal of older treatments, all of which are designed to create an injury at the base of the hemorrhoid, thereby strangling the blood vessels that feed it, said Dr. Gayle M. Randall, an assistant professor of medicine at the University of California at Los Angeles School of Medicine and the director of endoscopy at the West Los Angeles Veterans Hospital. Controlled injuries are deliberately produced with chemicals, freezing, laser and infrared light, rubber bands and, more recently, electric currents. . . .

The newest methods using electricity seem to produce the least tissue injury for the greatest effect, Dr. Randall said. Patients say the procedures are painless.

One device, the Bicap, is a probe device that places one second pulses of alternating current at the hemorrhoid's base. Each hemorrhoid requires four or five pulses to coagulate the tissue, Dr. Ramall said. "You hear a sizzle and the mucosa turns white" inside the rectum, she said. The hemorrhoid gradually shrinks over the next few weeks.

Electricity is conducted by moisture in the hemorrhoid, said Richard Kligus, Bicap's product manager at Circon ACMI in Stamford, Conn. When the hemorrhoid dries out, the current cuts itself off automatically.

SOURCE:

Blakeslee, Sandra. "Removing Hemorrhoids in Painless Office Visit." *The New York Times* (April 25, 1991): B7.

USE OF OVER-THE-COUNTER PRODUCTS

In 1980, the FDA convened an Advisory Panel on OTC hemorrhoid products to study the safety and efficacy of these ingredients. They were divided into nine categories. Six categories (protectants, astringents, counterirritants, local anesthetics, vasoconstrictors and keratolytics) contained some safe and effective ingredients. Three categories (antiseptics, anticholinergics, and wound healing agents) contained no ingredients with evidence of safety and effectiveness. Some ingredients were considered in more than one category. All ingredients were considered for appropriateness externally (for the anal and perianal areas) and intrarectally (in the rectum). . . .

The most widely used anti-hemorrhoidal product is Preparation H, which now holds an estimated 56 percent share of the more than $100 million hemorrhoid product market. Its producer, American Home Products' Whitehall Laboratories, spent $14.6 million in 1981 to convince people of Preparation H's ability "to shrink swelling of hemorrhoidal tissue." Despite its popularity, the product's active ingredients are unconvincing in their effectiveness.

The active ingredients in Preparation H are live yeast cell derivative and shark liver oil. Live yeast cell derivative is a purported wound-healing agent which has no evidence of effectiveness as such. Shark liver oil is neither a safe nor an effective wound-healing agent. However, in adequate amounts (more than currently found in Preparation H) it is an effective—though expensive—protectant. Preparation H contains only 3 percent shark liver oil; in order to be an effective protectant, shark liver oil would need to constitute 50 percent of the product. Preparation H, therefore, despite its price and popularity, is not recommended as a safe and effective product for hemorrhoids.

SOURCE:

"Hemorrhoids." *Public Citizen Health Research Group Health Letter* 7, no. 3 (March 1991): 3, 5.

RESOURCES

PAMPHLET

National Digestive Diseases Information Clearinghouse:

Fact Sheet: Hemorrhoids. NIH Pub. No. 89-3021. January 1989. 2 pp.

RELATED ARTICLES

"The Best Medicine for Hemorrhoids." *The Johns Hopkins Medical Letter* (January 1991): 3.

Guthrie, James F., and others. "Tips on Managing Anorectal Disorders." *Patient Care* 23 (December 15, 1989): 31–39.

"Hemorrhoids." *Health News* (University of Toronto) 8 (February 1990): 4–6.

"Review of Hemorrhoid Products." *FDA Consumer* 24 (November 1990): 2.

HEPATITIS

OVERVIEW

Viral hepatitis is the most common of the serious contagious diseases caused by several viruses that attack the liver. About 70,000 cases are reported to the Centers for Disease Control each year but this represents only a fraction of the cases occurring in this country.

Hepatitis means inflammation of the liver, usually producing swelling and tenderness and sometimes permanent damage to the liver. Hepatitis may also be caused by non-viral substances such as alcohol, chemicals, and drugs. These types of hepatitis are known respectively as alcoholic, toxic, and drug-induced hepatitis.

At least five types of viral hepatitis are currently known, each caused by a different identified virus.

- **Hepatitis A**—formerly called infectious hepatitis, is most common in children in developing countries, but is being seen more frequently in adults in the western world.
- **Hepatitis B**—formerly called serum hepatitis, is the most serious form of hepatitis, with over 300 million carriers in the world and an estimated one million in the United States.
- **Hepatitis C**—formerly called non-A, non-B hepatitis, is now the most common cause of hepatitis after blood transfusion. More than one percent of Americans are carriers of the virus.
- **Hepatitis D**—formerly called delta hepatitis, is found mainly in intravenous drug users who are carriers of the hepatitis B virus which is necessary for the hepatitis D virus to spread.
- **Hepatitis E**—formerly called enteric or epidemic non-A, non-B hepatitis, resembles hepatitis A, but is caused by a different virus commonly found in the Indian Ocean Area.
- Other viruses, especially members of the herpes virus family, including the cold sore virus, chicken pox, infectious mononucleosis virus and others can affect the liver as well as other organs they infect. This is particularly true when the immune system is impaired.

Hepatitis A and E viruses are excreted or shed in feces. Direct contact with an infected person's feces or indirect fecal contamination of food, the water supply, raw shellfish, hands and utensils may result in sufficient amounts of virus entering the mouth to cause infections.

Hepatitis B is spread from mother-to-child at birth or soon after birth, through sexual contact, blood transfusions or contaminated needles. Almost a quarter of the cases may result from unknown sources in the general population. In families the virus can be spread from adults to children.

Hepatitis C is spread directly from one person to another via blood or needles. While sexual transmission and mother-to-child spread may occur, the transmission of this disease is not clearly understood.

Hepatitis D is spread mainly by needles and blood. Hepatitis D infects only individuals infected with hepatitis B and may be transmitted by carriers of hepatitis D and B.

SOURCE:
American Liver Foundation. *Viral Hepatitis: Everybody's Problem?* pp. 1–3.

RISKS

The U.S. Public Health Service recommends getting the hepatitis B immunization if you. . .

- are in an occupation at risk, such as medical or public safety personnel
- are a client or staff member of an institution for developmentally disabled
- are a hemodialysis patient
- are a sexually active homosexual man
- are a user of illicit injectable drugs
- are a hemophilia patient or receive clotting factor concentrates
- have household and/or sexual contact with hepatitis B carriers
- are a native Alaskan or Pacific Islander or are from areas with high hepatitis B infection rates
- are heterosexual with multiple partners
- are an international traveler who lives in close contact or may have blood or sexual contact with groups heavily infected with hepatitis B. . . .

Suppose you have not been immunized but are exposed to a hepatitis B carrier. What do you do? First, assess the exposure. Casual contact among office workers or older students in a classroom does not usually constitute true exposure.

But if you perform CPR on a bleeding individual with hepatitis B or are forced to wrestle an infected crime suspect, then you have been exposed. If you have sex with a prostitute or if your spouse becomes infected, you are at risk for infection.

When exposed, act quickly to obtain an injection of hepatitis B immune globulin (HBIG). HBIG is a plasma product containing a high level of anti-hepatitis B antibody that affords immediate protection. Since HBIG dwindles over time, it is combined with hepatitis B vaccine for longer lasting defense. If the combination is given within 7 days of exposure (the sooner the better), 90% effectiveness is achieved.

SOURCE:
Guiteras, G. Patrick. "What You Should Know About. . .The Alphabet of Hepatitis." *Executive Health Report* (March 1991): 2–3.

SYMPTOMS

When they produce symptoms at all, which is by no means inevitable, each of the hepatitis viruses causes a flu-like illness, typically with fever, nausea and pervasive tiredness, sometimes accompanied by jaundice (yellowed skin, mucous membranes and eye-whites). The severity of viral hepatitis and its progress vary according to the virus involved and the age and immune defenses of the person infected. But whichever the triggering virus, hepatitis gives few or no warning signs. Many with viral hepatitis have a subclinical infection that goes totally unnoticed except for perhaps some fatigue and lassitude lasting four to six weeks. The fact that someone has viral hepatitis is often revealed only by blood tests.

Whether or not they cause any noticeable illness, hepatitis B, C and D viruses can linger on in the body, producing chronic, perhaps lifelong, infection. "Silent," symptomless carriers can infect others even though they feel perfectly well and they face serious risks of liver disease—cirrhosis (scarring) and liver cancer—perhaps 10 to 20 years down the road. A few of those infected develop a fulminant or fast-progressing, rapidly fatal form of hepatitis.

SOURCE:
"The ABCs of Viral Hepatitis." *Health News* (University of Toronto) (February 1991): 3.

EXPERIMENTAL THERAPIES

As yet there is no really effective treatment for any form of hepatitis. Shots of immune globulin, a short-acting product derived from blood plasma, can prevent the spread of hepatitis A during outbreaks. Highly effective, safe vaccines for hepatitis B are now available to all Canadians. Hepatitis B immune globulin (HBIg) is also provided, when circumstances warrant, for treating post-hepatitis B exposure. There are as yet no vaccines for the other forms of hepatitis. The best way to combat this infection is prevention: by getting hepatitis B shots (if in a risk-group) and practicing "safer sex"—using condoms—which prevents the spread of hepatitis B and probably also D.

Antivirals, such as alpha-interferon, are so far the most promising therapy for chronic viral hepatitis, giving remission in up to 50 per cent of hepatitis C sufferers and 30 percent of those with hepatitis B ("active" type). Interferon evidently works better against the C than the B hepatitis virus. But the improvement often vanishes once the drug is stopped. About half of those who try interferon develop side effects such as joint pains and headaches, which soon fade with repeated doses. Its long term effects aren't known.

Prostaglandin E (derived from a natural body component) shows some promise for very severe or rapidly advancing, fulminant hepatitis, of whatever form.

Liver transplants are a slowly increasing option for those with some types of hepatitis-caused liver disease. The liver is a very forgiving organ and can fulfill its vital function until almost two thirds of it is damaged. At this "end stage" of liver injury, selected chronic hepatitis sufferers may be offered a liver transplant but not usually those with chronic, active hepatitis B infection because of high chances of re-infection in the transplanted liver. Those with transfusion-acquired chronic hepatitis C can now often be offered liver transplants with apparently good results.

SOURCE:
"The ABCs of Viral Hepatitis." *Health News* (February 1991): 6.

HEPATITIS AND CHILDREN

Effective control of hepatitis B in the United States requires a change in vaccination strategy. To date, most vaccine usage has targeted health care personnel who are exposed to blood, staff and residents in institutions for the developmentally disabled, and staff and patients in hemodialysis units. Indeed, there has been some decrease in the proportion of hepatitis B cases involving health care personnel, and this may at least partially be attributed to vaccination; however, the populations most likely to have received vaccine account for only a small fraction of persons at increased risk of infection. The overall incidence of hepatitis B has not declined since the introduction of vaccine. Clearly, the vaccine is not being administered to most of the persons who need it. . . .

To be effective, the vaccine must be administered to susceptible persons before they engage in high-risk behavior such as sexual promiscuity or drug abuse. An argument can be made for mass immunization of adolescents. Because most of the reported cases of hepatitis B in the United States occur in the young adult population, the vaccination of adolescents should result in a fairly rapid decline in hepatitis B incidence. At present, however, there is no program in place that can deliver vaccine to this age group.

In the long term, hepatitis can be best controlled through universal vaccination of infants. Hepatitis B vaccine should be considered for inclusion in the standard battery of pediatric immunizations. One possibility would be to administer hepatitis B vaccine in conjunction with DTP (e.g., at 2, 4, and 6 months). Not only may it be possible to give a variety of pediatric vaccines at the same times, it also may be possible to develop a number of combined vaccine formulations (e.g., hepatitis B-DTP). Studies now are being done to evaluate these possibilities.

Continued efforts to vaccinate identifiable high-risk groups coupled with programs to effect widespread immunization of adolescents and infants could eliminate hepatitis B.

SOURCE:
West, David, and others. "Vaccination of Infants and Children Against Hepatitis B." *Pediatric Clinics of North America* 37, no. 3 (June 1990): 597–598.

RESOURCES

ORGANIZATION
American Liver Foundation. Cedar Grove, NJ 07009. (201)857-2626.

RELATED ARTICLES

Eddleston, Adrian. "Modern Vaccines: Hepatitis." *The Lancet* 335, no. 8698 (May 12, 1990): 1142–1145.

"Hepatitis C." *Mayo Clinic Health Letter* (June 1991): 7.

Hollinger, F. Blaine. "Factors Influencing the Immune Response to Hepatitis B Vaccine, Booster Dose Guidelines, and Vaccine Protocol Recommendations." *The American Journal of Medicine* 87 (Suppl. 3A) (September 4, 1989): 36S–40S.

Koretz, Ronald L. "Chronic Hepatitis." *American Family Physician* 39, no. 6 (June 1989): 197–202.

HERPES SIMPLEX VIRUS INFECTION

(*See also:* SEXUALLY TRANSMITTED DISEASES)

OVERVIEW

Herpes is the medical name for a group of similar viruses. This group includes the varicella-zoster virus, which causes chicken pox; the Epstein-Barr virus, which causes infectious mononucleosis (mono); cytomegalovirus (CMV), which is responsible for infections that usually afflict newborns and people with defective immune systems; and the herpes simplex virus, which causes genital and oral infections.

To most people, however, herpes is the common term for infections caused by the herpes simplex virus (HSV). HSV infections take the form of blisters or lesions that generally occur periodically, often causing itching and pain.

There are two types of herpes simplex virus. In most cases Type 1 (HSV-1) causes cold sores or fever blisters, and Type 2 (HSV-2) causes genital herpes. However, some genital herpes may be caused by HSV-1 virus, and some oral herpes may be caused by HSV-2. This cross infection can happen when sexual partners have oral-genital relations.

SOURCE:

Burroughs Wellcome Co. Herpes: *The Good News Is that It Can Now Be Controlled.* 1985. p. 2.

HERPES SIMPLEX TYPE 1

Called fever blisters or cold sores, HSV Type 1 infections typically take the form of tiny, clear, fluid- filled blisters on the face. Type 1 infections may also occur in the genital area after oral sexual exposure with an individual who has a herpes infection on the face.

Type 1 occurs on mucous membranes and may also develop in wounds on the skin. Nurses, physicians, dentists, and other health care workers sometimes contract a herpetic sore after HSV enters a break in the skin of their fingers.

There are two kinds of infections—primary and recurrent. Though most individuals contract the virus, only 10% or so will actually develop symptoms indicative of a primary, or first, infection. The primary infection lasts from seven to ten days and appears two to twenty days after direct exposure to an infected person.

The number of blisters varies, from one to a whole cluster. Before the blisters erupt, the soon-to-be-infected skin may itch or become very sensitive. The natural course of the blisters is to break spontaneously or as a result of minor trauma, allowing the fluid contents to ooze.

Eventually, scabs form and slough, leaving slightly red skin.

Though the primary infection heals completely, rarely causing a scar, the virus that caused it remains in the body, migrating to nerve cells where it remains in a dormant phase.

Many people will not experience another infection or recurrence. Others will be plagued with recurrences, either in the same location as the first infection or in a nearby location. The infections may recur every few weeks or infrequently.

Recurrent infections, which tend to be milder than primary infections, may be triggered by a variety of stresses including fever, exposure to the sun, and menstruation. However, for many individuals, the recurrences are unpredictable and have no recognizable precipitating cause.

SOURCE:
American Academy of Dermatology. *Facts about Herpes Simplex.* 1987. p. 2.

HERPES VIRUS INFECTIONS—FEVER BLISTERS

If fever blisters erupt, they should be kept clean and dry to prevent bacterial infections. A soft, bland diet is recommended to avoid irritating the sores and surrounding sensitive areas. Care should be taken to refrain from touching the sores and spreading the virus to new sites, such as the eyes and genitals. To prevent infecting others, kissing should be avoided as well as touching the sores and then touching others. . . .

Research on fever blisters is extensive. Several laboratories are developing and testing new antiviral drugs tailored to hamper or prevent blister outbreaks. Investigators are also trying to develop ointments that enable antiviral drugs to penetrate the skin more effectively. . . .

Acyclovir is a recently developed antiviral drug that in clinical studies lessened the symptoms and frequency of fever blister recurrences for some patients. This drug prevents the herpes virus from multiplying and is effective when taken in pill form prior to an outbreak of the virus. One study showed that during the 3-month period when they took 4 acyclovir pills daily, the majority of patients had no recurrences of fever blisters compared to having an average of one recurrence a month prior to taking the drug. Acyclovir creams applied to blisters or areas of the lip that tingle or itch prior to a blister outbreak were also tested but these topical applications were shown to be ineffective. The long-term effects of daily oral doses of acyclovir are not known, nor are the effects the drug might have on an unborn child.

SOURCE:
National Institutes of Health. *Fever Blisters and Canker Sores.* 1987. pp. 5, 6.

HERPES SIMPLEX TYPE 2—GENITAL HERPES

Genital herpes is a contagious viral infection that affects an estimated 30 million Americans. Each year as many as 500,000 new cases are believed to occur. The infection is caused by the herpes simplex virus (HSV). Two types of HSV can cause genital herpes: HSV type 2 and HSV type 1, which more commonly causes oral (on or near the mouth) herpes, known as fever blisters or cold sores, but can cause genital infections as well.

Most people who are infected with HSV never develop any symptoms. However, either type of virus can produce sores in and around the vaginal area, on the penis, and around the anal opening, buttocks, or thighs. Occasionally, sores also appear on other parts of the body that have come into contact with HSV type 1 or 2.

Genital herpes infection is usually acquired by sexual contact with someone who has an outbreak of herpes sores. People with oral herpes can transmit the infection to the genital area of a partner during oral-genital sex. In some cases, herpes infections can be transmitted by a person who has no noticeable symptoms. It is unlikely that the virus can be spread by contact with an object such as a toilet seat. . . .

During an active herpes episode, whether primary or recurrent, it is important to follow a few simple steps to speed healing and to avoid spreading the infection to other sites of the body or to other people:

- Keep the infected area clean and dry to prevent the development of secondary infections.
- Try to avoid touching the sores directly, and if unavoidable, wash hands afterwards.
- Avoid sexual contact from the first recognized symptoms until the sores are completely healed.

Until just a few years ago, there was no drug available for the relief of herpes sores. In 1982, acyclovir ointment was approved by the Food and Drug Administration for use in persons suffering from an initial episode of genital herpes. Investigators at the National Institute of Allergy and Infectious Diseases (NIAID) and elsewhere subsequently studied the use of an oral form of acyclovir, which proved to be successful in treating persons with primary and recurrent episodes of genital herpes. The oral form of the drug can speed healing time and limit the severity of a herpes outbreak. . . .

Genital herpes poses risks for babies born to women who have an active outbreak at the time of delivery. If a baby is infected during its passage through the birth canal, the virus may cause blindness, brain damage, or even death. Because the risk of infecting the infant is high if an outbreak occurs shortly before delivery, most doctors recommend that a woman with genital herpes be tested each week during the last weeks of her pregnancy. If these tests show no signs of the virus and if a careful examination immediately before delivery shows no sign of infection, most experts feel that vaginal delivery is safe. If there is any doubt, however, most doctors recommend that the infant be delivered by cesarean section.

SOURCE:
National Institute of Allergy and Infectious Diseases. *Genital Herpes.* NIH Pub. No. 87-909C. August 1987. pp. 1, 2-3.

PREVENTION

Genital herpes may have taken a backseat to the more serious sexually transmitted diseases of the day—AIDS and the human papilloma virus—but it has not gone away. According to the Centers for Disease Control (CDC) in Atlanta, thirty million Americans were infected with the virus in 1980, and each year since then, physicians have diagnosed about 450,000 new cases. More women (roughly 18 percent) are infected than men (about 14 percent). And while there's still no cure, researchers are making inroads with improved methods of diagnosis and treatment and, most promising, preventive vaccines.

"Safe sex may be getting a lot of press, but it's not being practiced on a steady basis," says Paul Zenker, M.D., medical epidemiologist for the CDC. As a result, he says, "the number of cases of all STDs is going up; herpes isn't an isolated phenomenon." . . .

Genital herpes symptoms aren't easy to pinpoint since not everyone develops visible blisters, but the infection risk to others is reduced by completely avoiding sexual contact whenever blisters or other symptoms are present. To help offset the risk of asymptomatic spreading, particularly for known carriers, using a condom along with a spermicide containing nonoxynol-9 or octoxynol may up the protection against transmitting the herpes virus. The bottom line: Anyone and everyone who's sexually active should know the symptoms (itching or burning in the genitals followed by painful, fluid-filled sores), examine herself regularly and see a physician when she has reason to be suspicious of a symptom or a partner's symptoms.

SOURCE:

Spence, Annette. "Herpes Update: Safe Sex Hasn't Slowed the Spread of this Virus, but Treatments Are on the Horizon." *Self* (September 1990): 262, 263.

RESOURCES

ORGANIZATIONS

American Academy of Dermatology. 1567 Maple Avenue, P.O. Box 3116, Evanston, IL 60204.

American Sexual Health Association. Herpes Resource Center. P.O. Box 13827, Research Triangle Park NC 27709.

PAMPHLET

March of Dimes:

Herpes: The Good News is That it Can Now Be Controlled. Burroughs Wellcome. 1985. 7 pp.

ADDITIONAL ARTICLES

"Cold Sores and Canker Sores." *Harvard Medical School Health Letter* (August 1989): 6-7.

Eknath, A. D., R. S. Smeeta. "Herpes Simplex Encephalitis." *American Family Physician* 37, no. 2 (February 1988): 184-188.

Rose, F. B., and C. J. Camp. "Genital Herpes: How to Relieve Patients' Physical and Psychological Symptoms." *Postgraduate Medicine* 84, no. 3 (September 1, 1988): 81-86.

Sagall, R. J. "Herpes and Pregnancy." *Pediatrics for Parents* (July-August 1988): 8.

HERPES ZOSTER (CHICKEN POX/SHINGLES)

OVERVIEW

Everyone who's had chicken pox has the potential to develop herpes zoster, or shingles. The reason: The same virus that causes chicken pox causes zoster. Ther virus remains in a dormant state in certain nerve cells of the body for months to many years and then reactivates, causing zoster. About 20 percent of the population is affected at some time during their lives.

What prompts the virus to "awaken" and cause problems in normal, healthy people is not clear. Most physicians believe there is a temporary decrease in the body's immune response, which somehow removes the shackles on the virus, allowing it to start reproducing and to move along nerve fibers toward the skin. The fact that the disease occurs more often in people older than age 50 (although children can get it, too) supports this concept, as the immune response is believed to wane in older people. Trauma or possibly stress may also trigger a zoster attack.

In a slightly different group are people who are "immuno suppressed," that is, whose immunological systems are weakened and unable to fight off disease normally. Such people are more prone to develop zoster and are more likely to have a serious form of it. This includes some people with cancer, such as leukemia or lymphoma, or who have undergone chemotherapy or radiation therapy for cancer; people who have had organ transplants and are taking drugs that ward off transplant rejection but depress the immune response; and people with diseases that affect the immunological system, such as AIDS.

SOURCE:
American Academy of Dermatology. *Herpes Zoster (Shingles).* 1988. p. 1.

PREVALENCE

Varicella zoster virus (VZV) causes substantial worldwide morbidity both in its primary (varicella) and reactivation (herpes zoster) forms. A member of the human herpesvirus family that now contains six siblings, VZV is responsible for the most prevalent exanthematous [characterized by a skin eruption or rash] disease of childhood in developed countries—chickenpox. Approximately 3.5 million cases of chickenpox occur in the United States annually, resulting in hospitalization of at least 4,000 children. Herpes zoster, the reactivation form of VZV infection, is also relatively common. Based on estimates by Ragozzino et al, about 300,000 cases of herpes zoster occur annually in the United States.

SOURCE:
Balfour H. H. "Varicella Zoster Virus Infections in Immunocompromised Hosts: A Review of the Natural History and Management." *The American Journal of Medicine* 85 (suppl. 2A) (August 29, 1988): 68.

MAIN FEATURES

Shingles or Herpes zoster (zoster for short) is an adult reactivation of a childhood chicken pox infection. However, the skin rash, instead of covering large parts of the body as in chicken pox, usually appears only on a small area of skin in rows like shingles on a roof. A typical shingles rash follows the path of certain nerves on one side of the body only—generally on the trunk, buttocks, neck, face or scalp—usually stopping abruptly at the midline. Shingles is common in the elderly, rare among the young. About two thirds of shingles cases occur in those over 50, afflicting both sexes equally. Most people suffer only one attack although repeat bouts occasionally occur, usually at the same site as the first eruption.

If shingles occurs on the face, the nose and cornea of the eye are often involved. This condition, known as zoster keratitis, can lead to blindness if left untreated, so anyone with shingles on the upper face no matter how mild should see a physician at once. A tingling at the tip of the nose may herald possible eye involvement. When the trigeminal facial nerve and the eyes are affected, people are more likely to experience prolonged post-shingles pain. And with advancing age, there's an increasing chance of being left with irritating discomfort, vision impairment or severe pain after the zoster rash heals.

An attack of shingles generally begins with feverish discomfort (chills, headache, upset stomach) perhaps accompanied by a preliminary itching or burning sensation. Pain may precede the rash by a few days (occasionally mistaken for a heart attack, lung infection or back problem) but the discomfort is more commonly felt only during and/or after the rash.

The rash, typically confined to one side of the body, starts as a series of raised red spots surrounded by a swollen area that turn into clear blisters, which become cloudy, dry out and crust over. The spots may bleed and become very itchy and painful. In a few, especially the immunosuppressed, attacks are severe, the rash covering a wide area. The rash may take three to four weeks to heal. Shingles pain occasionally occurs alone, without any rash—known as zoster sine herpete. Normally, once the herpetic rash fades, the area stops hurting and full recovery follows.

SOURCE:

"Shingles Is a Pain." *Health News* (University of Toronto) 7 (December 1989): 4.

TREATMENT WITH ACYCLOVIR

In 1990, FDA broadened the approved use of the anti-herpes virus drug acyclovir (Zovirax) to include treatment of acute shingles. The drug had previously been approved for use in genital herpes. Controlled clinical trials showed that acyclovir reduced the period during which new shingles lesions formed and shortened the times to scabbing, healing, and complete cessation of pain in patients with uncomplicated shingles. Patients receiving acyclovir were less likely to suffer pain and other discomfort during the acute phase of illness. Taken orally over a period of 7 to 10 days, acyclovir also lessened the time during which patients "shed" VZV and thus could infect people who had never had chickenpox. A person with active shingles can give chickenpox to someone who has not had the disease, but shingles itself is not contagious.

Although some drugs can reduce the pain, neither acyclovir nor any other treatment lowers the risk of postherapeutic neuralgia following an acute attack of shingles. But research over the last several years has focused attention on a drug that seems to offer pain relief for many patients afflicted by PHN. The drug is capsaicin, not a product of chemical conjuring, but a derivative of the plant family from which we get red pepper.

Capsaicin cream (Zostrix) has been reported by investigators at the pain clinic of Toronto General Hospital to reduce pain in a significant percentage of PHN victims. The researchers say that more than half (56 percent) of PHN patients who received capsaicin cream for four weeks had good or excellent pain relief, and that 78 percent noted at least some improvement in pain.

Although capsaicin is an over-the-counter drug sold for muscular aches and pains, patients should consult a physician before using it to treat PHN. The drug should not be applied until the lesions caused by shingles have completely healed.

The Canadian investigators pointed out that burning was a common adverse effect in most patients receiving capsaicin, about one-third of whom had to stop the treatment early because of an intolerable burning sensation. But other investigators have reported that the burning caused by capsaicin subsides if patients stay on the drug beyond 72 hours, by which time it has measurably lowered their sensitivity to both heat and pain.

Although the drug may seem to be merely a counterirritant, laboratory and clinical studies suggest that capsaicin directly reduces the amount of substance P, a chemical responsible for the transmission of pain impulses. It apparently depletes substance P from nerve fibers and prevents the nerves from taking up a fresh supply of the chemical. Without substance P, nerves can't pass pain signals to the brain. Ease of administration—the cream is applied to the skin three or four times a day—and the fact that capsaicin does not interact with other drugs makes it especially suitable for use in elderly patients.

SOURCE:

Flieger, Ken. "Shingles—Or Chickenpox, Part Two." *FDA Consumer* 25, no. 6 (July-August 1991): 39–40.

RESOURCES

RELATED ARTICLES

Carmichael, J. Kevin. "Treatment of Herpes Zoster and Postherpetic Neuralgia." *American Family Physician* 44, no. 1 (July 1991): 203–210.

Jolleys, J. V. "Treatment of Shingles and Post-Herpetic Neuralgia: Relieves Shingles but Does Not Prevent Neuralgia." *British Medical Journal* 298, no. 6687 (June 10, 1989): 1537–1538.

"Varicella-Zoster Virus Infections: Biology, Natural History, Treatment, and Prevention." *Annals of Internal Medicine* 108, no. 2 (February 1988): 221–237.

HIGH BLOOD PRESSURE (HYPERTENSION)

OVERVIEW

High blood pressure, or hypertension, is one of the most common medical problems in America. Between 15 and 30% of the adult American population—or about 60 million of us—have blood pressure high enough to require some treatment. Of that 60 million, only half know that they have high blood pressure—and of that half, only about a quarter are receiving adequate treatment. Left untreated, hypertension can damage the eyes, kidneys, heart, and brain. Indeed, high blood pressure is a factor in 68% of first heart attacks and 75% of first strokes. . . .

Blood pressure is the force that the blood exerts against the walls of the arteries as it circulates through the body. This pressure is determined by the amount of blood pumped by the heart, and the resistance of the peripheral arteries (those in your limbs) to that flow.

A blood pressure reading is given as two numbers; for example, 120/80. The first number represents the systolic pressure—the pressure exerted against the arterial wall when the heart contracts, pumping blood out through the arteries. The second number represents the diastolic pressure—the pressure exerted against the arterial wall as the heart relaxes between beats. Both numbers refer to the millimeters of mercury in a sphygmomanometer, the device used to measure pressure.

Blood pressure will rise if there is an increase in either the cardiac output or the arterial resistance. The pressure is regulated by a complex interaction of heart, kidneys, and the involuntary (or autonomic) nervous system. The output will increase, for example, if the force of the heart's contractions increases. The resistance will increase if the muscles in the walls of the small arteries (or arterioles) constrict in response to stimuli from the nervous system and cause the arteries themselves to constrict in turn.

Pressure normally varies during the day. So long as it is not consistently elevated, the system is able to accommodate the highs and lows. But if the blood pressure remains high, the strain on the system can cause damage.

What is too high? Clinicians differ on just how to define normal pressure, borderline hypertension, and high blood pressure. In general, however, the higher the pressure over 120/80, the higher the risk of developing cardiovascular complications. Most clinicians consider 140/90 the upper limit of normal in adults age 18 or over and will recommend some type of treatment in patients whose diastolic pressure (based on the average of two or more readings) is above 95 and/or whose systolic pressure is above 160. In patients with pressures immediately below those figures—systolic pressure between 140 and 160 and diastolic pressure between 90 and 95—physicians will take into account age and other individual factors before calling for any medical treatment.

SOURCE:
"How to Handle Hypertension." *The Johns Hopkins Medical Letter* (September 1989): 4.

AN OVERTREATED CONDITION?

Severe high blood pressure, defined as a diastolic reading of 115 or higher, affects one million Americans, the National Institutes of Health says. Moderate pressure, a reading of 105 to 114, affects 2.5 million people, and mild, from 90 to 104, affects 24 million. It is not clear how many of the remaining 16 million people might be counted in other groups or not need treatment. They are people younger than 18 or older than 74; those in the military or institutions, or people with blood pressure less than 140/90 but taking anti-hypertensive drugs.

Most newly diagnosed cases of high blood pressure fall in the mild category. Doctors who responded to the Institute's latest survey conducted in 1987 said they prescribed drugs for most people in the mild range.

Virtually all experts agree on the need for treatment of diastolic blood pressures above 100, but opinions differ for lower measurements. The debate is most intense over patients with diastolic pressures from 90 to 94; an estimated 14.5 million Americans fall in this category, the National Heart, Lung and Blood Institute says. But the Institute says it does not know how many people have lowered their pressure to this range and are included in the total.

Only the United States has set the lower limits at 90, other countries start at 95 or 100. The World Health Organization calls pressures from 90 to 94 borderline hypertension.

Dr. Lenfant and other experts say the aggressive American policy is driven in part by demands from patients. But critics say that because the American health system does not reward doctors for taking time to discuss nonpharmacological treatments, it is easier for them to reach for the prescription pad. Fear of malpractice suits is an additional factor.

At the heart of the dispute is the variable and unpredictable nature of the progression of mild high blood pressure. A large Australian study found that in untreated mild hypertensives the diastolic pressure fell to normal levels in almost half, continued to rise in about 12 percent, and stayed about the same in 40 percent after a five-year period.

But because doctors are unable to predict which patient's pressure will rise or drop, the general strategy is to treat everyone with high blood pressure, reserving drugs for those whose pressure cannot be controlled by other means.

SOURCE:

Altman, Lawrence K. "High Blood Pressure: An Overtreated Condition?" *The New York Times* (November 9, 1990): B25.

NONDRUG THERAPY

Although drug therapy is without doubt the most effective way to manage hypertension, there's good reason to try other ways to keep blood pressure under control. All blood pressure drugs can have bothersome side effects. Nondrug therapy may help some people with mild hypertension control their blood pressure without taking medication. Even if such therapy merely reduces the need for medication, it can help lessen the frequency and severity of drug side effects.

Here's what you can do in addition to, and perhaps instead of, taking drugs:

Lose Weight

Excess weight makes high blood pressure more difficult to control. And obesity—defined as 20 percent or more above one's "desirable weight"—is frequently associated with hypertension.

Studies dating back to the early 1920's have shown that reducing weight lowers blood pressure in many people. This effect is most marked in people who are obese, but it also occurs in those who are only moderately overweight. A 1988 review of more than 20 studies on obesity and hypertension confirmed that a loss of weight decreases blood pressure in most people, whether they have hypertension or not. The National Heart, Lung, and Blood Institute recommends that obese hypertensive adults reduce body weight to within 15 percent of their desirable weight.

However, as a strategy to control high blood pressure, weight loss has major limitations. First, not everyone can lose weight. In some studies, half the participants couldn't achieve significant weight loss even in a structured clinical setting. Second, the reduction in blood pressure persists only as long as the weight is kept off. Long-term success depends on a permanent change in lifestyle, which very few study participants typically manage to sustain.

Reduce Sodium

Although a high sodium intake may not cause hypertension, it can elevate blood pressure in those who are sodium sensitive. Sodium may also interfere with antihypertensive drug treatment.

In the 1940's, extreme low-sodium diets, bed rest, and sedation were used to reduce blood pressure. But few people could stick to a regimen of rice and fruit juices, phenobarbital, and inactivity. As blood pressure drugs were developed, they quickly proved more effective and, despite their side effects, more tolerable than a life without salt or savor.

Recent studies indicate that about half of those with hypertension can reduce their blood pressure by making modest reductions in dietary sodium. The National Heart, Lung, and Blood Institute suggests that people with hypertension restrict their sodium intake to under 2500 milligrams a day. Americans, on average, consume some 2300 to 6900 mg daily.

Effective ways to reduce sodium without drastic dietary changes include:

- Keep the salt shaker off the table. (Salt substitutes may help you do without. However, they often contain potassium, which can be harmful to some people.)
- Reduce or eliminate salt (and flavorings that contain salt) in cooking. You won't miss it as much if you substitute such flavorings as onion, herbs, or spices.

- Avoid obviously salty foods—bacon, dill pickles, hot dogs, potato chips, sauerkraut, soy sauce. Some high-salt foods—celery, cheese, instant pudding, canned soup—aren't so obvious. Processed (including frozen) and fast foods are often loaded with salt. Look for low-sodium versions. Check food labels and refer to books that list sodium content of foods.

Cut back on alcohol

More than 30 studies worldwide have shown an associations between high alcohol intake and elevated blood pressure. Between 5 and 11 percent of all cases of hypertension in men (far fewer in women) have been attributed to alcohol intake.

Most of the evidence about the alcohol connection comes from observation of the higher prevalence of hypertension among people who drink. Compared with rates in nondrinkers, the prevalence of hypertension is about 50 percent greater in people consuming three or four drinks a day and 100 percent greater in those consuming six or seven drinks a day.

The few well-designed clinical trials that have tested the effect of reducing alcohol consumption have indeed found corresponding reductions in blood pressure. However, these trials were small (10 to 48 people) and short (3 days to 6 weeks). Although the results so far are encouraging, more research is needed to demonstrate that this beneficial effect can be maintained.

The National Heart, Lung, and Blood Institute suggests a limit of one ounce of alcohol a day. That's equivalent to 2 ounces of 100 proof liquor, 8 ounces of wine, or 24 ounces of beer.

Less certain, perhaps risky

Medical evidence that other nondrug measures lead to sustained reductions in blood pressure is far less convincing.

Exercise. Various studies have suggested that exercise may lower blood pressure moderately. A study of about 15,000 Harvard alumni is often cited as support for the therapeutic effects of exercise. But that retrospective study noted a lower incidence of hypertension among those who exercised; it did not directly test the use of exercise as therapy for hypertensives.

Some studies have attempted to test exercise as therapy. Typically, participants begin an exercise program, discontinue after a number of weeks or months, and then resume. Blood pressure is monitored before the program begins and at each stage. Several small uncontrolled studies found blood pressure dropped during the exercise periods but reverted to original levels when exercise was discontinued.

Modify dietary fats. A few studies have suggested that diets high in unsaturated fat may lower blood pressure in people with hypertension. However, no study has yet been designed to isolate this one dietary change in order to note its effect on blood pressure.

Fish oil has been purported to lower blood pressure. But the link is not clear, and too much fish oil can increase the risk of hemorrhagic stroke in people with hypertension.

Increase calcium. Some studies have found a weak association between increased calcium intake and decreased blood pressure. Others have found just the opposite. Small studies of people taking calcium supplements have suggested some beneficial effect on blood pressure. One well-designed study reported modest decreases in the blood pressure of 48 people with mild hypertension who took a one-gram calcium supplement every day for eight weeks. Whether the slight benefit would persist in long-term use is unknown. While most people can consume that amount of calcium safely, a few may incur an increased risk for kidney stones.

Increase potassium. Some researchers theorize that humans naturally require a high-potassium, low-sodium diet. The low-potassium, high-sodium diet common in many industrialized countries leads to high blood pressure, they say. But studies suggesting that increased potassium consumption lowers blood pressure have involved few patients and have been of short duration. The benefit found has been modest, and the overall results have been inconsistent. Further, excessive potassium can be harmful to people with impaired kidney function and those taking certain antihypertensive drugs (potassium-sparing diuretics or ACE inhibitors).

Biofeedback and relaxation. Because stress and excitement can cause temporary elevations in blood pressure, it's long been theorized that reducing stress and inducing relaxation can lower blood pressure. In biofeedback, special instruments allow people to monitor their blood pressure, pulse rate, muscular tension, sweating, or body temperature while they try to consciously control those vital functions. Relaxation techniques—deep breathing, meditation, progressive muscle relaxation—are aimed at relieving muscular tension and achieving a calm, peaceful state of mind. Both strategies take time and practice.

Recent research supports the notion that some people with mild hypertension may achieve modest decreases in blood pressure through a combination of biofeedback and relaxation. But many people can't sustain the daily effort. And even for those who do, there's no proof that these methods will maintain a pressure-lowering effect.

SOURCE:

PHARMACOLOGIC THERAPY

Because of the large number and variety of antihypertensive drugs currently available and the rapid advances in our understanding of the pathophysiology of hypertension, it is now possible to individualize antihypertensive treatment. Since most hypertensive patients have mild BP elevations, most can be controlled with a single drug. The JNC [Joint National Committee on Detection, Evaluation and Treatment of High Blood Pressure] recommends initiating therapy with a single agent from one of four classes of antihypertensive drugs: diuretics, angiotensin-converting enzyme [ACE] inhibitors, calcium channel blockers, and β-adrenergic receptor blockers. The class of agents most likely to be effective in BP lowering and best tolerated for any given patient should be selected as initial therapy. If the initial agent is ineffective at maximal recommended therapeutic doses or has undue side effects, an alternative agent from another class should be tried. When monotherapy is unsuccessful, a second agent, usually of a different class, should be added. Additional agents should be added or substituted as necessary to provide effective and well-tolerated BP control.

SOURCE:
Oparil, Suzanne, and David A. Calhoun. "Hypertension." *DM—Disease-a-Month* 35, no. 3 (March 1989): 143.

MAJOR TYPES OF ANTIHYPERTENSIVES

Currently, doctors use four main types of drugs:

- Diuretics (thiazide, including hydroclorathyazide, chlorathalidone and indapamide). Relatively inexpensive, diuretics increase the elimination of salt and water through urination, thereby lessening blood volume and pressure. Physicians may prescribe them on their own or in combination with other drugs. Possible side effects include reduced libido, generalized weakness, muscle cramps and joint pain.
- Beta blockers (propranolol, atenolol, nadolol, pindolol, labetolol). Beta blockers lower blood pressure by reducing the amount of blood pumped by the heart. These drugs may also reduce the risk of a subsequent heart attack in patients who have already had one. Possible side effects include fatigue, impotence, abnormalities in fatty substances in the blood and interference with blood-sugar regulation.
- Angiotensin converting enzyme (ACE) inhibitors (captopril, enalapril, lisinopril). These medications lower blood pressure by blocking the production of a hormone known as angiotensin, which increases blood pressure. Although ACE inhibitors—which are relatively new on the market—are costly, they have fewer known side effects than other drugs; however, side effects can include a dry, hacking cough and palpitations.
- Calcium channel blockers (nifedipine, nicardipine, verapamil, diltiazem). Calcium channel blockers relax blood-vessel walls, thereby lowering pressure. They are also quite expensive and may cause side effects such as constipation and swollen legs.

SOURCE:
Gagliardi, Nancy. "How to Lower Your Blood Pressure." *Ladies' Home Journal* (February 1991): 106.

RESOURCES

ORGANIZATIONS

American Heart Association. 7320 Greenville Avenue, Dallas, TX 75231.

National High Blood Pressure Education Program. 120/80, 4733 Bethesda Ave., Bethesda, MD 20814.

PAMPHLETS

American Heart Association:

About High Blood Pressure. 1986. 16 p.

Feelin' Fine: Living with High Blood Pressure as We Grow Older.

National High Blood Pressure Information Center:

High Blood Pressure and What You Can Do about It. 1987. 32 pp. (By Marvin Muses.)

High Blood Pressure: Your Doctor's Advice Could Save Your Life.

BOOKS

Rees, Michael K. *The Complete Guide to Living with High Blood Pressure.* New York: Prentice Hall, 1988. 286 pp.

Sorrentino, Sandy, and Carl Hansman. *Coping with High Blood Pressure.* New York: Dembner Books, 1990. 208 pp.

ADDITIONAL ARTICLES

Cressman, Michael D., and Ray W. Gifford, Jr. "Pharmacologic Management of Hypertension: New Guidelines Based on Latest Studies." *Postgraduate Medicine* 85, no. 8 (June 1989): 259–268.

Gifford, Ray W., Jr., and Borazanian, Raymond A. "Traditional First-Line Therapy: Overview of Medical Benefits and Side Effects." *Hypertension* 13, no. 5, pt. 2 (May 1989): I119–I124.

"Hypertension: Lower Your Blood Pressure Without Drugs." *Mayo Clinic Nutrition Letter* (May 1990): 2–3.

Moser, Marvin. "Controversies in the Management of Hypertension." *American Family Physician* 41, no. 5 (May 1990): 1449–1460.

Moser, Marvin. "Relative Efficacy of, and Some Adverse Reactions to, Different Antihypertensive Regimens." *The American Journal of Cardiology* 63, no. 4 (January 17, 1989): 2B–7B.

1988 Joint National Committee. "The 1988 Report of the Joint National Committee on Detection, Evaluation, and Treatment of High Blood Pressure." *Archives of Internal Medicine* 148 (May 1988): 1023–1038.

Schwartz, Gary L. "Initial Therapy for Hypertension—Individualizing Care." *Mayo Clinic Proceedings* 65, no. 1 (January 1990): 73–87.

HOMEOPATHY

OVERVIEW

Homeopathy is a system of medical therapy that concentrates on care of the whole person by methods that are gentle and sympathetic to the body's needs. It developed from investigations carried out in the eighteenth and nineteenth centuries by a German physician, Dr. Samuel Hahnemann. This development has been generally independent of other kinds of therapy, but homeopathy is, in many ways, complementary to other systems of health care, including Western orthodox medicine. And although conventional doctors cannot explain exactly how homeopathy works, work it does—often with quite dramatic and remarkable results.

The word homeopathy was coined by Hahnemann from two Greek words, homoios (like) and pathos (suffering). The first syllable is pronounced to rhyme with Tom, and has nothing to do with the Latin homo (man). Hahnemann's word neatly sums up one of the basic principles of homeopathy, which had been expressed for centuries in medical treatises by the Latin tag *similia similibus curantur*, meaning 'like is cured by like'. In contrast, orthodox medicine is generally based on the principle of opposites, so Hahnemann coined the word 'allopathy', from the Greek allos (other) to describe its principles.

Together with the principle of 'like cures like' homeopathy couples a second, equally important, concept: the use of the minimum dose. The appropriateness of homeopathic medicines has been determined by monitoring the effects of various substances on healthy people. This is known as 'proving'. A patient who displays signs and symptoms similar to those produced by the large dose is given a minimum dose of the same substance, to stimulate his or her body's own defence systems. Briefly, the illness and the remedy that is prescribed to treat it produce a similar set of symptoms. The key word is 'similar', not 'the same'. Note that 'symptoms' are felt and detected by patients themselves, whereas 'signs' are the outward manifestations that a practitioner sees when examining patients.

One major advantage of homeopathy is its safety. While its medicines are powerful in action, working with the body's own defences, their actual measurable strength is too low to give rise to the undesirable side-effects that many modern drugs produce in orthodox medicine, which requires larger doses to be prescribed.

A central principle of homeopathic diagnosis and treatment concerns the signs and symptoms of a disease. Homeopathic practitioners regard them as expressions of the way in which the body itself is endeavoring to combat disease. They see them as positive indications of the body's attempt to maintain the status quo, rather than manifestations of the disease itself, which is the way that other medical systems tend to regard them.

This view of illness leads naturally to the way in which a homeopath looks upon somebody who is ill. Rather than seeing their patients as mere objects, exhibiting particular pathological symptoms, homeopaths look first at the person as a whole. This is because they recognize that, if symptoms reflect the patient's physical response to illness (rather than the illness itself), it is necessary to take account of everything about the patient before the symptoms can be correctly understood. A particular patient may exhibit different signs and symptoms in response to a disease such as a cold at different times. The signs and symptoms depend on the person's age, general health and vitality, previous medical history and even state of mind.

If you have a strong vitality and basic good health, then when you fall ill your body's ability to heal itself is likely to be good. You will quickly throw off the cold or whatever the complaint is. Typically, you experience temporary symptoms indicating that your system is attempting to return to health, but they follow a predictably improving course. This is especially so if you are able to rest, and take other appropriate steps to allow your immune system to do its job.

On the other hand, if you catch a cold when you are already feeling run down and depressed, the composite healing process is far more complicated—resulting in a cold that is much harder to shake off.

According to homeopathic principles, seeking help with this healing process is necessary only when your own self-healing mechanism fails, and is unable to complete the normal process of returning you to your usual state of health. That is when you need homeopathy.

SOURCE:
Richardson, Sarah. *Homeopathy: The Illustrated Guide*. New York: Harmony Books, 1988. pp. 8–9.

HOMEOPATHIC MEDICINES

Many homeopathic remedies now can be purchased in health food stores and corner pharmacies without medical consultation. The Food and Drug Administration, although aware of the surging sales of homeopathic medicines, has not yet examined them for safety and effectiveness.

Homeopathic remedies were permitted to be sold under the Food, Drug and Cosmetic Act of 1938. Since they were considered harmless, they have not been priority items for F.D.A. review. The agency, however, has issued a guide instructing manufacturers to sell only standard homeopathic remedies and restrict to prescription sale remedies intended for treating serious diseases. . . .

Homeopathic medicines are produced by combining an extract with water or water and alcohol in a 1-to-10 dilution. The mixture is vigorously shaken for a prescribed period of time, then diluted again 1 to 10 and shaken. The dilutions and shaking continue until the final solution may have not one molecule remaining of the original extract. This dilution is the usual homeopathic remedy.

How can something diluted this much be effective? Even advocates of homeopathy offer no demonstrable explanation and can only guess at a possible mechanism. The prevailing theory is that the shaking somehow imparts an energy, or "molecular memory," to the dilutant that triggers a therapeutic response.

Most physicians insist that this is nonsense and that solutions lacking active ingredients cannot have anything but a placebo effect.

SOURCE:
Brody, Jane E. "For Those Seeking Homeopathic Treatment or Remedies, a Caution on Course of Action." *The New York Times* 138 (March 2, 1989): B6(N).

EVALUATION OF EFFECTIVENESS OF HOMEOPATHIC REMEDIES

Homeopathic remedies have enjoyed renewed interest in the last 20 years. They're safe, relatively inexpensive, and as accessible as the nearest health food store. But do they work? Three Dutch physicians took this question seriously enough to conduct a comprehensive assessment of 107 published studies, many of which compared people given homeopathic remedies with those given a placebo (dummy pill). Their findings, published recently in the *British Medical Journal* (9 February 1991), indicate that "there is a legitimate case for further evaluation of homeopathy." The homeopathic remedies were shown to be more effective than placebo in the treatment of a variety of common problems, including migraine headaches, dry cough, and ankle sprains. . . .

The University of Limberg investigators, who are all epidemiologists, conducted an exhaustive search of the published medical literature to find evidence of homeopathy's efficacy regardless of implausibility. They found an astonishing 107 controlled studies. Many of them compared a homeopathic remedy with a placebo. While some studies were well designed, the doctors found that the methods used in the majority left much to be desired. But their findings were favorable enough toward homeopathy to suggest further evaluation. . . .

All in all, the University of Limberg investigators found that number of published studies to be impressive. "The amount of positive evidence even among the best studies came as a surprise to us." But they acknowledged that many questions remain. Chief among them is a plausible explanation for how homeopathic remedies work.

SOURCE:
"Homeopathic Remedies: Safe, Inexpensive . . . And They Seem to Work." *HealthFacts* 16, no. 143 (April 1991): 1, 2.

RESOURCES

ORGANIZATIONS

American Institute of Homeopathy. 1500 Massachusetts Ave NW, Washington, DC 20005.

Foundation for Homeopathic Education and Research. 5910 Chabot Crest, Oakland, CA 44018.

Homeopathic Educational Services. 2124 Kittredge Street, Berkeley, CA 94704.

BOOKS

Cummings, Stephen, and Dana Ullman. *Everybody's Guide to Homeopathic Medicines*. New York: St. Martin's, 1991.

Panos, Maesimund, and Jane Heimlich. *Homeopathic Medicine at Home*. Los Angeles: Tarcher, 1980.

RELATED ARTICLES

Arnall, Bradley, and Christina Casteris. "The Great Homeopathy Debate." *East West* 19 (February 1989): 42–47.

Furnham, Adrian, and Chris Smith. "Choosing Alternative Medicine: A Comparison of the Beliefs of Patients Visiting a

General Practitioner and a Homeopath." *Social Science and Medicine* 26, no. 7 (1988): 685–689.

"Homeopathy." *University of California, Berkeley Wellness Letter* (January 1990): 7.

Kleijnen, Jos, Paul Knipschild, and Gerben ter Riet. "Clinical Trials of Homeopathy." *British Medical Journal* 302 (February 9, 1991): 316–323.

HOSPITAL MORTALITY RATES

HCFA (Health Care Financing Administration) Data: 1990

The federal government's latest release of hospital mortality data contains refinements promised last year. But it remains the focus of grumbling by providers still worried that the public will see the statistics as a quality of care proxy. . . .

This is the fourth time HCFA has released statistics on mortality rates of patients treated at specific hospitals. The initial 1986 release angered hospital industry officials, because it came without warning and because they felt the data (released with little explanation) were misunderstood by the media and inaccurately reported to the public.

Patient confusion remains a concern, said John Kelly, MD, director of the AMA Office of Quality Assurance. "Mortality data are easily misinterpreted and are inadequate in judging a hospital's ability to treat patients. Such data should never be used as per se indicators of quality of care provided."

Dr. Wilensky, administrator of HCFA, reiterated that mortality data not be used by themselves as a quality indicator. But she defended the information's public release.

"I think consumers can use these data as a prompter for questions for their physician. The information can be a starting point for a discussion with the physician who is making the admission to a particular hospital."

Dr. Wilensky added that most hospitals performed well in the report. But 161 hospitals had overall death rates more than twice as high as predicted by the HCFA model, and 15 hospitals were labeled "mortality rate outliers" in each of the four data releases.

After the chaos of the first mortality report, subsequent data have been sent to hospitals in advance to brace them for public release. In the last two reports, hospitals have rebutted the data with an accompanying letter.

The advance release to hospitals, the rebuttals and increased explanatory information with the public release have lessened the concern that the data will be misused, said American Hospital Assn. policy expert Tom Granatir.

"One of our biggest concerns initially was that patients would use the raw data in the process of selecting a hospital, but that seems not to be the case," he said. Although the initial release garnered much media coverage, later reports drew less public attention.

Among the refinements in this year's data, Dr. Wilensky said, were shifts in reporting from calendar year to fiscal year; from mortality statistics for a single year to data from the three most recent years; and from deaths only within 30 days of admission to those at 30, 90, and 180 days.

Dr. Wilensky said expanding the reporting term to 180 days was an attempt to get a clearer picture of deaths from diseases that have a longer term of illness. But hospital administrators and quality experts say the new information is misleading.

"Patient deaths as long as 180 days after a hospital admission may be attributable to a variety of factors which have no relation to the quality of care provided during a particular hospital admission," said Dr. Kelly. . . .

Officials are reporting deaths for eight medical conditions and nine surgical procedures for the first time. Former reports had data for 16 diagnostic categories. This change has led to problems, says Granatir. "The data report actual and predicted mortality rates for each condition or procedure, but in many cases the number of cases in a given category is so small there is no confidence level in the expected mortality rate and no way to formulate a standard deviation. But the expected rate is still published alongside the actual rate, and there will be a tendency to compare the two numbers anyway."

Dr. Wilensky said the data were not perfect, but worthwhile. "This information is a valuable resource for the health care community, but especially for hospital administrators and medical staffs as they evaluate the quality of care in their facilities," she said.

SOURCE:
McCormick, Brian, and Laurie Jones. "Mortality Data, Round 4: HCFA's Refined Information Still Found Lacking." *American Medical News* (May 13, 1991): 27–28.

CONDITIONS AND PROCEDURES INCLUDED IN HCFA DATA

Mortality data to be released by the Health Care Financing Administration this spring will contain 30-, 90-, and 180-day mortality rates at every U.S. hospital for the following:

- **All Causes** (overall number)
- **Conditions**
  Acute myocardial infarction
  Congestive heart failure
  Pneumonia/influenza
  Chronic obstructive pulmonary disease
  Transient cerebral ischemia
  Stroke
  Hip fracture
  Sepsis
- **Procedures**
  Angioplasty
  Coronary artery bypass graft
  Initial pacemaker insertion
  Carotid endarterectomy
  Hip replacement/reconstruction
  Open reduction of hip fracture
  Prostatectomy
  Cholecystectomy
  Hysterectomy

SOURCE:
McCormick, Brian. "HCFA Refining Hospital Mortality Data: Providers: New Methods Still Flawed." *American Medical News* 34 (January 21, 1991): 36.

DATA INTERPRETATION

Wheeling, W.Va., has two hospitals: Ohio Valley Medical Center with 473 beds, and Wheeling Hospital, with 275. In 1988, 20.4 percent of the cancer patients over age 65 admitted to Ohio Valley Medical Center died. At Wheeling Hospital, 28.1 percent did. Not a big enough difference, by itself, to affect a cancer patient's choice. But 30.3 percent of the patients who came to Ohio Valley Medical Center with serious metabolic disorders such as diabetes died—more than three times Wheeling's rate. Such differences are not uncommon, and prospective patients should seek an explanation. "As a teaching hospital, we usually see much sicker diabetes patients," says Gary Colberg, Ohio Valley's chief operating officer.

The statistics on death rates in hospitals are available to anyone and are one measure of performance worth taking. Since 1986, the Federal Health Care Financing Administration (HCFA) has published annually its multivolume Medicare Hospital Mortality Information, a compilation of data about the death rates of medicare beneficiaries at about 6,000 U.S. hospitals. You can get the volume for your region, free, by calling (301) 966-1133. The rates, calculated on the percentage of patients who died within 30 days of admission, are broken down for 16 different causes of death. They are stacked up against a "predicted" death rate, which is derived from a formula that takes into account such factors as a hospital's mix of patients and—since death rates for many diseases vary by region—its location.

Experts generally agree that mortality rates should be read as only one barometer of quality. The hospital industry argues that the data do not adequately account for the population of sicker patients in some hospitals—teaching institutions and inner-city hospitals, for example—patients who will die in greater proportions no matter how expert their care. Smaller hospitals that treat relatively few patients with a given disease can have widely varying records from year to year based on chance alone. In the case of the Ohio Valley Medical Center, for example, deaths from metabolic disorders in 1987 and 1986 were half the 1988 rate. In 1987, Wheeling Hospital's rate was twice Ohio Valley Medical Center's. The data should be used as a source of pointed questions for your doctor: Why is the mortality rate of patients with your illness high? Or, why has it fluctuated from one year to the next?

The chief flaw in the data is that the range of predicted death rates is sometimes too broad to be useful. At Philadelphia's John F. Kennedy Memorial Hospital, for example, 12 of 48 people who were treated for cancer in 1988 died—a death rate of 25 percent. The predicted range of deaths for cancer patients: 12.5 to 46 percent. When only a handful of patients with a condition have been treated, the predicted range is given as 0–100 percent. Consumers should therefore look warily at hospitals whose actual death rates fall at the high end of the predicted range—especially when the rates tend toward the upper limits in more than one year. The HCFA volumes released during 1989 give data for the years 1986, 1987, and 1988.

Besides red-flagging a hospital, the data can help you spot institutions that consistently do better than predicted rates in a particular specialty. Several hospitals noted for cancer treatment, including M.D. Anderson Cancer Center in Houston and Roswell Park Cancer Institute in Buffalo, N.Y., for example, had lower-than-expected 1988 death rates due to cancer. Since the report stops short of breaking out results for different forms of cancer, however, this information, too, must be interpreted with care.

SOURCE:

Findlay, Steven. "What Mortality Rates Don't Tell You." *U.S. News & World Report* (April 30, 1990): 54–55.

RESOURCES

ORGANIZATIONS

American Hospital Association. 840 N. Lake Shore Dr., Chicago, IL 60611.

American Medical Association. Office of Quality Assurance, 535 N. Dearborn St., Chicago, IL 60610.

Health Care Financing Administration. 200 Independence Ave. SW, Washington, DC 20201.

RELATED ARTICLES

Berwick, Donald M., and David L. Wald. "Hospital Leaders' Opinions of the HCFA Mortality Data." *JAMA* 263 (January 12, 1990): 247.

"Death Rates Found High in Hospitals." *New York Times* (May 2, 1991).

Green, Jesse, Neil Wintfeld, and others. " The Importance of Severity of Illness in Assessing Hospital Mortality." *JAMA* 263 (January 12, 1990): 241.

McCormick, Brian. "Hospitals Find Inclusion on HCFA 'Hit List' Damaging." *AMA News* (May 27, 1991): 1, 30.

Park, Rolla Edward, Robert H. Brook, and others. "Explaining Variations in Hospital Death Rates: Randomness, Severity of Illness, Quality of Care." *JAMA* 264 (July 25, 1990): 484.

HYSTERECTOMY

(*See also:* UTERINE FIBROIDS)

OVERVIEW

Hysterectomy is the surgical removal of the uterus. . .

The uterus, or womb, is a pear-shaped, muscular organ that lies behind the urinary bladder, in front of the rectum, and above the vagina. It is connected to the vagina through the cervix, or neck, and it connects with the abdominal cavity through the fallopian tubes. The uterus serves four main functions: to prepare for the reception of a fertilized egg, to nurture and support the embryo during its development, to expel the baby when it has matured and is ready to be born, and, when a woman is not pregnant, to allow the egg, or ovum, that is produced on a monthly basis by one of her ovaries to pass into the fallopian tubes and out through the uterus to the vagina. Menstruation occurs approximately two weeks later if there is no pregnancy.

Symptoms and Conditions Necessitating Hysterectomy

There are a number of conditions that may lead your doctor to recommend hysterectomy.

1. Fibroid tumors. Fibroid tumors are the most common indication for hysterectomy, but there are two important facts to remember. First, if a fibroid tumor is present but you have no symptoms, you may not need to have an operation. Second, experts are of the opinion that fibroid tumors rarely turn into cancer. If you have a fibroid tumor and no symptoms, however, it is a good idea to see your doctor regularly so that he or she can keep close watch on the tumor and make sure that it does not begin to change rapidly.

The most frequently encountered symptoms caused by fibroid tumors that would indicate a need to have a hysterectomy are: intermittent, persistent, or uncontrollable uterine bleeding from the vagina; severe abdominal pain; a rapidly growing mass; and ongoing or increasing interference with bladder and bowel functions.

Fibroid tumors also can be the cause of sterility or repeated miscarriages. If you are anxious to preserve your ability to have children, your surgeon may propose that you undergo a myomectomy rather than a hysterectomy. In this operation, the fibroid tumor is "shelled out," leaving the uterus intact. Of course, your doctor will recommend the operation that he or she believes would be best for you based on your physical condition, your age, and your symptoms.

2. Excessive uterine bleeding. Some women experience persistent uterine bleeding that is not associated with fibroid tumors and that cannot be controlled by curettage—the scraping of the interior of the uterus with a surgical instrument called a curette. Conditions causing severe menopausal bleeding include hormone imbalances and a condition called adenomyosis in which the lining of the uterus has penetrated into the wall of the uterus, causing the heavy bleeding and sometimes severe cramps.

3. Precancerous conditions. If you have not gone through menopause and you experience persistent uterine bleeding, your doctor may recommend that you undergo diagnostic curettage. In this procedure, the surgeon will scrape out the interior of your uterus with a curette and send the tissue to a pathologist to be examined microscopically. If the pathologist finds cells that are precancerous—that is, they have the possibility of becoming cancerous—your doctor may advise you to have a hysterectomy so that you can avoid the possibility of developing cancer.

4. Cancer of the uterus. Although cancer may affect both the cervix and the body of the uterus, it is important to remember that in many cases it can be treated successfully, especially if it is detected in its early stages. The early stages of cancer of the cervix, which can be detected through routine Papanicolaou, or "pap" smears, can be treated by an extensive operation called a radical hysterectomy; in that operation, the surgeon removes all the pelvic organs and the surrounding lymph nodes and lymph channels. In other cases, cervical cancer is best treated with radium and X ray or with both radiation and surgical intervention. Cancer of the body of the uterus, which is most commonly found in older women, may cause abnormal bleeding shortly before or after menopause; sometimes it may cause sudden bleeding years after a woman has gone through menopause. This is a most important symptom and should never be ignored. In treating cancer of the body of the uterus, the surgeon removes both the body and the cervix of the uterus and possibly both ovaries and fallopian tubes.

5. Postdelivery hysterectomy. Although it does not happen very frequently, it occasionally may become necessary for the surgeon to remove the uterus just after a woman has given birth. A hysterectomy may be performed in this case if a large tear in the new mother's uterus has resulted in a life-endangering hemorrhage or if the afterbirth is in a diseased condition. Sometimes a surgeon may recommend a hysterectomy for a woman who has had several deliveries by cesarean section and whose uterus, as a result, has become impossible to repair or is in such a weakened condition that it would be dangerous for her to have more children.

About the Operation

Hysterectomy is one of the safest abdominal operations and is considered to have a low risk in otherwise healthy individuals.

Most often, the operation is performed through an incision a few inches long in the lower abdomen. Some surgeons use a vertical incision (top to bottom), while others prefer a horizontal (sometimes called a "bikini") incision just above the pubic hairline. A surgeon may also elect to perform a vaginal hysterectomy, which is the removal of the uterus through the vagina. The kind of hysterectomy your doctor recommends will depend on the condition of your organs. If your doctor recommends a total hysterectomy, he or she will remove the body and cervix of your uterus. Depending on your age, the condition of your ovaries, and the primary reason for the hysterectomy, your surgeon may not have to remove your ovaries. However, if either your tubes or your ovaries must be removed, your surgeon may also suggest that you have a hysterectomy, because the uterus serves no purpose without the ovaries and can develop problems such as abnormal bleeding or cancer.

You should know that your ability to have sexual intercourse will not be affected, and you will be able to resume sexual relations following the recovery period specified by your surgeon. You will, however, no longer be able to become pregnant.

Recovering from the Operation

In uncomplicated situations, the hospital stay following hysterectomy is five to 10 days. During the operation, a catheter, or tube, will be inserted into your bladder either through your urethra or through a small incision in the abdomen. The catheter will allow you to pass urine and usually will be removed the morning after your operation.

Having a hysterectomy does not necessarily bring on menopause, because menopause occurs when the ovaries cease to function and has nothing to do with the removal of the uterus. Thus, if one or both ovaries are left in place, menopause will not occur, although menstruation will cease.

Most patients experience no complications following the operation and can resume normal activities within four to six weeks.

SOURCE:

American College of Surgeons. *About Hysterectomy (Surgical Removal of the Uterus)*. n.d. pp. 1-6.

INCIDENCE

This year nearly 600,000 American women will undergo a hysterectomy, or removal of the uterus. About 45% of them will be castrated, the medical term for removing the ovaries—a practice that continues despite accumulating evidence that it may do more harm than good. Today, one American woman in three has had a hysterectomy by age 60. The number of operations totaled 578,000 in 1988, the last year for which data are available, and the influx of baby boom women into the 35-to-44 age range—when most hysterectomies are done—may soon mean more surgery than ever before. Using 1987 figures, the National Center for Health Statistics (NCHS) projects 783,000 operations in 1995 and 824,000 in 2005. Hysterectomy is now the second most frequent major operation for women in the U.S. Fibroid tumors and endometriosis account for half the operations. But there is increasing evidence that hysterectomy can lead to a variety of medical problems, including bone-mass loss, depression and loss of sexual desire. Although two states have laws requiring doctors to inform women of hysterectomy's health consequences and alternative procedures, the statutes may protect doctors more than patients. . . .

Are 600,000 hysterectomies a year really necessary? A look at the geographical data suggests that many women could be spared. Compared with women living in the Northeast, women are 78% more likely to have a hysterectomy if they live in the South; 41% more likely if they live in the Midwest; and 20% more likely if they live in the West. And the rate of hysterectomy in Great Britain is half that of the U.S.—with American women showing no health gains from this more aggressive treatment. According to Dr. Ruth Schwartz, a member of an American College of Obstetricians and Gynecologists (ACOG) task force on hysterectomy, European doctors do relatively few hysterectomies for "quality of life"—that is, on women with persistent discomfort or bleeding that isn't health threatening.

There are also local variations. An ongoing study in Maine has found striking differences in hysterectomy rates from community to community. The researchers attribute the disparities to different surgical styles. A 1988 New York State Department of Health study found similar differences in hysterectomy rates from county to county, with rates lowest in and around New York City. Rates for nonwhites throughout the state were 39% higher than for whites. The report also found 3.5% of the physicians surveyed did 100 or more hysterectomies each during the course of the three-year study, whereas the average for the state's physicians was 21 hysterectomies over the three years.

The American College of Obstetricians and Gynecologists task force attributed the geographical disparities partly to regional differences in gynecologists' training. Financial motives on the part of surgeons can't be discounted: Fewer hysterectomies are done under prepaid health plans than when doctors are directly compensated for surgery.

SOURCE:

Dranov, P. "An Unkind Cut." *American Health* (September 1990): 36, 39.

TYPES OF HYSTERECTOMY

There are several different hysterectomy techniques.

Total abdominal hysterectomy (TAH): Removal of the uterus and cervix through an incision in the lower abdomen. The fallopian tubes and ovaries are not removed.

Total abdominal hysterectomy and bilateral salpingo-oophorectomy (TAH and BSO): Removal of the ovaries (oophorectomy) and fallopian tubes (salpingectomy) along with the uterus and cervix through an incision in the lower abdomen.

"Complete Hysterectomy": A lay term sometimes used for removal of the ovaries in addition to the uterus, fallopian tubes, and cervix. "Complete hysterectomy" is the same as TAH and BSO.

Vaginal Hysterectomy: Removal of the uterus and cervix through an incision inside the vagina. The fallopian tubes and ovaries are usually not removed.

Subtotal hysterectomy: Removal of the uterus but not the cervix. The fallopian tubes and ovaries are not removed. This procedure is rarely used today except in emergency situations when the additional time and surgery steps needed for removal of the cervix are inadvisable because the woman's medical condition is so poor. Under normal circumstances most surgeons recommend total hysterectomy because they feel the cervix has no essential functions when the uterus is not present, and does pose a future risk of cervical cancer. However, this operation may become more popular in the future. In some situations, removal of the cervix is not an essential goal and Pap testing can provide good protection against future cervical cancer risk. The cervix plays a role in female sexuality, and its removal in "total" hysterectomy also involves some shortening of the vagina and may make intercourse uncomfortable for some women.

Pelvic repair (vaginal repair): Surgery to improve muscle and fibrous tissue support for the bladder and/or rectum. Pelvic repair may correct the vaginal bulges, cystocele and/or retocele that are caused by lax support of the bladder and/or rectum adjacent to the vaginal walls. Depending on the structural abnormalities that need correction, pelvic repair may involve abdominal and/or vaginal incisions that allow the surgeon to carry out one of the many surgical techniques developed for this purpose. The uterus is often removed at the time of repair, and in some cases the tubes and ovaries as well.

SOURCE:

Stewart, F. H., and F. Guest. *Understanding Your Body: Every Woman's Guide to a Lifetime of Health.* New York: Bantam, 1987. p. 862.

ALTERNATIVES

Despite all the talk these days about unnecessary hysterectomies, University of Michigan gynecologist George Morley, M.D., believes the number of hysterectomies has remained stable over the past 10 years—and that most are performed for good reason.

When the diagnosis is cancer, the issue is usually clear-cut. Removal of the uterus is necessary for uterine and ovarian malignancies and for advanced, invasive cervical cancer. (Early, non-invasive cervical cancers usually are treated by removing a small portion of the cervix while leaving the uterus intact.)

But some physicians come to a parting of the ways regarding hysterectomy for benign conditions. A small but vocal group claims as many as 90% of hysterectomies could be avoided and that the uterus should be removed only under the strictest of circumstances. (The U.S. Centers for Disease Control places the number of questionable operations at about 15%.)

This group promotes a variety of alternative procedures loosely grouped under the heading *female reconstructive surgery.* These procedures include removing fibroid tumors while saving the uterus, using lasers and/or drugs to eliminate non-malignant overgrowth of endometrial tissue and restoring a prolapsed uterus by rebuilding ligaments and repositioning organs.

But many gynecologists insist that female reconstructive surgery is nothing more than a fancy label for some techniques that have been performed for years and for others that are too experimental to be used at all outside a research setting.

For women troubled by excessive menstrual bleeding, laser destruction of the uterine lining can be a good alternative to hysterectomy. But if the diagnosis is *endometrial hyperplasia,* a form of uterine tissue overgrowth that can be pre-cancerous, the laser technique is too experimental, says Dr. Morley, who heads up a hysterectomy task force for the American College of Obstetricians and Gynecologists.

And though drug therapy has a role in treating fibroid tumors, drugs alone won't solve the problem. Powerful hormonal treatments can shrink uterine fibroids, but the drugs can have distressing side effects and tumors re-grow as soon as therapy is stopped. The drugs most helpful in shrinking large fibroids down to a size where they can be surgically removed through a *myomectomy* (a procedure that cuts away the tumors while leaving the uterus intact).

Myomectomy is usually reserved for younger women who may still want children. It's a bloodier operation than hysterectomy—and thus more patients require transfusions—and the risk of infection is higher. But if you're not ready to close to door on childbirth, you should ask your doctor whether myomectomy is an option. Similarly, women with endometriosis who still want to have children can be treated with laser surgery, cauterization and/or drugs.

As with any major surgery, if your doctor recommends hysterectomy, you should ask about alternative treatments and get a second opinion. Except in the case of malignancy or uncontrollable hemorrhage, hysterectomy is rarely an emergency procedure. Take time to explore the options. Make sure you understand why you need the operation, what it entails and what the possible complications are.

SOURCE:
"Hysterectomy: When is it Really Necessary?" *University of Texas Lifetime Health Letter* 1, no. 8 (September 1989): 4.

RESOURCES

ORGANIZATIONS
American College of Obstetricians and Gynecologists. 409 12th St. SW, Washington, DC 20024.

HERS Foundation (Hysterectomy Educational Resources and Services). 422 Bryn Mawr Avenue, Bala Cynwyd, PA 19004.

National Women's Health Network. 1325 E Street NW, Washington, DC 20005.

PAMPHLET
American College of Obstetricians and Gynecologists:

Understanding Hysterectomy. 1987.

BOOKS
Culter, Winnifred B. *Hysterectomy: After—A Comprehensive Guide to Preventing, Preparing for, and Maximizing Health after Hysterectomy*. New York: Harper & Row, 1988.

Hufnagel, V. *No More Hysterectomies*. New York: New American Library, 1989.

Morgan, L. *Coping with Hysterectomy: Your Own Choice, Your Own Solutions*. New York: New American Library, 1985.

Page, L. *How to Avoid a Hysterectomy: An Indispensable Guide to Exploring All Your Options*. New York: Random House, 1987.

RELATED ARTICLES
Gambone, J. C., J. B. Lench, and others. "Validation of Hysterectomy Indications and the Quality Assurance Process." *Obstetrics and Gynecology* 73, no. 6 (June 1989): 1045–1049.

"Hysterectomy and Its Alternatives." *Consumer Reports* (September 1990): 603–607.

Loffer, F. D. "Hysteroscopy with Selective Endometrial Sampling Compared with D&C for Abnormal Uterine Bleeding: The Value of a Negative Hysteroscopic View." *Obstetrics & Gynecology* 73, no. 1 (January 1989): 16–20.

Pokras, R., and V. G. Hufnagel. "Hysterectomy in the United States, 1965–84." *American Journal of Public Health* 78, no. 7 (July 1988): 852.

IMMUNE SYSTEM AND AUTOIMMUNE DISEASES

(*See also:* ACQUIRED IMMUNE DEFICIENCY SYNDROME [AIDS])

OVERVIEW

Every second of every day, the body engages in a fight for its life. It is constantly resisting assaults by enemies ranging from infectious organisms to harmful chemicals to cancerous cells. Fortunately, if healthy, it has the means to win these battles—the white blood cells and protein molecules of the immune system.

Phagocytes give the immunologic army much of its destructive force. (Their name means "eater cells.") The two chief types are neutrophils, short-lived fighters designed for the quick attack; and macrophages ("big eaters"), slower cells which wipe out invaders missed by neutrophils and which clean up the debris left after the battle.

These cells are the immune system's soldiers. They do combat with foreign invaders, attaching to them, killing them with toxic chemicals, and digesting them with proteins known as enzymes.

Some phagocytes, the Ia positive macrophages, also convey important information about the enemy to other blood cells called lymphocytes, which serve not only as fighters but as strategists, commanders and munitions manufacturers in the war against disease.

One of the two most important kinds of lymphocytes is the T cell. It gets its name from the thymus, an organ in the chest which influences its development.

T cells perform a vital role in health—ridding the body of diseased or abnormal cells. An example would be a respiratory cell in which a virus is reproducing. The T cell has the unique ability to recognize on the surface of the infected cell both the foreign characteristics (antigens) of the enemy and special molecules that identify the respiratory cell as a part of the body. These "self" molecules are called major histocompatibility (MHC) proteins.

Having selected the virus-containing respiratory cell for destruction, the T cell also makes sure that the job gets done. It may signal a cytotoxic T cell to divide and produce a battalion of other warriors like itself which will attack directly.

Or the T cell may get phagocytes to do the actual killing, using messenger proteins known as lymphokines to command them into action. An example of a lymphokine that stimulates macrophages is interferon. By means of such powerful chemicals, different types of lymphocytes control many immunologic events. For instance, by releasing particular lymphokines, helper T cells facilitate and suppressor T cells curb the action of the other major kind of lymphocyte, the B cell.

This blood cell is named after the organ which controls its development in birds, the Bursa of Fabricius. The part of the human body in which B lymphocytes begin to learn their special role, the equivalent of the thymus for T cells, has not yet been identified.

The ultimate mission of B cells is to eliminate enemies outside of cells. An example would be virus organisms that have multiplied in a respiratory cell, have burst the cell, and are circulating in the body seeking other healthy cells to invade.

The B cell recognizes a virus particle as a member of a particular enemy force with the help of an antibody, a highly sensitive "scout" molecule on its surface.

When stimulated by lymphokines released by a helper T cell, the B cell grows into a plasma cell, a factory turning out great numbers of identical antibodies. These patrol the blood stream, zero in on the viruses, and hook precisely into their antigens, signalling that the invaders must be destroyed.

This antibody-antigen linkage sets off still another important element of the immune system, a group of eleven proteins collectively known as complement. (The name derives from the fact that these molecules "complete" antibody's action.) In chain-reaction fashion, each of these protein molecules activates one or more others. This complicated, multi-part operation culminates when the last two complement components damage or destroy the target.

Complement, which is manufactured by macrophages, serves other important roles in the body's defense as well. It increases permeability of blood vessels so phagocytes can easily get to the battle site, attracts the fighter cells to the area, and gets them to join the fray. It sometimes may be able to respond directly to antigens, bypassing the usual activation by antibody.

Antibodies and complement exist as part of the fluids (or "humors") of the body, so the type of defensive campaign in which these molecules predominate is referred to as humoral immunity. The immunologic process involving mainly T lymphocytes and phagocytes is known as cellular immunity.

Scientists still are identifying the different parts of the immune system and learning what they do. For example, they are studying important classes of lymphocytes other than T and B cells such as the natural killer (NK) lymphocytes, which play a role in the body's defense against viruses and tumor cells.

SOURCE:
National Jewish Center for Immunology and Respiratory Medicine. *Understanding Immunology*. 1985. pp. 1-2.

STRATEGY AND TACTICS OF THE IMMUNE SYSTEM

Bringing all these forces to bear against an enemy requires both a grand strategy and ingenious tactics. Suppose, for example, that *Salmonella* bacteria have hitched a ride on your lunch. As the invaders make their way into the body, they scatter bits of themselves—antigens that can be recognized as foreign by the right lymphocyte. On their scavenging rounds, macrophages pick up these pieces of molecular debris and carry them about, rather like banners.

If you are resistant to this infection, the macrophage will soon, literally, bump into a T cell that recognizes this antigen. The T cell raises the alarm, emitting a shower of signaling chemicals, and the antibody response swings into action. The appropriate B cells, alerted by the signal, start churning out antibody, which makes its way through the bloodstream to the enemy. Appropriate T cells gather, to coordinate operations and give the B cells appropriate help. Complement molecules also converge and, in so doing, call in the macrophage clean-up squad. The antibody tackles the invaders, trying to pierce their outer membranes and disperse their fluids. The macrophages, spurred on by the complement, attempt to gobble the enemies up. Once the combined defensive forces have the intruders on the run, suppressor T cells give the all-clear, the immune response slows, and the system returns to its customary state of watchful readiness.

If the invader is a virus, however, a different strategy comes into play. These wily enemies work under cover and from within; they infiltrate the body's cells and commandeer them into producing more viruses. When a cold virus enters your body, for example, the immune system's task is to find and destroy "self" cells gone haywire. The same holds true when cells have become cancerous. The defending immune system must recognize both these types of turncoat cells by antibodies carried on their outer surfaces. Two classes of troops undertake the attack: (1) natural killer cells, lone hunters that roam the body on search-and-destroy missions; and (2) killer cells, T cells turned into killers under orders of a lymphokine called interleukin.

Given the crucial position of the T cells in both sounding the alarm and organizing the battle, a person without a proper T cell defense is clearly open to all kinds of dangerous diseases. And that is precisely what happens in AIDS (acquired immune deficiency syndrome). The AIDS virus kills T4 lymphocytes, which play a central role in initiating and coordinating the immune response. In ways not yet fully understood, the virus apparently also disables macrophages, leaving the body defenseless against the cancers and infectious diseases that eventually prove fatal to those with the disease.

SOURCE:
Burge, B. "The Immune System: Your Body's Department of Defense." *Healthline* (November 1990): 4-5.

DISORDERS OF THE IMMUNE SYSTEM—AUTOIMMUNE DISORDERS

The most common types of allergic reactions—hay fever, some kinds of asthma, and hives—are produced when the immune system responds to a false alarm. In a susceptible person, a normally harmless substance—grass pollen or house dust, for example—is perceived as a threat and is attacked. . . .

Sometimes the immune system's recognition apparatus breaks down, and the body begins to manufacture antibodies and T cells directed against the body's own constituents—cells, cell components, or specific organs. Such antibodies are known as autoantibodies, and the diseases they produce are called autoimmune diseases. (Not all autoantibodies are harmful; some types appear to be integral to the immune system's regulatory scheme.)

Autoimmune reactions contribute to many enigmatic diseases. For instance, autoantibodies to red blood cells can cause anemia, autoantibodies to pancreas cells contribute to juvenile diabetes, and autoantibodies to nerve and muscle cells are found in patients with the chronic muscle weakness known as myasthenia gravis. Autoantibody known as rheumatoid factor is common in persons with rheumatoid arthritis.

Persons with systemic lupus erythematosus (SLE), whose symptoms encompass many systems, have antibodies to many types of cells and cellular components. . . .

No one knows just what causes an autoimmune disease, but several factors are likely to be involved. These may include viruses and environmental factors such as exposure to sunlight, certain chemicals, and some drugs, all of which may damage or alter body cells so that they are no longer recognizable as self. Sex hormones may be important, too, since most autoimmune diseases are far more common in women than in men. . . .

Many types of therapies are being used to combat autoimmune diseases. These include corticosteroids, immunosuppressive drugs developed as anticancer agents, radiation of the lymph nodes, and plasmapheresis, a sort of "blood washing" that removes diseased cells and harmful molecules from the circulation.

SOURCE:
National Institutes of Health. Schindler, Lydia Woods. *Understanding the Immune System.* NIH Pub. No. 90-529. 1990. pp. 20-21.

IMMUNODEFICIENCY DISEASES

Lack of one or more components of the immune system results in immunodeficiency disorders. These can be inherited, acquired through infection or other illness, or produced as an inadvertent side effect of certain drug treatments.

People with advanced cancer may experience immune deficiencies as a result of the disease process or from extensive anticancer therapy. Transient immune deficiencies can develop in the wake of common viral infections, including influenza, infectious mononucleosis, and measles. Immune responsiveness can also be depressed by blood transfusions, surgery, malnutrition, and stress.

Some children are born with defects in their immune systems. Those with flaws in the B cell components are unable to produce antibodies (immunoglobulins). These conditions, known as agammaglobulinemias or hypogammaglobulinemias, leave the children vulnerable to infectious organisms; such disorders can be combatted with injections of immunoglobulins.

Other children, whose thymus is either missing or small and abnormal, lack T cells. The resultant disorders have been treated with thymic transplants.

Very rarely, infants are born lacking all the major immune defenses; this is known as severe combined immunodeficiency disease (SCID). Some children with SCID have lived for years in germ-free rooms and "bubbles." A few SCID patients have been successfully treated with transplants of bone marrow.

The devastating immunodeficiency disorder known as the acquired immunodeficiency syndrome (AIDS) was first recognized in 1981. Caused by a virus (the human immunodeficiency virus, or HIV) that destroys T4 cells and that is harbored in macrophages as well as T4 cells, AIDS is characterized by a variety of unusual infections and otherwise rare cancers. The AIDS virus also damages tissue of the brain and spinal cord, producing progressive dementia.

SOURCE:
National Institutes of Health. Schindler, Lydia Woods. *Understanding the Immune System.* NIH Pub. No. 90-529. 1990. p. 23.

IMMUNODEFICIENCY AND TRANSPLANTS

Since organ transplantation was introduced over a quarter of a century ago, it has become a widespread remedy for life-threatening disease. Several thousand kidney transplants are performed each year in the United States alone. In addition, physicians have succeeded in transplanting the heart, lungs, liver, and pancreas.

The success of a transplant—whether it is accepted or rejected—depends on the stubbornness of the immune system. For a transplant to "take," the body of the recipient must be made to suppress its natural tendency to get rid of foreign tissue.

Scientists have tackled this problem in two ways. The first is to make sure that the tissue of the donor and the recipient are as similar as possible. Tissue typing, or histocompatibility testing, involves matching the markers of self on body tissues; because the typing is usually done on white blood cells, or leukocytes, the markers are referred to as human leukocyte antigens (HLA). . . .

The second approach to taming rejection is to lull the recipient's immune system. This can be achieved through a variety of powerful immunosuppressive drugs. Steroids suppress lymphocyte function; the drug cyclosporine holds down the production of the lymphokine interleukin-2, which is necessary for T cell growth. When such measures fail, the graft may yet be saved with a new treatment: OKT3 is a monoclonal antibody that seeks out the T3 marker carried on all mature T cells. By either destroying T cells or incapacitating them, OKT3 can bring an acute rejection crisis to a halt.

Not surprisingly, any such all-out assault on the immune system leaves a transplant recipient susceptible to both opportunistic infections and lymphomas. Although such patients need careful medical follow-up, many of them are able to lead active and essentially normal lives.

SOURCE:
National Institutes of Health. Schindler, Lydia Woods. *Understanding the Immune System.* NIH Pub. No. 90-529. 1990. p. 25.

RESOURCES

RELATED ARTICLES

Haddy, R. I. "Aging, Infections, and the Immune System." *The Journal of Family Practice* 27, no. 4 (October 1988): 409–413.

Marwick, C. "As Immune System Yields Its Secrets, New Strategies Against Disease Emerge." *JAMA* 262, no. 20 (November 24, 1989): 2786–2787.

Nakamura, R. M., and W. L. Binder. "Current Concepts and Diagnostic Evaluation of Autoimmune Disease." *Archives of Pathology and Laboratory Medicine* 112, no. 9 (September 1988): 869–877.

Nossal, G. J. V. "The Basic Components of the Immune System." *The New England Journal of Medicine* 316, no. 21 (May 21, 1987): 1320–1325.

IN VITRO FERTILIZATION

OVERVIEW

For hundreds of thousands of years, there was only one way to make a baby, at least for humans. Either it worked or it didn't, and if it didn't there was little anyone could do about it. All that has changed dramatically. The growing problems of infertility—exacerbated by a generation of would-be parents who put off having babies until their 30s and 40s—and the early successes of in-vitro ("test tube") fertilization have laid the groundwork for a revolution in reproductive technology. Hardly a week goes by without news of a breakthrough to help nature take its course. [Fall 1990] produced two such announcements: one offers new hope to women with blocked Fallopian tubes; the other promises to extend women's fertility beyond their prime childbearing years—even past menopause.

Of all the barriers to pregnancy, menopause, which shuts down the release of eggs from the ovaries, was long considered the most insurmountable. But though the ovaries may shrivel like raisins, the other reproductive organs of postmenopausal women are still viable. These women can now become pregnant using someone else's eggs, according to a remarkable report in last week's *New England Journal of Medicine.* A team led by Dr. Mark Sauer of the University of Southern California impregnated six of seven postmenopausal women, ages 40 to 44, using eggs that were taken from younger women and fertilized with sperm from the older women's husbands. Four of these prematurely menopausal women gave birth to healthy offspring, one miscarried, and one had a stillborn baby—an outcome that Sauer said would have been considered normal with six younger women.

"The limits on the childbearing years are now anyone's guess," wrote Dr. Marcia Angell in an accompanying editorial. Theoretically, donor eggs could allow women whose ovaries have stopped functioning to bear children into their late 40s and 50s. Researchers believe that the new technique will have the biggest impact on women in their 40s who have not yet reached menopause but have failed to conceive. The new findings suggest that these women may be infertile not because their uteruses are too old but because their ovaries are, and that with eggs donated by younger women their chances of getting pregnant may be as good as those of the young women themselves. The hitch is, of course, that the children developing from such eggs have the genes of the female donor and are genetically unrelated to the mother who bears them—a fact that presents both legal and ethical problems as yet unresolved.

The other report . . . focuses attention on the Fallopian tubes, the narrow passages that carry eggs from the ovaries to the uterus. Women whose tubes are clogged with scar tissue or other obstructions cannot conceive by natural means because their eggs have no way of getting to the womb. In the past, such women had to undergo surgery to have their tubes cleared. Now the problem can be overcome in a doctor's office, according to an article in the *Journal of the American Medical Association.* With a tiny balloon similar to those used to clear blocked arteries, scientists were able to unclog the fallopian tubes in 64 of 77 women, 22 became pregnant within a year. Dr. Edmond Confino, who pioneered the technique at Mount Sinai Hospital Medical Center in Chicago, estimates that it could help nearly one-third of the 1 million American women who suffer from blocked tubes.

The new methods join an array of novel techniques that seem to multiply faster than test-tube babies. Most are variations on the pioneering procedure known as in-vitro fertilization [IVF]. In IVF, eggs are removed from the ovaries, mixed with sperm in a laboratory dish, allowed to develop into embryos and then inserted into the uterus. The technique has produced 20,000 offspring since 1978.

But even at well-run clinics, the original IVF procedure fails 75% to 85% of the time. The biggest snag comes when the embryo is inserted in the uterus, an operation that can be very disruptive to the womb. As a result, such embryos often fail to take root, or implant.

To increase the chances of implantation, many doctors are now inserting egg and sperm into the Fallopian tube, a procedure known as GIFT (for gamete intra-Fallopian transfer). Fertilization takes place not in a laboratory dish but in the Fallopian tube, as it would naturally, and the resulting embryo drifts gently into the uterus, where it is much more likely to be successfully received. In yet another variation, called ZIFT (for zygote intra-Fallopian transfer), the sperm are allowed to fertilize the eggs before transfer to the Fallopian tube. The advantage: only those eggs that are successfully fertilized need be transferred.

GIFT and ZIFT have turned out to be breakthrough procedures. Some doctors who have switched from standard IVF to the new techniques have doubled their success rates, which now approach 50%. As the odds have improved, the demand for IVF has surged, despite the high cost (up to $8,000 a try) and the uneven quality of the clinics offering the service.

SOURCE:
Elmer-Dewitt, Philip. "A Revolution in Making Babies: New Techniques Help Childless Couples—Even After Menopause." *Time* (November 5, 1990): 76–77.

DEFINITION OF TERMS

In vitro fertilization (IVF): In this procedure, a woman's eggs are retrieved and combined with sperm to fertilize in the laboratory. Any fertilized eggs, called embryos, are returned to the uterus.

The steps involved in IVF are:

Step 1 Egg Stimulation

Step 2 Egg Retrieval

Step 3 Fertilization

Step 4 Embryo Transfer

If all goes well, the next two steps are:

Step 5 Clinical Pregnancy

Step 6 Live Birth

Gamete intrafallopian transfer (GIFT): This procedure differs from IVF in that retrieved eggs and sperm are injected into a woman's fallopian tubes where fertilization can take place.

Because fertilization does not take place outside the body, there is no embryo transfer step in GIFT.

Egg Stimulation: This refers to the administration of fertility drugs to a woman to "stimulate" and increase egg production.

Egg Retrieval: This process involves the removal of an egg or eggs from the ovaries and follicles for subsequent fertilization through IVF or GIFT.

Fertilization: The retrieved egg is mixed with sperm, after which the egg becomes fertilized and forms what then becomes an embryo.

Embryo Transfer: After an egg and sperm fertilize in the laboratory, the newly formed embryo is transferred to the uterus.

Clinical Pregnancy: This is a pregnancy which has been confirmed by ultrasound or other clinical means. Prior to this point, a blood test or a urinary pregnancy test *may* indicate a pregnancy. Such tests look for human chorionic gonadotropin or hCG. If the blood or urinary tests indicate a positive reading, then the pregnancy is referred to as a "chemical pregnancy." Infertility service providers generally do not accept chemical pregnancies as anything more than an indicator because conditions other than pregnancy can account for a positive reading.

Live Birth: This refers to the actual live birth of one or more babies. In determining success-rate data using live births, the industry standard is to count a "live birth" as a single delivery, regardless of how many babies were born.

SOURCE:
Federal Trade Commission Office of Consumer/Business Education. "Infertility Services." *Facts for Consumers* (March 1990): 2.

GIFT (GAMETE INTRAFALLOPIAN TRANSFER)

GIFT stands for gamete intrafallopian transfer. A gamete is a male or female sex cell, a sperm, or an egg. During GIFT, sperm and eggs are mixed and injected into one or both fallopian tubes. After the gametes have been transferred, fertilization can take place in the fallopian tube as it does in natural, unassisted reproduction. Once fertilized, the egg or embryo travels to the uterus by natural processes.

As in IVF [in vitro fertilization], a GIFT treatment cycle begins with ovulation enhancement which is followed by egg harvest, usually by means of laparoscopy. But the similarity to IVF ends here. In IVF, an embryo is transferred. In GIFT, gametes are transferred.

Patients with normal, healthy fallopian tubes are candidates for GIFT. These include women who have unexplained infertility or mild endometriosis and couples whose infertility results from male, cervical, or immunological factors. Some doctors recommend that couples with male factor infertility proceed with GIFT only if it has been proven that the man's sperm can fertilize the woman's egg either by in vitro fertilization or by past pregnancies.

The basic steps of GIFT are ovulation enhancement, egg harvest, insemination, and gamete transfer. The eggs are usually harvested during laparoscopy. During this same laparoscopy procedure, lasting about an hour to an hour and a half, the eggs are mixed with semen, and the gametes are transferred. . . .

There are several differences between GIFT and IVF. The most important one is that GIFT requires healthy fallopian tubes, whereas IVF is appropriate treatment for women with tubal disease or even no fallopian tubes at all. At present, GIFT always requires laparoscopy for gamete transfer. Other techniques, still in experimental stages, are being developed to transfer gametes without laparoscopy. During IVF, the physician uses ultrasound guidance during the egg harvest procedure, instead of viewing through the laparoscope.

With GIFT, fertilization occurs unobserved inside the body. With IVF, fertilization takes place in a laboratory dish and can be confirmed visually with a microscope. Visual confirmation of fertilization is especially important in cases of male factor or unexplained infertility.

SOURCE:
American Fertility Society. *IVF & GIFT: A Patient's Guide to Assisted Reproductive Technology*. pp. 7–8, 9.

SUCCESS RATE

Since 1978, in vitro fertilization (IVF) and its newer cousin, gamete intrafallopian transfer (GIFT), have helped some 5,000 couples in the U.S. conceive and bear children, and the number of such births grows each year. But the successes have overshadowed the facts. The odds of giving birth to a test-tube baby are far slimmer, it now turns out, than many infertility clinics would have their patients believe.

The science of conceiving a baby outside the womb has led to a new commerce in treating infertile couples, and that commerce has resulted in heated competition. In 1978, only a handful of clinics in this country were experimenting with in vitro fertilization. Today, some 200 clinics offer IVF, GIFT, or both. About a third are for-profit ventures, charging as much as $8,000 for a single procedure. If it fails, each repeat effort generates new fees. In their zeal to pull in business, a recent congressional investigation has found, many clinics play fast and loose with the way their successes are defined.

Couples might expect to be told simply the number of births compared with the number of IVF or GIFT procedures. Yet clinics frequently tout success rates in achieving pregnancy rather than rates of babies born, without making clear what the numbers mean. Conception rates may run as high as 40 or 50 percent at some clinics. But since 30 percent of all pregnancies fail, it is highly misleading to imply that pregnancies represent births, critics charge.

Many newer clinics have limited experience; quite a few have yet to produce a baby. To get an idea of true success rates, the subcommittee and the American Fertility Society, and association of doctors who treat infertility, undertook the first nationwide survey of clinics. The results were released [in March 1989].

By analyzing data from 145 clinics on procedures performed in 1987, the researchers got a clearer sense of overall success rates for both IVF and GIFT. Couples who tried a single IVF procedure, in which a woman's eggs are surgically removed from the ovary, fertilized in a petri dish with sperm and placed in the womb, had a 1-in-9, or 11 percent, chance of having a baby. People who tried GIFT had about a 1-in-8, or 13 percent, chance. In GIFT the eggs are removed and mixed with sperm; the mixture is placed in the woman's fallopian tube, where a sperm can fertilize the egg much as it would under natural circumstances.

The contrasting birth rates in couples who use these procedures and those of, say, a couple in their 20s or early 30s with no infertility problems are significant. Couples without problems have about a 23 percent chance in any given month of conceiving and carrying a baby to term. While infertile couples may be able to afford only one or two procedures, other couples obviously can work at conceiving month after month.

SOURCE:
Findlay, S. "What Do Infertility Clinics Really Deliver? Too Often, Success Means Pregnancies Rather Than Babies." *U.S. News and World Report* 106, no. 2 (April 3, 1989): 74.

CRYOPRESERVATION

Techniques to unite the sperm and egg of consenting married adults outside of the body and to transfer the fertilized product into the wife's uterus are now widely accepted. Nevertheless, a number of religious, ethical, and legal issues remain.

The freezing and thawing of animal embryos to increase reproductive potential has been an established practice in agriculture for more than a decade. The freezing and thawing of human embryos, although still experimental, is slowly becoming part of the routine practice of in vitro fertilization around the world. The major advantage of cryopreservation is that retrieved oocytes (primordial or incompletely developed ova) that are not used during a particular cycle can be fertilized and stored for later use. It is speculated that the use of cryopreserved embryos could increase the rate of pregnancies per oocyte-retrieval procedure by 8 to 12 percent. Because the use of cryopreserved embryos in subsequent cycles does not require additional oocyte-retrieval procedures, the cost of attempting fertilization during these cycles is reduced. Successful pregnancies from frozen and thawed human embryos have been reported in the United States, Australia, and Europe. Because success rates after the freezing and thawing of embryos are similar to those achieved by conventional in vitro fertilization, the demand for cryopreservation is growing.

The main legal issues that surround cryopreservation concern the authority to dispose of the embryo, the length of storage, posthumous use, inheritance rights, and family relations after embryo donation and surrogacy. The primary ethical questions include whether the freezing and thawing of human embryos results in abnormal or defective births (no evidence thus far indicates that it does), whether the embryo itself has rights before implantation, and whether the freezing of embryos is an unacceptable intrusion into the natural process of reproduction. The Ethics Committee of the American Fertility Society has determined that although embryos deserve special respect, they do not themselves have the rights or status of persons and, therefore, cannot be wronged.

SOURCE:

Seibel, M. M. "A New Era in Reproductive Technology: In Vitro Fertilization, Gamete Intrafallopian Transfer, and Donated Gametes and Embryos." *The New England Journal of Medicine* 318, no. 13 (March 31, 1988): 833–834.

SELECTING AN INFERTILITY SPECIALIST

You may want to begin your search for fertility specialists by asking your gynecologist, obstetrician, family doctor, or friends and relatives for recommendations. Ask your local hospital or medical society for names. In addition, you may want to contact local infertility support groups, which can provide you with both information and emotional support.

Plan to talk with several providers of infertility services before taking any particular course of action. By doing so, you can compare programs, gain more information about the field, and learn about different treatments applicable to your situation.

You may want to contact infertility programs first by telephone, study any literature sent to you and, then, visit those that most interest you. Try to select an infertility provider that you feel comfortable with and is convenient for you. Here are some questions to ask providers.

What is your infertility service's success rate and how is it calculated? *For established programs:* What is your live birth rate per egg stimulation attempted? *For new programs:* What is your live birth rate plus ongoing pregnancies past 26 weeks per egg stimulation?

You will want to examine how each infertility service tabulates its success rate and consider how meaningful these figures are.

What is your success rate with couples who have problems similar to ours?

Most importantly, find out how successful an infertility service has been in helping couples with your specific problems. Tell the staff your individual circumstances. Then ask: "Given our particular medical history, what are our chances of having a baby after undergoing a single egg-stimulation procedure?"

How long has your infertility service been in existence? How many patients have you treated? What is the specific training of your medical personnel?

You probably will want to select a program that is well-established, has worked with many patients, and has a highly-trained medical staff.

Is your infertility service associated with a medical board specializing in infertility?

You may wish to determine whether the infertility service has a doctor who is board-certified by the American Board of Obstetrics and Gynecology in the subspecialty of Reproductive Endocrinology. This board certification provides recognition of tested expertise in IVF and GIFT procedures.

Can you send me written material about the particular procedure you are recommending?

It is helpful to get written information about any medical procedures you may undergo. IVF and GIFT treatments should be explained to you in detail so that you fully understand the nature of these procedures.

What are the fees for these procedures? How much will drugs cost? What is typically covered by insurance?

Costs for infertility procedures are relatively expensive, and coverage by health insurance plans varies. Ask the cost of each step in the IVF or GIFT procedure. Most infertility services charge you as you advance through each step of the procedure rather than require a payment-in-full prior to the start of a treatment. You should review your health insurance to see which parts, if any, of the IVF or GIFT procedures are covered and discuss the matter with the provider of your choice.

Can we talk with several former or current patients who have had problems similar to ours?

Talking with a provider's patients can help in confirming your impressions of an infertility program, particularly the way in which patients are treated. You frequently can get an idea of a program's strengths and weaknesses from those who have participated in it.

SOURCE:

Federal Trade Commission Office of Consumer/Business Education. "Infertility Services." *Facts for Consumers* (March 1990): 2–3.

RESOURCES

ORGANIZATIONS

American Fertility Society. 2140 11th Ave. S, Suite 200, Birmingham, AL 35205.

Resolve, Inc. Five Water St., Arlington, MA 02174.

Serono Symposia USA. 100 Longwater Circle, Norwell, MA 02061.

PAMPHLETS

American College of Obstetricians and Gynecologists:

"Infertility: Causes and Treatments." *Gynecologic Problems,* AP002. October 1989. 11 pp.

American Fertility Society:

Questions to Ask about an IVF/GIFT Program. 1989.

California Medical Association:

"In-Vitro Fertilization." *HealthTips* index WH-47 (May 1989): 2 pp.

"Infertility." *HealthTips* index 136 (July/August 1988): 2 pp.

Serono Symposia USA:

GIFT: Gamete Intra-Fallopian Transfer. 1990. 13 pp.

In Vitro Fertilization and Embryo Replacement. 1990. 12 pp.

BOOKS

Becker, Gay. *Healing the Infertile Family.* New York: Bantam, 1990.

Harkness, Carla. *The Infertility Book—A Comprehensive Medical and Emotional Guide.* San Francisco: Volcano Press, 1987. 324 pp.

Liebmann-Smith, Joan. *In Pursuit of Pregnancy.* New York: Newmarket Press, 1987. 193 pp.

Silbo, Sherman. *How to Get Pregnant with the New Technology.* New York: Wane, 1991.

RELATED ARTICLES

Frey, Keith A., Morton A. Stenchever, and Michelle P. Warren. "Helping the Infertile Couple." *Patient Care* 23 (May 30, 1989): 22–31.

"Frozen Pre-Embryos." *JAMA* 263, no. 18 (May 9, 1990): 2484–2487.

Griffith, Carolyn S., and David A. Grimes. "The Validity of the Postcoital Test." *American Journal of Obstetrics and Gynecology* 162 (March 1990): 615–620.

"In-Vitro Fertilisation: On the Receiving End." *The Lancet* (January 5, 1989): 342.

Nero, Filomena A. "When Couples Ask about Infertility." *RN* 51 (November 1988): 26–33.

Page, H. "Calculating the Effectiveness of In-Vitro Fertilization. A Review." *British Journal of Obstetrics and Gynecology* 96, no. 3 (March 1989): 334–339.

Wagner, M. G., and P. A. St. Clair. "Are In-Vitro Fertilisation and Embryo Transfer of Benefit to All?" *The Lancet* 2, no. 8670 (October 28, 1989): 1027–1030.

INFLAMMATORY BOWEL DISEASE

OVERVIEW

Inflammatory bowel disease is a name given to a group of chronic digestive diseases of the small and large intestines. Your doctor may refer to your particular condition by any one of several terms including colitis, proctitis, enteritis, and ileitis. Most often, doctors divide IBD into two groups: Ulcerative colitis and Crohn's disease.

Ulcerative colitis causes ulcers and inflammation of the lining (mucosa) of the colon (large intestine). It almost always involves the rectum and usually causes a bloody diarrhea.

Crohn's disease is an inflammation that extends into the deeper layers of the intestinal wall. The disease either is limited to one or more segments of the small intestine (30 percent), usually the ileum (ileitis), or involves both the ileum and the colon (ileocolitis) (50 percent). In the remaining 20 percent, Crohn's disease is confined to the colon (Crohn's colitis). Sometimes, inflammation may also affect the mouth, esophagus (gullet), stomach, duodenum, appendix, or anus.

Both ulcerative colitis and Crohn's disease are chronic conditions and may recur over a lifetime. On the other hand, many people will have long periods—sometimes years—when they will be free of symptoms. Unfortunately, doctors cannot predict with certainty when the disease will go into remission or when the symptoms will return.

The most common symptoms of IBD are diarrhea and abdominal pain. Ulcerative colitis usually causes rectal bleeding as well. Crohn's disease also may cause rectal bleeding, but less often than does ulcerative colitis. In either disease, inflammation, fever, and bleeding may be serious and persistent, leading to weight loss and anemia (low red blood cell count). Children may also suffer stunted growth and delayed development.

There are many theories about what causes IBD, but none has been proven. The current leading theory suggests that some agent, possibly a virus or an atypical bacterium, interacts with the body's own immune defense system to trigger an inflammatory reaction in the intestinal wall. Although there is much scientific evidence that patients with IBD have abnormalities of the immune system, doctors do not know whether these abnormalities are a cause or a result of the disease. Doctors do believe, however, that there is little basis for the idea that Crohn's disease and ulcerative colitis are caused by emotional distress or are the product of an unhappy childhood.

It is estimated that between 1 and 2 million Americans suffer from IBD. Men and women are affected about equally. Some people seem to be more likely targets for these diseases. For instance, IBD seems to be more common among Jews than non-Jews and more prevalent among whites than blacks, Orientals, Hispanics, or Native Americans, although no population group is immune from attack. Also, the number of people who get Crohn's disease has been increasing steadily over the last several decades. The incidence has, in the past, been highest in North America, the British Isles, and northwestern Europe and Scandinavia. In recent years, an increase in frequency has been observed in developing nations throughout the rest of the world. Doctors cannot yet explain why these changes are occurring. . . .

Ulcerative colitis is usually relatively easy for the doctor to recognize. If bloody diarrhea is what caused you to go to the doctor's office, the doctor will probably examine your rectum with an instrument called a proctoscope or sigmoidoscope. In many cases, the doctor will obtain a culture of the stool and order a barium enema x-ray.

Crohn's disease is not so easily diagnosed because the symptoms are not always so dramatic, and because the affected part of the intestine may not be within the easy reach of a sigmoidoscope. However, if you have experienced chronic abdominal pain, diarrhea, fever, weight loss, and anemia, the doctor will examine you for signs of Crohn's disease. The diagnosis can almost always be established by a good medical history and a thorough x-ray examination of the digestive tract, including an upper gastrointestinal (GI) series, a careful small bowel study, and a barium enema.

No medicine has yet been found to cure Crohn's disease or ulcerative colitis, but several drugs are helpful in controlling the disease processes and symptoms.

Abdominal cramps and diarrhea may be alleviated by drugs. The drug sulfasalazine often lessens the inflammation. More serious cases may require cortisone-related medication.

Some cases of IBD have improved with certain very potent anti-infective agents or with drugs that suppress the body's immune system. These are relatively new treatments for IBD and, because they sometimes produce severe reactions, they are not used routinely. It is very important that you take only those medications your doctor has prescribed for you.

No special diet has been proven effective for preventing IBD or helping most IBD patients. Some patients find their symptoms are made worse by milk, alcohol, hot spices, or roughage. But there are no hard and fast rules for the majority of IBD patients. Let your common sense tell you if you need to avoid any foods that seem to make your symptoms worse. Maintaining good general nutrition and adequate caloric intake is far more important than emphasizing or avoiding any particular food. Also, large doses of vitamins are useless and may even produce harmful side effects. . . .

Surgery can cure ulcerative colitis. Although most patients cope effectively with this disease for many years, about one-third will eventually require the removal of the colon. In the standard form of this operation the entire colon and rectum are removed. A small opening (stoma) is made in the front of the abdominal wall and the tip of the lower small intestine (ileum) is then brought through. The stoma is fitted with a pouch to collect waste products. This external opening to the intestine is called an ileostomy.

Cosmetically more appealing options to this standard procedure have recently been developed, but they are controversial because they are more prone to complications. One such procedure is called a continent ileostomy. In this operation, a pouch is created out of the ileum inside the wall of the lower abdomen. The pouch is emptied regularly through a valve on the outside of the abdomen and a small tube.

In an even newer operation, ileoanal anastomosis, only the diseased inner lining of the rectum is removed, leaving the outer muscle coats of the rectum intact. The ileum is then inserted inside the rectum (a procedure sometimes called a "pull-through") and attached just above the anus. Because the rectal muscles are left intact, stool can be passed normally.

Your doctor will explain the possibilities and recommend which form of surgery is best for you. The most important thing to remember, however, is that removal of the colon and rectum provides a total and permanent cure for ulcerative colitis, regardless of the type of procedure performed.

Crohn's disease can be helped by surgery, but it cannot be cured by surgery. The inflammation tends to return in areas of the intestine immediately next to the area that had been removed. Even so, about two-thirds of Crohn's disease patients require surgery, either to provide relief from chronic disability or to correct specific complications. Unfortunately, neither the continent ileostomy nor the ileoanal anastomosis can be used in Crohn's disease patients because of the likelihood or recurrence of the disease.

SOURCE:

Sachar, David. B. *Inflammatory Bowel Disease.* National Digestive Diseases Education and Information Clearinghouse (December 1985): pp. 1–4.

ULCERATIVE COLITIS

Ulcerative colitis is a chronic disease in which the lining of the colon (large bowel) and rectum becomes inflamed. When this happens, the bowel tries to empty itself frequently, causing diarrhea. As cells on the surface of the lining of the colon die and slough off, ulcers (tiny open sores) form, causing pus, mucus, and bleeding.

Some patients with ulcerative colitis experience little more than frequent bowel movements that are softer and looser than normal. More common symptoms are abdominal cramps, straining to move the bowels, and bloody diarrhea. Patients may also suffer fatigue, weight loss, and loss of body fluids and nutrients. Severe bleeding can result in anemia. Sometimes patients also have skin ulcers, joint pain, inflammation of the eyes, or liver disorders. . . .

Most patients are able to manage their disease most of the time. While there is no special diet for ulcerative colitis, patients may be able to control mild symptoms simply by avoiding foods that seem to upset their bowels. In some cases, the doctor may advise avoiding highly seasoned foods or milk sugar (lactose) for a while. When treatment is necessary, it must be tailored for each case, since what may help one patient may not help someone else. The patient also should be given needed emotional and psychological support.

Less than a quarter of patients with ulcerative colitis have symptoms severe enough to require hospitalization. In these cases, the doctor will try to correct malnutrition and to stop diarrhea and loss of blood, fluids and mineral salts. In order to accomplish this, the patient may need a special diet, feeding through a vein, medications, or, sometimes, surgery.

Patients with either mild or severe colitis are usually treated with the drug sulfasalazine. This drug can be used for as long as needed, and it can be used along with other drugs. Side effects such as nausea, vomiting, weight loss, heartburn, diarrhea, and headache occur in a small percentage of cases. Patients who do not do well on sulfasalazine often do very well on related drugs known as 5-ASA agents.

SOURCE:

National Digestive Diseases Information Clearinghouse. *Ulcerative Colitis.* (October 1989): pp. 1–2.

CROHN'S DISEASE

A troublesome ailment of the intestinal tract.

At one time or another, you've probably experienced a sudden bout of abdominal cramps and diarrhea. A bacterial or viral infection of the gastrointestinal tract often is the culprit. But if you have Crohn's disease, these symptoms may be part of a more serious constellation of problems.

Normal bowel function.

Throughout its length, your intestine digests and absorbs the food and liquids you consume. Different segments have specific jobs. For example, the beginning of your small intestine, the duodenum (du-o-de'num), absorbs most of the calcium in your diet. The end of your small bowel, called the terminal ileum, is where vitamin B-12 is absorbed. Your colon (large intestine) regulates removal of water from the intestinal contents.

When disease interrupts these important functions, the consequences can be serious.

Inflammatory bowel disease.

Crohn's disease falls within the broad category of disorders called inflammatory bowel disease. The cause of Crohn's disease remains unknown, but genetics, infection, altered immunity and psychological factors all may play a role. The disease is more common in Caucasians and it can affect more than one member of a family.

While both viruses and bacteria can cause acute colitis (inflammation of the colon), little evidence suggests that infections actually lead to Crohn's disease.

Some people with Crohn's also have arthritis. Because a malfunction in the immune system also can cause certain types of arthritis, a problem in the immune system also may play a role in the development of Crohn's disease.

Flare-ups of Crohn's may occur at times of emotional stress, but there is no convincing evidence that psychological factors cause the illness.

The symptoms.

Involved segments may be interspersed between apparently normal bowel. Abnormal segments are called "skip lesions."

Diarrhea, abdominal pain and fever are the most common symptoms. But symptoms depend on the region of bowel that is affected by Crohn's disease.

For example, the greater the involvement of the small bowel, the greater the loss of nutrient absorption. This can result in significant weight loss. If the terminal ileum is involved, failure to absorb vitamin B-12 can lead to anemia.

Crohn's disease involves the entire thickness of the bowel wall. As inflammation progresses, the involved portion of bowel can become thickened and narrowed. Sometimes this can obstruct the flow of intestinal contents.

Because of this extensive involvement of the entire thickness of the bowel wall, an opening or tract (fistula) can develop between different areas of the bowel and other organs or the skin.

The diagnosis.

Crohn's disease can be difficult to distinguish from other forms of inflammatory bowel disease. Specialists in disorders of the intestinal tract often use several diagnostic techniques. Included are X-ray examination and colonoscopy. In colonoscopy, the doctor uses a flexible, lighted tube to examine directly the inside of the intestine.

The doctor also may remove tissue for examination under a microscope to help confirm the diagnosis.

The treatment.

For 40 years, the mainstay of treatment for Crohn's disease has been a drug called sulfasalazine. This medication contains an aspirin-like compound (salicylate) that helps reduce inflammation.

In some people, steroids (derivatives of cortisone) are used to suppress the immune response. Other drugs that inhibit the immune system, such as 6-mercaptopurine or azathioprine, also are used to treat some people with Crohn's disease.

Metronidazole may be another helpful option. Even though this antibiotic kills bacteria, its beneficial effect in the treatment of Crohn's disease is yet to be understood.

Despite advances in the medical treatment of Crohn's, surgery may be necessary to remove the diseased segment of bowel. Surgery is reserved for those people in whom medical treatment has been ineffective.

Other indications for surgery include:

- Permanent narrowing or an obstruction of the bowel.
- Development of a fistula between an involved segment and the bladder, vagina or skin.

- Infection in the area of the anus.
- Perforation of the bowel.
- Abscess (localized infection) within the abdomen.
- Extreme widening (toxic dilation) of the colon.

Crohn's disease can recur after surgery, even if the surgeon removed all traces of the disease.

If the colon and rectum are extensively diseased, the surgeon may have to perform an ileostomy (il'eos'-tome). This is an opening on the surface of the abdomen through which intestinal contents may drain. A disposable plastic bag is sealed to the skin to collect the drainage.

Despite the serious nature of the disease, treatment often permits the person with Crohn's disease to lead an active and productive life.

SOURCE:

"Crohn's Disease." *Mayo Clinic Health Letter* (November 1990): 4–5.

TREATMENT

The urgency that afflicts patients with inflammatory bowel disease is being matched in the search for effective treatment.

"There is a lot of reason to be optimistic," though much of the hope stems from unconfirmed trials, says Stephen Hanauer, MD, codirector of the University of Chicago's outpatient gastrointestinal clinic.

Current treatments for ulcerative colitis and Crohn's disease are as unsatisfactory as these two somewhat similar diseases are unpredictable. Sulfasalazine cannot be tolerated by one third of patients, and neither it nor steroids are proven to maintain remission.

But with the consensus that some immune malfunction is involved in the etiology of these diseases, several existing agents and one new class of drugs are being tried, according to reports at a Digestive Disease Week program in San Antonio, Tex. Among others, the following treatments were reported:

The sun may shine on 5-aminosalicylic acids (5-ASAs), effective now as enemas, with the report of remission with oral mesalamine.

A drug used to prevent malaria, plaqenil, shows promise.

Immune modulators such as methotrexate and cyclosporine, tried in many suspected autoimmune disorders, show efficacy.

Fish oil, also tried in other chronic inflammatory diseases, provides some benefit but not in control of bleeding, cramps, and frequent bowel movement.

And a new drug, a 5-lipoxygenase inhibitor, which works the side of the arachidonic pathway ignored by traditional anti-inflammatories, beat placebo in its first double-blind human trial.

SOURCE:

Cotton, P. "New Approaches May Aid Patients with Inflammatory Bowel Disease." *JAMA* 263, no. 23 (June 20, 1990): 3121-3122.

RESOURCES

ORGANIZATIONS

Crohn's and Colitis Foundation of America. 444 Park Avenue South, New York, New York 10016.

Ileitis and Colitis Educational Foundation. Central DuPage Hospital, 23 North Winfield Road, Winfield, Illinois 60190.

International Association for Enterostomal Therapy. Suite 290, 2081 Business Center Drive, Irvine, California 92715.

United Ostomy Association. Suite 120, 36 Executive Park, Irvine, California 92714.

PAMPHLETS

National Digestive Diseases Clearinghouse:

IBD and IBS: Two Very Different Problems. 1987.

Ulcerative Colitis. 1990.

What is Irritable Bowel Syndrome? 1989.

National Foundation for Ileitis and Colitis:

Questions and Answers about Crohn's Disease & Ulcerative Colitis. n.d. 15 pp.

BOOKS

Brandt, L. J., and P. Steiner-Grossman. *Treating IBD: A Patient's Guide to the Medical and Surgical Management of Inflammatory Bowel Disease*. New York: Raven Press. 1989.

Steiner, P., and others (eds.). *People Not Patients: A Source Book of Living with Inflammatory Bowel Disease*. National Foundation for Ileitis and Colitis. 1985.

RELATED ARTICLES

Farley, D. "Living with Inflammatory Bowel Disease." *FDA Consumer* (April 1988): 9–15.

Jagelman, D. G. "Surgical Alternatives for Ulcerative Colitis." *Medical Clinic of North America* 74, no. 1 (January 1990): 155–167.

Neufeldt, J. "Helping the I.B.D. Patient Cope with the Unpredictable." *Nursing* 87, 7 (August 1987): 47–49.

Nord, H. J. "Complications of Inflammatory Bowel Disease." *Hospital Practice* (November 30, 1987): 67, 70–72, 75, 78, 80, 82.

Pepperman, M. A. "Advances in Drug Therapy for Inflammatory Bowel Disease." *Annals of Internal Medicine* 112, no. 1 (January 1990): 50–60.

Sachar, D. B. "Cyclosporine Treatment for Inflammatory Bowel Disease." *New England Journal of Medicine* 321, no. 13 (September 28, 1989): 894–896.

Schuman, B. M. "Inflammatory Bowel Disease: Options in Office Management." *Postgraduate Medicine* 83, no. 4 (March 1988): 291–294.

Sutherland, L. R. "Medical Treatment of Inflammatory Bowel Disease: New Therapies, New Drugs." *Canadian Medical Association Journal* 137 (November 1, 1987): 799–802.

"Ulcerative Colitis and Crohn's Disease." *Harvard Medical School Health Letter* 13, no. 8 (June 1988): 4–8.

INFORMED CONSENT

OVERVIEW

Information is power, and because information sharing inevitably results in decision sharing, the doctrine of informed consent has helped transform the doctor-patient relationship. This is why informed consent is the most important legal doctrine in both the doctor-patient relationship and treatment in health care facilities. Not only is it important because of its implications for power and accountability, but it is also important because many of the other rights patients have are either derived from or enhanced by the doctrine of informed consent. The basic concept is simple: a doctor cannot touch or treat a patient until the doctor has given the patient some basic information about what the doctor proposes to do, and the patient has agreed to the proposed treatment or procedure. The overwhelming majority of Americans agree with this proposition, and the foundation on which it stands: people have a right not to have their bodies invaded without their approval because of their interests in bodily integrity and self-determination. Put more simply, it is the patient's body. The patient is the one who must experience invasion and live with the consequences. There is no obligation to accept any medical treatment, and it is remarkable that anyone ever considered it acceptable practice to treat a person without that person's informed consent. Physicians have no roving mandate to treat whoever they believe is in need of their services.

As one court summarized the law at the dawn of the twentieth century: "Under a free government at least, the free citizen's first and greatest right which underlies all others—the right to the inviolability of his person, in other words, his right to himself, is the subject of universal acquiescence, and this right necessarily forbids a physician. . .to violate without permission the bodily integrity of his patient by a major or capital operation."

In the most important study of informed consent to date, the President's Commission for the Study of Ethical Problems in Medicine concluded that informed consent has its foundations in law, [and] is an ethical imperative as well. It also concluded that "ethically valid consent is a process of shared decision making based upon mutual respect and participation, not a ritual to be equated with reciting the contents of a form that details the risks of particular treatments." Its foundation is the fundamental recognition "that adults are entitled to accept or reject health care interventions on the basis of their own personal values and in furtherance of their own personal goals." . . .

The doctrine of informed consent, simply stated, is that before a patient is asked to consent to any treatment or procedure that has risks, alternatives, or low success rates; the patient must be provided with certain information. This information includes at least the following, which must, of course, be presented in language the patient can understand:

1. A description of the recommended treatment or procedure.

2. A description of the risks and benefits of the recommended procedure, with special emphasis on risks of death or serious bodily disability.

3. A description of the alternatives, including other treatments or procedures, together with the risks and benefits of these alternatives.

4. The likely results of no treatment.

5. The probability of success, and what the physician means by success.

6. The major problems anticipated in recuperation, and the time period during which the patient will not be able to resume his or her normal activities.

7. Any other information generally provided to patients in this situation by other qualified physicians. . . .

All information must, of course, be presented in language the patient can understand, and treatment should not proceed until the health care provider is satisfied that the patient actually does understand the information presented.

SOURCE:

Annas, George J. "Informed Consent." In *The Rights of Patients*. Carbondale, Illinois: Southern Illinois University Press, 1989. pp. 83–84, 86–87.

A SHARED THERAPEUTIC ALLIANCE

Physicians must view informed consent as not just a legal doctrine justifying a form of defensive medicine to protect the doctor from legal liability. Rather, informed consent must be viewed as an essential feature of a shared therapeutic alliance between physician and patient. Such a restructuring of the doctor-patient relationship will discourage overly technical legal claims inspired by patient dissatisfaction. The patient must be allowed to share in the medical decision-making process if he wishes to do so. Alternative courses of treatment may be chosen by a patient even if they are not medically preferable. In policing the doctor-patient relationship through the informed consent doctrine, courts should be sensitive to the realities of medical decision-making and analyze the entire communication process, the dynamics of the relationship, and overall medical care.

A practical doctrine of medical-legal informed consent must weigh the importance of the two often conflicting goals of individual self-determination and health. The variability of each patient-doctor encounter, however, prevents formulation of firm rules to define clearly the importance of each of those goals. Flexibility is necessary because of the diverse spectra of medical settings, physician-patient relationships, patient illnesses, treatments and procedures, and patient personalities, educational levels, values, abilities, and needs.

SOURCE:

Sprung, Charles L., and Bruce J. Winick. "Informed Consent in Theory and Practice: Legal and Medical Perspectives on the Informed Consent Doctrine and a Proposed Reconceptualization." *Critical Care Medicine* 17, no. 12 (December 1989): 1346–1354.

RESOURCES

ORGANIZATIONS

American Civil Liberties Union. 132 West 43rd St., New York, NY 10036.

People's Medical Society. 462 Walnut Street, Allentown, PA 18102.

PAMPHLET

American College of Surgeons:

When You Need an Operation . . . Giving Your Informed Consent.

BOOKS

President's Commission for the Study of Ethical Problems in Medicine and Biomedical and Behavioral Research. *Making Health Care Decisions: The Ethical and Legal Implications of Informed Consent in the Patient-Practioner Relationship. The Patient's Role in Medical Decisionmaking.* 3 volumes. Washington, DC: Government Printing Office, 1982.

RELATED ARTICLES

Appelbaum, Paul S., and Thomas Grisso. "Assessing Patients' Capacities to Consent to Treatment." *The New England Journal of Medicine* 319, no. 25 (December 22, 1988): 1635–1638.

Hollander, Rachelle D. "Changes in the Concept of Informed Consent in Medical Encounters." *Journal of Medical Education* 59, no. 10 (October 1984): 783–788.

Hunt, Morton. "Patients' Rights." *The New York Times Magazine* (March 5, 1989): 55–56.

Marcelo, Ana. "Patient's Orders." *Health* (September 1990): 52, 54.

IRRITABLE BOWEL SYNDROME

(*See also:* CONSTIPATION; DIARRHEA)

OVERVIEW

Irritable bowel syndrome or IBS is a chronic disorder of the colon. Its cause and cure are as yet unknown. Doctors call it a functional disorder because there is no sign of disease when the colon is examined by x-ray or other diagnostic methods. However, IBS causes a variety of symptoms including lower abdominal pain, gas, bloating, constipation or diarrhea, or alternating constipation and diarrhea.

Through the years, IBS has been called by many names—mucous colitis, spastic colon, colitis, spastic bowel, and functional bowel disease. Most of these terms are inaccurate. Colitis, for instance, means inflammation of the colon. IBS, on the other hand, causes no inflammation and should never be confused with the more serious disorder—ulcerative colitis.

Though IBS can cause a great deal of discomfort, it is not serious and does not lead to any serious disease. With attention to proper diet, stress management, and sometimes medication prescribed by their physician, most people with IBS can keep their symptoms under control.

It is important to remember that normal bowel function varies widely from person to person. Doctors generally agree that normal bowel function ranges from three stools a day to three each week. A normal movement is one that is formed but not hard, contains no blood, and is passed without cramps or pain.

People with IBS, on the other hand, usually have some combination of constipation and diarrhea as well as pain, gas, and abdominal bloating. Most people with IBS have episodes of lower abdominal pain and constipation, sometimes followed by diarrhea. Others may have pain and mild constipation and no diarrhea. The rarest form of the disorder is severe, painless diarrhea. People in this group have watery bowel movements after breakfast almost every day. These may be followed by episodes of diarrhea after other meals, following stressful events, or for no apparent reason. Although IBS is usually a mild annoyance, for some people it can be disabling. Patients in the latter group may be afraid to go to dinner parties, seek employment, or travel on public transportation.

Because doctors have been unable to pinpoint its organic cause, IBS often has been considered to be caused by emotional conflict or stress. While stress may certainly be a factor, recent studies indicate that other factors may be involved.

Most IBS symptoms are related to an abnormal motility (movement) pattern of the colon. The colon connects the small intestine with the anus. Approximately 6 feet long, the colon has two major functions: it absorbs water and salts from digestive products that enter from the small intestine. Two liters of liquid matter enter the colon from the small intestine each day. This material may remain there for several days until most of the fluid and salts are absorbed back into the body. The stool then passes through the colon by a delicate pattern of movements to the rectum where it is stored until a bowel movement occurs.

Movements of the colon are controlled by nerves and hormones and by electrical activity in the colon muscle. The electrical activity serves as a "pacemaker" similar to the mechanism that controls heart function. Movements of the colon propel the contents slowly back and forth, but mainly toward the rectum. Segments of the colon also contract periodically to promote the absorption of water from feces.

In people who have IBS, the muscle of the lower portion of the colon contracts abnormally. An abnormal contraction—or spasm—may be related to episodes of crampy pain. Sometimes the spasm delays the passage of stool, leading to constipation. At other times, the spasm leads to more rapid passage of feces and the result is diarrhea.

IBS is a diagnosis that doctors reach after more serious organic diseases have been excluded. This process is necessary because IBS offers doctors no signposts to help identify the disorder. A complete medical history that includes a careful description of the symptoms, a physical examination, and specific laboratory tests will be done. Also, your doctor will probably order some diagnostic tests such as x-rays or endoscopy to eliminate organic causes of your symptoms. Unless your symptoms change, you will not need to undergo these tests again.

SOURCE:

National Digestive Diseases Information Clearinghouse. *What Is Irritable Bowel Syndrome?* NIH Pub. No. 90-693. October 1989. pp. 1-2.

PSYCHOLOGICAL ASPECTS

Although recent studies on irritable bowel syndrome have focused more on colon motility than psychological influences, some people have underlying psychiatric disturbances that somatize or show up as intestinal symptoms. Two U.S. studies recently showed that approximately 50 per cent of those reporting IBS also have signs of psychiatric illness—such as depression or anxiety disorders. By comparison, only one-fifth of patients with organic gastrointestinal diseases (such as colitis) had accompanying depression or anxiety syndromes. These results suggest that in some people a psychiatric disorder unrelated to IBS may manifest itself as a bowel problem. On the other hand, people with chronic abdominal pain due to intestinal problems may develop psychological imbalances. Yet others exhibit "learned illness behaviour" and complain about physical problems to gain attention denied them by other means. Thus, IBS is a benign condition handled differently by different sufferers—some just ignoring it, others (who may be anxious, uncertain or fear "loss of control") seeking medical attention and still others focussing on it because of underlying depression or other psychological disturbances. The impact of IBS may be exaggerated if sufferers shun social gatherings or avoid activities such as air-travel because of their unpredictable bowel habits. While not all patients with IBS are psychologically disturbed, many share the following features:

- a tendency to regard minor illnesses (e.g., a common cold) as very serious;
- more frequent visits to physicians than others;
- a history of being pampered as children, given treats when sick and allowed to stay home from school more often than other children;
- other family members with IBS—suggesting "learned illness behaviour."

SOURCE:

"Bowel Trouble Examined: Irritable Bowel Syndrome." *University of Toronto Health News* 8 (April 1990): 13.

TREATMENT

Successful management of irritable bowel syndrome usually includes dietary modification. Diets must be individualized, but for most irritable bowel syndrome patients, a high-fiber, low-fat diet is recommended. Because fiber shortens intestinal transit time, dietary bran or bulk laxatives consisting of hydrophilic psyllium seed (Effer-Syllium, Metamucil), in a daily dose of 15 to 25 g, may be effective in treating patients with constipation; they may also decrease symptoms in patients with diarrhea. As previously mentioned, patients may need to avoid caffeinated beverages and nondigestible but fermentable carbohydrates such as beans and cabbage. Milk and milk products need to be avoided only by patients with lactose intolerance.

Many patients with irritable bowel syndrome also have irregular bowel habits, and the physician should discuss how these can be regulated. For example, the patient with constipation should schedule regular meal times and routine toilet visits.

Pharmacologic intervention may be considered for the patient who does not respond well to more conservative modes of therapy. No one agent has been proved effective for irritable bowel syndrome. Anticholinergic medications may reduce colonic spasm and relieve pain in patients with constipation. However, a clear relationship between symptoms and motor response of the intestines has not been established.

If improvement is needed in the patient's response to stressful circumstances, tranquilizers, particularly benzodiazepines, may be used for a brief period. These tranquilizers have no effect on colonic motility but may temporarily "take the edge off" the psychologic factors exacerbating the symptoms of irritable bowel syndrome. Antidepressants may help patients with signs of major depression (weight loss, fatigue and sleep disturbance). These agents may have independent actions on the intestines. Studies suggest improvement in symptoms of irritable bowel syndrome with the use of these drugs, but constipation may increase in some patients.

Loperamide (Imodium) is an antidiarrheal agent that has been shown to be effective in the treatment of diarrhea, urgency and fecal soiling in patients with irritable bowel syndrome. This opioid-like drug, which appears to act via peripheral receptors in the intestines, may be safer than narcotics, since it does not cross the blood brain barrier. Other drugs to consider include metoclopramide (Reglan), 10 mg four times daily, for patients with predominant nausea and vomiting associated with delayed gastric emptying. Dextromethorphan (Delsym), 15 to 30g four times daily, may relieve pain symptoms.

Psychologic and behavioral treatments are a rational form of adjunctive therapy for patients with irritable bowel syndrome. Simple forms of relaxation or exercise (e.g., baths, golf, tennis, rest periods) may reduce tension and enable the patient to feel more in control. This is important, because many patients with irritable bowel syndrome come to the physician already feeling a loss of control over their lives. In selected patients, insight or cognitive psychotherapy can lead to emotional and symptomatic improvement. Finally, hypnotherapy, biofeedback or other structured relaxation techniques can be considered.

SOURCE:

Drossman, Douglas A. "Irritable Bowel Syndrome." *American Family Physician* 39, no. 6 (June 1989): 163.

USE OF MEDICATIONS

At present, drugs are likely to be prescribed for irritable bowel syndrome, if only because patients will continue imploring their physicians for relief from symptoms they find so distressing. Are there any rational guidelines for the sensible use of medications when irritable bowel syndrome is severe? Here are some observations about the major kinds of drug likely to be prescribed:

- **Antispasmodics (anticholinergics).** These agents, atropine and its relatives, act by inhibiting the action of acetylcholine, the nervous system's signal to stimulate bowel contractions. The main indications for antispasmodics are cramping pains, excessive gurgling, and diarrhea provoked by eating. Side effects include dryness of the mouth and sluggishness of bladder and bowel.
- **Bulking agents.** Fiber preparations, most commonly derived from psyllium seeds but also including bran, retain liquid within feces and thus promote a softer and bulkier stool. Bulking agents help relieve constipation. Lower abdominal cramping and gas may worsen for a while after bran is begun, but this reaction is unlikely to persist beyond a month or so and eventually may subside completely.
- **Stool softeners.** Various brands of docusate (Colace, Dialose, Kasof, Modane Soft, and others) soften feces by promoting retention of water in the stool. When excessively hard stools cause discomfort, a docusate preparation may provide relief, but increasing intake of liquids and bulking agents should accomplish the same goal.
- **Opiates.** When diarrhea becomes disabling, opiates can be helpful if used in moderation. They act directly on the bowel to decrease motility. In low doses, opiates have few systemic effects, but a sense of bloating can be unpleasant. Used habitually or at high doses, opiates have a range of side effects from nausea to disorientation and dependency.
- **Tranquilizers.** If periods of high stress clearly trigger exacerbations, medication to relax the psyche can be helpful in calming the gut. This is not to advocate tranquilizers as the automatic solution to all of life's vexations, but temporary relief has its value and its place.
- **Antidepressants.** Not all depressions are obvious. Various physical symptoms, including an irritable bowel, can be the principal manifestation of depression. So antidepressants may have a role in treating irritable bowel by helping with an underlying depression. As a bonus, they have antispasmodic properties of their own and are capable of reducing bowel spasm independent of any mood-elevating action.
- **Cholestyramine.** This resin, which binds bile salts in the bowel, is a long shot, but worth a try for people with chronic diarrhea that is not accompanied by cramping, constipation, or gas. Rarely, such diarrhea is due to a faulty ability of the bowel to absorb bile salts. By binding them, cholestyramine (Questran) keeps these irritating substances from provoking diarrhea when they reach the colon. Cholestyramine can, however, prevent drugs from being absorbed.
- **Charcoal.** It may be a bit of wishful thinking, but activated charcoal does seem, sometimes, to help control excessive flatus (see the HMS Health Letter, February 1987). Expect no improvement in any other symptom. Fairly large amounts are necessary, and much like cholestyramine, charcoal can trap drugs within the bowel, preventing them from being absorbed.

Still other agents, not enumerated here, have been employed from time to time in this domain of medicine, which is long on art and short on science. Anecdotal reports give hope to the beleaguered. But nobody with irritable bowel syndrome ought to be deluded into believing that a final answer to his or her problem is as simple as coming up with just the right medicine or diet—or doctor, for that matter.

SOURCE:

"Irritable Bowel Syndrome—Can Medication Help?" *Harvard Medical School Health Letter* 14 (January 1989): 7–8.

RESOURCES

ORGANIZATIONS

National Digestive Diseases Information Clearinghouse. Box NDDIC, Bethesda, MD 20892.

National Foundation for Ileitis and Colitis. 444 Park Avenue South, New York, NY 10016.

PAMPHLET

National Digestive Diseases Information Clearinghouse:

IBD and IBS: Two Very Different Problems. NIH Pub. No. 90-3079. November 1989. 2 pp.

RELATED ARTICLES

Bayless, Theodore M., and Mary L. Harris. "Inflammatory Bowel Disease and Irritable Bowel Syndrome." *Medical Clinics of North America* 74, no. 1 (January 1990): 21–28.

Bayless, Theodore M., and others. "Help Your IBD Patient Help Himself." *Patient Care* 22 (October 15, 1988): 139–148.

Camilleri, Michael, and Matteo Neri. "Motility Disorders and Stress." *Digestive Diseases and Sciences* 34, no. 11 (November 1989): 1777–1786.

Walker, Edward A., Peter P. Roy-Byrne, and Wayne J. Katon. "Irritable Bowel Syndrome and Psychiatric Illness." *American Journal of Psychiatry* 147, no. 5 (May 1990): 565–572.

JET LAG

OVERVIEW

Interruption of the sleep/wake cycle, fatigue, and other symptoms caused by disturbance of normal body rhythms as a result of flying across different time zones.

Each person has an "internal clock" that determines when the desire to sleep, wake, and eat, the release of various hormones, and many other bodily functions take place in every 24-hour period. The near 24-hour cycle of each activity is called a circadian rhythm. When an air traveler crosses several time zones, his or her day (as timed by an external clock) is longer or shorter than 24 hours, depending on the direction of the flight. Most of the traveler's circadian rhythms are unable to adjust to this shorter or longer day, resulting in jet lag when the flight is over. Jet lag is the desire to sleep during the local day, wakefulness at night, general fatigue, reduced physical and mental activity, and poor memory.

Jet lag tends to be worse after an eastward flight (which shortens the traveler's day) than after a westward one. It is most likely to affect people over 30 who normally follow an established daily routine.

The symptoms of jet lag can be minimized by drinking plenty of nonalcoholic fluids during the flight and avoiding heavy meals. Also, people flying east should go to bed earlier than usual for a few days before the journey; people flying west should do the opposite. If possible, try to arrive in the new time zone in the early evening and go to bed early.

It may take several days to adjust to a new time zone (about half a day to one day for each time zone crossed). The adjustment can be eased by breaking up a long journey with a stopover and by resting after the flight.

SOURCE:
Clayman, Charles B. (ed.). "Jet Lag." In *The American Medical Association Encyclopedia of Medicine.* New York: Random House, 1989. pp. 611, 613.

THE ANTI-JET-LAG DIET

The Anti-Jet-Lag Diet was developed by Charles Ehret, a senior biologist at Argonne National Laboratory's Division of Biological and Medical Research who is now retired. The diet works by quickly synchronizing the traveler's circadian rhythms to the new time zone. It actually resets your body clock. The alternation of meals that stimulate alertness and that induce sleep, followed by days in which the body's carbohydrate stores are depleted, facilitates a faster resetting of the circadian rhythms. All you need to do to avoid jet lag is:

Three days before your flight eat according to the "feast" schedule. This means a high-protein breakfast and lunch and a high-carbohydrate dinner. Suitable protein meals include high-protein cereals, beans, eggs, milk products, tofu, tempeh, fish and poultry. Carbohydrate meals include pasta, rice, bread, potatoes, winter squashes and sweet desserts. If you drink caffeinated beverages, drink them only between 3 P.M. and 5 P.M.; this is the only period during which they will not disrupt your circadian rhythms.

Two days before your flight eat according to the "fast" schedule. This means low-carbohydrate, low-protein, low-calorie foods. Suitable foods include bouillon soups, simple salads with low-calorie dressings, fruits, vegetables, and fruit and vegetable juices. You can drink caffeinated beverages between 3 P.M. and 5 P.M.

One day before your flight return to the "feast" schedule.

On the day of your flight begin on the "fast" schedule. Reset your watch to the current time at your destination. Try to sleep until breakfast time at your destination; do not sleep past the normal waking hour there. Eat a high-protein breakfast when you wake up. Force yourself to stay awake, eating "feast" meals according to the correct time at your destination. Your body clock should now be reset for the new time zone.

SOURCE:
Bloyd-Peshkin, Sharon. "Beating Jet Lag." *Bestways* 17 (December 1989): 45.

EFFECTIVENESS OF THE THE ANTI-JET-LAG DIET

"Eat a HIGH-PROTEIN breakfast, a HIGH-PROTEIN lunch, and a HIGH-CARBOHYDRATE supper... a daily total of 800 calories is ideal.... Shortly after six o'clock at night, no matter where you are or what you are doing, whether you are still in the airplane or not, DRINK TWO TO THREE CUPS of black coffee or strong, plain tea. Now RESET YOUR WRISTWATCH TO DESTINATION TIME." So goes the advice of Charles F. Ehret, PhD, and Lynne Waller Scanlon in their book *Overcoming Jet Lag*. The tips are part of one of their several dietary plans to help minimize the fatigue as well as impaired mental and physical ability that strikes many travelers who fly across several time zones at once. And a good number of them have bought into it.

More than 200,000 copies of *Overcoming Jet Lag* have been put into print since it was first published in 1983. Moreover, such notables as former President Ronald Reagan and his wife Nancy reportedly followed it for a time, and at least one airline has offered meals based on it. The plan even piqued the interest of Pentagon officials looking for a way to combat jet lag among military troops who must be able to respond to emergencies at a moment's notice, even after traveling long distances. The problem is that the so-called jet lag diet has undergone little, if any, scientific scrutiny—until now.

The U.S. Army recently put it to the test on a group of 23 marines. After placing the men in isolation for 15 straight days and manipulating their sleeping and waking hours in order to simulate a New York-to-Paris flight on the seventh night, researchers found that, overall, those put on the "jet lag diet" before the "flight" experienced no fewer symptoms of jet lag than those who ate as they typically did. In fact, all the marines, whether they followed the diet or not, reportedly felt less alert, less happy, more sleepy, more weary, and less able to perform routine activities with ease after the "flight" according to the scientists at the U.S. Army Natick Research, Development and Engineering Center who conducted the study in conjunction with the New York Hospital-Cornell University Medical Center. If anything, the researchers say, the jet lag diet actually interfered with the marines' sleep during the flight presumably because the plan calls for the inflight drinking of caffeinated coffee or tea.

The lesson here? If you're planning on traveling overseas anytime soon, don't count on a special eating regimen to ease your shift to a new time zone. The only surefire way to overcome jet lag remains the tried and true way—tough it out.

SOURCE:
"Diet for Jet Lag Lacks Scientific Fuel." *Tufts University Diet and Nutrition Letter* (August 1990): 2.

CIRCADIAN RHYTHMS

The new research on circadian rhythms suggests certain strategies that people working the night shift or flying across time zones can try.

The following advice is based on that research as well as tips from sleep specialists.

Night workers can:

- Work in the light. Keep your work area as bright as you can. If you do close work in a small area, fix bright light on that spot.
- Sleep in the dark. Use dark blinds or curtains to keep light out.
- Keep a regular schedule. Ideally, you'd go to bed and rise at about the same time every day. But if you want to spend more daylight time awake on your days off, work out a compromise that doesn't upset your normal sleep pattern entirely. On those days, go to bed at your accustomed time in the morning and sleep for a few hours. Later in the day, you could get a little more sleep.

For jet lag, try these strategies:

- Adjust your schedule. Begin shifting your sleep routine before you leave home. That's feasible mainly for people flying east, where the day starts earlier.

Here's how you might prepare for a trip from New York to Rome, where morning comes six hours earlier. Five weeks before the trip, start moving your bedtime and your morning alarm 10 minutes earlier every other day. That would gradually reset your sleep time about three hours earlier and give your body clock a major head start on its adjustment.

- Get outside. When you arrive at your destination, spend time outside to get as much exposure as possible to the local rhythms of light and darkness.

SOURCE:
"Resetting the Body's Clock." *Consumer Reports Health Letter* 2 (September 1990): 66.

USE OF MELATONIN TO ALLEVIATE JET LAG

The loss of wellbeing which is often experienced after transmeridian flights is related to the traveller's need to resynchronise his circadian rhythmicity with that of the new environment. Malaise, loss of appetite, tiredness during the day, and disturbed sleep are common complaints. Indeed, some people react very unfavourably to intercontinental flights; this may be more likely in middle age when sleep is less restful, although sleep deprivation caused by sleep disturbance during the flight or by the delay in the first rest period may sometimes lead to improved sleep over the first couple nights.

However, displacement of the timing of the rest period from that of the home time zone often leads to problems while the new pattern is being established. Difficulty in sustaining sleep after westward flights is usual, although adaptation appears to be fairly rapid since the requirement to lengthen the day is aided by the innate circadian period, which is longer than 24 h. Adaptation after an eastward flight is likely to be slower, apparently because of the difficulty in trying to shorten the day; delay in re-adaptation eastward may lead to sleep disturbance over the whole night, starting several days after the flight.

There is much interest in the possibility that drugs could have a part to play in the management of jet lag. It is possible that a drug could modulate directly the oscillatory mechanism which controls rhythmicity, so that circadian rhythms would be advanced or delayed to synchronise more rapidly with the new environment. Conversely, if ingested at the appropriate time, it could induce some activity, such as sleep, which would then, in turn, influence the basic mechanism. A drug could also alleviate some adverse effect during the process of adaptation, such as sleep disturbance.

In the context of altering the basic oscillatory mechanism attention has lately focused on melatonin, secretion of which is linked to the dark part of the cycle and suppressed by light. The proposal is that, if melatonin is given at an appropriate time preceding the sleep period, the cycle will be advanced, and in this way the endogenous oscillator will be altered and with it the observed circadian rhythms. This sequence of events would resemble the modulation of circadian rhythmicity by changes in illumination. But this claim needs careful consideration. Unequivocal evidence is required that melatonin has not simply distorted the observed rhythm, and that this has not been inadvertently interpreted as a shift in phase. For these reasons it is desirable that rhythms are recorded during the days after treatment has ceased, and that it can be shown that the effect is not an evoked phenomenon, but is indeed a genuine phase shift. . . .

In the absence of convincing evidence that melatonin shifts circadian rhythms, together with its effects on the endocrine system, it may be more appropriate to use hypnotics in the management of sleep disturbance after transmeridian flights. Hypnotics could reinforce the rest and activity cycle at the new local time, and this could bring about more rapid entrainment by influencing the deep oscillator. Indeed, reinforcement of the rest-activity cycle is an interpretation of recent studies in animals which claim phase shifts with benzodiazepines. In any event, a hypnotic would assist sleep at an unusual time of the day, and it would reduce nocturnal wakefulness during the adaptation phase. In this way, even if it did not have a powerful entraining effect, it might improve daytime function by avoiding undue sleep loss. Nevertheless, the activity of a hypnotic used in this way must be restricted in the sleep period, and be free of residual effects on daytime function and of accumulation with daily ingestion. It must also have the potential to sustain sleep overnight; after both westward and eastward flights individuals who react unfavourably to transmeridian journeys may experience difficulty in staying asleep. Indeed, the judicious and occasional use of a low dose of hypnotic would appear, at least for the moment, to be the preferred approach, although adequate attention must always be given to sleep habits and day-to-day life.

SOURCE:
"Jet Lag and Its Pharmacology." *The Lancet* (August 30, 1986): 493, 494.

RESOURCES

BOOK
Ehret, Charles F., and Lynne Waller Scanlan. *Overcoming Jet Lag*. New York: Berkley, 1986. 160 pp.

RELATED ARTICLES
Petrie, Keith, and others. "Effect of Melatonin on Jet Lag after Long Haul Flights." *British Medical Journal* 298 (March 18, 1989): 705–707.

Wooldridge, W. E. "Medical Complications of Air Travel." *Postgraduate Medicine* 87, no. 7 (May 15, 1990): 75–77.

KIDNEY DIALYSIS

OVERVIEW

Dialysis is a procedure that replaces some of the kidney's normal functions and is performed when a person's own kidneys can no longer function adequately to maintain life. In the United States today more than 100,000 individuals undergo dialysis treatments to stay alive.

Treatment with dialysis is necessary when a person experiences kidney failure—usually when more than 95 percent of normal kidney function is gone in both kidneys.

Like healthy kidneys, dialysis keeps the body in balance by: 1) removing waste products, including salt, and excess fluids that build-up in the body; 2) maintaining a safe level of blood chemicals in the body, such as potassium, sodium and chloride; and 3) controlling blood pressure.

Some forms of kidney failure are temporary and get better on their own. This is called acute kidney failure.

Dialysis may be necessary for a short period of time until the kidneys recover. Chronic or end-stage kidney failure is the result of an irreversible scarring process which results in kidney shutdown.

Chronic kidney failure does not get better and patients need dialysis treatments for the rest of their lives, or if they are medically eligible, they may choose to be placed on a waiting list to receive a kidney transplant. . . .

Dialysis can be performed in a hospital, a free-standing dialysis unit, or at home. The location is determined by the patient's medical condition and personal desires. The patient, working with the physician, determines the best location for treatment.

SOURCE:
National Kidney Foundation, Inc. *Dialysis*. 1989. pp. 1–2.

TYPES OF DIALYSIS

There are two types [of dialysis]—hemodialysis and peritoneal dialysis. In hemodialysis, the patient's bloodstream is diverted to an external machine that continuously filters the blood, corrects its chemistry, and returns it to the body.

Usually, hemodialysis patients are treated about three times a week. The procedure can be carried out in a hospital, a dialysis center, or at home. Home dialysis can be more convenient for the patient, but it requires that the patient or care-giver be thoroughly familiar with the dialysis procedure and equipment and the critical importance of measures to prevent contamination of the blood supply. At home or in a health-care facility, each dialysis treatment lasts about five hours.

In continuous ambulatory peritoneal dialysis the patient's blood is not shunted outside the body. Instead, a catheter placed in the patient's abdomen allows the abdominal space to be slowly filled with a solution—the dialysate—used to clean and re-balance the chemistry of blood flowing through vessels in the abdomen. After about four or five hours, the dialysate is allowed to drain through the catheter and a fresh supply is introduced. The procedure is repeated several times a day while the patient goes about normal activities.

Cycling peritoneal dialysis is basically identical. It, however, requires an external machine and is usually done for about an hour and a half at night while the patient sleeps. Intermittent peritoneal dialysis is a hospital procedure that takes 10 to 12 hours. The oldest form of dialysis, it is often used in emergencies or as the first dialysis procedure following total kidney failure.

SOURCE:
Flieger, Ken. "Kidney Disease: When Those Fabulous Filters Are Foiled." *FDA Consumer*. March 1990. p. 29.

HEMODIALYSIS

In hemodialysis, an artificial kidney (hemodialyzer) is used to remove waste products from the blood and restore the body's chemical balance. In order to get the patient's blood to the artificial kidney, it is necessary to make an access to the patient's blood vessels. This requires surgery on an arm or a leg. The surgical procedure connects an artery to a vein underneath the skin. The joining of an artery to a vein creates an enlarged vessel known as a fistula. Once healing occurs, two needles are placed, one in the artery side and one in the vein side of the fistula. Plastic tubing connects the patient to the artificial kidney. . . .

The time required for each hemodialysis treatment is determined by the patient's amount of remaining kidney function, fluid weight gain between treatments and the build-up of harmful chemicals between treatments. On the average, each hemodialysis treatment lasts approximately 3-4 hours and is usually necessary three times per week.

A new treatment called high flux, or short-time dialysis is being used in some units. The exact time is determined by the person's body size, blood chemistries, food intake and urine output. It is important to stress that high-flux dialysis is not available everywhere. If treatment is available, the doctor will determine whether it is suitable for the patient.

SOURCE:
National Kidney Foundation, Inc. *Dialysis*. 1989. pp. 2-4.

PERITONEAL DIALYSIS

The three types of peritoneal dialysis are—Continuous Ambulatory Peritoneal Dialysis (CAPD); Continuous Cycling Peritoneal Dialysis (CCPD); and Intermittent Peritoneal Dialysis (IPD).

Continuous Ambulatory Peritoneal Dialysis (CAPD) is the only type of peritoneal dialysis that is done without the use of machines. Patients perform this procedure themselves, usually four or five times a day at home and at work. The patient drains a bag of dialysate into his/her peritoneal cavity by way of the catheter. The dialysate remains there for about 4-5 hours. After an exchange is complete, the patient drains the used dialysate back into the bag. The patient then repeats the procedure using a new bag of dialysate. While the dialysate remains inside the peritoneal cavity, the patient can go about his/her daily activities.

Continuous Cycling Peritoneal Dialysis (CCPD) differs from CAPD in that a machine (cycler) delivers and then drains the cleansing fluid rather than you adding and draining the fluid. The treatment usually is done at night when you sleep.

Intermittent Peritoneal Dialysis (IPD) is the oldest form of dialysis and is usually done in the hospital for 10-12 hours, three times each week. This treatment is often done in emergency situations or as a first dialysis treatment. The patient is hooked up to a machine during treatment, as in CCPD.

SOURCE:
National Kidney Foundation, Inc. *Dialysis*. 1989. pp. 5-6.

RESOURCES

ORGANIZATIONS

National Institute of Arthritis, Diabetes, and Digestive and Kidney Diseases. Westwood Building, Room 657, Bethesda, MD 20205.

National Kidney Foundation. 30 East 33rd Street, New York, NY 10016.

PAMPHLET

Cleveland Clinic Foundation:

Kidney Dialysis: What Are Your Options? August 1989. 15 pp.

RELATED ARTICLES

Berger, Edward E., and Edmund G. Lowrie. "Mortality and the Length of Dialysis." *JAMA* 265 (February 20, 1991): 909-910.

Copley, John B. "Dialysis." *Diabetes Forecast* (June 1990): 30, 32-35.

Maher, John F., and Andrew T. Maher. "Continuous Ambulatory Peritoneal Dialysis." *American Family Physician* 40, no. 5 (November 1989): 187-192.

Miller, Lisa Anselme. "At-Home Help for the CAPD Patient." *RN* (August 1990): 77-80.

Parfrey, P. S., H. Vavasour, and others. "Symptoms in End-Stage Renal Disease: Dialysis v. Transplantation." *Transplantation Proceedings* 19, no. 4 (August 1987): 3407-3409.

KIDNEY STONES

OVERVIEW

Renal stone disease (nephrolithiasis) accounts for about seven to ten of every 1000 hospital admissions in the United States and has an annual incidence of seven to 21 cases per 10,000 persons. Four of every five patients with stones are men, and in both sexes the peak age of onset is between 20 and 30 years, so people are affected during the years of prime adult life. The majority of stones, 70% to 80%, are composed of calcium oxalate crystals; the rest are composed of calcium phosphate salts, uric acid, struvite (magnesium, ammonium, and phosphate), or the amino acid cystine. Occasionally, stones injure kidneys and reduce their function by causing infection or obstruction, but many patients with stones suffer only from the pain of stone passage, urinary infection, and bleeding that is worrisome though not in itself dangerous, and from the inconvenience of hospitalization and the discomfort of urologic procedures. In essence, nephrolithiasis is a common cause of morbidity rather than of death or renal failure.

SOURCE:
"Prevention and Treatment of Kidney Stones." (Consensus Conference.) *JAMA* 260, no. 7 (August 19, 1988): 977-981.

* * *

A kidney stone develops when the salt and mineral substances in urine form crystals that stick together and grow in size. In most cases, these crystals are removed from the body by the flow of urine, but they sometimes stick to the lining of the kidney or settle in places where the urine flow fails to carry them away. These crystals may gather and grow into a stone ranging in size from that of a grain of sand to a golf ball. Most stones start to form in the kidney. Some may travel to other parts of the urinary system, such as the ureter or bladder, and grow there.

Kidney stone disease is an important medical problem in the United States. More than 1 million people are hospitalized each year for treatment of kidney stones. An equal number may be treated outside the hospital setting. About one fourth of those treated in hospitals have surgery as part of their treatment. An estimated 12 percent of men and 5 percent of women will have symptoms from a kidney stone at least once during their lifetime. Stones tend to occur in multiple numbers. They often recur even after spontaneous passage or surgical removal. Effective treatment depends upon finding the specific reasons why stones form.

Kidney stones tend to form when several factors work together in a susceptible person. The following factors may influence stone formation: age—more common during middle age; sex—three times more common in men than in women; activity—more common in people who are immobilized, or after excessive fluid loss through sweating; climate—more common in hot climates or during summer months; reduced water intake; during sleep; travel; genetic disorders such as gout, cystinuria, primary hyperoxaluria; metabolic disturbances, such as bowel, endocrine and kidney problems that increase blood and urine calcium and oxalate; diet—oxalate and calcium containing foods in excessive amounts can promote the tendency to stone formation in susceptible people; misuse of medications; urinary infections; and urine stagnation resulting from blockage give crystals a chance to grow.

Although a fair amount is known about kidney stones, the exact process leading to stone formation is still unclear. For instance, we know that urine normally contains chemicals that inhibit the formation of crystals. However, no one knows why these inhibitors do not work for everyone. Nor is it understood why stones form in some people, but not in others who have the same predisposing factors.

Kidney stones may form in some people without causing any symptoms. Some "silent" stones may cause only some blood in the urine or a persistent urinary infection. More often, a stone moves and irritates the lining of the urinary system or blocks the flow of urine. This can cause severe pain which usually starts suddenly and may last from minutes to hours, followed by long periods of relief. Nausea and vomiting may occur with the pain. Kidney stone pain usually starts in the kidney or lower abdomen and later may move to the groin. Burning and the urge to pass urine often may occur as the stone moves near the bladder. Cloudy or foul-smelling urine, fever, chills, and weakness may indicate the presence of an infection, which could result in a more serious illness.

Since 90 percent of stones contain calcium, x-rays can usually identify their presence and verify the cause of symptoms. A special dye is often injected into the patient before x-rays are taken to better assess the size and location of the stone and the relative function of the kidneys. Such x-rays are especially useful when a patient's stone contains little or no calcium. "Silent" stones—those not causing symptoms—usually are found during x-ray examination of the abdomen for other reasons. All stones associated with blockage or chronic infection should be removed to prevent further kidney damage.

When a diagnosis has been made, samples of the patient's blood and urine are tested for anything that might cause stone disease. Patients are questioned about their diet, use of medications, lifestyle and family history to learn about other factors that might contribute to stone formation.

SOURCE:
National Kidney Foundation, Inc. *About Kidney Stones*. 1988. pp. 1-4.

TREATMENT—USE OF EXTRACORPOREAL SHOCK WAVE LITHOTRIPSY

New instruments and techniques have improved and simplified the treatment of stones in the kidney or urinary tract. Percutaneous techniques permit surgeons to extract or disintegrate stones that as recently as five years ago could be treated only by conventional surgery. Open surgery now is required for the treatment of less than 5% of patients. The extracorporeal shock-wave lithotriptor was introduced into US practice in 1984; it can disrupt stones into fragments that can be passed with the urine, eliminating the need for most invasive surgery. Worldwide, over 500,000 patients have been treated with this instrument since 1980. These breakthroughs have reduced the risk of stone removal and have affected the public assessment of the benefits of medical stone prevention, complicating the question of what is the best way to evaluate and treat patients.

SOURCE:
"Prevention and Treatment of Kidney Stones." (Consensus Conference.) *JAMA* 260, no. 7 (August 19, 1988): 977-978.

* * *

Extracorporeal Shock Wave Lithotripsy (ESWL) is a nonsurgical technique for treating stones in the kidney and urinary tract. The procedure uses high energy shock waves to crush the stones into small particles the size of grains of sand, which can then be passed with the urine.

The major advantage of ESWL is that, in many patients, it avoids the need for invasive surgical procedures. As a result, complications, hospital stays, recovery period and costs are reduced with ESWL. Unfortunately, not all types of kidney stones can be treated by ESWL. Sometimes stone fragments may be left behind with ESWL.

The patient is placed in a stainless steel tub of comfortably warm water and positioned so that the stones are precisely targeted with the assistance of x-ray monitors. Typically, 1,000 to 2,000 shock waves are needed to crush the stones. The complete treatment takes about 45 to 60 minutes. ESWL technology is continuing to develop, and new variations may be introduced in the future.

Either local, regional or general anesthesia may be used. This reduces the movement of the patient's body and thus insures that the shock waves are focused on the stone.

Most patients are hospitalized for 1 to 2 days. In some cases, the procedure may be performed entirely on an outpatient basis. In contrast, patients undergoing comparable surgery for kidney stones typically remain in the hospital for 5 to 7 days, followed by 2 to 5 weeks of recuperation at home.

SOURCE:
National Kidney Foundation. *New Techniques for Treating Kidney Stones: Extracorporeal Shock Wave Lithotripsy*. 1987.

LASER TREATMENT

Doctors are increasingly turning to lasers to treat a painful and common ailment: kidney stones.

The procedure, which was approved by the Food and Drug Administration three years ago, has grown rapidly in use and is now one of the most common methods of treating stones in the lower ureter, the narrow passageway between the kidney and the bladder.

While just a few hundred of the more than 350,000 cases of kidney stones were treated with the laser when it was first introduced, nearly 25,000 kidney stone patients received the therapy last year. . . .

To treat kidney stones, a doctor inserts a hair-thin optical fiber into the patient's ureter until it reaches the stones. The laser is then triggered, releasing a burst of energy in the form of green light that breaks up the stone but leaves the surrounding tissue unharmed.

Many kidney specialists say laser therapy is the safest, simplest and least invasive method of treating stones in the lower ureter. About 20 percent of kidney stone cases involve stones in this area.

"With this method, we can get access to stones we could not see before," said Dr. Stephen P. Dretler, a urologist at Massachusetts General Hospital who helped developed the laser technique there in 1986.

About 180 hospitals around the world now have the laser machines, which can cost up to $200,000 each. . . .

After the laser impulses are transmitted through the fiber and smash the stone, the pieces are then either passed through the urine or pulled out using a miniature basket inserted through a catheter. The entire procedure takes about 35 minutes and requires a hospital stay of just two to three days.

SOURCE:
"Laser Treatment Coming of Age for the Removal of Kidney Stones." *The New York Times* (August 3, 1989): B5.

RESOURCES

ORGANIZATIONS
National Institute of Arthritis, Diabetes, and Digestive and Kidney Diseases. Westwood Building, Room 657, Bethesda, MD 20205.

National Kidney Foundation. 30 East 33rd St., New York, NY 10016.

PAMPHLET
American Kidney Fund:

Facts About Kidney Stones. 1987.

RELATED ARTICLES
LaPorte, Joann, and Neil Baum. "Kidney Stones: How to Identify the Cause and Prevent Recurrence." *Postgraduate Medicine* 87, no. 5 (April 1990): 219–225.

Lingeman, James E., and others. "Kidney Stones: Acute Management." *Patient Care* (August 15, 1990): 20–41.

Lingeman, James E., and others. "The Role of Lithotripsy and Its Side Effects." *Journal of Urology* 141 (March 1989): 793–797.

Motola, Jay A., and Arthur D. Smith. "Therapeutic Options for the Management of Upper Tract Calculi." *Urologic Clinics of North America* 17, no. 1 (February 1990): 191–206.

Peckrel, Kerry. "Say Goodbye to Kidney Stones: New Nonsurgical Treatments and Dietary Changes Can Rid You of Painful Kidney Stone for Good." *Prevention* (September 1989): 58–61.

LACTOSE INTOLERANCE

OVERVIEW

Lactose intolerance is the inability to digest significant amounts of lactose, which is the predominant sugar of milk. Close to 50 million American adults are lactose intolerant. Certain ethnic and racial populations are more widely affected than others. As many as 75 percent of all African-American, Jewish, Native American, and Mexican-American adults, and 90 percent of Asian-American adults are lactose intolerant. The condition is least common among persons of northern European descent.

Lactose intolerance results from a shortage of the enzyme lactase, which is normally produced by the cells that line the small intestine. Lactase breaks down milk sugar into simpler forms that can then be absorbed into the bloodstream. When there is not enough lactase to digest the amount of lactose consumed, the results, although not usually dangerous, may be very distressing.

Common symptoms include nausea, cramps, bloating, gas, and diarrhea, which begin about 30 minutes to 2 hours after eating or drinking foods containing lactose. Many people who have never been diagnosed as lactose intolerant or "lactase deficient" may notice that milk and other dairy products cause problems that don't occur when eating other foods. The severity of symptoms varies depending on the amount of lactose each individual can tolerate.

Some causes of lactose intolerance are well known. For instance, certain digestive diseases and injuries to the small intestine can reduce the amount of enzymes produced. In rare cases, children are born without the ability to produce lactase. For most people, though, lactase deficiency is a condition that develops naturally, over time. After about the age of 2 years, the body begins to produce less lactase. The reasons for this are unclear and still under study.

The most common tests used to measure the absorption of lactose in the digestive system are the lactose tolerance test, the hydrogen breath test, and the stool acidity test. A doctor can tell you where to go for these tests, which are performed on an outpatient basis at a hospital or clinic. . . .

Fortunately, lactose intolerance is relatively easy to treat. No known way exists to increase the amount of lactase enzyme the body can make, but symptoms can be controlled through diet.

Small children born with lactase deficiency should not be fed any foods containing lactose. Most older children and adults need not avoid lactose completely, but individuals differ in the amounts of lactose they can handle. For example, one person may suffer symptoms after drinking a small glass of milk, while another can drink one glass but not two. Others may be able to manage ice cream and aged cheeses, such as cheddar and Swiss, but not other dairy products. Dietary control of the problem depends on each person's knowing, through trial and error, *how much* milk sugar and *what forms* of it his or her body can handle.

For those who react to very small amounts of lactose or have trouble limiting their intake of foods that contain lactose, lactase additives are available from drug stores without a prescription. One form is a liquid for use with milk. A few drops are added to a quart of milk, and after 24 hours in the refrigerator, the lactose content is reduced by 70 percent. The process works faster if the milk is heated first, and adding a double amount of lactase liquid produces milk that is 90 percent lactose free. A more recent development is a lactase tablet that helps people digest solid foods that contain lactose. One to three tablets are taken just before a meal or snack.

At somewhat higher cost, shoppers can buy lactose-reduced milk at most supermarkets. The milk contains all of the other nutrients found in regular milk and remains fresh for about the same length of time.

Milk and other dairy products are a major source of nutrients in the basic American diet. The most important of these nutrients is calcium. Calcium is needed for the growth and repair of bones throughout life, and in the middle and later years, a shortage of calcium may lead to thin, fragile bones that break easily (a condition called "osteoporosis"). A concern, then, for both children and adults with lactose intolerance is how to get enough calcium in a diet that includes little or no milk.

Although the RDA (recommended dietary allowance) for calcium, set in 1980, is 800 mg per day, many experts in bone disease believe this is too low. The results of a 1984 conference at the National Institutes of Health (NIH) suggest that women who have not yet reached menopause and older women who are taking the hormone estrogen after menopause should consume about 1,000 mg of calcium daily (routhly the amount in a quart of milk). Pregnant women and nursing mothers need about 1,200 mg of calcium per day. Postmenopausal women not taking estrogen may need as much as 1,500 mg of calcium per day. The RDA for adult men is 1,000 mg per day and 1,500 mg per day for men in their later years.

It is important, therefore, in meal planning to make sure that each day's diet includes enough calcium, even if the diet does not contain dairy products. Quite a few foods are high in calcium and low in lactose. Many green vegetables and fish with soft, edible bones are excellent examples. . . .

Recent research has shown that yogurt may be a very good source of calcium for many lactose intolerant people, even though it is fairly high in lactose. There is evidence that the bacterial cultures used in making yogurt produce the lactase required for proper digestion.

Although milk and foods made from milk are the only noteworthy natural sources, lactose is often added to prepared foods. It is important for people with very low tolerance for lactose to know about the many foods that may contain lactose, even in small amounts. Grocery items that may contain lactose include:

- Bread and other baked goods.
- Processed breakfast cereals.
- Instant potatoes, soups, and breakfast drinks.
- Margarine.
- Lunch meats (other than kosher).
- Salad dressings.
- Candies and other snacks.
- Mixes for pancakes, biscuits, cookies, etc.

Some so-called nondairy products such as powdered coffee creamer and whipped toppings also may include ingredients that are derived from milk and therefore contain lactose.

Smart shoppers learn to read food labels with care, looking not only for *milk* and *lactose* among the contents but also for such words as whey, curds, milk byproducts, dry milk solids, and nonfat dry milk powder. If any of these are listed on a label, the item contains lactose.

SOURCE:
National Digestive Diseases Information Clearinghouse. *Important Information for You and Your Family: Lactose Intolerance.* 1991. pp. 1-4.

CHILDREN AND LACTOSE INTOLERANCE

Children have complained about stomach aches for ages. Figuring out what is causing the problem is tricky, even for doctors. Abdominal pain is a constituent of so many diseases and situations from stress and fear to flu and urinary tract infection. During the early 1960s, studies were done on children who had frequent tummy aches, as often as once a month for several months in a row. Scientists believe that as many as 15 percent of children who see pediatricians suffer with pain in the abdomen this frequently. This syndrome has been called "recurrent abdominal pain" (RAP).

Some of the common factors seen in RAP are children who look pale, suffer from headaches, were usually very colicky babies, and complain of stomach pain often.

Studies of these children revealed that some actually suffered from peptic ulcers. A few had urinary tract infections. Follow-up showed that some of them grew up to develop inflammatory bowel disease. It is important to note that 40 percent of these children were found to be lactose intolerant. It is also interesting to realize that for so many children, the diagnosis of lactose intolerance was missed because they did not show the classic symptoms of distention and diarrhea. Pediatricians more often attributed the abdominal pain in these children to psychogenic factors, and unfortunately did not remove milk and other dairy products from their diet.

These studies should have a great bearing on the way children with abdominal pain are treated by their doctors and parents. Do not assume that pain in the absence of diarrhea or disease is always stress-related. Lactose intolerance may be the culprit.

You should ask your pediatrician to check with a breath hydrogen test that has been modified for children. Or, you may do a challenge test at home. Simply eliminate all dairy products and lactose sources from your child's diet for at least four weeks. Keep a daily diary listing the foods your child is eating and note tummy ache complaints. After two weeks you should know whether lactose intolerance could be a factor.

Sometimes it is frustrating to live with a child who complains about stomach aches often. Parents may feel that the child is using his pain to manipulate the family or avoid life situations. But, we shouldn't automatically assume that this is the case when children complain about abdominal pain. Be sure to check all possible physical causes. Then, if a psychological problem is diagnosed, don't stop there. Help your child with professional guidance.

SOURCE:
"Abdominal Pain in Dairy-Fed Children." *Nutrition Health Review* (Winter 1990): 11.

* * *

Children with a milk intolerance lack the enzyme lactase so they can't break down lactose (milk sugar) into the simple sugars glucose and galactose. Many children with a lactase deficiency find they can eat yogurt without any problems. Yogurt contains bacteria that make beta-galacto-sidase, an enzyme that breaks down lactose. This enzyme is not found in unfermented products such as acidophilus milk, cultured milk, or pasteurized yogurt.

Unflavored yogurt caused the least problems, while flavored yogurts caused a few more problems. Frozen yogurt was similar to sherbert and ice cream in terms of the problems it caused.

SOURCE:
Sagall, Richard J. "Yogurt and Milk Intolerance." *Pediatrics for Parents* 9 (January 1988): 7.

USE OF LACTAID, LACTRASE

The lactose-intolerant individual may well benefit from commercially available lactase (LactAid, Lactrase). When added to whole or skim, fresh, canned, or reconstituted dry milk, cream, or infant formula, it reduces the lactose to glucose and galactose. The liquid form—a yeast-derived β-D-galactosidase in a glycerol carrier—calls for four or five drops per quart of milk. After shaking or mixing, the milk is refrigerated for 24 hours, during which time about 70% of the lactose is hydrolyzed. For someone who cannot tolerate even that small amount of lactose, have him add twice the amount of enzyme; this will reduce the lactose by more than 90%. This treated milk, which has an unchanged shelf-life, can be used for drinking, cooking, baking, making cheese and yogurt, and formula. The only change in its taste is a slight increase in sweetness due to the sweeter monosaccharides. Hydrolysis adds merely a trace to the caloric and carbohydrate value of the milk, but diabetics should be aware of its higher content of rapidly absorbed simple sugars.

Tablet and capsule forms of commercial lactase are also available. One or two of these taken with milk products usually allow the lactose-intolerant individual to consume the equivalent of a serving of milk without developing symptoms. Alternatively, the contents of the capsule form can be sprinkled on lactose-containing foods at the table.

SOURCE:
Bayless, Theodore, Irwin H. Rosenberg, and others. "When to Suspect Lactose Intolerance." *Patient Care* (September 30, 1987): 136–141, 144–145, 147.

RESOURCES

ORGANIZATIONS

American Dietetic Association. 216 West Jackson Blvd., Chicago, IL 60600.

National Digestive Diseases Information Clearinghouse. 1255 23rd St. NW, Suite 275, Washington, DC 20037.

BOOKS

American Dietetic Association. *Lactose Intolerance: A Resource Including Recipes*. Food Sensitivity Series. Chicago: American Dietetic Association, 1985.

Catper, Steve. *No Milk Today: How to Live With Lactose Intolerance*. New York: Simon and Schuster, 1980.

Zukin, Jane. *Dairy-Free Cooking*. New York: St. Martin's, 1989.

RELATED ARTICLES

Bayless, Theodore M., Irwin H. Rosenberg, and others. "When to Suspect Lactose Intolerance." *Patient Care* 21 (September 30, 1987): 136–141, 144–145, 147.

Murray, E. B. "The Acceptability of Milk and Milk Products in Populations With a High Prevalence of Lactose Intolerance." [Review] *American Journal of Clinical Nutrition* 48 (4 Suppl.) (October 1988): 1079–1159.

Vankineni, P. "Relative Efficiency of Yogurt, Sweet Acidophilus Milk, Hydrolyzed-Lactose Milk, and a Commercial Lactase Tablet in Alleviating Lactose Maldigestion." *American Journal of Clinical Nutrition* 49, no. 6 (June 1989): 1233–1237.

LASER SURGERY

OVERVIEW

As early as 1917, Albert Einstein had developed the theoretical basis for lasers. The term L-A-S-E-R is an acronym for Light Amplification by Stimulated Emission of Radiation (radiation here meaning light radiation). However, it was only in 1960, following much work by Soviet and U.S. scientists, that an American team of researchers finally overcame the technological hurdles and assembled the first rudimentary but workable laser. Since then, lasers have undergone a rapid advance. Surgeons were quick to recognize the potential for a highly focused cutting beam. By 1965, the first laser was in use for treating certain eye problems, such as a torn retina. Although the early machines were cumbersome and impractical, by the early 1970s argon lasers were being used experimentally for several medical procedures, including the treatment of diabetic eye problems and removal of small skin growths. Today the instruments are ubiquitous—contributing to areas as diverse as Beatlemania light shows, removing hemorrhoids and eradicating birthmarks. Laser technology has found its way into a broad range of medical specialties: from gynecology, gastroenterology, dentistry, dermatology, urology, ophthalmology, and neurology to ear, nose, and throat surgery and cancer treatment. Lasers can seal off bleeding blood vessels, kill malignant cells and vaporize away small growths in inaccessible parts of the body, such as the bowel and vocal cords, avoiding the need for surgery.

As the machines become cheaper, more manageable and "user friendly," small hospitals and clinics are acquiring their own laser centres. Their rapidly expanding repertoire brings significant benefits, in some cases almost replacing conventional therapy. The laser hasn't yet quite usurped the surgeon's knife, but if present trends continue, the surgical scalpel may ultimately retire to medical museums, along with leech jars and cupping basins.

Although new lasers are continually being developed, those most prevalent in medicine today are: the carbon dioxide (CO_2) laser, the neodymium-yttrium-aluminum-garnet solid state laser (Nd:YAG) and the argon laser. Lasers recently introduced for medical uses include the excimer laser and the tunable dye laser.

SOURCE:

"Lasers Revolutionize Medicine." *Health News* (October 1990): 7–8.

APPLICATIONS

For treating certain eye disorders. Since ophthalmologists first adopted lasers to treat retinal eye disorders in the mid-1960s, their use has been extended to treat many eye problems, enabling surgeons to work with local anesthesia. Argon lasers are widely used for treating diabetic retinopathy—a major cause of blindness (due to an abnormal collection of retinal blood vessels which become leaky). The argon laser beam penetrates the clear watery cornea without harming it and photocoagulates the bleeding vessels at the back of the eye, halting disease progression, although it can't always restore any vision already lost. Lasers are also invaluable for spot-welding tiny tears/holes that may lead to retinal detachment. Similarly, argon lasers are sometimes used for age-related macular degeneration (a major cause of vision loss in those over age 60). Both argon and Nd:YAG lasers can zap tiny holes in the eye's iris to alleviate the fluid build-up and pressure of glaucoma and to promote the flow of fluid away from the eye in open angle glaucoma. Contrary to popular misconception, lasers are not used in cataract surgery, although the Nd:YAG is sometimes employed after cataract surgery, to clear a cloudy layer behind the lens implant.

For gastrointestinal/digestive tract problems. Fibreoptic delivery systems have revolutionized the use of lasers in stomach and intestinal problems. The attachment of argon and Nd:YAG lasers to long fibreoptic cables enables doctors to see and reach otherwise inaccessible parts of the body, which formerly required major surgery. In diagnosing and treating digestive system problems, a surgeon can watch the laser's progress through the endoscope as it travels along the digestive tract on a video screen and accurately coagulate or vaporize away small tumors, ulcers or other lesions deep within the body. Endoscopic laser therapy is now often used to shrink large cancerous colorectal tumours that obstruct bowel function, making patients more comfortable.

For removal of gynecological growths. Both CO_2 and YAG lasers are now widely used to eradicate lesions of the vulva, vagina and cervix (opening of the uterus/womb) and for vaporizing away genital warts. Done easily and rapidly, on an out-patient basis, laser vaporization of non-cancerous cervical growths leaves the cervix in considerably better shape than conventional therapy—with less scarring, stenosis (constriction, narrowing) and post-operative pain or discharge.

SOURCE:
"Lasers Revolutionize Medicine." *Health News* (University of Toronto) (October 1990): 10.

USE IN REMOVAL OF ATHEROSCLEROTIC PLAQUE

Perhaps the most exciting prospect for laser surgery involves the removal of atherosclerotic plaque, the fatty deposits that plug up coronary arteries, causing heart attacks. Short of bypass surgery, the best current method of dealing with plaque is balloon angioplasty, in which a catheter is slid up an artery from thigh to heart, where a balloon at its tip is expanded. The expanded balloon flattens the lump of plaque against the vessel wall and makes more room for blood to flow, but in 30 to 40 percent of patients, the plaque gradually regains its obstructing shape. If instead of a balloon a laser fiber were in the catheter, it could melt or burn away the plaque altogether.

In fact, such laser treatment for plaque has been tried experimentally in animals, and later in humans. But the heat generated in the plaque would often spread to the artery wall, damaging it or even burning through it. Recently, however, doctors at Cedars-Sinai Medical Center in Los Angeles began using the ultraviolet light of an excimer laser, delivered in extremely short bursts; the heat generated in the plaque by each burst dissipates before it can affect the artery wall. In September of last year, Frank Litvack, M.D. of Cedars-Sinai reported to a cardiology conference that his group has used this method successfully on 110 patients, with no arterial perforations or deaths, and with only a 2.8 percent emergency surgical bypass rate, comparable to that of balloon angioplasty.

SOURCE:
Hunt, Morton. "Beams of Life." *Longevity* (December 1989/January 1990): 54.

RESOURCES

RELATED ARTICLES

"Cool Laser Zaps Plaques Without Char." *Medical World News* 29 (April 25, 1988): 96.

Gallagher, Maureen T., and Claudia Kahn. "Lasers: Scalpels of Light." *RN* 53 (May 1990): 46.

Hall, Laura T. "Cardiovascular Lasers: A Look Into the Future." *American Journal of Nursing* 90 (July 1990): 27.

"Lasers Battle Blindness." *Consumer Reports Health Letter* 2 (December 1990): 96.

LEAD POISONING

OVERVIEW

Lead is a neurotoxin. Although it often does not produce any physical symptoms, it can interfere with the development of a child's brain. In starker terms, lead is a killer of intelligence.

The metal has been known to be a health hazard since at least Roman times. But it wasn't until the early 1970's, when lead poisoning among poor children living in substandard housing made headlines, that the deadly nature of lead became widely appreciated in the United States. In many cases, children who ate chips or flakes of paint suffered convulsions and mental retardation, and some lapsed into comas.

Two decades later the problem persists, despite a ban on the residential use of lead paint. Fifty-five percent of poor black children have high enough levels of lead in their blood by the age of 6 to cause adverse effects, according to Dr. Herbert L. Needleman, a professor of psychiatry and pediatrics at the University of Pittsburgh School of Medicine.

But a growing body of evidence indicates that the risk of lead poisoning cuts across all socioeconomic groups. "Being financially comfortable offers no protection," says Dr. Needleman, who is one of many experts who believe that lead poisoning is the most common preventable serious disease of childhood.

The Federal Government estimates that 57 million houses and apartments—three-quarters of all occupied housing units built before 1980—contain lead paint. And it doesn't take home renovations to put people at risk. Peeling, chipping or cracking paint can release lead-contaminated dust—dust that can be ingested by young children, who constantly put their hands and their toys in their mouths. Children as well as adults can also be exposed to lead in soil, drinking water, some canned foods and even some ceramic dishes and cookware.

Many studies now show that lead is potentially harmful to children at much lower levels than previously thought. So experts say that exposure to small amounts of the metal, whether from paint dust or other sources, can pose an unacceptable risk.

"Lead at remarkably low concentrations has an awesome capability to rob children of some of their potential for the rest of their lives," says Dr. John F. Rosen, a professor of pediatrics at the Monteflore Medical Center in the Bronx.

A person's lead level is measured in micrograms per deciliter (about a fifth of a pint) of blood. A microgram is a millionth of a gram. Under the current Federal guideline, set by the Centers for Disease Control, a child with a level of 25 micrograms or more is considered to be at risk for neurological problems. (The standard for adults is 40.)

Studies of children have shown that lead at levels below the guideline can lower intelligence, cause memory loss, slow reaction time and shorten attention span. Most ominously, a child can suffer damage even before birth, since a woman can pass the toxin on to her fetus.

As a result of the new research on the dangers of low lead levels, the C.D.C. will most likely issue a lower Federal guideline—20 micrograms per deciliter—this summer, says Dr. Sue Binder, chief of the agency's lead poisoning prevention branch. Many researchers believe that millions of children already exceed that level.

SOURCE:

Yulsman, Tom. "Lead Hazards at Home." *The Good Health Magazine (New York Times)* (April 28, 1991): 28, 46.

HOME PRECAUTIONS

Children should be tested for lead poisoning unless they live in areas where widespread screening has revealed no problem, according to the Centers for Disease Control's advisory committee on lead. It recommends screening at 12 months and then again at 24 months. High-risk kids (from older run-down homes) should be tested earlier and more often. Make sure doctors use the "blood-lead test" instead of the FEP (Free Erythrocyte Protoporphyrin) test, which is extremely inaccurate. If results show elevated levels, get a confirmation test because even the blood-lead test are inexact. The blood-lead test should cost about $30.

Many doctors mistakenly believe that a blood-lead level under 25 micrograms per deciliter (written "25 mcg/dl") is safe. But the CDC is about to establish 10 mcg/dl as the level above which some sort of action should be taken. A child with a blood-lead level of 10–15 mcg/dl is not in imminent health danger but should be tested again three months later. If the lead level has not declined, the family should take steps to pinpoint and remove hazards by cleaning thoroughly and testing paint, drinking water and other potential sources. Make sure your child gets enough iron and calcium. If the level is more than 15 mcg/dl check with a doctor for a nutritional and medical assessment.

If your home was built before 1950, your probably have some lead paint, but others may have it, too. The Northeast, Midwest, and Western states have more lead than the South.

If your local health department won't test, two home kits have been rated by Consumers Union to be effective tests for highly leaded painted surfaces. LeadCheck Swabs are sold by HybriVet Systems Inc. (800-262-LEAD). Frandon Lead Alert Kit is sold by Frandon Enterprises, Inc. (800-359-9000).

If your child's blood-lead level is below 10 mcg/dl and the house has no cracking, peeling paint, don't panic. Odds are, renovations to remove the paint will just increase the dust level. Scrutinize windowsills, baseboards and doorframes, where friction grinds up the paint layers and creates lead dust. Watch for dust, not just peeling. To remove the dust, damp-mop or wipe with a high-phosphate detergent. Ask for trisodium phosphate washes (TSP) at paint or hardware stores. (It may not be available in some states.) Consider joining with other tenants or homeowners to buy a HEPAvac (High Efficiency Particulate Air Filtered Vacuum), which costs about $1,000, for an occasional superscrubbing, or check with the health department to see if one can be rented. Other experts recommend scrubbing with a TSP-drenched sponge. Or use a wet-and-dry or shop vacuum with this procedure: sponge down all smooth surfaces with TSP soap twice. Wet-mop the same surfaces using a solution of diluted high-phosphate soap. Make sure the surfaces are plenty wet and then clean with the shop vacuum.

Do not attempt a full-scale abatement yourself. If tests show you have a major hazard, hire a qualified contractor. An improperly done abatement will make things worse. The safest approach is encapsulating, covering or removing painted structures entirely. Scraping or using a heat gun can be trouble if done improperly. Power sanding and open-flame burning are almost always dangerous. Complete removal can cost thousands of dollars, but you might significantly reduce the hazard by replacing doors, window frames or contaminated carpeting, or by putting up wallpaper or paneling. Consult the health department about what to do with the leaded waste.

If your local health department doesn't have a list of recommended contractors, try the regional office of the U.S. Department of Housing and Urban Development. On the East Coast, call the Massachusetts Department of Labor and Industry (617-727-1932), or Maryland's Department of Environment (301-631-3859). Some contractors may be listed in the phone book under lead, others under asbestos. Grill them to ensure they're qualified: Have they been through a special lead-paint-abatement training program? What kind of cleanup do they do? What kind of precautions do they take for workers?

If you have lead-based paint, the safest approach [to doing renovations] is to send kids away from home until work is done and the house has been thoroughly cleaned. If that's impossible, seal off the rooms being renovated and clean well.

Exterior paint: Watch out during warm weather when children play on the porch or in a front yard. People can also track lead dust into the house.

Buying a house: Most inspections do not test for lead paint. Try to test and abate before you move in.

Ask your local water supplier for the names of EPA-certified laboratories that will test your water for $15 to $35. EPA considers water safe if it has less than 15 parts per billion of lead, although some doctors and advocacy groups call for less than 10. You should test if you have water from a drinking well, pipes with lead solder or water known to be very corrosive. EPA has a safe-drinking-water hot line that may help answer questions (800-426-4791). If water has too much lead, reduce risk by running the faucet for a minute. When cooking or washing vegetables use cold water, which is less likely to pick up lead. Be wary of water-filter scam artists; most filters don't work on lead.

Some imported ceramic dishes have lead in them. Test with a home kit. Don't store liquids in lead crystal; the lead may leach out. It's fine to use it for serving.

SOURCE:

Waldman, Steven. "Lead and Your Kids." *Newsweek* (July 15, 1991): 46–47.

REDUCING EXPOSURE TO LEAD-BASED PAINT

If you have lead-based paint, you should take steps to reduce your exposure to lead. You can:

1. Have the painted item replaced.
   - You can replace a door or other easily removed item if you can do it without creating lead dust. Items that are difficult to remove should be replaced by professionals who will control and contain lead dust.
2. Cover the lead-based paint.
   - You can spray the surface with a sealant or cover it with gypsum wallboard. However, painting over lead-based paint with non-lead paint is not a long-term solution. Even though the lead-based paint may be covered by non-lead paint, the lead-based paint may continue to loosen from the surface below and create lead dust. The new paint may also partially mix with the lead-based paint, and lead dust will be released when the new paint begins to deteriorate.
3. Have the lead-based paint removed.
   - Have professionals trained in removing lead-based paint do this work. Each of the paint-removal methods (sandpaper, scrapers, chemicals, sandblasters, and torches or heat guns) can produce lead fumes or dust. Fumes or dust can become airborne and be inhaled or ingested. Wet methods help reduce the amount of lead dust. Removing moldings, trim, window sills, and other painted surfaces for professional paint stripping outside the home may also create dust. Be sure the professionals contain the lead dust. Wet-pipe all surfaces to remove any dust or paint chips. Wet-clean the area before re-entry.
   - You can remove a small amount of lead-based paint if you can avoid creating any dust. Make sure the surface is less than about one square foot (such as a window sill). Any job larger than about one square foot should be done by professionals. Make sure you can use a wet method (such as a liquid paint stripper).
4. Reduce lead dust exposure.
   - You can periodically wet mop and wipe surfaces and floors with a high phosphorous (at least 5%) cleaning solution. Wear waterproof gloves to prevent skin irritation. Avoid activities that will disturb or damage lead based paint and create dust. This is a preventive measure and is not an alternative to replacement or removal.

SOURCE:
U.S. Consumer Product Safety Commission. "What You Should Know about Lead-Based Paint in Your Home." *Consumer Product Safety Alert* (September 1990): 3.

FEDERAL GUIDELINES

Dr. William Roper, director of the Federal Centers for Disease Control, said: "We believe that lead poisoning is the No. 1 environmental problem facing America's children. Therefore, it will take a major societal effort to eliminate it." . . .

The Department of Health and Human Services has drawn up guidelines for taking action on lead in the blood. It will start at 10 micrograms of lead for each deciliter of blood, at which level local officials are to be alerted so they may consider setting up programs to check lead levels in children living in high-risk areas.

It is believed that four to six million children already have lead in their blood at this level or above, at which damage to the nervous system may begin.

At 15 to 20 micrograms, the Government will recommend that a child be tested again, and that his parents consider cleaning up the lead in the house or changing the child's diet.

At 20 to 24 micrograms, the Government guidelines recommend that a child be closely monitored by the local health agency, with public health officials visiting the home to test for lead, and to recommend a clean up of lead in the home, and to offer help in changing a child's diet.

At 25 to 50 micrograms, medical treatment for lead poisoning will begin. Under the current Federal guidelines, no action is taken until a child's blood tests at 25 micrograms or higher, a level at which experts say damage to a child's nervous system has probably already begun.

The Government's goal is to get the highest level of lead in children to 10 micrograms by the end of the decade.

SOURCE:
Hilts, Philip J. "U.S. Opens a Drive on Lead Poisoning in Nation's Young." *The New York Times* (December 10, 1990): A1, A16.

HAZARDS OF LEAD CRYSTAL CONTAINERS

A recent study reported that wine and spirits can leach lead from crystal, and while no one is suggesting that $150 lead crystal goblets or $2,000 decanters be discarded, the Food and Drug Administration is recommending that people rethink the way they use lead crystal containers for food and beverages.

Lead is a chronic hazard that can damage the nervous system, the kidneys and bone marrow. Fetuses and small children are particularly sensitive to lead.

Jerry Burke, the director of the F.D.A.'s Office of Physical Science, made these recommendations:

- Do not use lead crystal every day. Occasional use is all right, but if you have a daily glass of wine, don't drink it from a crystal goblet.
- Don't store foods or beverages for long periods in crystal. This is particularly true for acidic juices, vinegar and alcoholic beverages. Mr. Burke defines a week or two as long. Others say overnight is the maximum.
- Women of child-bearing age should not use crystal ware.

• Don't feed children from crystal bottles or tumblers.

The current Federal limit for lead in water is 50 micrograms per liter, but that is expected to drop to 20 micrograms later this year.

There are no Federal standards for the amount of lead that is permitted to leach from crystal, but the F.D.A. says that standards for ceramic ware can be used as a benchmark for crystal. A large piece of ceramic holloware—one that will hold 1.1 liters or more—is permitted to leach 2,500 micrograms per liter in a 24-hour period when it contains a solution similar in acidity to white distilled vinegar. Smaller holloware pieces can leach 5,000 micrograms per liter. The F.D.A. is reviewing changes in the standards for large ceramic pitchers that would drastically reduce the permissible lead to 100 micrograms.

In the study, recently published in *The Lancet*, a British medical journal, Dr. Joseph H. Graziano and Dr. Conrad Blum at Columbia University discovered large amounts of lead in wine that had been stored in crystal decanters. Many but not all of the crystal pieces leached lead.

They also found that tiny amounts of lead begin to migrate to wine from crystal goblets and decanters within minutes of contact. After four months of storage in crystal decanters, the lead levels ranged from 2,162 to 5,333 micrograms per liter.

Mr. Burke suggests that people test their crystal with the Frandon Lead Alert Kit. "At this stage of the game it is a conservative measure," he said. The Frandon kit is available for $29.95, plus $3.50 shipping, from Frandon Enterprises, P.O. Box 300321, Seattle, Wash. 98103; (800) 359-9000.

SOURCE:

Burros, Marian. "F.D.A. Reacts to Peril of Lead in Crystal." *The New York Times* (February 20, 1991): B5.

RESOURCES

ORGANIZATIONS

Consumer Product Safety Commission. 5401 Westbard Ave., Bethesda, MD 20207.

Environmental Protection Agency (EPA). 401 M St., SW, Washington, DC 20460.

Food and Drug Administration (FDA). 5600 Fishers Lane, Rockville, MD 20857.

National Institute for Occupational Safety and Health (NIOSH). 1600 Clifton Rd., NE, Atlanta, GA 30333.

Occupational Safety and Health Administration (OSHA). 200 Constitution Ave., Washington, DC 20210.

RELATED ARTICLES

Agency for Toxic Substances and Disease Registry. *The Nature and Extent of Lead Poisoning in Children in the United States: A Report to Congress*. 1988.

Greeley, Alexandra. "Getting the Lead Out of Just about Everything." *FDA Consumer* (July/August 1991): 26–31.

Jaroff, Leon. "Controlling a Childhood Menace: Lead Poisoning Poses the Biggest Environmental Threat to the Young." *Time* (February 25, 1991): 68–69.

Needleman, H. L., and others. "The Long-Term Effects of Exposure to Low Doses of Lead in Childhood." *The New England Journal of Medicine* 322 (1990): 83–88.

"Plumb Brandy." *Harvard Health Letter* (April 1991): 7.

LEUKEMIA

OVERVIEW

Leukemia affects the production of white blood cells, causing them to reproduce uncontrollably, crowding out existing healthy cells. These abnormal white cells "overpopulate" the bone marrow—often with immature, nonfunctioning blasts—and spill over into the bloodstream. Hence the term leukemia, which is derived from the Greek, and literally means "white blood."

The bone marrow becomes severely impaired and is unable to maintain production of sufficient levels of red blood cells and platelets, while white cell production becomes so rapid that these cells do not reach the level of maturity necessary to perform their infection-fighting functions.

Leukemic cells infiltrate all the major organs of the body, sometimes causing these organs to malfunction or fail. The kidneys may become impaired. The liver may become enlarged, as may the spleen—particularly characteristic of CML [Chronic Myelogenous Leukemia]—causing it to become overactive, a condition known as hypersplenism. Normally, the spleen acts as a filter for the blood, screening out aging red cells and platelets. When the spleen becomes enlarged, it can actually start doing its job too well, removing perfectly healthy red cells and platelets—further reducing the number of these already decreased cells.

As leukemia progresses, the entire blood system becomes flooded with useless, immature blast cells. If this disease is left untreated, a person with leukemia becomes increasingly susceptible to fatigue, excessive bleeding and infections until, finally, the body becomes virtually defenseless—making every minor injury or infection very serious.

Leukemia, itself, rarely kills. People may die, instead, from internal bleeding which would have been prevented by the platelets. Or, more often, they may die from infections which may start with a minor virus or bacteria, and which would have ordinarily been quickly wiped out by healthy white blood cells.

The exact course leukemia takes, and the speed with which it takes that course, varies with the type and age of the white cells initially affected.

There are two major types of leukemia: lymphocytic leukemia which involves lymphoid committed cells which form and mature in the lymphatic system, and myelogenous leukemia which affects myeloid committed cells which form and mature in the bone marrow. In medical terminology, the root "myelo" always refers to bone marrow.

Each of these types can occur in either the acute or chronic form. The acute form affects young cells still involved in the growth process which divide quickly and hasten the progress of the disease. The chronic form involves more mature cells which have stopped dividing or do so at a relatively slow rate.

Chronic myelogenous or granulocytic leukemia specifically involves the overproduction of granulocytes which evolve from the myeloid "committed" cell. Since granulocytes are among the most mature white cells produced in the bone marrow, CML is considered to be a slowly-progressing disease. It does progress, however, and—if left undiagnosed or untreated—will reach its advanced leukemic stage, with far too much discomfort and in far too little time.

SOURCE:
Leukemia Society of America. *Chronic Myelogenous Leukemia.* 1988. p. 4.

CHRONIC LYMPHOCYTIC LEUKEMIA

The leukemias represent the ninth most prevalent fatal cancer in the United States. The most common type of leukemia in Western countries is chronic lymphocytic leukemia (CLL), which accounts for 25 to 40 percent of all leukemias. The average annual age-adjusted incidence of CLL in the United States is 24.6 cases per 100,000 in males and 12.3 cases per 100,000 in females. This incidence is approximately the same as the incidence of multiple myeloma, malignant melanoma and central nervous system cancers.

CLL is defined as a sustained, malignant proliferation of monoclonal, immunologically incompetent lymphocytes, leading to lymphocyte accumulation in the bone marrow, spleen, liver and superficial and deep lymph nodes. In over 95 percent of patients, the abnormal cell is a B-lymphocyte (B-CLL); in only a few patients are the T-cells affected.

CLL is a disease of the elderly. Ninety percent of all cases occur in persons over age 50; nearly 70 percent of patients are older than 60 years. Males are affected twice as often as females. Signs and symptoms of the disease often develop so insidiously that the onset cannot be identified. In 25 percent of cases, the disease is discovered on routine clinical examination.

SOURCE:
Johnson, L. E. "Chronic Lymphocytic Leukemia." *American Family Physician* 38, no. 6 (December 1988): 167.

LEUKEMIA—CAUSES

Known exogenous [originating outside the body] causes of leukaemia in human beings are ionising radiation, mutagenic drugs and chemicals, and the HTLV-1 retrovirus. There are several examples of radiation-induced leukaemogenesis [producing leukemia], including the atomic bomb survivors, people exposed to diagnostic X-rays in utero, and people who have received radiation for malignant or non-malignant conditions. Data about non-ionising radiation are controversial. The leukaemogenic effects of drugs and chemicals are most evident in people with cancer (usually Hodgkin's disease or ovarian cancer) who are receiving chemotherapy, and in those exposed to benzene. HTLV-1 is associated with the development of adult T-cell leukaemia (ATL) predominantly in Japan but also in other areas. In addition, several host factors increase the likelihood that leukaemia will develop, including congenital disorders associated with chromosomal imbalances or instability such as Down syndrome and Fanconi's anaemia.

SOURCE:
Butturini, Anne, and Robert P. Gale. "Age of Onset and Type of Leukaemia." *The Lancet* (September 30, 1989): 789.

THE PHILADELPHIA CHROMOSOME

Chromosomal studies are becoming more important in diagnosing chronic myelogenous leukemia and monitoring its progression. A bone marrow sample is used for these studies.

One of the chromosomal abnormalities found in leukemic cells is an exchange of genetic information between chromosome pairs 9 and 22. This swapping of genetic information can be traced to the disease process itself; it's not an inherited trait that causes leukemia. Because it was first identified at the University of Pennsylvania School of Medicine in Philadelphia, this genetic abnormality has come to be known as the Philadelphia chromosome. It's found in 90% of patients with chronic myelogenous leukemia. (The Philadelphia chromosome may also be found in some patients with chronic lymphocytic leukemia and the acute leukemias, but it's less common.)

SOURCE:
Konradi, D., and P. Stockert. "A Close-Up Look at Leukemia." *Nursing89* (June 1989): 37.

TREATMENT

The initial treatment of choice for all types of leukemia is chemotherapy. Its purpose is to destroy the leukemic cells in the bone marrow. Unfortunately, healthy cells are destroyed, too. But destruction of the leukemic cells gives the body a chance to replenish the marrow with new, healthy cells.

The leukemia patient will receive combinations of chemotherapeutic drugs. Depending on the type of leukemia, complete remission is possible in 50% to 90% of patients. Complete remission means no evidence of leukemia will be found in serum studies, and the bone marrow will return to normal.

The usual chemotherapy protocol is divided into three stages—induction, consolidation, and maintenance. During the induction stage, the patient receives intensive chemotherapy in an attempt to induce a complete remission. The largest number of leukemic cells are destroyed at this time.

Once remission has been induced, the consolidation stage begins. The purpose of this stage is to eliminate any remaining leukemic cells. It involves intermittent cycles of chemotherapy, using the same drugs as in the induction stage.

These first two stages last about 2 to 3 months, depending on the patient's response to treatment. If a complete remission is achieved, the patient enters the maintenance stage, which is designed to keep him in remission by preventing leukemic cells from returning to the bone marrow. During this stage, low doses of chemotherapeutic agents are given in various combinations every 3 to 4 weeks. The chemotherapy schedule is set up so that the patient can continue to receive treatments while maintaining as near-normal a life-style as possible.

Besides chemotherapy, a bone marrow transplant is another treatment option for patients with acute leukemia. The procedure remains investigational, however, and is performed only at select major medical centers. It's usually not considered unless chemotherapy has proven ineffective.

The major complications association with bone marrow transplants are infection and acute or chronic graft-versus-host disease (GVHD). Both forms of GVHD usually result from the donated marrow's rejection of the recipient's tissue. (The recipient's immune system may also reject the donated marrow.) Success rates for bone marrow transplants vary, depending on the medical center and patient-selection criteria. A survival rate of 10% to 15% is considered average.

SOURCE:

Konradi, D., and P. Stockert. "A Close-Up Look at Leukemia." *Nursing89* (June 1989): 39–40.

ELECTROMAGNETIC FIELDS AND LEUKEMIA

Preliminary results of a new scientific study show that childhood leukemia is not associated with household exposure to electromagnetic fields. But, in a finding that scientists say is baffling, the cancer is associated with proximity to power lines and the use of certain appliances like hair dryers.

In a break from normal scientific protocol, an industry group, the Electric Power Research Institute, made a summary of the study public today despite objections from the scientist who led it.

The scientist, Dr. John Peters, a professor of epidemiology at the University of Southern California, said in a written statement that he was not ready to discuss the study publicly because it has not yet been routinely reviewed for accuracy by other scientists before publication in a journal. Such publication is expected in about four months. . . .

In the study, Dr. Peters examined the lives of 464 children under the age of 10. Half had leukemia and half did not. Each leukemia patient was compared with a healthy child of the same age, sex, race, and geographic area. Parents were interviewed by telephone about occupation, household use of chemicals, smoking, drug use and daily activities, including exposure to electrical appliances.

Unlike those who conducted earlier studies, Dr. Peters's group entered homes and took direct measurements of the electric and magnetic fields. A recording device was placed in each child's bedroom to measure such fields every minute for 24 hours. Measurements were made with a field meter at several locations in and around the house both when most appliances were turned on and when they were off.

Finally, power lines in the neighborhood as well as the thickness of the wires and their distance from the house, were examined.

According to the institute, there was no association between childhood leukemia and measures of exposure to electric fields.

Like previous studies, however, there was an association between neighborhood power lines and the risk of childhood leukemia. The normal risk of childhood leukemia is 1 in 20,000 a year, the institute said, and the children with the greatest exposure to power lines had a risk of 2.5 in 20,000.

SOURCE:

Blakeslee, Sandra. "Electric Currents and Leukemia Show Puzzling Links in New Study." *The New York Times* (February 8, 1991): A11.

RESOURCES

ORGANIZATIONS

American Cancer Society. 90 Park Avenue, New York, NY 10017.

Leukemia Society of America. 733 Third Avenue, New York, NY 10017.

National Cancer Institute. Community Clinical Oncology Program, Blair Building, Room 7A07, Bethesda, MD 20892-4200.

National Cancer Institute. Office of Cancer Communications, Building 31, Room 10A24, Bethesda, MD 20892.

PAMPHLETS

Leukemia Society of America:

Leukemia: The Nature of the Disease. 1988. 5 pp.

National Cancer Institute:

What You Need To Know About Adult Leukemia. 1988. 21 pp.

What You Need To Know About Childhood Leukemia. 1988. 21 pp.

RELATED ARTICLES

Cheson, Bruce D., and others. "Report of the National Cancer Institute-Sponsored Workshop on Definitions of Diagnosis and Response in Acute Myeloid Leukemia." *Journal of Clinical Oncology* 8, no. 5 (May 1990): 813–819.

Poplack, D. G., and G. Reaman. "Acute Lymphoblastic Leukemia in Childhood." *Pediatric Clinics of North America* 35, no. 4 (August 1988): 903–932.

Stein, R. S. "Review: Advances in the Therapy of Acute Nonlymphocytic Leukemia." *American Journal of the Medical Sciences* 297, no. 1 (January 1989): 26–34.

Stevens, W., D. C. Thomas, and others. "Leukemia in Utah and Radioactive Fallout from the Nevada Test Site: A Case-Control Study." *JAMA* 264 (August 1, 1990): 585–589.

LIPOSUCTION

(*See also:* OBESITY)

OVERVIEW

Since its debut in the early 1980s, liposuction has been the No. 1 means of reshaping the body. Although the craze is slowing down now, more than 100,000 people every year have fat vacuumed from their tummies, hips and thighs.

Liposuction takes a minimum of 40 minutes to perform and is done under general or local anesthesia. Up to two quarts of fat (about a pound) can be removed from each thigh; if more than one area is being treated, doctors may vacuum off as much as three pounds of fat. (Following surgery, the patient wears a long-leg girdle for up to six weeks to contour the area.) The cost ranges from $800 to $4,000 and up, depending on the size and number of areas treated. (Like most cosmetic procedures, liposuction is not covered by medical insurance.)

The fat is dislodged with an instrument called a cannula, explains Eugene Courtiss, M.D., assistant clinical professor of plastic surgery at Harvard Medical School. A cannula is a long, hollow tube that is inserted through a small incision; with it, the doctor loosens fat, then hooks the instrument to a device that vacuums out the fat.

Some side effects are still common with liposuction; virtually every patient experiences numbness for up to eight months as a result of nerves being bumped by the cannula. There is a small risk of fat clots being loosened into the bloodstream, which can have serious health consequences. The surgery also leaves small, permanent scars where the cannulas were inserted. One potential side effect may be more welcome; a recent study showed that for unknown reasons, some women may gain in breast size after liposuction of their belly or thighs.

The Breakthrough: A shift to smaller, more versatile cannulas—some are pencil-thin, a mere 1/20" wide. The chief advantage of using the smaller instruments is that the risk of some side effects—such as rippled skin—is greatly reduced. (The larger cannulas removed fat in chunks, and were more likely to leave permanent indentations under the skin.) According to Simon Fredricks, M.D., clinical professor of plastic surgery at Baylor College of Medicine in Houston, the new tools also allow surgeons to contour areas of the body—ankles, knees, cheeks and under the chin—that were previously off-limits. Finally, the combination of tiny tools and improved techniques allows doctors to suction more than one area at a time, sparing patients repeated procedures.

Even so, liposuction is not a substitute for weight loss. The ideal candidate is lean, with one or two areas of fat that won't budge with diet and exercise. Women with heavier builds—a more common body type—tend to have fat distributed over their entire bodies, and are thus often not good candidates for the spot-treatment liposuction provides. Neither are women whose abdomens have been permanently stretched by pregnancy; the only procedure that works here is an abdominoplasty (tummy tuck), in which fat is surgically removed, muscles are sewn together and extra skin is cut away to create a flat stomach. This surgery costs roughly $4,000 and leaves a large scar.

While surgeons tend to dismiss postoperative pain of liposuction as minimal, patients often tell a different story.

SOURCE:

Rohlfing, Carla. "Cosmetic Surgery Breakthroughs: Lifts, Tucks, Implants." *Family Circle* (July 24, 1990): 53–54.

RISKS

In the early years of liposuction in this country, surgeons used slightly different techniques and larger cannulas, and also attempted to remove more fat during a single procedure. Results were sometimes mixed, leaving some patients with a rippled or corrugated area where the fat was removed. More seriously, some patients suffered nerve damage, infections, lost sections of skin, and even death.

Surgeons modified liposuction techniques as the procedure became more popular. Physicians screen patients carefully for health problems before surgery. The procedure is now limited to removing smaller amounts of fat, and is most commonly done under the safer local anesthesia. Preoperative antibiotics are used to help prevent infection.

Even so, liposuction carries some risk. "The most common side effect," according to Dr. Thomas Spicer, M.D. [a plastic surgeon in Rock Spring, Wyoming], "is abnormal firmness or lumpiness in the area." Numbness or a decreased sense of touch may also affect the area, but this condition is temporary. "I don't even know of a case of permanent nerve damage," said Dr. William P. Coleman III [Associate Clinical Professor of Dermatology at Tulane University School of Medicine]. He noted that normal sensation usually returns within two to three months.

In 1987, the American Society of Plastic and Reconstructive Surgeons issued a report stating that of over 100,000 liposuction procedures between 1982 and 1987, there were 11 deaths. A study of about 9,500 patients who underwent liposuction showed no deaths, but did show seven cases of severe illness due to blood loss or post surgery infection.

Most deaths involving liposuction were caused by blood or fat clots that dislodged during surgery and blocked arteries to the lungs. Seven of the 11 deaths occurred when liposuction was done in conjunction with other procedures, primarily abdominoplasty (the "tummy tuck"). During this procedure, excess skin and fat are removed from the abdomen, and simultaneous liposuction increases the chances of a clot dislodging. . . .

In addition to the risks specific for liposuction, there are the risks that are inherent in any surgery, such as allergic reaction to the anesthesia or to the antibiotics used. Even though the benefits of cosmetic surgery—improved appearance and better self image—can outweigh the risks for some people, these risks must be carefully considered.

SOURCE:
DeBenedette, Valeri. "Liposuction: Getting the Fa(c)ts." *Priorities* (Winter 1990): 16–17.

CHOOSING A PLASTIC SURGEON FOR LIPOSUCTION

Choosing a good plastic surgeon is not easy. The patient-to-be can expect to hear claims that may be misleading, and the lack of government and peer control is worrisome. Board-certified plastic surgeons John Sherman, M.D., Norman Cole, M.D., Garry Brody, M.D., and other authorities have provided us with suggestions on how to make that critical decision. Their guidelines:

- Ask physicians about their precise credentials, training and field of expertise. If advertisements say "board certified," find out which board and whether it is accredited by the American Board of Medical Specialties. Be aggressive in your questioning. Cole says, "I am amazed at how few questions people usually ask me about my training and credentials."
- Ask physicians about the hospitals where they have operating privileges. Contact those hospitals and ask if the physician has privileges to perform the specific operation you are considering (even if it is being done in a private office).
- If a physician "guarantees" results in cosmetic surgery, avoid that doctor. "There are no guarantees" is the uniform opinion of top plastic surgeons.
- Obtain recommendations from a physician's former patients. Your family doctor also may be able to provide background on a plastic surgeon you are considering.
- Be wary of physicians who promote liposuction as a weight-loss technique. It is for body contouring only. Brody says, "If you take out more than four pounds, you begin to challenge the body's fluid balance and it is dangerous. It is not a solution for obesity."
- Get a second and even third opinion on the procedure, asking about risks and benefits and whether it will benefit you in particular.

SOURCE:
Sherman, William. "Special Report: Medicine's New Cash Cow: The Cosmetic Surgery Free-for-All." *Longevity* (February 1990): 24.

RESOURCES

ORGANIZATIONS

American Board of Plastic Surgery. 1617 John F. Kennedy Blvd., Suite 860, Philadelphia, PA 19103.

American Society of Plastic and Reconstructive Surgeons. 444 E. Algonquin Rd., Arlington Heights, IL 60005.

RELATED ARTICLES

Berggren, Ronald B. "Liposuction: What It Will and Won't Do." *Postgraduate Medicine* 87, no. 6 (May 1, 1990): 187–195.

Daigneault, Lorraine. "Getting a Handle on Spare Tires." *American Health: Fitness of Body and Mind* 10 (March 1991): 20.

Drake, Lynn A., Roger I. Ceilley, and others. "Guidelines of Care for Liposuction." *Journal of the American Academy of Dermatology* 24, no. 3 (March 1991): 489–494.

"Liposuction: Body Recontouring Can Be Satisfying and Safe—If You Have the Right Attitudes and Doctor." *Mayo Clinic Health Letter* 7 (July 1989): 4–5.

LIVING WILLS

OVERVIEW

In an effort to implement patients' exercise of autonomy, many states have enacted right-to-die laws, the first being the California Natural Death Act of 1976. The provisions of these laws vary from state to state, but they have in common their recognition of the "living will" as a legal document; they also protect doctors acting in accordance with a living will from legal action by families or others. Even in those states where it is not valid (as of March 1988, eleven did not recognize it), the living will provides important though not binding evidence of an individual's wishes.

A living will is a statement made by a mentally competent person as to what he or she wants done in terms of health care if mental incapacitation occurs. An individual can draw up his or her own will, or can use a standard form, which will vary somewhat in different states. (These forms can be obtained from Concern for Dying, 250 West 57 Street, Room 83, New York, NY 10107, 212-246-6962.)

Typically, a living will expresses an individual's wish that, when the terminal phase of illness is reached, doctors should not use any life-sustaining measures that would serve only to prolong dying, and that he or she should be allowed to die with dignity. The wording is necessarily imprecise, since the will is intended to cover unknown future circumstances, but the individual's general intentions and desires will be unmistakable. It is incumbent on those to whom the directive is addressed to ensure that any treatment given conforms with those intentions, whether or not they would have chosen this course themselves. Some of the living will statutes provide for the appointment of a proxy, whose role is similar to that of a person acting under a durable power of attorney.

The living will is not without problems. It may reflect the values and expectations of a person's middle years, values that are likely to change with age. Unless it has been regularly reviewed and revised, the consent given may not be valid at the time the will comes into effect. This, together with inconsistencies in the law, may make doctors and hospitals reluctant to honor it.

Moreover, it may not be clear what treatments are to be thought of as life-sustaining or life-prolonging, and therefore to be withheld. For example, giving antibiotics to fight an infection is not generally considered life-sustaining—but it is a treatment that someone in great pain from terminal cancer, and with a newly developed pneumonia, might prefer to forgo. On the other hand, many people would be reluctant to think of food and water as treatment; they seem, rather, basic to care. But both the courts and the medical profession are increasingly accepting the tube-feeding of terminally ill or comatose patients as a life-prolonging measure. To make a living will truly effective, it would be necessary to be very specific—but the unknowns of the future prohibit this.

Despite problems with timeliness and lack of precision, however, the living will is a powerful tool. In drawing up the document, individuals secure the realization of their wishes for a time when, by definition, they no longer have the ability to make their wishes known.

SOURCE:

Rothman, David J., and Donald F. Tapley. "Evidence of Patients' Wishes." In *The Columbia University College of Physicians and Surgeons Complete Home Medical Guide*. 2d ed. New York: Crown, 1989. pp. 43–44.

RECOMMENDED PROVISIONS IN LIVING WILLS

While the field of living-will law remains in flux, you can take measures to better the odds that your living will holds firm once you no longer can make decisions. Besides signing the standard form, you can attach a statement of your feelings about specific treatments, such as cardiac resuscitation, mechanical respiration and artificial feeding. Two advocacy groups, the Society for the Right to Die and Concern for Dying, recommend these steps:

- Have a heart-to-heart talk with your doctor and be sure he or she understands and supports your wishes. If the doctor is dubious or opposed, you may want to switch physicians. Have the will placed in your medical file.
- Be as specific and detailed as possible when describing treatments you may or may not want and at what point you no longer want them.
- Designate a person to make health care decisions for you. This person should be familiar with your personal philosophy and feelings about terminal care, support them and be likely to make the same decisions for you that you yourself would make. A friend may be more persuasive with a judge than a relative who is also your heir. You should take this step even if you live in a state that does not yet provide for proxies or durable power of attorney for health care. It will make your doctor feel more comfortable and, in all likelihood, will be supported by a judge.
- Sign your living will before two witnesses and a notary. It must be notarized if you choose to execute the durable power of attorney. Give copies to your next of kin, your clergyman, lawyer and anyone else who might eventually act in a decision-making capacity for you.
- Store your living will where your family can easily get at it. Best to keep it out of a safe-deposit box, since you might be the only one who could put your hands on the key.
- Sign and date the document again every two or three years; do the same before a notary and witnesses every five years. The more recent the date, the more likely your doctor or a court will honor the living will. A carefully crafted document is no guarantee that you will end your life in peace, but it should help to fend off tubes and lawyers.

SOURCE:
Carey, Joseph. "The Faulty Promise of 'Living Wills.'" *U.S. News and World Report* 107 (July 24, 1989): 64.

DURABLE POWER OF ATTORNEY AND LIVING WILLS

In some states (for example, California and New York) a living will should be backed up with a Durable Power of Attorney for Health Care (DPAHC). This legally binding document empowers a designated person to make health-care decisions on your behalf. Choose someone to whom you've thoroughly explained your beliefs and who shares your philosophical position or at least clearly understands it. (You'll also need a back-up, in case your first choice is unable to act for you.) This person will have the authority to see that your wishes are carried out.

None of us is exempt from calamity or serious illness: everybody needs a living will and, if required, a DPAHC. The elderly, the chronically ill, and anyone about to undergo major surgery should certainly execute these documents. Most important: no document can substitute for frank discussions with your family, doctor, religious adviser, or friends who might be directly involved if you were critically ill. Besides ensuring that your wishes will be honored, a comprehensive living will and a DPAHC may help your family through some tough decisions.

SOURCE:
"Why You Need a Living Will." *The University of California, Berkeley Wellness Letter* 6, no. 6 (March 1990): 1–2. Excerpted from *The University of California, Berkeley Wellness Letter,* Copyright Health Letter Associates, 1990.

PITFALLS

Having a living will does not guarantee a passing free of turmoil. It is impossible for any statement of intent (of which a living will is one form) to cover every conceivable combination of events that might occur. There is usually enough ambiguity in any living will to leave any disagreement between physician and family unsettled.

For example, there is always a question of when to activate the living will. Is it when the patient becomes incompetent? If so, who defines incompetence? Is it when the patient goes into a coma, or when he is deemed terminally ill? What if the patient is not terminally ill but is severely brain-damaged, without hope for neurological recovery? If the circumstances under which a will is activated are not defined very clearly, the document may be more trouble than help.

Another pitfall is the definition of "heroic" measures. Antibiotics, feeding tubes, oxygen, and intravenous fluids are part of everyday hospital care. If the use of these will prolong life, do they automatically become "heroic"? Again, an explicit statement as to what is meant by treatment and what is to be avoided can help to limit the uncertainties of interpretation.

One argument against living wills is that they may discount the future. Some critics contend that a healthy person cannot predict the frame of mind when illness becomes a reality. The argument has also been made that a patient may, at the last minute, wish to change his instructions but, because of intermittent delusions, be declared incompetent and thus not permitted to do so.

A measure that can help circumvent some of these criticisms is to delegate to a friend or family member durable power of attorney. This role differs from normal power of attorney in that it does not lapse after a specified period of time, or when the person granting it becomes incompetent. The person with power of attorney can help interpret the patient's probably wishes when the circumstances are not covered in the will.

SOURCE:
Bennett, William I., and others (eds.). *Your Good Health: How To Stay Well, and What To Do When You're Not.* Cambridge, Mass.: Harvard University Press, 1987. pp. 483-484.

AN ALTERNATIVE TO LIVING WILLS—THE MEDICAL DIRECTIVE

Living wills have been strongly endorsed in principle. Unfortunately, existing living wills are rarely used in clinical practice because they are vague and difficult to apply. To remedy this, we propose a new advance care document: the Medical Directive. The Medical Directive delineates four paradigmatic scenarios, defined by prognosis and disability of incompetent patients. In each scenario, patients are to indicate their preferences regarding specific life-sustaining interventions. The Medical Directive also provides for the designation of a proxy to make decisions in circumstances where the patient's preferences are uncertain. Finally, there is a section for a statement of wishes regarding organ donation. The Medical Directive provides an opportunity for significant improvement in the documentation of patients' preferences regarding life-sustaining care in states of incompetence. As an expression of a patient's wishes, the Medical Directive should be honored by courts and should facilitate physician-patient discussions of critical and terminal care options. . . .

The four illness scenarios are as follows: when the patient is in an irreversible coma or a persistent vegetative state but with no terminal illness (situation A); when the patient is in a coma with a small and uncertain chance of recovery (situation B); when the patient has some brain damage causing mental incompetence and is terminally ill (situation C); and when the patient has some brain damage causing mental incompetence without any terminal illness (situation D). . . .

In each of these paradigmatic scenarios, the patient is to indicate whether he or she would want or not want interventions in 12 treatment categories, ranging from resuscitation and ventilation to artificial feeding and simple diagnostic procedures. These categories encompass the typical range of diagnostic and therapeutic interventions for incompetent patients.

SOURCE:
Emanuel, Linda L., and Ezekiel J. Emanuel. "The Medical Directive: A New Comprehensive Advance Care Document." *JAMA* 261 (June 9, 1989): 3288-3293. Copyright 1989, American Medical Association.

RESOURCES

ORGANIZATIONS
Concern for Dying. 250 West 57th St., New York, NY 10107.

Society for the Right to Die. 250 West 57th St., New York, NY 10107.

PAMPHLET
Concern for Dying:

A Living Will. 1984. 4 pp.

BOOK
Colen, B. D. *An Essential Guide to the Living Will.* New York: Pharos, 1987.

RELATED ARTICLES
"Avoiding a Prolonged Death: A Living Will or a Proxy Can Help Keep Machines from Pointlessly Prolonging the Process of Dying." *Consumer Reports Health Letter* 2, no. 8 (August 1990): 57–58.

Bullock, Carole. "Creating a Living Will." *Weight Watchers Women's Health and Fitness News* (September 1989): 2–3.

Emanuel, Linda L., and others. "Advance Directives for Medical Care: A Case for Greater Use." *The New England Journal of Medicine* 324 (March 28, 1991): 887–895.

Stolman, Cynthia J., and others. "Evaluation of Patient, Physician, Nurse, and Family Attitudes Toward Do Not Resuscitate Orders." *Archives of Internal Medicine* 150 (March 1990): 653–658.

LUNG CANCER

(*See also:* SMOKING)

OVERVIEW

Lung cancer is the most common form of cancer diagnosed in the United States and also the major cause of cancer death, accounting for about 15 percent of all cancer cases and 25 percent of all cancer deaths—more than 142,000 deaths annually. Two-thirds of lung cancer cases and deaths occur in men. Lung cancer has now surpassed breast cancer as the number one cause of cancer mortality in American women as well. The age at time of diagnosis for both sexes is usually over 45, with a peak during the seventies.

For many years, new lung cancer cases in the United States increased rapidly, about 240 percent in the 5 years from 1983 to 1988. Recently, however, there has been a decrease in incidence among white men but essentially no change in mortality. This decrease in incidence is associated with a reduction in cigarette smoking since 1965. It is hoped that, when rates are adjusted to take age into account, lung cancer incidence will reach a plateau and begin to drop during the next few years.

Lung cancer is also the leading cancer in many other countries, particularly in western Europe and other parts of North America. At present, the incidence is comparatively low in China, India, and several Latin American and African countries. Yet, even in these areas of the world lung cancer ranks as one of the three most common types of cancer in men. In large part, the worldwide variation can be attributed to differences in tobacco use.

SOURCE:
National Cancer Institute. *Cancer of the Lung: Research Report.* NIH Pub. No. 90-526. 1989. p. 9.

MAJOR TYPES OF LUNG CANCER

Lung cancers are generally divided into two types: small cell lung cancer and nonsmall cell lung cancer. The tumor cells of each type grow and spread differently, and they are treated differently.

Small cell lung cancer is sometimes called oat cell cancer because the cancer cells look like oats when they are viewed under a microscope. This type of lung cancer makes up about 20 to 25 percent of all cases. It is a rapidly growing cancer that spreads very early to other organs. It is generally found in people who are heavy smokers.

There are three main kinds of nonsmall cell lung cancer, and they are named for the type of cells found in the cancer.

- Epidermoid carcinoma, which is also called squamous cell carcinoma, makes up about 33 percent of all lung cancer cases. (Carcinoma is a cancer that begins in the lining or covering tissues of an organ.) This type of lung cancer often begins in the bronchi and may remain in the chest without spreading for longer periods than the other types. It is the most common type of lung cancer.
- Adenocarcinoma accounts for about 25 percent of all lung cancers. It often grows along the outer edges of the lungs and under the tissue lining the bronchi.
- Large cell carcinomas make up about 16 percent of all lung cancer cases. These cancers are found most often in the smaller bronchi. . . .

Lung cancer may cause a number of symptoms. A cough is one of the more common symptoms and is likely to occur when a tumor grows and blocks an air passage. Another symptom is chest pain, which feels like a constant ache that may or may not be related to coughing.

Other symptoms may include shortness of breath, repeated pneumonia or bronchitis, coughing up blood, hoarseness, or swelling of the neck and face.

In addition, there may be symptoms that do not seem to be at all related to the lungs. These may be caused by the spread of lung cancer to other parts of the body. Depending on which organs are affected, symptoms can include headache, weakness, pain, bone fractures, bleeding, or blood clots.

Sometimes symptoms may be caused by hormones that are produced by lung cancer cells. For example, certain lung cancer cells produce a hormone that causes a sharp drop in the level of salt (sodium) in the body. A decrease in sodium level can produce many symptoms, including confusion and sometimes even coma. Like all cancers, lung cancer can also cause fatigue, loss of appetite, and loss of weight.

These symptoms may be caused by a number of problems. They are not a sure sign of cancer. However, it is important to see a doctor if any of these symptoms lasts as long as 2 weeks. Any illness should be diagnosed and treated as early as possible, and this is especially true for cancers.

SOURCE:
National Cancer Institute. *What You Need To Know about Lung Cancer.* NIH Pub. No. 90-1553. 1989. pp. 6, 7.

RISKS FROM SMOKING

Smoking appears to cause all types of lung cancer, although it is most strongly associated with epidermoid carcinoma and SCLC [small cell lung cancer]. Overall, smokers are 10 times more likely to die from lung cancer than are nonsmokers, and it is clear that the risk of developing lung cancer increases with the number of cigarettes smoked. However, this risk gradually begins to level off upon cessation of smoking, and after 15 to 20 years the ex-smoker's risk of dying from lung cancer is similar to that of an individual who has never smoked. Persons who smoke filtered, low-tar cigarettes generally have a lower lung cancer risk than those who smoke nonfiltered, high-tar cigarettes. But, there is evidence that people often smoke more cigarettes if the nicotine is reduced. Furthermore, the cancer risk for such smokers is still far greater than for nonsmokers.

Still, not all heavy smokers develop lung cancer, and not all people with lung cancer are heavy smokers. About 10 to 15 percent of all cases of lung cancer occur in nonsmokers. Occupational hazards, exposure to cigarette smoke in the environment, air pollution and other environmental factors such as radon gas in the soil have been implicated.

Recent evidence indicates that involuntary exposure of nonsmokers to tobacco smoke is associated with lung cancer. Nonsmokers inhale environmental tobacco smoke, which consists of a combination of sidestream smoke (from the burning end of a cigarette as it smolders) and exhaled mainstream smoke (smoke that is breathed out by a smoker). Scientists believe that the risk for lung cancer in non-smokers increases about 30 percent if they are married to a person who smokes; the risk increases to 70 percent if the spouse is a heavy smoker. Additional studies are needed to investigate other factors that may influence nonsmokers' risk of developing cancer.

Workers who are exposed to carcinogens face an even greater chance of developing lung cancer if they smoke cigarettes. For example, epidemiologic studies show that workers in the asbestos industry who have been exposed to large concentrations of asbestos dust have a risk of lung cancer that is three to four times greater than that of workers who have not been exposed to asbestos. For asbestos workers who smoke cigarettes the risk increases to 30 times that of nonsmoking workers, and 90 times that of workers who neither smoke nor work with asbestos.

SOURCE:
National Cancer Institute. *Cancer of the Lung: Research Report.* NIH Pub. No. 90-526. 1989. pp. 7-8.

RISKS FROM RADON

The risk associated with radon is an estimated 6-11 times higher in smokers than in nonsmokers. Risk is also higher in asbestos workers who smoke than in those who do not smoke. Although information on the population prevalence of exposure to radon and asbestos (and to each in combination with cigarette smoking) is preliminary, mortality attributable to these causes can be estimated. Exposure to radon in homes is associated with 5,000-20,000 lung cancer deaths annually; an estimated 85% of these deaths are due to the combined exposure of radon and cigarette smoke. Approximately 5500 lung cancer deaths in the United States in 1987 were expected among persons with occupational exposure to asbestos.

SOURCE:
Center for Disease Control. "Chronic Disease Reports: Deaths from Lung Cancer—United States, 1986." *JAMA* 262, no. 9 (September 1, 1989): 1170, 1172.

* * *

People whose houses have very high radon concentrations may be concerned about their risk of lung cancer. Alarming levels of risk are projected for the concentrations already measured in many houses. For example, the "Citizen's Guide" projects 270 to 630 deaths from lung cancer per 1000 persons with a continuous exposure to 3700 Bq per cubic meter (100pCi per liter). Such people should be advised that these projections are theoretical and highly uncertain. Cigarette smokers should be reminded that the cessation of smoking reduces the risk of lung cancer in any case, and that much of the risk attributed to radon reflects a synergism with smoking.

The presence of radon inside houses is an unprecedented, although evidently a longstanding, environmental health problem. Most sources are natural ones, and radon is present in every dwelling. We lack experience in considering, let alone controlling, risks of this type. In view of present scientific uncertainty and our naivete with regard to policy, a thoughtful and ongoing evaluation of the evolving national strategy with respect to radon is needed. We encourage the creation of an effective mechanism for such a review.

SOURCE:
Samet, Jonathan M., and Anthony V. Nero, Jr. "Sounding Board: Indoor Radon and Lung Cancer." *New England Journal of Medicine* 320, no. 9 (March 2, 1989): 593.

TREATMENT

Standard treatments for patients with lung cancer are of limited effectiveness in all but the most localized tumors. For this reason, patients are encouraged to consider participating in clinical trials (research studies) that are designed to evaluate new approaches to therapy. . .

Surgery, radiation therapy, and chemotherapy, alone or in various combinations, may be used to treat lung cancer. The choice of treatment depends on many factors, including the type of tumor, the extent of the disease when it is diagnosed, the age and general health of the patient, and other variables.

Surgical procedures that may be employed include wedge or segmental resection (removal of a portion of the affected lungs), lobectomy (removal of the entire lobe of the lung), or pneumonectomy (removal of the entire right or left lung).

Radiation therapy is usually given by external beam, using machines located outside the body that deliver x-rays or electrons to the location of the tumor. The radiation dose is based on the size and location of the tumor. Some patients first receive external therapy to a wide area that includes the primary tumor and surrounding tissue. After the initial treatments, a smaller area is treated, with a final treatment area that may be quite small; radiation here is referred to as a "boost." Like surgery, radiation therapy is called local treatment because it affects only the cells in the area being treated.

Chemotherapy (treatment with anticancer drugs) is a systemic treatment; the drugs enter the bloodstream and travel through the body, affecting cancer cells outside the lung area.

SOURCE:
National Cancer Institute. *Cancer of the Lung: Research Report.* NIH Pub. No. 90-526. 1989. p. 17.

RESOURCES

PAMPHLETS
American Cancer Society:

Facts on Lung Cancer. 1987. 12 pp.

Environmental Protection Agency:

A Citizen's Guide to Radon: What It Is and What to Do about It. DHHS Pub. No. (EPA) 86-004. 1986.

RELATED ARTICLES
Janerich, Dwight T., W. Douglas Thompson, and others. "Lung Cancer and Exposure to Tobacco Smoke in the Household." *New England Journal of Medicine* 323, no. 10 (September 6, 1990): 632-636.

Screening for Lung Cancer. *American Family Physician* 41 (June 1990): 1763-1766.

Wynder, Ernst L., and Geoffrey C. Kabat. The Effect of Low-Yield Cigarette Smoking on Lung Cancer Risk. *Cancer* 62, no. 6 (September 15, 1988): 1223-1230.

LUPUS

OVERVIEW

Lupus is a Latin term meaning "wolf." In earlier times, people thought the shape and color of skin lesions common to this disorder resembled the bite of a wolf.

Today, physicians understand more about lupus, but its cause and cure remain unknown. Lupus affects nearly one person in 800, placing it among the more common rheumatic diseases. Besides the skin, this disease can affect joints and muscles, the kidneys, nervous system, heart and lungs.

Lupus frequently strikes women of childbearing years, but it can affect both sexes from youth to old age. Each person's case is different, ranging from mild to disabling.

Here are the most common types of lupus.

- **Systemic lupus erythematosus (SLE)**—This is the most common form of lupus. "Systemic" means it can affect several parts of your body. SLE is a chronic disorder, the course of which can vary over a person's lifetime. Symptoms may be mild; remissions can last for months or years.

There is no single pattern of symptoms to announce the onset of SLE. Weight loss, fatigue and fever may be early signs. Erythematosus refers to redness. A reddish "butterfly" rash may develop on the nose and cheeks. Skin changes may appear on the arms, neck or scalp. Exposure to sunlight can worsen the rash. Your fingers may turn bluish and become sensitive to cold. You may notice pain in the joints of your ankles, knees, elbows, wrists and hands. Muscle aches, swollen glands, nausea and loss of appetite are common.

SLE can cause kidney damage, anemia and inflammation of the membranes that line the surface of the heart and lungs. The disease can lead to excessive bleeding and an increased susceptibility to infections.

In rare cases, SLE can affect the brain, leading to convulsions.

- **Discoid lupus erythematosus (DLE)**—DLE involves inflammation of the skin only. Individual patches come together to form lesions over the bridge of the nose and cheeks, and sometimes on the scalp. Lesions dry into scales that fall off the body, leaving scars.
- **Drug-induced lupus**—Some medications uncommonly used for high blood pressure, heart disease and tuberculosis can cause many symptoms of SLE. Eliminating the medication almost always stops the problem.

An individual test to diagnose lupus is unavailable. After obtaining a detailed medical history and performing a complete physical examination, doctors often order many tests to confirm a diagnosis.

A blood test, called the anti-nuclear antibody (ANA) exam, tells whether the antibody associated with SLE is present in the blood. Additional blood and urine tests assess the involvement of organs such as the kidneys and bone marrow. A chest x-ray may indicate if the lungs are involved. An electrocardiogram or echocardiogram will help your doctor determine heart involvement.

Because lupus has so many forms, it may take some time for your doctor to find the best balance of treatments.

If you have lupus, follow your treatment program carefully. Altering medications on your own can make you seriously ill and hinder your doctor from analyzing your condition. Alert your doctor to any change in symptoms.

If you're a woman with lupus, consult your doctor if you are considering having children. Many pregnancies are uneventful, but lupus can increase your chance of miscarriage, and the symptoms of lupus can be more severe after delivery.

Here are the leading methods for treating lupus:

- **Aspirin**—If you have mild lupus, aspirin may be the only medication your doctor prescribes.
- **NSAIDs**—This abbreviation stands for non-steroidal anti-inflammatory drugs. They work like aspirin and are easier to tolerate.
- **Corticosteroids**—Among the strongest anti-inflammatory drugs available, corticosteroids can ease pain and swelling in just a few hours. Corticosteroids inhibit the immune system and any part it might play in the development of lupus.

Your doctor may use corticosteroids either in the form of pills or as a topical cream. Potential side effects, more common with pills, include weight gain, puffiness in the face, easy bruising, thinning of the bones, depression, high blood pressure and cataracts.

- **Immunosuppressive drugs**—When the medications above fail to resolve the symptoms, or vital organs, such as the kidneys, are involved, doctors may turn to other medications capable of further impeding the immune system.
- **Anti-malarial medications**—There is no known link between lupus and malaria, but antimalarial drugs sometimes are used to treat lupus. They help prevent rashes resulting from exposure to the sun's ultraviolet light.
- **Skin creams**—Because exposure to sunlight can aggravate the skin of sun-sensitive people with lupus, they should limit outside activities between 10 A.M. and 2 P.M.; and use a sunscreen with a protection factor of 15.

Chronic disorders like lupus cause emotional and social challenges, as well as physical discomfort. But because lupus varies so widely, many people can expect long periods when symptoms are mild or no problem.

SOURCE:
"Lupus: Coping With a Chronic Rheumatic Condition." *Mayo Clinic Health Letter* 8, no. 12 (December 1990): 3.

DIAGNOSIS

According to the Lupus Foundation of America there is no single test that can definitively say whether a person has lupus. But the following tests can aid in diagnosis by examining the status of the patient's immune system.

- The anti-nuclear antibody test determines if the person has autoantibodies that react with components in cell nuclei. Over 90 percent of lupus patients will have a positive reaction to this test. However, positive results occur with a variety of other illnesses and in up to 10 percent of the normal population.
- The anti-DNA antibody test determines if the patient has antibodies to DNA.
- The anti-Sm antibody test looks for antibodies to a protein that was first discovered in the blood of a lupus patient (whose initials were S.M.). While many lupus patients do not have anti-Sm antibodies, they are rarely found in people without lupus.
- Tests for the presence of immune complexes (the combination of antibodies and the substances with which they react) in the blood are valuable both for diagnosing and monitoring the disease.
- An analysis of the serum complement level, which tends to fall when the disease is active, is also useful for both diagnosis and monitoring. The serum complement is a group of proteins involved in the inflammation that can occur in immune reactions.

"It should be stressed that because patients with other diseases may also have immune complexes and low serum complement, the diagnosis of [lupus] can only be made by examining all the features of the person's illness and by excluding a number of other illnesses that [lupus] may mimic," writes Ronald I. Carr, M.D., in the Lupus Foundation of America's *Lupus Handbook*.

The interpretation of the results of these tests is made even more difficult by the unpredictability of the disease. A test may be positive one time and negative the next, depending, in part, on whether the disease is active or in remission.

Kidney and skin biopsies can also help with diagnosis. A kidney biopsy may show deposits of antibodies and immune complexes, and a sample of skin tissue may reveal deposits of antibodies and complement proteins.

SOURCE:
Stehlin, Dori. "Living With Lupus." *FDA Consumer* (December-January 1990): 10.

DRUG-RELATED LUPUS

Systemic lupus erythematosus is one of the connective-tissue diseases whose specific cause or causes remain undetermined. However, it is known that drugs and other agents can produce a lupuslike syndrome: drug-related lupus. . . .

The implicated drugs can be divided into three major groups. The first includes drugs for which there is definite proof of association and of which controlled prospective studies have been completed. Drugs in this category include hydralazine, procainamide, isoniazid, methyldopa, chlorpromazine, and quinidine. The second group comprises drugs that are probably associated with the syndrome. They include many anticonvulsant agents, antithyroid drugs, penicillamine, sulfasalazine, the beta-blockers, and lithium. The third group includes drugs for which anecdotal reporting has suggested a possible association with drug-related lupus. Among them are para-aminosalicylic acid, estrogens, gold salts, penicillin, griseofulvin, reserpine, and tetracycline.

SOURCE:
Hess, Evelyn. "Drug-Related Lupus." *The New England Journal of Medicine* 318, no. 22 (June 2, 1988): 1460.

TREATMENT

Because the symptoms of lupus vary not only in type but also severity, the treatment may also need to vary. It may take time to find the right combination of treatments for each individual. Medication is necessary for almost all people with lupus but the type and amount may change as the course of the disease changes. Your doctor will help you alter the schedule of any medication you are taking. Getting plenty of rest is also important, especially during periods when the symptoms flare up, or get more severe. For many people with lupus, skin rashes are made worse by excessive sun exposure. Just how much sun is excessive will vary from person to person, but people with lupus should use a good sunscreen when they spend time outdoors.

Aspirin may be the only medication your doctor prescribes, though perhaps in high doses. Besides being a pain-killer, aspirin is an anti-inflammatory drug, especially helpful in treating the joint pain of lupus. Other anti-inflammatory drugs may also be prescribed.

Corticosteroid drugs are also commonly used to treat lupus. They are the strongest anti-inflammatory drugs available. They can dramatically reduce many symptoms of lupus. Unfortunately, corticosteroids also have side effects. Common side effects include weight gain, puffiness (especially in the face), and easy bruising. Serious side effects can include bone thinning, high blood pressure, cataracts and depression. These drugs must be carefully monitored by your physician, and you should tell any physician or dentist who is treating you if you are taking steroids.

There are other medications which may be prescribed to treat lupus. Antimalarial drugs are sometimes helpful, although there is no known relationshop between malaria and lupus. Rarely, people with lupus are given immunosuppressive drugs. These drugs weaken, or suppress, the cells that cause the inflammation and immune response, but they can have very serious side effects. Other medications may be given to treat particular symptoms as they occur.

SOURCE:
"Systemic Lupus Erythematosus." *HealthTips* (December-January 1988): 3.

RESOURCES

ORGANIZATIONS

American Lupus Society. 3200 N. Summit Ave., Milwaukee, WI 53211.

Lupus Foundation of America. 1717 Masachusetts Ave. NW, Suite 203, Washington, DC 20030.

PAMPHLET

Arthritis Foundation:

Systemic Lupus Erythematosus. 1986.

BOOKS

Aladjem, Henrietta, and Peter H. Scher. *In Face of the Sun: A Woman's Courageous Victory Over Lupus*. New York: Scribner's, 1988.

Phillips, Robert H. *Coping With Lupus: A Guide to Living With Lupus For You and Your Family*. Wayne, NJ: Avery, 1984.

Radziunas, Eileen. *Lupus: My Search For a Diagnosis*. New York: Hunter House, 1989.

RELATED ARTICLES

Klippel, John H. "Systemic Lupus Erythematosus: Treatment-Related Complications Superimposed on Chronic Disease." *JAMA* 263, no. 13 (April 4, 1990): 1812–1815.

Roberts, Donna M., and W. Michael Hughes. "Systemic Lupus Erythematosus: How to Manage This Chronic, Complicated Disorder." *Postgraduate Medicine* 86, no. 8 (December 1989): 191–200.

Watson, Rosemarie. "Cutaneous Lesions in Systemic Lupus Erythematosus." *Medical Clinics of North America* 73, no. 5 (September 1989): 1091–1111.

LYME DISEASE

OVERVIEW

In 1975, Lyme disease was discovered in Old Lyme, Connecticut. Parents were perplexed by the high incidence of arthritis among their children and called for an investigation; this revealed that the children were suffering from a "new" disease. Today, Lyme disease is the most common tick-transmitted disease in the world, with about 5,000 cases reported in the United States in 1988. Most cases are concentrated in the coastal Northeast, Wisconsin, Minnesota, northern California, and Oregon. In the east coast, 80 percent of the cases occur between May and August—July is the peak month of incidence. In California, the disease occurs throughout the year, with a slight increase in the summer months.

Lyme disease is a spirochetal infection acquired through tick bites. The two species of ticks that are known to transmit the disease are *Ixodes pacificus* (the Western Black-legged Tick) and *Ixodes dammini* (in the east). Ticks live in wooded and grassy areas and survive by attaching to animal hosts and sucking their blood. They attach to deer, field mice, other wild animals, and humans as well. The Western Black-legged Tick also feeds on birds and cold blooded animals such as lizards. Recent research indicates that the spirochete has also been found in horse flies, deer flies, mosquitoes and fleas, but it is not yet clear whether they can transmit the disease to humans like the tick can. Other ticks, such as the common dog tick, do not transmit Lyme disease.

Known as "The Great Imitator," its numerous disguises may allow it to slip through medical exams without being detected. The list of symptoms it is known to cause has been expanding, as researchers get a better understanding of the short and long-term effects of this deceptive disease.

The first sign of Lyme disease usually occurs several days or a month after the tick bite, and consists of a small red pimple that later expands to form a ring-shaped rash—"bull's eye"—a bright red ring encircling the bite and a clear area at the center. This rash varies in size—it can be as small as a dime or it can cover a person's entire back; it may mark the site of the bite or it can appear with several others throughout the body. Flu-like symptoms, such as headaches, stiff neck, muscle aches and fatigue may also be present. About half of the infected people never develop the rash, thus making it more difficult to diagnose the illness.

The second stage of the disease, which occurs within the next several weeks, involves joint pain and may bring about complications in the nervous system or the heart. Neurologic complications, such as inflammation of the brain and its covering membranes, inflammation of the nerve roots, and facial paralysis, occur in about 15 percent of the patients. Symptoms may last several months but usually disappear completely. Heart disease symptoms occur in about 8 percent of the patients, and include dizziness, shortness of breath, and an irregular heart rhythm. Generally, they disappear completely within weeks.

Arthritis may progress in stage 3 of the disease. Joint pain may appear weeks or even years after the rash, and it affects more than 50 percent of the patients. The large joints—knees, shoulders, elbows, ankles, and wrists—are usually involved. They become swollen and painful. The first attack usually lasts about a week, but recurrent attacks are quite common. At this stage, a small number of people may also develop neurologic abnormalities such as somnolence (drowsiness), loss of memory, mood swings, and inability to concentrate.

Due to this variety of symptoms, a diagnosis cannot always be made quickly and accurately. If the patient knows that he or she has been bitten by a tick recently, a straightforward diagnosis can be made, and the most difficult part is over. Unfortunately, the bite often goes undetected. If Lyme disease is suspected, the physician can order a blood test to check for infection. The blood test, however, may be negative during the early phases of the disease, and false positives have been known to occur.

Antibiotics usually offer effective treatment. The physician chooses the appropriate antibiotic and dosage, depending on the severity of the symptoms. Tetracycline or ceftriaxone is usually recommended for adults, and penicillin for pregnant women and children. The earlier the disease is treated, the shorter and less severe the symptoms will be.

The best way to prevent Lyme disease is to avoid areas that are known to contain ticks, specially during the summer months. If you are going into wooded or grassy areas, wear light-colored clothing that fits tightly around the ankles and wrists, and tuck the pants into boots or socks. Spray your clothing with tick repellant. When you return, examine your body and clothing for ticks—they are very small, so look carefully. Brush off the ones that are not attached and use tweezers to remove those that are. To remove them, grasp the tick's mouthparts as close to the skin as possible, and use a slow steady pressure while pulling straight out. Don't attempt to jerk the tick out. Try not to squeeze the tick's body or tear the skin, and always wash the area immediately with soap and water, alcohol or antiseptic. Pets should also be checked as they come into the house.

Many ticks are disease free, so a tick bite does not mean you will automatically develop Lyme disease. If any possible symptoms develop, however, report them promptly to your physician.

SOURCE:

California Medical Association. Lyme Disease. *HealthTips* index 524. (July/August 1989): 1-2.

LYME ARTHRITIS

Myalgias and arthralgias are common symptoms of early Lyme disease. A quite common—and diagnostically helpful—symptom is temporomandibular joint pain (which is rare as an early feature of chronic arthritic disorders). In contrast, frank arthritis is quite uncommon during the early weeks. However, 60% of untreated Lyme disease patients in the United States eventually develop inflammatory arthritis. The mean time from the onset of Lyme disease (in those who have erythema chronicum migrans at the onset) to the development of frank arthritis is six months (range, four days to two years).

The most common arthritic presentation is an intermittent inflammatory arthritis of one or a few large joints, particularly the knee. Large effusions and Baker's cysts occur frequently. Individual attacks of acute joint inflammation remit spontaneously in most patients after a few days to a few months but may recur for several years. Longitudinal follow-up of patients with untreated Lyme arthritis has demonstrated that the prognosis is generally good, with 10% to 20% per year achieving spontaneous long-term remission. . . .

Lyme arthritis can be treated successfully in most patients by a number of alternative antibiotic regimens. A month-long course of doxycycline or of amoxicillin plus probenecid will cure Lyme arthritis in about 70% of patients. Response, however, is often delayed until many weeks after completion of the course, which suggests that noninfectious inflammatory mechanisms (perhaps involving uncleared antigenic material) can contribute to the perpetuation of arthritis in many patients. Another 10% or 15% respond to a second course of a different oral antibiotic or to a course of parenteral antibiotic therapy.

SOURCE:

Rahn, Daniel W., and Stephen E. Malawista. "Clinical Judgment in Lyme Disease." *Hospital Practice* (March 30, 1990): 48, 52.

TREATMENT

Treatment of Lyme Disease continues to evolve, and current therapies share only one common element: administration of antibiotics. Currently, with more than 15 years of experience in the United States, there is a certain consensus as to specific antibiotics, duration of treatment, and follow-up treatment for recurring symptoms, although specialists sometimes prefer one regimen over another. The choice of drug and duration of therapy are equally important, and therapy should be individualized because patient response varies considerably.

Doxycycline hyclate (Doryx, Vibramycin, Vibra-Tabs, etc.) has come to be widely prescribed for the *Borrelia burgdorferi* infection, in a dosage of 100 mg po bid for 14–21 days, for stages 1 and 2 of Lyme disease. A large patient may require the same dosage three times a day. For the arthritis of stage 3, a 28-day course is recommended. Doxycycline is not appropriate for children younger than 8 years or for pregnant women, and it may provoke photosensitivity rashes. Nausea can be reduced if doxycycline is taken with meals.

Amoxicillin (Amoxil, Trimox, Wymox, etc.) is also a good choice, at 500 mg po tid for 14-21 days in stage 1, and amoxicillin in the same dosage plus probenecid (Benemid), 500 mg po tid, for 28 days for the arthritis of stage 3. In pediatric cases, the dosage of amoxicillin should be determined by the child's weight, 20–40 mg/kg/d.

An alternative to doxycycline or amoxicillin in the early disease is erythromycin, 250 mg qid for 28 days, especially for patients who cannot take tetracycline or penicillin. Another option is penicillin G, 500 mg po qid for 28 days. If the patient has facial palsy with abnormal CSF in stage 2, prescribe ceftriaxone sodium (Rocephin), 2 g/d IV, given in one or two doses, for 14–21 days, or cefotaxime sodium (Claforan), 3 g IV bid, for the same period.

Arthritis in advanced Lyme disease requires doxycycline, 100 mg po bid for 28 days; amoxicillin, 500 mg po tid, plus probenecid, 500 mg po tid for 28 days; or ceftriaxone, 2 g/d IV, in one or two doses, for 14–21 days. The addition of corticosteroids to the regimen is not recommended. If an arthritic patient fails to respond to oral medication, IV antibiotic therapy should be considered.

IV [intravenous] therapy is appropriate for late disease with advanced features such as heart block and CNS involvement as well as severe arthritis. Options include ceftriaxone, 2 g/d for 21–28 days, or cefotaxime, 3 g bid for 21–28 days.

SOURCE:
Duffy, Joseph, Robert T. Schoen, and Leonard H. Sigal. "1991 Update on Lyme Disease." *Patient Care* (June 15, 1991): 39, 45.

PREVENTION

If you're in an area where infected ticks are found, these steps can help keep you safe:

Know the risk. Ask your state or local health department about the presence of Lyme disease in your area. Find out when it's peak season. In northeastern and north-central states, for example, most infections occur from May to August. On the Pacific Coast, most cases are reported between January and June, although they occur year-round.

Respect the tick's turf. Ticks tend to be found in grass, bushes, or woods. You're most likely to pick up ticks when you sit or lie on the ground or brush up against tall grass or bushes.

Dress smart. Don't go barefoot or wear sandals. Long pants cinched at the ankle (perhaps with rubber bands) or tucked into socks are best. And wear light-colored clothing so ticks are easier to spot.

Use repellent. Research published in May supports the common assumption that insect repellents reduce the risk of Lyme disease. A study of nearly 700 workers for the New Jersey Department of Environmental Protection found that repellents cut the risk of Lyme disease in half.

Most repellents contain deet—the nickname for N,N-diethyl-meta-toluamide. Some products are 100 percent deet. That's probably too much of a good thing. Pure deet may pose a greater risk of skin reactions than diluted deet and offers little, if any, advantage over repellents that contain about 50 percent deet.

Repellent lasts longer if you apply it to your clothes. Be sure to use some on the areas most accessible to ticks: shoe tops, socks, and pants cuffs. (Deet can be safely applied to cotton, wool, and nylon. But it can damage synthetics such as acetate, rayon, and spandex, as well as plastic items such as eyeglasses or watch crystals.)

Before applying deet to your skin, make sure you're not allergic by trying a "patch test" a day or so in advance: Apply a small amount to your forearm or thigh and check the spot for redness over the next day or two. If there's no reaction, apply repellent sparingly to any exposed skin (but not your face).

While deet repels ticks, the chemical permethrin—applied only to clothing—actually kills them. Studies have shown permethrin to be a more effective tick repellent than deet. The Environmental Protection Agency sanctions permethrin's use in various pesticide products. According to an agency source, its approval for use in repellents is expected by midsummer. Permanone, an aerosol spray that contains permethrin, should be available in all 50 states by the end of the year.

In April, the Environmental Protection Agency warned that R-11, an ingredient in some repellents, had caused birth defects, ovarian shrinkage, and certain benign tumors in test animals. Products containing that ingredient—listed as 2,3,4,5-Bis(2-butylene)tetrahydro-2-furaldehyde—should have been withdrawn from the market or reformulated by now. To be safe, though, check the label before you buy a repellent.

Search and destroy. Check yourself periodically when you're outside in a possibly infested area. Look carefully: A young deer tick, responsible for most Lyme disease in humans, is smaller than a sesame seed. (After gorging on blood for several hours, ticks are many times larger and easier to spot.) Brush off any ticks you find on your clothes, or that are still crawling on your skin and thus haven't bitten yet.

Taking a shower when you come inside may dislodge any hangers-on that haven't bitten. If a tick does bite you, you probably won't feel it. So get in the habit of inspecting yourself and any young children or pets each night during tick season. Although ticks may feed anywhere on the body, they prefer sites on or near the trunk, particularly the armpits and groin.

If you're bitten by a tick, the chances are still good that you won't contract Lyme disease. Even in a high-risk region of Connecticut, for example, at most one-third of deer ticks are actually infected. If you remove a tick soon after it bites you, you'll probably avoid the disease even if the tick is infected; it may take a tick as long as 24 to 48 hours to transmit the disease. In a study of that same high-risk Connecticut region, only one of 29 people developed the disease after being bitten.

Have tweezers ready in case you find a tick. Grasp the insect as close as possible to the spot where its mouth enters the skin, and pull upward steadily. Grasping too far back on the body may actually squeeze disease microbes from the tick into the wound.

Other popular tick-removal tactics—such as butter, fingernail polish, gasoline, kerosene, petroleum jelly, rubbing alcohol, and lit matches or cigarettes—are usually ineffective and can even be hazardous.

SOURCE:
"Lyme Disease Is on the Rise: But You Can Cut the Risk." *Consumer Reports Health Letter* 2, no. 6 (June 1990): 41, 43.

RESOURCES

ORGANIZATIONS

Arthritis Foundation. 1314 Spring St. NW, Atlanta, GA 30309.

Lyme Borreliolis Foundation. 39 Anderson Rd., Tolland, CT 00084.

National Institute of Allergy and Infections Diseases. NIH Building 31, 9000 Rockville Pike, Bethesda, MD 20892.

National Institute of Arthritis and Musculoskeletal and Skin Diseases. NIH Building 31, 9000 Rockville Pike, Bethesda, MD 20892.

PAMPHLETS

American Council on Science and Health:

Lyme Disease. June 1988, 21 pp.

National Institute of Arthritis and Musculoskeletal and Skin Diseases:

NIAMSD Research Update: Lyme Disease. July 1989. 6 pp.

RELATED ARTICLES

Rahn, Daniel W. "Treatment of Lyme Disease: Best Use of Antibiotics." *Postgraduate Medicine* 87, no. 6 (May 1, 1990): 159–164.

Seligmann, Jean. "Tiny Tick, Big Worry." *Newsweek* (May 22, 1989): 66–72.

Steere, Allen C. "Medical Progress: Lyme Disease." *New England Journal of Medicine* 321, no. 9 (August 31, 1989): 586–596.

Thomas, Patricia. "Lyme Disease: Tick Terror." *Harvard Health Letter* 16, no. 9 (July 1991): 1–4.

Wallace, Jean. "Update on Lyme Disease: Here's How to Avoid Ticks When You're Out on Nature's Trail this Summer." *Parents* (July 1990): 118–120.

Williams, David N. and Eric S. Schned. "Lyme Disease: Recognizing Its Many Manifestations." *Postgraduate Medicine* 87, no. 6 (May 1, 1990): 139–146.

MACULAR DEGENERATION

OVERVIEW

As the eye looks straight ahead, the macula is the point of the retina upon which the light rays meet as they are focused by the cornea and the lens of the eye. Similar to the film in a camera, the retina receives the images that come through the "camera-like" lens. If the macula is damaged, the central part of the images are blocked as if a blurred area had been placed in the center of the picture. The images around the blurred area may be clearly visible.

Macular degeneration is damage or breakdown of the macula. The eye still sees objects to the side, since side, or "peripheral," vision is usually not affected. For this reason, macular degeneration alone does not result in total blindness. However, it can make reading or close work difficult or impossible without the use of special low vision optical aids.

The retina is the delicate layer of tissue that lines the inside wall of the back of the eye. The macula is a very small area in the center of the retina. In size, the macula is about the same as a capital "O" in the type of this [book]. This small area is responsible for our central "straight ahead" sight used for reading and other fine tasks.

Although macular degeneration most often occurs in older people, aging alone does not always result in central visual loss. Nevertheless, macular degeneration is the leading cause of impairment of reading and fine "close-up" vision in the United States.

The most common form of macular degeneration is called involutional macular degeneration. This form accounts for 70% of all cases, and is associated with aging. It is caused by a breakdown or thinning of the tissues in the macula.

About 10% of macular degeneration falls into a category called exudative macular degeneration. Normally, the macula is protected by a thin tissue that separates it from very fine blood vessels nourishing the back of the eye. Sometimes these blood vessels break or leak and cause scar tissue to form. This often leads to the growth of new abnormal blood vessels in the scar tissue. These newly formed vessels are especially fragile. They rupture easily and may leak. Blood and leaking fluid destroy the macula and cause further scarring. Vision becomes distorted and blurred, and dense scar tissue blocks out central vision to a severe degree.

Other types of macular degeneration are inherited, may occur in juveniles (juvenile macular degeneration), and are not associated with the aging process. Occasionally, injury, infection, or inflammation may also damage the delicate tissue of the macula.

If only one eye is affected, macular degeneration is hardly noticeable in the beginning stages, particularly when the other eye is normal. This condition often involves one eye at a time, so it may be some time before a patient notices visual problems.

Macular degeneration can cause different symptoms in different people. Sometimes only one eye loses vision while the other eye continues to see well for many years. If both eyes are affected, however, reading and close-up work may become extremely difficult. Macular degeneration alone does not cause total blindness. Since side vision is usually unaffected, most people can take care of themselves quite well.

Color vision may become dim and these other visual symptoms can develop due to macular degeneration.

Many patients do not realize they have a macular problem until blurred vision becomes obvious. Your ophthalmologist can detect macular degeneration in the early stages. The ophthalmologist examines the macula carefully by viewing it with an instrument called an ophthalmoscope to see if damage is present.

The examination will usually include a few more tests:

- A grid test, in which the patient looks at a test page (similar to graph paper), will be used to check for the extent of sight loss spots.
- A color vision test will show whether a patient can tell color differences, and additional tests will help to discover conditions that may be causing the macula to deteriorate.
- Sometimes a fluorescein angiogram is done. The ophthalmologist injects a dye into the patient's arm, and then takes photos of the retina and macula. The dye helps to clarify any blood vessel abnormality that might be present.

Macular degeneration can be detected and diagnosed early by an ophthalmologist if periodic eye examinations are part of health care. Early detection is important since people may not realize their vision is impaired. Having your eyes checked is especially appropriate if other family members have a history of retinal problems. For patients with macular degeneration, early diagnosis by an ophthalmologist may prevent further damage or aid the individual in making a visual adjustment with low vision aids.

SOURCE:
American Academy of Ophthalmology. *Macular Degeneration: Major Cause of Central Vision Loss.* April 1987. pp. 1-6.

TREATMENT

At present the only treatment proven effective for any stage of macular degeneration is the use of laser photocoagulation for patients with well-defined neovascularization. This includes neovascularization involving the very center of the macula as long as that neovascularization is two disc areas in extent or less. It is still true that most neovascularization associated with age related macular degeneration is poorly defined so that treatment cannot be considered using existing guidelines.

Studies are currently under way to evaluate the potential role of laser treatment and other treatment for poorly defined areas of neovascularization.

SOURCE:
Fine, Stuart L. Letter to publisher. December 9, 1991.

USE OF ARGON LASERS IN TREATMENT

A different type of laser—the argon laser—is used to treat some patients with the more severe form of an eye disorder called macular degeneration. Although this disease doesn't cause total blindness, it is a leading cause of loss of both central and reading vision. Macular degeneration is particularly common in people over 65.

The macula is the portion of the light-sensing retina that light rays strike to provide the sharp, straight-ahead vision needed for driving and reading small print. In the less common but more severe form of macular degeneration, for no known reason, new blood vessels grow beneath the macula. These abnormal vessels leak fluid and blood, destroying nearby macula cells. If the leakage and bleeding continue, much of the macula may be damaged irreparably within a few weeks or months. The resulting dense scar tissue blocks out central vision, much like an opaque smudge does in the center of one's glasses.

With early detection, severe vision loss from this type of macular degeneration can usually be prevented with argon laser treatment. This relatively low-energy laser heats rather than vaporizes, tissues, acting essentially like a welder. A study conducted by the National Eye Institute showed that argon laser treatment can slash by more than half the chances of experiencing severe vision loss from macular degeneration.

The green beams of the argon laser are only absorbed by red objects, so it selectively heats up and seals blood vessels (because they contain red blood cells) and leaves most other parts of the eye undisturbed. The narrowness of the beam enhances laser precision, allowing the ophthalmologist to target only diseased blood vessels.

This type of surgery generally takes only a few minutes and may be done with the aid of a local anesthetic to prevent discomfort. Soon afterwards, the patient is able to return home and resume normal daily activities.

A fungal disease called ocular histoplasmosis can cause faulty blood vessels to grow and damage the macula. This is a significant cause of vision loss in the southeast and midwest United States, where this particular fungus is prevalent. Experts estimate that laser treatment of the abnormal vessels can prevent up to 2,000 cases of serious vision loss due to the disease each year if treatment is given early, before extensive damage has occurred.

SOURCE:
Patlak, Margie. "Lights for Sight: Lasers Beginning to Solve Vision Problems." *FDA Consumer* 24 (August 1990): 15-16.

USE OF DIFFUSE LASER BEAMS IN TREATMENT

Macular degeneration is a painless, progressive eye disorder that most often affects older people. It's the most common cause of irreversible blindness in the U.S. In severe cases, leakage from blood vessels scars the macula, a small area near the center of the retina that distinguishes fine detail.

Lasers are sometimes used to seal off those leaky vessels. But the lasers can damage small parts of the retina and leave blind spots, so they're currently used only when the leaks are few or close together, where they can be fixed with just a few laser pulses. Now, however, researchers at Johns Hopkins University are developing a technique that fires a diffuse scatter-burst of fine laser beams to seal leaks in a wider area of the retina, leaving it largely intact.

Based on preliminary data, the researchers, Susan B. Bressler, M.D., and Neil M. Bressler, M.D., report that the new technique appears to staunch vessel leakage without damaging the retina. Once they've determined whether the technique preserves vision, the researchers hope to launch a multi-center study.

SOURCE:
"Lasers Battle Blindness." *Consumer Reports Health Letter* 2 (December 1990): 96.

USE OF ZINC IN TREATMENT

Daily zinc supplements have been shown in a preliminary study to be the only effective means of retarding the severe visual loss from macular degenerations. There is no known cause for this condition that produces a slow or sudden painless loss of central vision due to deterioration of the central part of the retina. People with macular degeneration usually retain good peripheral vision, but they are often defined as "legally blind," requiring low vision devices and services due to loss of the central vision. It is the leading cause of severe visual loss in people over the age of 55.

In the study conducted by David A. Newsome, M.D., of the Louisiana State University School of Medicine, 151 people, aged 42 to 89, with macular degeneration were assigned randomly to receive identical-appearing tablets containing either 100 mg zinc sulfate or a lactose/fructose combination that served as a placebo (*Archives of Ophthalmology*, February 1988). All participants were told to take a tablet with food twice daily. Their vision was checked by a team of physicians at six-month intervals for one to two years. "Although some eyes in the zinc-treated group lost vision," reported the investigators, "this group had significantly less visual loss than the placebo group after a follow-up of 12 to 24 months."

There is no effective drug treatment for macular degeneration, and laser surgery can benefit only a small minority who develop an additional complication. (In about one in 20 cases, abnormal blood vessels grow into the macula, where they rupture, bleed, and form scar tissue that further obscures vision.) The Louisiana State study was prompted by numerous published studies showing high concentrations of zinc in ocular tissue. The high incidence of zinc deficiency among older people and the mineral's key role in the metabolism of the retina were cited by the investigators as motivating factors for their study. Retinal abnormalities have been observed in humans who are zinc deficient due to gastrointestinal malabsorption.

While the reported side effects were minimal for the study participants (one dropped out because zinc aggravated preexisting peptic ulcer symptoms), the investigators warned that any recommendation of widespread use of oral zinc would be premature. Potentially serious adverse reactions, such as anemia and worsening of cardiovascular disease, from long-term, high dose zinc therapy have been identified by other researchers. Yet the Louisiana State results clearly merit additional research, and plans for a larger study are already in the works. "This is the first controlled oral intervention study to show a positive, if limited, treatment effect in macular degeneration, a major public health problem," stated the investigators.

SOURCE:
"Zinc Retards Macular Degeneration." *HealthFacts* 13 (April 1988): 5.

RESOURCES

ORGANIZATIONS

American Academy of Ophthalmology. P.O. Box 7424, San Francisco, CA 94120.

National Eye Institute. Age-Related Eye Disease Study Center, NIH Building 31, 9000 Rockville Pike, Bethesda, MD 20892.

BOOK

Neal, Helen. *What You Can Do To Preserve—and Even Enhance—Your Usable Sight*. New York: Simon and Schuster, 1987.

RELATED ARTICLES

"Do We Have a Nutritional Treatment for Age-Related Cataract or Macular Degeneration?" *Archives of Ophthalmology* 108 (October 1990): 1403–1405.

Farber, Matthew E., and Andrew S. Farber. "Macular Degeneration: A Devastating but Treatable Disease." *Postgraduate Medicine* 88, no. 2 (August 1990): 181–183.

"Macular Degeneration: Early Treatment Vital to Preventing Permanent Loss of Central Vision." *Mayo Clinic Health Letter* (September 1990): 5.

Newsome, David A., and others. "Oral Zinc in Macular Degeneration." *Archives of Ophthalmology* 106 (February 1988): 192–198.

MAGNETIC RESONANCE IMAGING (MRI)

(*See also:* CAT SCANS [COMPUTED TOMOGRAPHY])

OVERVIEW

In less than a decade, advances in technology have revolutionized the way doctors look into the human body.

One of the most dramatic examples is magnetic resonance imaging (MRI). Considering the views of the human body that this remarkable technology provides, and its wide-ranging uses, MRI clearly is one of the most important developments in medical imaging since X-rays were discovered in 1895.

MRI is an amazing new tool for diagnosis—but not for treatment. The device houses a powerful magnet.

When you undergo this procedure, the force of the magnet causes nuclei of hydrogen atoms within your body to align themselves with the magnet's field. (The magnet's field is 25,000 times stronger than the earth's magnetic field.) A radio signal alters this alignment for an instant. As these hydrogen nuclei realign themselves with the magnetic field, signals are produced. The signals are characteristic for each body tissue.

A computer uses information from the signals to create an image that represents a thin slice (cross section) of the area under investigation. Slices can be obtained in any direction or plane. This gives a previously unobtainable perspective of organs and other tissues.

No single imaging technique is appropriate for all situations. For example, MRI is not particularly good at recording the appearance of moving organs, such as those of the abdomen. For this purpose, computer tomography (CT) is the better choice.

Specifically, MRI offers these advantages:

- It's convenient—MRI is painless, non-invasive and can be performed on an outpatient basis. Unlike CT or X-rays, MRI does not use ionizing radiation. MRI has no harmful side effects, so it is helpful if you need multiple or periodic scans.
- New views—MRI creates previously unavailable views of blood vessels, blood flow, cartilage, bone marrow, muscles, ligaments, the spinal cord and fluid in the brain and spine.
- Analyzes tissue health—MRI's crisp images allow physicians to distinguish between healthy and diseased tissue. MRI can chart the progress of disease, such as cancer of the cervix or endometrium, and spot a recurrence that demands immediate, aggressive treatment.
- Limits need for other techniques—MRI offers early diagnosis of multiple sclerosis, other neurologic diseases and certain tumors. Accurate identification of these conditions may eliminate the need for additional testing.

Sharp MRI images of blood vessels, walls and chambers of the heart can sometimes make heart catheterization unnecessary. This can be especially helpful for children who have congenital heart disease.

MRI is not appropriate if your body has been implanted with certain electronic devices, such as a pacemaker or a cardiac stimulator.

If you are extremely obese or exceptionally uncomfortable when confined to small spaces (claustrophobic), this test probably is not for you.

SOURCE:

"Magnetic Resonance Imaging: Important New 'Window' to Your Body's Interior." *Mayo Clinic Health Letter* (September 1990): 6–7.

USE IN VISUALIZING BRAIN AND SPINAL CORD

MRI has become the standard of care in the diagnosis of most abnormalities involving the brain and spine.

About 90% of all MRI scans are ordered for the diagnosis of suspected cranial and spinal disorders. Its major advantages over CT in these areas are better soft-tissue contrast, direct multiplanar images, and freedom from streak artifacts caused by bone and implanted metal devices. In general, these attributes permit superb visualization of the brain and spinal cord in areas that may be obscured on CT, particularly in regions of dense bone or adjacent to dense bone: the middle and posterior fossae, the sella turcica, the auditory canal, the orbit, and the entire spinal canal. MRI also provides exquisite delineation of extra-axial tumors such as acoustic neuromas (especially when enhanced with contrast), and beautifully demonstrates the pituitary gland.

MRI's excellent visualization of the intrinsic structure of the brain and spinal cord permits detection of many abnormalities when they are still very small or at an early stage of development. This is true, for instance, in multiple sclerosis, infarcts, tumors, and infection, among other problems.

MRI has proven extremely useful in the diagnosis of multiple sclerosis, but while MRI is much more sensitive than CT to abnormal changes associated with multiple sclerosis, an abnormal study result is not synonymous with disease; the diagnosis remains a clinical one. Furthermore, the ability of MRI to support a diagnosis of multiple sclerosis declines with increasing patient age because the prevalence of similar nonspecific changes in brain white matter increases with age.

Although CT often yields no more than equivocal findings in the first 24-48 hours following cerebral infarction, MRI can detect the definitively localized cerebral infarction within hours of the event. MRI is also assuming a wider role in the rapid diagnosis of focal viral encephalitis and other cerebral infections in both normal and immunocompromised populations.

SOURCE:
Cushmore, Frederick N., Walter Kucharczyk, and David L. Rodibaugh. "MRI: When You Can't Afford Not To." *Patient Care* 23 (February 28, 1989): 29–30.

HAZARDS OF MAGNETIC RESONANCE IMAGING

Despite the relative safety of MRI, two basic risks are associated with the procedure. The first risk relates to the immediate environment of the magnetic resonance imaging suite, where appliances and other magnetic materials may become high-speed projectiles in the presence of powerful magnetic forces. The second risk involves patients who have metallic implants, including pacemakers, prosthetic cardiac valves, surgical clips, orthopedic appliances, penile implants, cochlear implants, intravascular filters, stents, coils, dental materials and shunt connectors.

Materials that are dangerous in the radiographic suite include oxygen bottles, stretchers and wheelchairs made of magnetic materials. Emergency carts also contain such materials. If carts are left in the imaging area, they may act as missiles against either the machine itself or the patient. Stretchers for use in imaging suites should be made of aluminum, plastic or stainless steel, since these materials do not have magnetic attraction. Emergency carts should be kept outside the suite. Imaging personnel must be properly instructed about avoiding patient injuries in MRI suites.

Metallic implants in patients can contraindicate MRI examinations and should therefore be documented by careful histories. Cardiac pacemakers, for example, would be dangerous in MRI examinations. Two forces act on the pacemaker—the magnetic field and the gradient field. MRI may result in asynchronous pulsing of the numerous magnetic and electronic parts of the pacemaker when the pacemaker is exposed to these fields. Radio frequency pulses also can cause difficulty with pacemaker electrical systems. In addition, problems may result from pacemaker position shifts within the chest wall.

Although the magnetic fields affect prosthetic valves, they are not of sufficient force to dislodge such valves and do not interfere with valve function. . . .

Many patients cannot tolerate the closed-in space of the MRI machine. The resultant anxiety sometimes necessitates stopping or cancelling the examination. Anxiolytic medication may help but may not be sufficient. The noise of the radiofrequency pulses also can be so disturbing to patients that the examination must be stopped.

SOURCE:
Deluca, Salvatore A., and Frank P. Castronovo, Jr. "Hazards of Magnetic Resonance Imaging." *American Family Physician* 41, no. 1 (January 1990): 145–146.

RESOURCES

BOOK
Stark, D. D., and W. G. Brudley. *Magnetic Resonance Imaging.* St. Louis: C.V. Mosby, 1988.

RELATED ARTICLES
Consensus Conference. "Magnetic Resonance Imaging." *JAMA* 259, no. 14 (April 8, 1988): 2132–2138.

Hinshaw, David B., Jr. "Magnetic Resonance Imaging Versus X-Ray Computed Tomography: Which Is the Appropriate First Imaging Examination?" *The Western Journal of Medicine* 151 (November 1989): 569–570.

"MRI: Judged Comparable To and Safer Than the CT Scan." *HealthFacts* 14 (February 1989): 3.

Plankey, Elaine Deutsch, and James Knauf. "What Patients need to Know about Magnetic Resonance Imaging." *American Journal of Nursing* 90 (January 1990): 27–28.

Randal, Judith E. "NMR: The Best Thing Since X-Rays?" *Technology Review* 91 (January 1988): 58–65.

MAMMOGRAMS AND BREAST BIOPSY

(*See also:* FIBROCYSTIC BREAST DISEASE)

OVERVIEW

The objective of breast screening is to reduce the number of deaths by detecting cancerous tumors at an early stage when therapies are most effective. Therefore, the criteria for a screening test should include sensitivity, availability, simplicity, and safety. A cancer screening test needs to be sensitive enough to detect unsuspected disease accurately in its early stages when treatment is most effective. An effective screening test should be easy to perform and not too time-consuming, so that many women can be examined in a short period of time. In addition, the test should be readily available to a wide range of women: availability includes low cost, convenience, and adequate supply. Finally, a screening test should be safe so that it does not cause more illness than it was designed to detect.

Currently, there are three principal methods of screening for breast cancer that meet most of these criteria: mammography, clinical breast exam (a manual physical exam by a trained individual), and the breast self-exam. Other methods of imaging the breast for cancer, including transillumination, ultrasound and thermography, are not recommended for screening purposes. Mammography in combination with a clinical breast exam is the most effective means of detecting breast cancer.

Of the three breast screening methods, mammography is the most sensitive. It can detect breast tumors when they are small and localized before they have a chance to grow and become invasive or to spread to other parts of the body. Mammography can detect tumors as small as a quarter of an inch in diameter. The other methods detect lumps about a half inch across, at the point that can be felt or palpated. By the time a lump is large enough to be felt in a physical exam, it contains billions of cancer cells, some of which can break away and spread to other organs.

The sensitivity of mammography increases with women's age. As women grow older, their breasts become less dense, making it easier for radiologists to detect tumors in their mammograms. For example, studies have found that among women younger than 50, mammography detects breast cancer tumors only about 50 percent of the time. In contrast, for women over 50 mammography can detect existing breast cancers almost 90 percent of the time. This level of detection, however, can only be achieved if proper equipment is used, meticulous attention is given to technical considerations, and the radiologist is familiar with and can recognize the early and indirect signs of malignancy. In addition, radiologists must regularly check the results of pathology reports of patients they recommend for biopsy in order to determine their rate of accuracy in identifying suspicious mammograms.

Although screening mammography is a simple procedure for most women, there are risks associated with it. Unfortunately, advocates of mammography screening rarely inform women of these risks. Presumably, they fear that if women knew what the risks were, they might be less inclined to have a mammogram. While this may be true in some cases, it discounts women's ability to make rational decisions about their own bodies and health. HRG believes that women should be informed about the benefits and risks of mammography so that they can make their won decisions about using this procedure.

The major concern about screening mammography is that because x-rays are used there is an increased risk of developing radiation-induced breast cancer. The estimated lifetime risk of radiation-induced breast cancer is between 0.8 and 4.9 additional cases of breast cancer among a million women each year per rad of dose. This risk is greater for women under age 50, for whom the additional years of exposure carry a small but real additional risk of radiation-induced cancer.

Another risk is that the radiologist will fail to see a tumor, when one is actually present: the "false negative" result. If this happens, the tumor may spread to other organs before it is detected, at which point the likelihood of successful treatment will be significantly reduced. The failure to detect breast tumors is more likely among women with dense breast tissue, which is common in younger women. A reason why mammographers sometimes miss tumors is that mammograms of dense breast tissue are harder to read; images of normal dense tissue may mask abnormal growths such as cancer tumors which are also composed of dense tissue. Other reasons why tumors are missed on mammograms include poor technique, lack of recognition of subtle radiographic signs, and absence of radiographic criteria for cancer.

Women with breast implants are also at greater risk of being misdiagnosed because the implants and the fibrous dense tissue which often surrounds them may interfere with the accurate reading of the mammogram.

SOURCE:
Public Citizen Health Research Group. "HRG Report on Screening Mammography: Part I." *Health Letter* (August 1991): 2–3.

DEFINITION

Mammography uses radiation (X-rays) to create an image of the breast on film or paper called a mammogram. It can reveal tumors too small to be felt by palpation. It shows other changes in the structure of the breast which doctors believe point to very early cancer. A mammographic examination usually consists of two X-rays of each breast, one taken from the top and one from the side.

SOURCE:
National Cancer Institute. *Breast Exams: What You Should Know*. NIH Pub. No. 86-2000. August 1986. p. 5.

GUIDELINES

According to the American Cancer Society (ACS) and the National Cancer Institute, all asymptomatic women who are at average risk for breast cancer should undergo screening mammography by age 40. Mammography should be repeated every 1–2 years for women aged 40-49 and annually thereafter. A clinical breast examination is recommended every three years for women aged 20–40 and every year after age 40. The ACS also advocates monthly breast self-examination for women age 20 and older.

These guidelines are endorsed by 10 professional and research groups, including the American Medical Association, and for the most part have become the standard of care. Those for routine screening mammography in 40–49-year-old women continue to be controversial, however; and because randomized studies have shown an insufficient benefit, they are not endorsed by the American Academy of Family Physicians, the American College of Physicians, the International Union Against Cancer, or the U.S. Preventive Services Task Force.

No doubt remains that routine screening mammography reduces mortality from breast cancer in women older than 50. The Health Insurance Plan (HIP) of Greater New York study of 62,000 women and other controlled, randomized studies in Europe have conclusively demonstrated it. The HIP study has now shown a delayed benefit for women aged 40–49 as well, although the major contribution was from clinical breast examination. In another large study, the Breast Cancer Detection Demonstration Project, participants in their 40s and those in their 50s have been found to have similar survival rates. These studies, the incidence of breast cancer in women younger than 50, and the need for early detection of cancers before they become palpable have persuaded the groups endorsing the ACS guidelines that routine screening mammography for women in their 40s is warranted.

Some experts in breast disease prefer that women in their 40s have mammography every year and suggest beginning as early as age 35 if risk factors for breast cancer other than sex and age are present. Of the women who develop the disease, however, 75% have none of the three high-risk factors, and 25–33% of breast cancers occur in women younger than 50. Conceivably, the incidence would be higher if more women were routinely screened in their 40s.

SOURCE:
"Screening the Average-Risk Woman." *Patient Care* (August 15, 1990): 84.

MAMMOGRAPHY QUALITY CONTROL

According to recent data, the radiation dose you may be exposed to can vary by a factor of 10, and image quality of the picture of your breast can also vary significantly between units.

In fact, an accreditation process carried out over the past several years flunked almost one-third of the mammography practices evaluated. According to data collected by the American College of Radiology (ACR) Mammography Screening Accreditation Program, as of February 1990, of the 1,348 units evaluated, 442 failed the first attempt at accreditation.

Dr. R. Edward Hendrick, Chief of the division of radiologic sciences at the University of Colorado in Denver, has been involved in the ongoing accreditation process. He writes:

> At the heart of the observed variations in image quality and breast dose is the lack of standardized quality control practices in mammography sites with-

in the United States. The majority of mammography units that are in hospitals undergo annual inspection of x-ray-producing equipment by a physicist as part of an ongoing quality assurance program. . . however, more than 50% of mammographic screening sites are located outside of hospitals and therefore are not necessarily subject to mandated annual inspections. To my knowledge, no accurate statistics exist on the fraction of mammography units located outside of hospitals that are evaluated annually.

When you go for a mammogram, try to go to a facility that has been accredited. You can find them by calling your state's division of the American Cancer Society or by calling the National Cancer Institute at 1-800-4-CANCER.

SOURCE:
Wolfe, Sidney M., and Rhoda Donkin Jones. *Women's Health Alert*. Reading, MA: Addison-Wesley, 1991. pp. 14–15.

BREAST BIOPSY

You have a lump or some other change in your breast. Most breast lumps or other changes are not cancer. However, to be sure, your doctor tells you that a biopsy must be done.

A biopsy is minor surgery to take out all or part of a breast lump or the tissue in question. A doctor called a pathologist looks at the biopsy tissue under a microscope to see if cancer is present. A biopsy is the only way to know for sure if a breast change is benign (not cancer) or malignant (cancer).

You have a choice between two procedures for your biopsy. The most common is the two-step procedure. For this procedure, the biopsy is done first. Then if cancer is found, treatment begins a week or two later. Some women choose a one-step procedure. When this is used, the woman is treated immediately if cancer is found.

Your doctor can use several biopsy methods to remove tissue for the pathologist to examine. The choice depends on such things as the size and location of the bump or suspicious area and your general health. Ask your doctor which of these methods will be used for your biopsy:

- Aspiration. The use of a needle and syringe to try to drain the lump. If the lump is a cyst (a fluid-filled sac that is not cancer), removing the fluid will collapse it. No other treatment is needed.
- Fine-Needle Aspiration. The use of a thin needle and syringe to collect cell clumps or single cells from the lump.
- Needle Biopsy. The removal of a small piece of breast tissue using a needle that has a special cutting edge; also called a core needle biopsy.

If cancer is not found using fine-needle aspiration or needle biopsy, the doctor will most likely do an excisional or incisional biopsy. The doctor uses these test to make sure cancer cells were not missed by the needle.

- Excisional Biopsy. The removal of all of the lump. Used most often, it is the current "standard" procedure for small (less than about an inch in diameter) lumps. Also called a lumpectomy.
- Incisional Biopsy. The removal of part of the lump. This method may be used if the breast lump is large.
- Mammographic Localization With Biopsy. Used when a breast change can be seen on a mammogram (an x-ray of the breast) but cannot be felt. In this procedure, the doctor uses the mammogram as a guide for placing small needles (needle localization) at the site of the breast change. Sometimes dye is used instead of needles to mark the site. The suspicious tissue then can be removed for examination by the pathologist.

SOURCE:
National Cancer Institute. *Breast Biopsy: What You Should Know*. NIH Pub. No. 90-657. July 1990. 1, 3, 5.

* * *

As late as the mid-1970s, women with suspicious breast lumps were routinely given general anesthesia for biopsy tests. In the event that malignancy was found, a radical mastectomy (involving removal of the breast tissue, the chest muscles, and all chest and underarm lymph nodes) or a modified radical mastectomy (which leaves some chest muscles intact) was performed while the patient was still under anesthesia. Today, biopsies and treatment are usually scheduled as two separate steps, thereby allowing women to be active decision makers in the treatment process.

Specific techniques in the breast biopsy itself have also improved. Such improvements are especially significant because the growing use of mammography has resulted in a marked increase in suspicious findings that require surgical diagnosis. Because 70% to 80% of such mammographic findings are benign, the goal of excising a minimal amount of tissue becomes even more important.

Needle-directed biopsy, one technique used when suspected abnormalities are not easily felt, has a high success rate of lesion removal while excising only a small specimen (often no more than the diameter of a quarter). In this procedure, the suspicious area is pinpointed by a radiologist using mammography. He or she then positions a needle to serve as a localizing device. The precise area indicated by the needle is then removed by a surgeon. This needle-directed biopsy, although still allowing for thorough pathologic examination, can often be performed with the patient under local anesthesia, minimizes trauma to the patient, and causes little cosmetic change.

SOURCE:
Tinklenberg, Mae, R.N. "Reducing the Fear of Breast Cancer." *Healthline* (October 1990): 2–3.

RESOURCES

ORGANIZATIONS

American Cancer Society. 40 Park Avenue, New York, NY 10016.

Encore Program. YWCA, 726 Broadway, New York, NY 10003.

National Cancer Institute. Office of Cancer Communications, Building 31, Bethesda, MD 20892. (800)4-CANCER.

PAMPHLET

National Cancer Institute:

Smart Advice for Women 40 and Over. NIH Pub. No. 90-1581. January 1991. 15 pp.

RELATED ARTICLES

"Breast Cancer Screening Guidelines Agreed On by AMA, Other Medically Related Organizations." *JAMA* 262, no. 9 (September 1, 1989): 1155.

"The Clear Case for Mammograms." *The Johns Hopkins Medical Letter: Health After 50* (December 1990): 2-3.

"Mammography: The New Boom Business?" *People's Medical Society Newsletter* 8, no. 5 (October 1989): 1, 6.

NCI Breast Cancer Screening Consortium. "Screening Mammography: A Missed Clinical Opportunity." *JAMA* 264, no. 1 (July 4, 1990): 54-58.

"Not Everyone Agrees with New Mammographic Screening Guidelines Designed to End Confusion." *JAMA* 262, no. 9 (September 1, 1989): 1154-1155.

U.S. Preventive Services Task Force. "Screening for Breast Cancer." *American Family Physician* 39, no. 6 (June 1989): 89-96.

MEASLES

(*See also:* VACCINES)

OVERVIEW

Once a common disease, measles was almost considered a medical curiosity for many years. In fact, many young pediatricians had never even seen a case of measles. Until recently, that is. Measles has now made its presence felt on college campuses and almost all major cities have reported outbreaks. According to current thinking, the vaccine, once thought to be protective for life, seems to lose its protective effect some time during the second decade. Because of this, major reimmunization programs have been instituted to attempt to prevent further outbreaks. However, it has become important for parents as well as health care providers to familiarize themselves with this disease as it is bound to show up in every part of the country.

Measles is caused by a paramyxovirus. The virus has an incubation period of 10–12 days and usually begins with a fever, fatigue and a general feeling of ill health. Fever will rapidly increase to 104–105 degrees over a 4-5 day period and then rapidly return to normal. Physicians like to talk about measles in terms of "the three C's." These are cough, conjunctivitis and coryza. The cough of measles will start early in the illness and can become quite severe. The virus invades the lining of the trachea and bronchi, producing a cough that can persist for about 10 days.

Conjunctivitis, which refers to redness and watering of the eyes, is always present during the illness. The eyes may also be painful and sensitive to light. Coryza refers to severe nasal irritation and discharge. This will begin on the second day of the illness and disappear by day five or six.

Measles is particularly noted for its rash. However, the first rash of measles does not occur on the skin. Early in the course of the illness small white spots surrounded by a reddened area can be found on the inner surface of the cheeks. Known as Koplik's spots, they are only found in measles. Soon after the appearance of the Koplik's spots the skin rash of measles begins. This rash begins on about the third day, first appearing on the scalp and face. Red and blotchy, it soon spreads down the body and may cover it completely. It begins to fade by the seventh or eighth day of the illness. The skin may peel in the more severely reddened areas.

Children with measles can be severely ill. In the early sixties prior to the development of the vaccine there were 400–500,000 cases annually with about 500 deaths. Currently there are about 10–15,000 cases per year. Most children with measles will have an uneventful recovery. However like most viral illnesses, it is not treatable. During the course of the illness treatable bacterial complications can occur, including ear, sinus and lung infections. Other complications can occur such as encephalitis which is an infection of the brain by the virus. This can cause paralysis, deafness or death.

The vaccine used today is a live virus product. Prior to its development a killed virus vaccine was used, up until 1967. Today's adults who may have received this vaccine as children can get a disease called atypical measles if they come in contact with a person with measles. This illness is characterized by a rash, fever, swelling of the extremities, pneumonia and accumulation of fluid in the lungs called an effusion. Physicians caring for adults must be aware of the entity especially in light of the current measles resurgence.

The importance of using measles vaccine cannot be overemphasized. The vaccine is effective and safe and should be given at 15 months of age. We now know that a repeat dose should be given after 10 years of age. It has few side effects. Some children will experience a fever and a skin rash five to ten days after receiving the first dose of the vaccine.

Measles can be confused with some other viral infections such as roseola and infectious mononucleosis. It can also be confused with an allergic skin reaction. However, if one has a good grasp of the natural progression of the disease the differentiation should not be difficult.

SOURCE:
"Measles." *Parents Pediatric Report* 7, no. 4 (April 1990): 22.

IMMUNIZATION

For the past several years, measles outbreaks have tended to fit into two patterns: (1) unvaccinated preschool children, usually inner-city minority populations, and (2) previously vaccinated school-age children and college students. The first type of outbreak illustrates a failure to implement current immunization recommendations. The second type illustrates the ability of measles to spread in fully or nearly fully immunized populations.

Official recommendations regarding measles vaccination have been revised periodically. The dramatic increase in the number of cases in 1989 prompted the Immunization Practices Advisory Committee of the Centers for Disease Control to recommend, for the first time, a second dose of measles vaccine prior to school entry. (This recommendation is endorsed by the American Academy of Family Physicians.) Unfortunately, this recommendation is not fully consistent with that of the American Academy of Pediatrics (AAP). While recognizing the legitimacy of other dosing schedules, the AAP recommends that the second dose be given at the time of entry into middle or junior high school. . . .

Measles vaccine comes in both a monovalent form and polyvalent combinations of measles-rubella (MR) and measles-mumps-rubella (MMR). Use of MMR is preferred in all cases except in children from six to 11 months of age.

SOURCE:
Campos-Outcalt, D. "Measles Update." *American Family Physician* 42, no. 5 (November 1990): 1278.

PUBLIC HEALTH SERVICE RECOMMENDATIONS

Concerned about the growing number of measles cases in the United States, the Public Health Service recently recommended that two doses of measles vaccine be given to all children, preferably as combined MMR (measles, mumps, rubella vaccine). Previously, only one dose was recommended routinely.

While the tally is not yet complete for 1989, about 14,000 measles cases were reported to the federal Centers for Disease Control in the first 48 weeks of the year, compared with the previous post-vaccine era high of 6,282 cases for all of 1986.

The new PHS recommendations specify that in most localities, the first dose of vaccine should be given at 15 months of age and the second one at 4 to 6 years, when the child starts school. However, in counties with more than five cases among preschool-aged children during each of the preceding five years, with recent outbreaks among unvaccinated preschool-aged children, or with large inner-city populations, the first dose should be given at 12 months.

Students entering college and medical personnel with direct patient care who are beginning employment should present documentation of having received two doses of measles vaccine no less than a month apart after their first birthday, or other evidence of immunity. If resources are available, PHS suggests that institutions may want to extend this recommendation to all medical personnel. Because some medical workers born before 1957 have acquired measles in medical facilities, institutions may consider also requiring at least one dose of measles vaccine for older employees who may be exposed to the disease during their work.

In outbreaks involving children under 1 year, children as young as 6 months of age can be vaccinated. However, children initially vaccinated before their first birthday should be revaccinated at 15 months. In institutional outbreaks, all students and their siblings and all school personnel born after 1956 who do not have documentation of immunity should be revaccinated.

Persons who received immune globulin at the same time as live "further attenuated" [Swarz or Moraten] vaccine should consider themselves unimmunized. The practice of giving immune globulin with measles vaccine was particularly common in 1967–69 when both the live "attenuated" (weakened) Edmonston B vaccine, recommended to be used with immune globulin, and the newer "further attenuated" vaccines, not requiring immune globulin, were in use. People vaccinated in 1967–69 who know they also received immune globulin but don't know which vaccine they received should consider themselves unimmunized and should receive two vaccinations more than one month apart.

SOURCE:
New Recommendations for Measles Immunizations. *FDA Consumer* 24 (April 1990): 3.

RESOURCES

RELATED ARTICLES

American Academy of Pediatrics Committee on Infectious Diseases. "Measles: Reassessment of the Current Immunization Policy." *Pediatrics* 84, no. 6 (December 1989): 1110–1113.

Brunell, P. A. "Measles One More Time." *Pediatrics* 86, no. 3 (September 1990): 474–478.

Holtan, N. R. "Measles: Forgotten But Not Gone." *Postgraduate Medicine* 88, no. 1 (July 1990): 95–98.

"Measles Revaccination." *Medical Letter on Drugs and Therapeutics* 31, no. 797 (July 28, 1989): 69–70.

Rosenthal, Elisabeth. "Measles Resurges, and with Far Deadlier Effects." *The New York Times* (April 24, 1991): A1.

Snyder, R. C., S. E. Gaskins and others. "Rubeola." *American Family Physician* 37, no. 2 (February 1988): 175–178.

MEDICAL MALPRACTICE

OVERVIEW

The major trend in medicine in the past two decades has been toward the transformation of the physicians' primary goal from treating patients in the best way they know how to the goal of treating patients in a way that minimizes their potential exposure to a medical malpractice suit. This risk-aversive movement is characterized by use of "defensive medicine" (tests and procedures ordered not to help the patient but to protect the physician in the event of a lawsuit), almost constant complaining about the price of liability insurance and the "medical malpractice crisis," and the rise of "risk management" as a health care industry specialty. Many physicians feel that the medical profession has lost control over its own destiny, and that regulators, lawyers, and insurance companies have stripped them of their professional autonomy. Physicians have a point: public policy over the past decade has been driven by the desire to contain and reduce costs rather than the desire to increase access to medical care or to improve its quality. This emphasis has tended to limit physician income and hurt physician morale. There is no magic solution to the "medical malpractice insurance problem."

Medical malpractice denotes the basis for a lawsuit by a patient against a health care provider for injuries suffered as a result of the provider's negiligence. The method for compensating victims of medical malpractice is a fault-and-liability system through which the person at fault is responsible to pay for the harm inflicted on an innocent victim. Whether the health care provider is at fault is determined in an adversary proceeding in which the provider and the patient are each represented by legal counsel. The trier of fact, usually a jury, must decide if the health care provider is responsible for the injury.

Primarily because they are usually decided by lay juries in public, physicians have deplored malpractice lawsuits for almost a century and a half. In 1845, for example, physicians indicated alarm at the increase in malpractice lawsuits and suggested alternatives to jury trials, such as committees made up of physicians, to judge such claims. In 1872, the American Medical Association recommended that physicians be appointed independent arbiters by the court to judge their peers. Physicians have also historically hated the term "malpractice" itself, a term that denotes "evil" or "bad" practice. In fact, it refers simply to a physician who has not lived up to the customary professional standard set by the actions of the "average competent physician" in the same or similar circumstance. Today, more than 80 percent of all malpractice suits are brought on the basis of an incident that occurred in a hospital. About 15 percent involve doctors' offices, and the rest occur in nursing homes, HMOs, surgical centers, and other settings. Our society permits malpractice suits for three basic reasons: 1) to control quality by holding health care providers accountable for their actions, 2) to compensate patients for injury, and 3) to give patients an opportunity to express dissatisfaction with the care they have received.

A valid malpractice claim against a health care provider must have four elements: duty, breach, causation, and damages. Each element must be proven by a "preponderance of the evidence" (that it is more likely than not that it is true). Duty to a patient requires the prior establishment of a provider-patient relationship and is defined by the standard of care. The standard by which a provider's actions are measured is that of a reasonably prudent practitioner under the same or similar circumstances. Breach of that duty by specific conduct on the part of the practitioner, by action or inaction, is measured by the applicable standard of care. Proximate cause denotes a causal connection between provider's conduct and the damages alleged by the patient; that is, the provider's breach of duty must be the cause of the patient's harm. The plaintiff cannot recover any money damages for improper conduct on the part of the defendant if the breach of duty itself produced no harm or injury. The final element is the actual injury or damages suffered by the patient, and these are measured in monetary terms.

SOURCE:
Annas, George J. *The Rights of Patients: The Basic ACLU Guide to Patient Rights.* 2nd ed. Carbondale, IL: Southern Illinois University Press, 1990. pp. 239-241.

CONTINGENCY FEES

Most lawyers handle medical malpractice cases on a contingency fee. Under this fee system, a lawyer is paid only for out-of-pocket expenses unless the suit is won, in which case the lawyer takes about 25 to 50 percent of the award as payment for services. This payment system is often blamed for contributing to the number of malpractice claims. It is argued that contingency fees encourage lawyers to pursue claims of doubtful merit or to require unjustifiably large amounts in terms of potential damages for legitimate claims, in the hope of achieving recovery through settlement or awards from sympathetic juries.

Legislation has been enacted in many states to regulate plaintiff-attorney fees. These have taken various forms. One requires that the court review an attorney's proposed fees and approve what it considers "reasonable fees." Several set a fixed percentage ceiling for contingency fees in malpractice actions. Others adopt a sliding scale, most often expressed in terms of a percentage of the final reward. Under this arrangement, as the amount recovered increases, the lawyer's percentage decreases.

In attempting to establish reasonable guidelines for the amount that a plaintiff's attorney can receive from the injured patient's award, these statutory provisions perform a needed service. But to the extent that they reduce the number of claims brought by diminishing the willingness of attorneys to handle certain meritorious claims, they are a disservice to those injured patients who cannot otherwise afford legal counsel.

The contingency fee structure also compels lawyers to screen out claims that are spurious, or for which recovery appears less than probable, and to refuse claims for which damages would not amount to enough to cover their expenses. Since the attorney, rather than the plaintiff, bears the financial risk of losing the suit, the attorney has no incentive to invest any time or money in a claim for which recovery appears doubtful. In addtion, with the average unregulated fee rate approximately one-third of recovery, many lawyers decline malpractice cases that will probably achieve settlements or awards of less than $25,000, because the expected compenstion for time expended is not seen as worthwhile. The threshold value for acceptance of cases for which recovery is less than probable would, on the average, be higher, perhaps as much as $250,000.

SOURCE:
Annas, George J. *The Rights of Patients: The Basic ACLU Guide to Patient Rights.* 2nd ed. Carbondale, IL: Southern Illinois University Press, 1990. pp. 244-245.

THE NATIONAL PRACTITIONER DATA BANK

The scheduled opening of the National Practitioner Data Bank on September 1 is a major step in strengthening the credentials review process for health care professionals and improving the quality of health care for Americans. The data bank was established by Congress to encourage professional peer review and restrict the ability of incompetent physicians and dentists to move from state to state without discovery of previous substandard performance or unprofessional conduct.

The Health Resources and Services Administration (HRSA), an agency of the US Public Health Service in the Department of Health and Human Services (DHHS), administers the data bank. The bank was developed and is operated under contract with Unisys Corp, an information systems company. Federal officials and representatives of numerous organizations, including the American Medical Association and the Council of Medical Specialty Societies, serve on the executive committee that advises Unisys.

The bank is a nationwide database and alert system used to facilitate and guide a more comprehensive and critical review of professional credentials. The data are intended to supplement other sources of information that are traditionally used to evaluate the credentials of physicians and dentists.

Actions that must be reported to the data bank include the following:

- Anyone who makes a medical malpractice payment on behalf of a licensed health care practitioner must submit a Medical Malpractice Payment Report when payment is made.
- Hospitals and other health care entities are required to file an Adverse Action Report when a professional review action is taken that adversely affects the clinical privileges of a physician or dentist for more than 30 days. The action must be related to professional competence or conduct. Such a report also must be filed when a practitioner voluntarily gives up or restricts clinical privileges while under investigation for professional competence or professional conduct.
- Professional societies must file an Adverse Action Report when an adverse action is taken against the membership of a physician or dentist for reasons related to professional competence or conduct.
- State medical and dental boards are required to file an Adverse Action Report when certain licensure

disciplinary actions are taken against a practitioner for reasons related to professional competence or conduct.

There are stringent penalties for failure to file.

When a hospital or health care entitiy lifts restrictions on privileges or a state professional board reinstates licensure, the actions must be reported to the data bank.

To ensure confidentiality, the information in the data bank is accessible only to authorized parties and is to be used for actions relating to licensure, clinical privileges, and professional society membership.

Hospitals must query the bank every 2 years regarding physicians and other licensed health care practitioners on the medical staff or who hold clinical privileges. Hospitals also must query when considering an applicant for a medical staff appointment or for clinical privileges. Other health care entitities may query when considering extending privileges to physicians or dentists. Licensing boards also may query. In very limited circumstances, a plaintiff's attorney may query the data bank.

SOURCE:
Harmon, Robert G. "The National Practitioners Data Bank." *JAMA* 264 (August 22, 1990): 945.

RESTRICTED ACCESS TO THE NATIONAL PRACTITIONER DATA BANK

October 14, 1989 will be a bittersweet day for medical consumers, a reminder of the medical disclosure that almost came within our grasp—only to be torn away by powerful anti-consumer groups.

On that Saturday a national computer system, mandated by Congress in 1986, begins to track malpractice suits and disciplinary actions taken against all physicians as well as other licensed health care practitioners: dentists, physical therapists, and nurses. The system will store critical records about misdiagnoses, mistreatment, and professional misconduct—just the sort of information the public needs to shop around for fair, honest, and competent medical care.

But now for the bitter pill: Consumers won't have access to one word of those records. All this crucial data has been snatched from us and locked in secret files. It's a slap in the face of consumerism and the consumer groups—PMS [People's Medical Society] and all the others—who have worked long and hard for medical disclosure. . . .

The way the medical system has always operated is that all kinds of doctors, dentists, therapists, and nurses can pile up a long list of black marks on their professional records and then escape their records by relocating. . . .

Enter the "National Practitioner Data Bank," as it's called—the new, much-needed legislation designed to track incompetent practitioners. When a practitioner moves around the U.S., the data bank insures that disciplinary records follow. If the individual has a clean record, no files will be kept for that person.

Key sources will feed data into the National Practitioner Data Bank. Health care providers, as well as insurance companies, must report settlements or payments on malpractice lawsuits. State medical and dental licensing boards must report whenever they revoke, suspend or restrict a practitioner's license or otherwise censure or reprimand the practitioner. Reports will also come from other medical "entities"—such as licensed hospitals, health maintenance organizations, group medical practices, and certain professional societies that follow formal peer review processes. . . .

Right now, the National Practitioner Data Bank is stamped "Top Secret—Consumers Keep Out." The only way to remedy that glaring injustice is to ply members of Congress with the demand for public access to all relevant records on doctor competence.

SOURCE:
"New Physician Tracking System Says 'Consumers Keep Out.'" *People's Medical Society Newsletter* 8, no. 2 (April 1989): 1, 5.

RESOURCES

BOOKS

Edwards, Frank John. *Medical Malpractice: Solving the Crisis.* New York: Holt, 1989.

Inlander, Charles B., and Eugene I. Pavalon. *Your Medical Rights: How to Become an Empowered Consumer.* Boston: Little, Brown and Company, 1990.

RELATED ARTICLES

Jacobson, Peter D. "Medical Malpractice and the Tort System." *JAMA* 262 (December 15, 1989): 3320–3327.

Weinstein, Louis. "Malpractice—The Syndrome of the 80s." *Obstetrics & Gynecology* 72, no. 1 (July 1988): 130–135.

MEDICAL RECORDS

CONTENTS

A physician's office records are required to conform to "accepted medical practice." Accepted practice is to maintain a record that documents the patient's history, physical findings, treatment, and course of disease. Sufficient information should be included in the record to document the diagnosis and course of treatment. If a patient accuses a physician or nurse of malpractice or incompetence, the medical record will usually be the provider's best defense. This is because it was made contemporaneously with the treatment and is generally much more reliable than the memory of either the patient or the provider. It is important for both patient and provider that complete and accurate records be maintained.

Requirements regarding the maintenance and content of health care facility records are usually found in state statutes or regulations that govern licensure. These requirements fall into three groups: 1) those that simply mandate the maintenance of records that are accurate, complete, or adequate; 2) those that set forth broad categories of information that must be included; and 3) those that provide specific requirements for information that must be included. Provisions for the signing and retention of records are often contained in such regulations as well.

Although it is unlikely that a health care facility would actually lose its license for failure to comply with record-keeping requirements, licensing bodies do scrutinize the facility's compliance procedures. Moreover, hospitals can and do impose sanctions such as temporary suspension of the operating or admitting privileges on those physicians who fail to meet their record-keeping requirements.

Additional requirements concerning the contents of hospital records have been promulgated by the JCAH. They include:

1. Identification information
2. Patient's medical history
3. Report of patient's physical examination
4. Diagnostic and therapeutic orders
5. Evidence of appropriate informed consent or indication of the reason for its absence
6. Observations of patient condition, including results of therapy
7. Reports of all procedures and tests, and their results
8. Conclusions at the end of the hospital stay or after evaluation or treatment.

SOURCE:
Annas, George J. *The Rights of Patients: The Basic ACLU Guide to Patient Rights*. 2d ed. Carbondale, IL: Southern Illinois University Press, 1989. pp. 161–162.

RIGHTS

The medical records kept by doctors and hospitals have long been shared—with patients' permission—with health insurance companies and, in some cases, government payers, law enforcement agencies, credit bureaus, schools, and employers. But, ironically, these records have been kept from the patients themselves. Recently, medical organizations and state legislatures have been insisting that medical records be made available to patients, too.

Why would you want to see your records? According to the American Medical Record Association, seeing your records can help you become "a more involved and informed patient, more attentive to your health, and more in control of your own health care. It will establish a more open, equal, and therefore improved physician-patient relationship. It will provide you with continuity of care when you change doctors, and help you protect your privacy by allowing you to inspect and correct information about you that will be released to others."

While it is true that much of the material in your medical records may be couched in incomprehensible technical terms (and written in indecipherable handwriting), other materials, such as laboratory reports on blood tests, are easy to read. And, should you learn of new research on, say, advisable cholesterol levels, you can check your own records to see whether you should bring something to your doctor's attention.

In the past, doctors and other health-care providers have argued that a patient's right of unlimited access to medical records could cause the patient to draw wrong and alarming conclusions on the basis of their new, and incomplete, knowledge—or even attempt to treat themselves. In particular, people with psychiatric problems might be harmed by learning details about their diagnoses.

Those who favor disclosure of medical records argue, however, that access will encourage patients to seek better understanding of their medical profiles, to ask good questions, and be better able, when necessary, to provide informed consent for specific medical procedures. . .

Despite the demand, patients' access to their medical records is restricted in nearly half of the states of the U.S. In some states, patients are allowed access to hospital records, but not to those of their physicians—although a recent poll of physicians in one area of the country where laws do not require them to open their records showed that almost 75% of them would be pleased to turn over records if their patients asked for them.

If you have trouble obtaining prompt and complete access to your medical records, there are several things you can do. The first, and usually easiest, course is to ask another doctor who is willing to share the information with you to request your records. Most states have laws that oblige hospitals and doctors to turn records over to a succeeding physician. Moreover, the rules of professional conduct of the American Medical Association oblige a physician to transfer records when a patient requests it.

If, for some reason, this fails, you may want to contact patients' rights groups in your area. If you don't know of such a group, contact a Public Interest Research Group or Citizen Action Group in your state for a referral. Or you may ask your lawyer to make the request in your name, since some states mandate access to records if they are requested by a lawyer. If a polite request does not suffice, some legal clout usually will.

If you still have trouble, write or call the American Medical Record Association.

SOURCE:
"Your Right to Have Your Medical Records." *The Johns Hopkins Medical Letter* 2, no. 8 (October 1990): 3.

CONFIDENTIALITY

Patient files, formerly a symbol of security as inviolate as the confessional, are beginning to look more like a lending library for a mixed bag of browsers. Employers, insurers, and utilization reviewers are all gaining wider access to medical records—and to more detailed information within those documents. Using computer banks, telephone inquiries, and "blanket" release forms, they are making a mockery of the very concept of patient confidentiality, say critics of the trend.

"It's almost as if nothing is truly confidential," said Dr. Russell H. Patterson of New York, who chairs the AMA's Ethical and Judicial Affairs Committee.

But aside from cries of alarm and some legal action, not much has been done to challenge the record rummagers or install greater safeguards. In fact, the patient's best protection against unwarranted release of medical records may be the physician who wrote those records.

"There's virtually no confidentiality left anymore," University of Houston law professor Mark Rothstein said of the situation. He's been tracking the spread of "blanket" release forms, which may appear harmlessly routine but carry fine print authorizing broad access to all kinds of information, regardless of its relevance to a patient's fitness for work or to an insurance claim or application.

For instance, the forms can use language permitting the release of "any knowledge" of the person who signs the form. Some specifically cover "any nonmedical information."

"There should be no such thing as blanket consent," said Joan Banach, communications director of the Chicago-based American Medical Record Association. "Every request for medical information should be specific, limited in terms of time, clear about the purpose of the release of information, and have very specific identification of who should have it and how much of it."

Yet blanket releases are now "very widespread, practically (the only type) I see," said Banach, and some insurance companies deny coverage if applicants won't sign them. "That's a real pressure threat. I brought the issue to the Health Insurance Association of America a year ago and after several months they responded that they don't dictate policy to members."

SOURCE:

Cotton, Paul. "Confidentiality: A Sacred Trust Under Siege." *Medical World News* 30 (March 27, 1989): 54, 55.

RESOURCES

BOOKS

Annas, George G. *The Right of Patients: The Basic ACLU Guide to Patient Rights.* Carbondale, IL: Southern Illinois University Press, 1989.

Greenberg, Allen. *Medical Records: Getting Yours.* Washington DC: Public Citizen Health Research Group, 1986.

RELATED ARTICLES

Burnum, J. F. "The Misinformation Era: The Fall of the Medical Record." *Annals of Internal Medicine* 110, no. 6 (March 15, 1989): 482–484.

Halpern, Sue. "Your Medical Records: They're Not As Private As You Think." *Glamour* (September 1990): 104, 109–110.

Klop, Renata, Frans C. B. van Wijmen, and Hans Philyosen. "Patients' Rights and the Admission and Discharge Process." *Journal of Advanced Nursing* 16 (1991): 408–412.

"Your Medical Record May Be Fundamentally Flawed: Fact or Fiction." *People's Medical Society Newsletter* 8, no. 4 (August 1989): 1, 4–5.

MEDICARE

(*See also:* HEALTH INSURANCE; HEALTH MAINTENANCE ORGANIZATIONS [HMOs])

OVERVIEW

The Medicare program is a Federal health insurance program for people 65 or older and certain disabled people. It is run by the Health Care Financing Administration of the U.S. Department of Health and Human Services. Social Security Administration offices across the country take applications for Medicare and provide general information about the program.

There are two parts to the Medicare program. Hospital Insurance (Part A) helps pay for inpatient hospital care, some inpatient care in a skilled nursing facility, home health care and hospice care. Medical Insurance (Part B) helps pay for doctors' services, outpatient hospital services, durable medical equipment, and a number of other medical services and supplies that are not covered by the hospital insurance part of Medicare.

Part B of Medicare has premiums, deductibles, and coinsurance amounts that you must pay yourself or through coverage by another insurance plan. Part A has deductibles and coinsurance, but most people do not have to pay premiums for Part A. The amounts you pay are set each year, according to formulas established by law. New payment amounts begin each January 1. When amounts increase, you will be notified. . . .

Generally, people age 65 and over can get premium-free Medicare hospital insurance (Part A) benefits, based on their own or their spouses' employment. You can get Medicare Part A if you are 65 or over and:

- receive benefits under the Social Security or Railroad Retirement system,
- could receive benefits under Social Security or Railroad Retirement system but did not file for them, or
- you or your spouse had certain government employment.

If you are under 65 you can get premium-free Medicare hospital insurance (Part A) benefits if you:

- have been a Social Security or Railroad Retirement Board disability beneficiary for more than 24 months.

Certain government employees and certain members of their families can also get Medicare when they are disabled for more than 29 months. They should apply with the Social Security Administration as soon as they become disabled.

Or, you may be able to get premium-free Medicare hospital insurance (Part A) benefits if you receive continuing dialysis for permanent kidney failure or had a kidney transplant.

No one needs to have worked more than 10 years to be able to get premium-free Medicare hospital insurance benefits. Check with Social Security to see if you have worked long enough under Social Security, Railroad Retirement, as a government employee, or a combination of these systems to be able to get Medicare hospital insurance benefits.

Any person who can get premium-free Medicare hospital insurance benefits as described above can enroll for Part B, pay the monthly Part B premiums, and get Part B benefits.

If you do not have enough work credits to be able to get Medicare hospital insurance benefits and you are 65 or over, you may be able to buy Medicare hospital and medical insurance- by paying monthly premiums. Check with Social Security or Railroad Retirement to find out about buying into Medicare.

SOURCE:

The Medicare Handbook. 1990. Published by the U.S. Department of Health and Human Services. Health Care Financing Administration. Pub. No. HCFA 10050. 1990. p. 1.

MEDICARE COORDINATED CARE PLANS

What Are Coordinated Plans?

More and more Medicare beneficiaries are joining coordinated care plans. These coordinated care plans are prepaid, managed care plans, most of which are health maintenance organizations (HMOs) or Competitive Medical Plans (CMP). Both HMOs and CMPs contract with Medicare and follow the same contracting rules. In this [section], HMOs will be used to illustrate the benefits for both.

Many beneficiaries find that coordinated care plans are a good way to get more health care for their dollar. HMOs provide or arrange for all Medicare covered services, and generally charge you fixed monthly premiums and only small copayments. This means that if you join a coordinated care plan and get all of your services through the HMO, your out-of-pocket costs are usually more predictable. Also, depending on your health needs, those costs may be less than you would pay if you were liable for the regular Medicare deductible and coinsurance amounts.

Coordinated care plans may also offer benefits not covered by Medicare for little or no additional cost. Benefits may include preventive care, dental care, hearing aids and eyeglasses.

Who Can Enroll in Coordinated Care Plans?

Most Medicare beneficiaries are eligible to enroll in HMOs. HMOs cannot screen their applicants to find whether they are healthy, or delay coverage for preexisting condition. The only enrollment criteria for Medicare HMOs are:

- You must be enrolled in Medicare Part B and continue to pay the Part B premiums (you do not need to be able to get Part A, but the HMO has the right to charge you for Part A services you get from the plan. The plan can charge you a monthly premium for Part A coverage, or actual charges for the Part A services you get);
- You must live in the plan's service area;
- You cannot be receiving care in a Medicare-certified hospice; and
- You cannot have chronic kidney disease.

If you develop chronic kidney disease or choose hospice coverage after joining a coordinated care plan, the plan will provide or arrange for your care.

Joining a Coordinated Care Plan

To join a coordinated care plan, contact plans in your area that have a contract with Medicare. All HMOs have an advertised open enrollment period at least once a year. Once you join, you may stay with the plan as long as you wish. And you may return to regular Medicare at any time.

If you enroll in a coordinated care plan you will usually be required to get all care from the plan. In most cases, if you get services that are not authorized by the HMO (unless they are emergency services, or services you urgently need when you are out of the plan's service area) *neither the plan nor Medicare will pay for the services.*

When you join an HMO, be sure to read your membership materials carefully to learn your rights and coverage.

Ending Enrollment in a Coordinated Care Plan

To end your enrollment in a coordinated care plan, send a signed request to your plan or to your local Social Security or Railroad Retirement Board Office. You return to regular Medicare the first day of the following month.

SOURCE:
Health Care Financing Administration. *The Medicare Handbook. 1992.* Pub. No. HCFA 10050. 1992. p. 9.

MEDICARE SUPPLEMENT INSURANCE

Medicare supplement (Medigap) insurance policies generally pay for a high proportion of services and expenses that are not completely covered by Medicare. These expenses can include Medicare deductibles or co-payments, and other health services not covered by Medicare at all. It is important to compare closely various policies that provide Medicare supplemental coverage. All states have minimum standards for Medicare supplement policies and some publish comparisons of policies offered in the state to help you make a sound decision. Contact your State or local Area Agency on Aging or State Insurance Office for this information. Their phone numbers and addresses can be found in the telephone directory.

Medicare supplement- or Medigap-insurance is available through commercial insurance companies and through Blue Cross and Blue Shield plans. Health maintenance organizations (HMOs) also offer benefits that supplement Medicare. You may purchase a Medigap policy on an individual basis or through group plans, such as those available from a religious, aging or fraternal organization.

Medicare supplement policies can differ as to coverage and cost. Examine any policies you are offered carefully to be sure that the features most important to you are included.

Also, make sure you are not overinsured. If you buy more than one policy, you may be paying premiums for policies that duplicate or overlap coverage.

If you are considering replacing your existing policy with a new one, you should be aware that there will be a break in your coverage if you cancel your old policy, since most policies carry a "pre-existing condition" clause. For Medicare supplement policies, this means there may be no reimbursement during the first six months of the new policy for expenses connected with a medical condition existing at the time of enrollment. For other policies, the "pre-existing condition" clause depends on the policy itself and may last anywhere from six months to two years. Before you purchase any policy, be sure you are familiar with the conditions of enrollment and the date on which coverage will begin.

Don't be misled by the phrase "no medical examination required." If you have had health problems, the insurer might not cover expenses connected with that problem.

SOURCE:
American Council of Life Insurance, Health Insurance Association of America. *Health Care and Finances: A Guide for Adult Children and Their Parents*. December 1987. p. 7.

HOW TO PURCHASE MEDIGAP INSURANCE

Medicare covers "reasonable" costs for "necessary" service. That approach is helpful, but can leave you with significant expenses. In response, many newer insurance policies help bridge the gap between Medicare coverage and the amount of your medical bill.

Filling the gap

When looking for supplemental insurance, keep these points in mind:

- *Shop carefully*—Yearly premiums vary widely in price, so choose a policy that reflects your individual needs.

If you travel frequently outside the United Stares, consider a supplemental policy with international coverage. But don't pay a premium for minor benefits like discount coupons for over-the-counter medications.

Ask a respected financial advisor for an impartial opinion as you review a policy's costs and benefits. Compare several policies before making a decision.

- *Know your seller*—Don't believe claims that a Medicare supplement is a government-sponsored program. Federal and state governments don't sell or service supplemental insurance policies. Ask for proof that a company is licensed by your state to sell such insurance.

Don't be pressure into making a decision. And if you want a policy, don't pay in cash. Write a check, money order or bank draft payable to the insurance company, not to the agent or any other individual.

Claim service is important. How easy is it to file a claim? How quickly—and accurately—are claims processed?

- *Avoid duplication*—A single comprehensive policy is less expensive and easier to work with than several overlapping policies. If you want to switch policies, remember that the new plan may impose a waiting period (usually 30 days) before coverage begins.
- *Check for 'pre-existing' exclusions*—Don't be misled by the advertising phrase, "No medical exam required." Many policies wait six months until covering conditions for which you received prior medical advice or treatment.
- *Know your maximum benefits*—Most policies limit payment for a condition or the number of days of care you receive. Some policies pay less than Medicare—or nothing at all—for treatment in a doctor's office or hospital outpatient service.
- *Check your right to renew*—Policies with automatic or guaranteed renewal offer extra protection. Your premiums may go up, but the company can't cancel your policy. Beware of companies that renew your coverage on an individual basis. Most policies cannot be canceled because of claims you make or disputes you might have with the company.
- *Look beyond the limits*—Remember that supplements fill only the gaps in Medicare's coverage. You'll still pay for charges beyond the Medicare allotment.
- *Complete the application carefully*—Some companies ask for detailed medical information. Provide it. Otherwise, the firm could deny coverage for any unlisted conditions or cancel your policy.

SOURCE:
"Medicare Supplemental Insurance." *Mayo Clinic Health Letter* (February 1991): 4-5.

DRGs—PROSPECTIVE PAYMENT TO HOSPITALS

The DRG [Diagnosis-Related Groups] system is Medicare's current method of prospective payment. It was developed originally by the Yale School of Organization and Management and became law for hospitals in the state of New Jersey before Congress made it nationwide for Medicare. Using sophisticated statistical techniques, Medicare cases were analyzed to see how payments should be set to cover as many cases as possible. This research showed that the main or primary diagnosis of the patient, secondary diagnoses, age, and operations performed predicted costs for the majority of patients quite well. The billions of possible combinations of these factors were reduced to 467 diagnosis-related groups (DRGs), which are best understood as the overall condition of a patient. Congress understood that these 467 groups would not cover every case, and they made provisions for outliers—people who needed more days in the hospital, or more expensive hospital stays, because they had illnesses, or needed operations, that fell outside the DRGs. Hospitals can be granted payment for cases that require more hospital days than predicted by the DRG, provided the continued stay is medically necessary. Cases that do not exceed the length of stay criteria, but are more costly than predicted by a certain amount, are paid more if the hospital applies for additional payment.

The DRG system was phased in over several years, and as of October 1, 1987, virtually every general, acute-care hospital in the country was paid with DRGs. The way it works is as follows: You are admitted to the hospital as a

Medicare patient. Your DRG cannot be assigned when you come in, because your diagnosis may be unknown or wrong. Also, the operation(s) that you will have cannot be predicted in advance, especially if you are admitted for a diagnostic workup. Once everything has been done, and you are ready to be discharged (dead or alive), the hospital prepares a fact sheet for your hospital chart which indicates your DRG. The DRG will probably have been assigned by a computer program that was purchased by the hospital and designed to pick the highest-paid DRG possible, based on your combination of age, diagnoses, operations, and other factors. The Medicare intermediary pays the hospital the DRG rate, after a computer review of the hospital's DRG coding.

Note that the hospital couldn't assign the DRG when you came in, and therefore could not predict the cost of your care or how much it would be paid. The result is that on some admissions the hospital will lose money and on some admissions it will make money. On the average, hospitals that are generally as "good"—measured by their use of resources on patients, not by the results they produce—as the average hospital will break even. Those that are better, in this sense, will make money, and they are allowed to keep their profits. Those that are worse will lose money, and they will have to swallow their losses.

The important point is this: there is no guarantee from Medicare that the hospital will not lose money, or make money, on your case. Its loss or gain, under the DRG system, is supposed to have nothing to do with your care.

SOURCE:
Inlander, Charles B., and Charles K. MacKay. "The Diagnosis-Related Groups (DRG) System." In *Medicare Made Easy*. Reading, Mass.: Addison-Wesley, 1989. pp. 100–101.

HOW TO APPEAL MEDICARE DECISIONS

If you disagree with a decision on the amount Medicare will pay on a claim or whether services you received are covered by Medicare, you have the right to appeal the decision. The notice you receive from Medicare tells you the decision made on the claim and also tells you exactly what appeal steps you can take. If you ever need more information about your right to appeal and how to request it, call Social Security, or the Medicare intermediary or carrier in your state. If you need more information about your right to appeal a Peer Review Organization (PRO) decision, you can call the PRO in your state. (The number of the Medicare intermediary or carrier is listed on the notice explaining Medicare's decision on the claim.)

Appealing Decisions Made by Providers of Part B Services

In many cases the first written notice of noncoverage you receive will come from the provider of the services (for example, a hospital, skilled nursing facility, home health agency or hospice). This notice of noncoverage from the provider should explain why the provider believes Medicare will not pay for the services. This notice is not an official Medicare determination, but you can ask the provider to get an official Medicare determination. If you ask for an official Medicare determination, the provider must file a claim on your behalf to Medicare. Then you will receive a Notice of Utilization, which is the official Medicare determination. If you still disagree, you can appeal by following the instructions on the Notice of Utilization.

Appealing Decisions Made by Peer Review Organizations (PROs)

When you are admitted to a Medicare participating hospital, you will be given a notice called *An Important Message From Medicare.* The notice contains a brief description of PROs, and the name, address, and phone number of the PRO in your state. Also, it describes your appeal rights.

PROs make determinations mainly about inpatient hospital care and ambulatory surgical center care. The PROs decide whether care provided to Medicare patients is medically necessary, provided in the most appropriate setting, and is of good quality. When you disagree with a PRO decision about your case, you can appeal by requesting a reconsideration. Then, if you disagree with the PRO's reconsideration decision, and the amount remaining in question is $200 or more, you can request a hearing by an Administrative Law Judge. Cases involving $2,000 or more can eventually be appealed to a Federal Court.

If you belong to a Medicare health maintenance organization (HMO), the HMO will usually make decisions about the medical necessity, the appropriateness of setting and the quality of your care. Although you do not have the right to appeal to the PRO, you do have the right to register complaints about the quality of your hospital care to the PRO.

NOTE: In the case of elective (non-emergency) surgery, either the hospital or the PRO may be involved in preadmission decisions. If the hospital believes that your proposed stay will not be covered by Medicare, it may recommend, without consulting the PRO, that you not be admitted to the hospital. If this is the case, the hospital must give you its decision in writing. If you or your physician disagree with the hospital's decision, you should make a request to the PRO for immediate review. If you want an immediate review, you must make your request, by telephone or in writing, within three calendar days after receipt of the notice.

Appealing Decisions of Intermediaries on Part A Claims

Appeals of decisions on most other services covered under Medicare Part A (skilled nursing facility care, home health care, hospice services, and a few inpatient hospital matters not handled by PROs) are handled by

Medicare intermediaries. If you disagree with the intermediary's initial decision, you have 60 days from the date you receive the initial decision to request a reconsideration. The request can be submitted directly to the intermediary or through Social Security. If you disagree with the intermediary's reconsideration decision and the amount remaining in question is $100 or more, you have 60 days from the date you receive the reconsideration decision to request a hearing by an Administrative Law Judge. Cases involving $1,000 or more can eventually be appealed to a Federal Court.

Appealing Decisions Made by Carriers on Part B Claims

Your doctor must provide you with a written notice if he or she knows or believes that Medicare will not consider a particular service reasonable and necessary and will not pay for it. This written notice must be given to you before the service is performed and must clearly state the reasons your doctor believes Medicare will not pay. If your doctor does not give you this written notice and you did not know that Medicare would not pay for the services you received, you cannot be held liable to pay for them. However, if you did receive written notice and signed an agreement to pay for the services yourself so you could be treated, you will be held liable to pay.

This written notice is not an official Medicare determination. If you disagree with it, you may ask your doctor to submit a claim for payment to the Medicare carrier to get an official Medicare determination. . . . If you receive an adverse decision from Medicare and you still disagree, you have the right to appeal that decision. You have six months from the date of the decision to ask the carrier to review it. Then, if you disagree with the carrier's written explanation of its review decision and the amount remaining in question is $100 or more, you have six months from the date of the review decision to request a hearing before a carrier hearing officer. You may combine claims that have been reviewed or reopened within the past six months, to meet the $100 requirement.

If you disagree with the carrier hearing officer's decision and the amount remaining in question is $500 or more, you have 60 days from the date you receive the decision to request a hearing before an Administrative Law Judge. You may combine claims that have had a hearing decision within the past sixty days to meet the $500 requirement. Cases involving $1,000 or more can eventually be appealed to a Federal Court.

Appealing Decisions Made by Health Maintenance Organizations (HMOs)

If you have Medicare coverage through an HMO, decisions about coverage and payment for services will usually be made by your HMO. When your HMO makes a decision to deny payment for Medicare covered services or refuses to provide Medicare covered supplies you request, you will be given a *notice of initial determination.* Along with the notice, your HMO is required to provide a full, written explanation of your appeal rights.

If you believe that the decision your HMO made was not correct, you have the right to ask for a reconsideration. You must file your request for reconsideration within 60 days of the *notice of initial determination.* Your request must be in writing. You may mail it or deliver it personally to your HMO or to a Social Security Office (or the Railroad Retirement Board if you get Medicare through Railroad Retirement).

Your HMO is responsible for reconsidering their initial determination to deny payment or services. If your HMO does not rule fully in your favor, the HMO must send your reconsideration request to the Health Care Financing Administration (HCFA) for a review and determination.

If you disagree with HCFA's decision, and the amount in question is $100 or more, you have 60 days from receipt of HCFA's decision to request a hearing before an Administrative Law Judge. Cases involving $1,000 or more can eventually be appealed to a Federal Court.

SOURCE:

Health Care Financing Administration. *The Medicare Handbook. 1992.* Pub. No. HCFA 10050. 1992. pp. 37-38.

RESOURCES

ORGANIZATIONS

AARP. 1909 K Street NW, Washington, DC 20049.

Health Care Financing Administration. 6325 Security Blvd., Baltimore, MD 21207.

Social Security Administration. 6401 Security Blvd., Baltimore, MD 21235.

BOOKS

National Association of Insurance Commissioners, and the Health Care Financing Administration. *1991 Guide to Health Insurance for People with Medicare.* Pub. No. HCFA-02110.

Oshiro, Carl, Harry Snyder. *Medicare/Medigap: The Essential Guide for Older Americans and Their Families.* Fairfield, OH: Consumer Reports Books, 1990.

RELATED ARTICLES

Pearson, Linley E. "Medigap Sellers Mislead Many Elderly." *The Journal of State Government* 111-113.

Radovsky, Saul S. "U.S. Medical Practice Before Medicare and Now—Differences and Consequences." *The New England Journal of Medicine.* 322, no. 4 (January 25, 1990): 263-267.

Rossiter, Louis F., Kathryn Langwell, and others. "Patient Satisfaction Among Elderly Enrollees and Disenrollees in Medicare Health Maintenance Organizations: Results from the National Medicare Competition Evaluation." *JAMA* 262, no. 1 (July 7, 1989): 57-63.

MENOPAUSE

(*See also:* ESTROGEN REPLACEMENT THERAPY; MENSTRUATION; OSTEOPOROSIS)

OVERVIEW

Generations past called it "change of life." Today we're more apt to call it what it is: menopause. Yet our understanding of this change in a woman's childbearing status may still be clouded by myth and mystification.

Natural menopause is the end of menstruation and childbearing capability that occurs in most women somewhere around age 50. Today women can expect to live about a third of their lives after menopause.

Technically, the term "menopause" refers to the actual cessation of menstrual periods. When a woman has not had a period for a year, then the date of her last menstrual period is retrospectively considered the date of her menopause. However, the term "menopause" has come to be used in general sense in place of the more proper terms, "climacteric" or "peri-menopause," which encompass the years immediately preceding and following the last menstrual period.

To cut through some of the myth and mystery surrounding the hormonal changes that accompany menopause, it is necessary first to understand what happens in the cycle of a normally menstruating woman.

The menstrual cycle, averaging 28 days, is divided into two phases. The first is called the follicular, or pre-ovulatory, phase and lasts to 10 to 17 days. The second is the luteal, or post ovulatory, phase lasting 13 to 15 days. . . .

Usually sometime in a woman's early to mid 40s—two to eight years before actual menopause—her menstrual cycle begins changing. Notably, levels of hormones such as estrogen, produced by the ovaries, decrease; ovulation (release of eggs from the ovaries) stops or becomes more infrequent; and the pattern of the menstrual cycle changes.

Initially this may mean heavier and/or more frequent periods. Later, periods may be scantier and less frequent. Lack of ovulation may cause some light bleeding or spotting between periods. However, not all women follow this pattern exactly. Some may experience simply a wide variability in the time and quantity of flow, and a few may have little or no change in menstrual cycle. For some women, the unpredictability of menstrual pattern changes is unsettling because social activities can no longer be planned around a specific cycle, and there is no period due date to help determine pregnancy status. And indeed, because most women continue to ovulate at least in some cycles, pregnancy is possible until a woman has actually passed menopause. In fact, in some cultures where women bear many children, it is not uncommon for a woman to give birth to her last child and never menstruate again.

In the vast majority of cases, menstrual irregularities in the years before menopause are simply manifestations of the normal transition in the woman's hormonal status. Sometimes, if these irregularities cause too many problems or if a woman's doctor suspects that the uterine lining is not being shed completely during menstruation as happens during a normal period, the doctor may suggest treatment with a synthetic progesterone, called a progestin, to make the cycle more regular. In cases of extremely heavy bleeding, the doctor may recommend surgery.

The age at which a woman has her last period is not known to be related to race, body size, or her age when she began to menstruate.

The average age for menopause in American women is 50 to 52. But it is not abnormal for it to occur several years earlier or later. Some studies show that women who have had many children reach menopause earlier.

And smokers may experience menopause an average of one to two years earlier than nonsmokers.

Even after menopause, women's bodies continue to produce estrogen, but far less of the hormone is made in the ovaries. Most postmenopausal estrogen is produced in a process in which the adrenal gland makes precursors of estrogen, which are then converted by stored fat to estrogen. However, far less estrogen is produced in this manner than is produced in the ovaries before menopause.

The most common symptom of menopause, the hot flush or flash, may begin before a woman has stopped menstruating and may continue for a couple of years after menopause. Although it is known that the hot flash (or "vasomotor flush," as doctors sometimes call it) is related to decreased estrogen levels, exactly how this occurs is not completely understood.

Many women describe the hot flash as an intense feeling of heat. Some say it actually feels like the temperature in the room has risen. Most commonly the sensation starts in the face, neck or chest and may extend to other parts of the body. It is usually accompanied by perspiration and may last a few seconds to several minutes. Increased heart rate and finger temperature have been documented during hot flashes.

About half of the women who have hot flashes visibly blush or have a patchy reddish flush of the face, neck and chest. For some women, the feeling of heat is followed by a feeling of being chilled. The hot flash may be particularly disturbing when it occurs during sleep.

This problem, often involving profuse sweating, can awaken the women and is credited for much of the insomnia sometimes associated with menopause.

Up to 75 percent to 85 percent of women have hot flashes, but less than half of all women experiencing a natural menopause have symptoms severe enough to warrant medication. Obese women tend to have a lower incidence of hot flashes, possibly because they have higher levels of estrogen, converted from stored fat.

Many women find they can cope with hot flashes by dressing in layers that can be removed, wearing natural fabrics, drinking cold rather than hot beverages, keeping rooms cooler, and sleeping with fewer blankets.

For women who cannot get sufficient relief without drugs, hormone replacement therapy may be prescribed. The length of time that a woman is advised to continue taking hormones may vary from several months to several years, depending on her symptoms.

SOURCE:
Willis, Judith. "Demystifying Menopause." *FDA Consumer* 22 (July-August 1988): 24–27.

DIAGNOSIS

You may want to know how your doctor diagnoses your entry into the climacteric. It is difficult to confirm, if you have not yet become menopausal. There are some telltale symptoms, however, such as the changes in your menstrual pattern and the onset of hot flashes, which offer diagnostic clues.

We suspect menopause when there is a long interval without periods in a woman over the age of fifty, particularly if she has hot flashes or a low estrogen profile. The low estrogen profile can be discovered during a physical examination by means of an atrophic vaginal smear, the absence of vaginal mucus, or an atrophic endometrium, diagnosed by a biopsy.

In younger women, if the menses have been absent for one year, there may be a strong reason to diagnose menopause. FSH [Follicle-Stimulating Hormone] levels in the blood can be measured, and if they are elevated, then you are beyond menopause. Ideally, you should not wait this long without a period before seeking medical advice.

Diagnostic difficulties can come from several sources. When a woman in her thirties or forties loses her period, she is often referred to a gynecologic endocrine unit to search for reasons other than premature menopause. Another diagnostic challenge arises when an older woman on oral contraceptives asks if she can stop taking the pill without fear of pregnancy. Answering this question requires that she stop the pill and then have her FSH level monitored before she can be assured that ovulation has, indeed, stopped. After hysterectomy, hot flashes are the most frequent signal of menopause, but the diagnosis of menopause is conclusively determined by measurement of the FSH levels in the blood.

Once menopause is confirmed, and if hormones are prescribed, you must see your gynecologist at least once every six months. This schedule is important to assess your general health and to determine your response to HRT [Hormone Replacement Therapy], if you are taking it. It is up to you to assure your continued good health and fitness by following the treatment program that you and your gynecologist devise. If you are under any other physician's treatment, you should visit that physician twice a year, in addition to your gynecologist. Be sure that each doctor knows what the other is prescribing or recommending for you, so that they both can work together to bring you maximum benefits.

SOURCE:
Utian, Wulf H., and Ruth S. Jacobowitz. *Managing Your Menopause.* New York: Prentice Hall, 1990. pp. 81–82.

VAGINAL SYMPTOMS

Like other menopausal effects, vaginal changes are individual: sudden and severe in some women and so gradual they practically go unnoticed in others. When estrogen is withdrawn, vaginal walls may become thinner and lose moisture, making them more vulnerable to irritation. Some women report itching and burning; intercourse may cause bleeding and pain. Menopausal hormone changes also disrupt the delicate pH of the vagina, creating a hospitable environment for yeast and bacterial infections. At the same time, the muscles supporting the vagina, uterus and bladder may become lax.

But don't get discouraged. While vaginal changes may be inevitable to a certain extent, they don't have to become troublesome if you follow these suggestions:

Choose personal hygiene products with care. Use mild (nondeodorant and fragrance-free) soap or cleansing bars. Avoid personal hygiene sprays, which can irritate dry, sensitive vaginal tissues.

Dry thoroughly after shower or bath. If your perineal area remains damp, bacteria could multiply and invade vulnerable vaginal tissues. To be safe, use a blow-dryer on a cool (not hot) setting to remove excess moisture between your legs. Also, always wear cotton-crotch pantyhose and underwear. Cotton "breathes" better than nylon, allowing moisture to evaporate.

Think twice about using antihistamines. Antihistamines don't discriminate; they dry mucous membranes in the nose and in the vagina. If you need to treat an allergy or nagging cold, ask your pharmacist or your doctor to suggest an alternative medication.

Strengthen pelvic muscles. Specially designed Kegel exercises zero in on crucial muscles: Use the same motion you would to stop a stream of urine to contract the pelvic muscle. Do 10 contractions a day: five fast, plus five held for three to five seconds. Build up to a total of 50 or 100 contractions a day.

Keep sex alive. Regular sexual activity helps keep natural moisture flowing and maintains pelvic muscle tone. Gloria A. Bachmann, M.D., gynecology professor at Robert Wood Johnson Medical School in New Brunswick, New Jersey, recommends that women indulge in a relaxing, warm (not hot) bath before sex to relieve tension arising from meddlesome menopausal symptoms. And don't forget birth control. No matter how erratic your menstrual cycles, you're not pregnancy-safe until you've put an entire year between you and your last period.

Replace lost lubrication. If dryness becomes a problem, you may want to try a brand-new nonprescription lubricant, called Replens. It comes in single-dose, tamponlike dispensers, used every three days to provide continuous lubrication. Dr. Bachmann and a colleague tested Replens on 89 menopausal women who said the product stayed in place better than a standard water-soluble lubricant applied with a dispenser. Another advantage: The lubricant helps normalize vaginal acidity, thus reducing the risk of infections. One note of caution: If you have a history of allergic reactions to medications, use this product only under a doctor's care.

Consider hormone replacement therapy. Experts say that even the most severe vaginal symptoms can be reversed with estrogen in doses lower than are needed to resolve hot flashes. Sometimes, too, estrogen cream applied directly to the vagina can alleviate the itching and dryness with fewer potential side effects than oral estrogen. Discuss hormone options with your doctor.

SOURCE:

McVeigh, Gloria. "Mastering Menopause: A Plan of Action for Every Symptom and Side Effect." *Prevention* 42 (April 1990): 51–52.

SEXUAL DYSFUNCTION

The capacity for orgasm with coitus also decreases in the postmenopausal years. As Hallstrom reported, in the 38-year-old age group, 12% said they didn't experience orgasm with coitus; in the 50-year-old age group, 16% reported this; and in the 54-year-old age group, 24% reported no orgasm with coitus.

Other changes in the sexual response cycle postmenopausal women experience include:

- decreased incidence of skin flushing,
- decline in muscle tension,
- lack of increase in breast size during sexual stimulation,
- slowing or absence of Bartholin's gland secretions,
- delayed or absent vaginal lubrication,
- decreased vaginal expansion and lengthening,
- shorter transcervical width,
- decreased congestion in the outer third of the vagina, and
- fewer and occasionally painful uterine contractions with orgasm.

Perhaps not surprisingly, overall sexual responsiveness is often dulled in the postmenopausal woman. . . .

The physician can frequently offer information on how to alter unsatisfactory sexual practices. Some examples include:

- Oil-based lubricants may be necessary if water-based ones do not provide sufficient lubrication in women with severe atrophic vaginitis.
- Performance may be enhanced by engaging in sexual activity in the morning rather than in the evening. Identifying what time of day the couple feels at their peak may be beneficial for those who suffer from arthritis or back pain.
- A hot bath before intercourse may enhance physical enjoyment of sexual exchange.
- The use of erotic literature or films can help the older couple become sexually stimulated, if the partners seem inclined to consider such advice.

It is of extreme importance that physicians only give information to their patients that they feel comfortable discussing. If a situation occurs that the physician is not at ease discussing, consideration of patient referral to another health care provider who deals with that medical area should be given.

SOURCE:
Bachmann, Gloria A. "Patterns of Sexual Activity in Postmenopausal Women." *Geriatrics* 43, no. 11 (November 1988): 80–81, 83.

MENTAL HEALTH

Most women have a healthy outlook throughout the menopause process and afterward feel "in their prime," glad to no longer be menstruating.

Mood changes may occur during menopause. Other symptoms commonly reported are fatigue, nervousness, excess sweating, breathlessness, headaches, sleeplessness, joint pain, depression, irritability, and impatience. These symptoms may be due in part to shifting hormonal balances or other factors such as heredity, general health, nutrition, medications, exercise, life events, and attitude. More research is needed on the role hormones play and how they interact with these other factors.

There is no specific mental disorder associated with menopause, and research shows that women experience no more depression during these years than at other times during life. Tension or depression can occur at any stage, but when these states occur during menopause, there is a tendency to blame the menopause process. Thus women with emotional problems are on occasion tagged "menopausal," sometimes long after menopause has taken place.

Important life changes often coincide with the menopause years: perhaps grown children are leaving home, aged parents need more attention and assistance, or a woman's life is taking on new directions. This is a time when many women think about growing older and the changes it will bring.

Developing positive attitudes toward menopause and aging is an important part of adjusting to life changes. As long as menopause is regarded as simply a normal life change and a woman goes on to participate in satisfying activities, coping with the transitions and body changes becomes easier. But viewing menopause as the end of a useful life only makes the transition difficult—so that if a crisis develops, such as a divorce or the need to care for parents who are ill, menopause is likely to seem an added burden.

Supportive friends and satisfying activities help ease any transition or crisis. Emotional support can come from a variety of sources: a friend, your husband, or relatives. Various types of support groups exist which can provide opportunities for you to talk with other people who are going through similar experiences. When coping is difficult, it may be useful to consult a gynecologist or seek the services of a social worker, psychologist, psychiatrist, or other mental health professional.

SOURCE:
National Institute on Aging. *The Menopause Time of Life*. NIH Pub. No. 86-2461. July 1986. pp. 13–15.

PREGNANCY AFTER MENOPAUSE

Time was, when a woman went through "the change" she lost her ability to conceive naturally. That is still a fact. But a recent study in which a group of postmenopausal women bore babies has generated a lot of interest. Doctors at the University of Southern California (USC) in Los Angeles used a variation of in vitro fertilization to implant donor eggs in five women age 40 to 44 who had experienced early menopause. All delivered healthy babies.

While news of the procedure has prompted more than 1,000 women in their 40s and 50s to contact the researcher, it isn't for everyone. Nor is it likely to rewrite the chapter on the birds and the bees. It will, however, give women who've experienced premature menopause a chance at a different ending. "Up to 10 percent of women in their 40s, many of whom are reproductively active, go through early menopause. It's tragic for these women when they haven't yet had families," says Mark V. Sauer, M.D., assistant professor of obstetrics and gynecology at the USC Medical Center, who headed the study.

According to Sauer, conventional wisdom blames the high rate of miscarriages in women over 40 on aging eggs and an aging uterus. He claims his study illustrates that, with proper hormonal treatment, the uterus of an older woman is capable of maintaining a pregnancy with donor eggs. Still, many doctors say the technology is best reserved for younger women who have gone through premature menopause, in part because the older woman is at greater risk for many pregnancy-related complications.

"Older patients can have problems with gestational diabetes, hypertension, intrauterine growth retardation, hemorrhage risk, premature labor and other abnormalities," says Anne Colston Wentz, M.D., president of the Society for Assisted Reproductive Technologies and professor of obstetrics and gynecology at Northwestern University School of Medicine. But for women who were once told they were infertile or too old for conventional in vitro fertilization, Sauer remains cautiously optimistic.

SOURCE:
Kase, Lori Miller. "The Mythology of Menopause." *Health* (March 1991): 95.

RESOURCES

ORGANIZATION

American College of Obstetricians and Gynecologists. 600 Maryland Ave. SW, Suite 300 East, Washington, DC 20024.

BOOKS

Burnett, Raymond G. *Menopause: All Your Questions Answered*. Chicago: Contemporary Books, 1987. 140 pp.

Greenwood, Sadja. *Menopause Naturally: Preparing for the Second Half of Life*. San Francisco: Volcano Press, 1984. 201 pp.

RELATED ARTICLES

Brenner, Paul F. "The Menopausal Syndrome." *Obstetrics & Gynecology* 72, no. 5 (suppl.) (November 1988): 6S–11S.

"Facing Menopause with Hope." *Scripps Personal Health Letter* (October 1990): 7.

"New Directions in Menopause: A Chronic Disease or a Stage of Life." *HealthFacts* 14, no. 126 (November 1989): 1, 4–6.

Weinstein, L. "Hormonal Therapy in the Patient with Surgical Menopause." *Obstetrics & Gynecology* 75, no. 4 (suppl.) (April 1990): 47S–50S.

Young, D. D. "Some Misconceptions about the Menopause." *Obstetrics & Gynecology* 75, no. 5 (May 1990): 881–883.

MENSTRUATION

(*See also:* ENDOMETRIOSIS; MENOPAUSE; PREMENSTRUAL SYNDROME; TOXIC SHOCK SYNDROME)

OVERVIEW

The length of a woman's menstrual cycle, for example, is highly variable and individual. Cycle length is defined as the number of days from the start of one period to the start of the next. For most women, this number repeats itself monthly like clockwork.

Traditionally, a normal menstrual cycle has been defined as 28 days, the length of the lunar cycle. This correspondence has taken on almost mythic proportions, and many women whose cycles are longer or shorter feel slightly abnormal, or out of sync. But studies fail to substantiate the poetry of women and the moon. In fact, only one out of six women has a 28-day cycle. The average cycle length is 29.1 days, and anywhere between 23 and 35 days is considered normal.

Some totally normal women do not have a regular interval at all—irregularity is their pattern. As long as each cycle falls somewhere within the normal range, 23 to 35 days, they need not worry. And many women who are within a few years of menarche (their first period) or menopause (their last period) find that their cycles are even more erratic.

Although irregular cycles can be normal, they are inconvenient. How can you be prepared if you don't know when your next period is coming? Fortunately, there is a way for many women to predict their next menstruation.

Let's review the normal menstrual cycle. To begin with, the uterus, or womb, cleans itself out. Soon the ovaries begin to make estrogen, a hormone that signals the uterus to start rebuilding a lining. Simultaneously, an egg begins to develop in the ovary. Within 10 days to three weeks, the lining and the egg are ready for conception and the egg is released in a process called ovulation. This is when pregnancy can occur. After ovulation, the ovary begins to secrete another hormone called progesterone. Progesterone stimulates the uterine lining to complete its development, in preparation for nourishing a possible pregnancy. Within two weeks, the body will know if pregnancy has occurred. If it has not, the ovary will drastically reduce its hormone output, and the lining of the uterus will shrink and eventually shed.

Doctors now know that variation in cycle length is almost always related to how long it takes the body to get ready for ovulation. In other words, the time from a period to the next ovulation is what changes or varies from woman to woman. The time from ovulation to the next menstrual period, on the other hand, is almost always exactly 14 days.

If you know when you ovulate, you can predict that your next period will be in 14 days. Not all women can tell when the egg leaves the ovary, but many feel a sharp pain in the side. Others, especially those who use natural family planning, will recognize a change in mucus, from thin and slippery to thick and white, as a sign that ovulation has occurred. So learning to know when you ovulate is useful not only in planning pregnancy but also in planning for your periods.

When I was in medical school, I chuckled during the first part of our lecture on menstruation. I couldn't believe that my mostly male cohorts didn't know what color menstrual blood was, or how often women have to change a tampon.

Then the professor asked the class how much blood the average woman loses during her period, and I realized that I had no idea.

Most women are surprised to learn that with the average menses they lose only two tablespoons to one half cup of blood. It seems like more, partly because not all of what a woman sees is blood. Almost two thirds of the discharge is fluid released from cells that have either shrunken or died as the lining of the uterus breaks down.

Only if you pass more than a half cup of blood are you in danger of losing too much, and becoming anemic. But it's notoriously difficult for any woman to estimate the amount of blood on her tampons or pads. Fortunately, there are some signs that often accompany truly heavy bleeding.

The uterus and vagina contain substances known as fibrinolytics, which prevent blood from clotting. In an ordinary period, a woman should see only small clots or none at all. Passage of many or large clots indicates that you have passed more blood than the fibrinolytics can work on, and you are probably bleeding to excess. Another sign of an inordinately heavy flow is passage of bright-red blood for more than a few hours.

If you feel your periods are unusually heavy, you should see your doctor. A pelvic examination may reveal the cause, and you can be treated accordingly. Some of the more common causes of excessive bleeding are abnormal growths in or on the uterus, and hormone imbalances that interfere with ovulation.

SOURCE:
Shepherd, Janet E. "Your Menstrual Period: As Unique as You Are." *Vibrant Life* 6 (March-April 1990): 22-23.

MENSTRUAL DISORDERS (AMENORRHEA IN ATHLETES)

A minority of female athletes participating in ballet, gymnastics, distance running, rowing, and cycling, as well as other sports activities, occasionally experience menstrual and associated physiologic changes. Women competing in the sports of ballet and gymnastics have been reported to have particularly increased incidence of primary and secondary amenorrhea [absence of menstruation], decreased bone density, stress fractures, and symptoms of anorexia nervosa. Results of several studies have indicated decreased levels of circulating estrogen as well as other metabolic changes.

Research designed to determine the etiology of the amenorrhea and the associated changes has shown mixed results.

Low body fat cannot be linked in a causative fashion to hormonal changes or decreased levels of circulating estrogen. Early studies linking minimum body fat and menarche, as well as maintenance of regular menstrual cycles, have not been replicated. However, measurement of percentage of body fat may be helpful in assessing the nutritional status of athletes.

Ballet and gymnastics are perceived by some to be activities that are stressful psychologically. Although stress has been shown to cause amenorrhea, studies to date have not demonstrated the presence of significantly increased levels compared with age-matched girls not participating in ballet and gymnastics.

Some authors have postulated that tall, thin athletes who may be genetically at risk for delayed maturation are naturally attracted to these sports. Some of the delays may relate to preselection. However, no evidence currently exists proving a definite relationship between preselection and the physiologic changes in these athletes.

There is an increased emphasis by athletes, coaches, judges, and spectators on a slender physique for female gymnasts and ballet dancers. Several investigators have shown dietary intakes of adolescent ballerinas that are inadequate in calories, nutritional components, vitamins, and minerals. The most common findings demonstrated in amenorrheic athletes are high intensity of exercise combined with poor nutritional status. Fasting and purging may be encouraged and anorexia nervosa or bulimia hidden in all athletic populations. Coaches need to be educated regarding the seriousness of these behaviors.

SOURCE:
Committee on Sports Medicine. "Amenorrhea in Adolescent Athletes." *Pediatrics* 84, no. 2 (August 1989): 394.

TREATMENT FOR MENSTRUAL CRAMPS

Menstrual cramps (dysmenorrhea) can be caused by specific medical problems such as endometriosis, pelvic infection, fibroid tumors (benign leiomyoma of the uterus), or ovarian cysts. Cramps associated with these conditions typically appear for the first time when a woman is in her 20s or 30s. Your clinician will call this condition secondary dysmenorrhea, for the cramps are secondary to (caused by) another medical problems. An IUD (intrauterine device) can also cause secondary dysmenorrhea.

Most women who have menstrual cramps don't have any underlying illness, however. Severe, disabling cramps without underlying illness is called primary dysmenorrhea. In addition to cramps, primary dysmenorrhea can cause backache, leg pain, nausea, vomiting, diarrhea, headache, and dizziness. As many as 70% of women experience at least some cramping pain during menstrual flow, and 15% of women have cramps severe enough to be disabling. Typically, a young woman may begin menstrual periods with somewhat irregular cycles and little pain during the first year or two, and then begin to have serious cramps when ovulation patterns and her regular cycle become established. Young women with severe cramps may be unable to manage normal daily activities for the first 24 to 36 hours of each menstrual period. Primary dysmenorrhea symptoms rarely last more than two days with each cycle, and severe cramps often subside somewhat on their own when a woman reaches her later 20s or has a full term pregnancy.

Prostaglandin hormone is the cause of cramps in primary dysmenorrhea. . . .

For mild, normal cramps of primary dysmenorrhea, your best home therapy may be all you need. Aspirin or acetaminophen may provide good relief, and low-dose antiprostaglandin pain relievers are available without a prescription. . . .

Also, avoid prolonged standing or walking on hard pavement, and try back massage, a heating pad, tub soaks, exercise to put endorphins—your brain's natural pain relievers—to work, and rest. One stiff drink may help, because alcohol relaxes the uterine muscle. Orgasm also helps relax the uterine muscle, and will decrease congestion in your pelvis. Warning: Pennyroyal, an herbal "remedy," can cause serious and even fatal poisoning.

If cramps are bothersome despite your own efforts, then by all means talk to your clinician about a prescription for antiprostaglandin medication.

Overall, at least 80% of women treated for cramps with antiprostaglandin medication can expect good relief. There are several closely related drugs called prostaglandin synthetase inhibitors that have similar effects. All of them decrease production of prostaglandin within normal body cells, including uterine lining cells. For most women any of the commonly used antiprostaglandin drugs is likely to be effective. They are not identical, however, so if one is not effective or side effects are a problem, then trying an alternative is reasonable. Many studies of antiprostaglandin drugs used for cramps have been published, and reported success rates for relieving pain range from about 60% to more than 90% for various products in various studies. Unfortunately, results are not comparable from one study to another because of differences in study design, so the relative effectiveness of different products is not yet clear.

These drugs belong to a large drug family called nonsteroidal anti-inflammatory drugs (NSAIDs). Aspirin is a member of the NSAID family, and many of the NSAIDs were originally developed for treatment of arthritis as alternatives to aspirin. Arthritis treatment often requires prolonged use of medications at quite high daily doses, so research evidence on possible risks and complications for NSAIDs is fairly extensive; generally they have side effects and adverse effects similar to those for aspirin.

SOURCE:

Stewart, Felicia H., Felicia Guest, and others. *Understanding Your Body: Every Woman's Guide to a Lifetime of Health.* New York: Bantam, 1987. pp. 559, 560, 562.

RESOURCES

ORGANIZATIONS

American College of Obstetricians and Gynecologists. 600 Maryland Avenue SW, Suite 300 East, Washington, DC 20024.

National Women's Health Network. 1325 G Street NW, Washington, DC 20005.

PAMPHLETS

American College of Obstetricians and Gynecologists:

Growing Up: Being a Teenager: You and Your Sexuality.

Gynecologic Problems: Dysmenorrhea. 1985. 11 pp.

National Institute of Child Health and Human Development:

Facts About Dysmenorrhea and Premenstrual Syndrome. n.d. 10 pp.

BOOKS

Nourse, A. *Menstruation: Just Plain Talk.* New York: Franklin Watts, 1990.

Weller, Stella. *Pain Free Periods: Natural Ways to Overcome Menstrual Problems.* Rochester, VT: Thorson Publishing Group, 1987. 192 pp.

RELATED ARTICLES

Cumming, David C., Ceinwen E. Cumming, and Dianne K. Dieren. "Menstrual Mythology and Sources of Information about Menstruation." *American Journal of Obstetrics and Gynecology* 164 (February 1991): 472–476.

Mansfield, M. Joan, and S. Jean Emans. "Anorexia Nervosa, Athletics, and Amenorrhea." *Pediatric Clinics of North America* 36, no. 3 (June 1989): 533–549.

MULTIPLE SCLEROSIS

OVERVIEW

Our bodies contain a fatty substance called myelin which surrounds and protects nerve fibers of the brain and spinal cord (the central nervous system) in the same way that insulation protects electrical wires. When any part of this myelin sheathing, or insulation, is destroyed, nerve impulses to the brain are interrupted and distorted.

The result is multiple sclerosis—multiple because many scattered areas of the brain and spinal cord are affected; sclerosis because sclerosed or hardened patches of scar tissue form over the damaged myelin.

We know how multiple sclerosis happens. We still don't know why. That is one of the questions researchers are investigating.

Symptoms of multiple sclerosis vary greatly depending upon where the sclerosed patches are formed in the central nervous system. They may include tingling sensations, numbness, slurred speech, blurred or double vision, muscle weakness, poor coordination, unusual fatigue, muscle cramps, spasms, problems with bladder, bowel and sexual function, and paralysis. Occasionally, there may be such mental changes as forgetfulness or confusion. These symptoms may occur in any combination and can vary from very mild to very severe.

There is no way at present to predict when or even if attacks of the disease will recur. Symptoms vary greatly from person to person and from time to time in the same person. In general, however, the typical pattern of multiple sclerosis is marked by periods of active disease called exacerbations and quiescent, or symptom-free periods called remissions.

Some people may have an initial attack and no recurrence afterward. Others have what is called "relapsing-remitting disease." This means they have exacerbations, whch may take place on an average of one every two or three years, followed by periods of remission, which may last months—even years. Still others may experience a chronic progressive form of multiple sclerosis. Thus, the complete spectrum can range from very mild to intermittent to a rapidly progressive form of the disease.

Because multiple sclerosis affects people so differently, it is difficult to make generalizations about the extent of disability. Statistics, however, have shown that two out of three people with multiple sclerosis remain ambulatory over their lifetimes. Multiple sclerosis is not contagious and it is rarely fatal.

Multiple sclerosis most often strikes people who are in their twenties or thirties—young adults "just as they're starting to live."

Women develop it more frequently than men, whites more frequently than blacks or Orientals. The reasons are not yet understood.

The disease is also most frequently found among people in the colder climates, both north and south of the Equator. Scientists don't understand why this is so, but studies strongly suggest that where you were born and lived during the first 15 years are more important than later residencies.

Studies also indicate certain genetic factors within individuals may make them more receptive to the disease, but there is no evidence that multiple sclerosis is directly inherited.

Multiple sclerosis is not always easy to detect or diagnose because early symptoms can be so spotty, because other diseases of the central nervous system have some of the same warning signs, and because we do not yet have a definitive neurological or laboratory test that can confirm or rule out MS. However, recent advances in the technology of imaging the brain are helping to clarify diagnosis.

In order for a conclusive diagnosis of multiple sclerosis to be made, two factors must be clearly shown: (1) there must be evidence of many patches of scar tissue in different parts of the central nervous system, and (2) there must have been at least two separate attacks (exacerbations) of the disease. A diagnosis can take several months, sometimes even years.

SOURCE:
National Multiple Sclerosis Society. *What is Multiple Sclerosis?* 1988. pp. 1–3.

TREATMENT

At least partial recovery from acute exacerbations can reasonably be expected, but further relapses may occur without warning, and there is no means of preventing progression of the disorder. Some disability is likely to result eventually, but about half of all patients are without significant disability even 10 years after onset of symptoms.

Recovery from acute relapses may be hastened by treatment with corticosteroids, but the extent of recovery is unchanged. A high dose (eg, prednisone, 60 or 80 mg) is given daily for 1 week, after which medication is tapered over the following 2 or 3 weeks. Long-term treatment with steroids provides no benefit and does not prevent further relapses.

Several recent studies have suggested that intensive immunosuppressive therapy with cyclophosphamide or azathioprine may help to arrest the course of chronic progressive active multiple sclerosis. Further clinical trials are in progress. There is some evidence that plasmapheresis [removal of plasma from withdrawn blood] may enhance any beneficial effects of immunosuppression in some patients with chronic progressive multiple sclerosis, at least for a time, but its role in the management of the various clinical forms of multiple sclerosis is uncertain. The findings in a recent trial of systemic interferon therapy suggested some benefit in patients whose disease was characterized by relapses and remissions rather than by steady progression. Further studies to evaluate this form of treatment in selected patients are proceeding. Finally, preliminary studies suggest that Cop 1 (a random polymer-simulating myelin basic protein) may be beneficial in patients with the exacerbating-remitting form of multiple sclerosis, and further evaluation of this approach seems warranted.

Treatment for spasticity and for neurogenic bladder [dysfunctional urinary bladder caused by lesion of the nervous system] may be needed in advanced cases. Excessive fatigue must be avoided, and patients should rest during periods of acute relapse.

SOURCE:
Schroeder, Steven A., and others. (eds.). *Current Medical Diagnosis and Treatment 1991.* Norwalk, CT: Appleton & Lange, 1992. pp. 752–753.

* * *

Aspirin, acetaminophen, and other painkillers may relieve the occasional pain some multiple sclerosis patients experience. If the pain stems from muscle spasms, an anticonvulsive such as carbamazepine or muscle relaxants such as diazepam and dantrolene sodium may also help. The constant pain that afflicts some people with severe multiple sclerosis is more difficult to relieve. Tricyclic antidepressants such as amitriptyline may be helpful. Drugs that relax the bladder, such as amitriptyline, can help alleviate urinary frequency and urgency in patients with these problems.

Preventive measures are also beneficial. Overexhaustion, emotional stress, viral infections, and a rise in body temperature (from a hot bath or hot and humid weather, for example) are thought to trigger or worsen symptoms and should therefore be avoided. Patients should also follow a well-balanced and nutritionally sound diet and maintain a desirable weight.

Patients with muscle stiffness may be aided by physical therapy, and moderate exercise can help keep limbs supple and maintain muscle function. Certain exercises can also alleviate muscle spasms.

SOURCE:
Patlak, Margie. "The Puzzling Picture of Multiple Sclerosis." *FDA Consumer* (July-August 1989): 21.

USE OF BACLOFEN IN TREATMENT

Baclofen for infusion into the spinal canal is now available under the Treatment IND (investigational new drug) Program for persons with multiple sclerosis or spinal cord injury suffering from severe and chronic spasticity who cannot tolerate or who do not respond to oral baclofen. The drug is infused into the spinal cord using a pump called the Medtronic SynchroMed Infusion System.

Under regulations enacted in 1987, providing certain safeguards are in place, drugs in controlled clinical trials can be made available outside these trials to treat patients with serious or immediately life-threatening diseases for which no comparable or satisfactory alternative-therapy exists.

Oral baclofen has been used to treat spasticity for 12 years. But about 20,000 patients with painful chronic spasticity either do not get sufficient relief with the oral preparation or they suffer unacceptable side effects.

The infusion pump containing baclofen is implanted beneath the skin in the patient's abdomen. The pump is programmed via radio signals to dispense the drug into the spine through a small catheter inserted into the spinal canal. The device is refilled every four to eight weeks by injection with a hypodermic needle through the skin and a self-sealing rubber cover on the pump. The number of patients treated to date is small. At least one death not explained by any other cause has occurred with infused baclofen. The informed consent required of patients makes note of this, and FDA is requiring close and careful monitoring by both physicians and the sponsor, Medtronics Inc.

SOURCE:

"Drug to Treat Spasticity Available Under Treatment IND." *FDA Consumer* 24 (June 1990): 5.

RESOURCES

ORGANIZATION

National Multiple Sclerosis Society. 205 East 42nd Street, New York, NY 10018.

BOOKS

Rosner, Louis J., and Shelley Ross. *Multiple Sclerosis.* Englewood Cliffs, NJ: Prentice-Hall, 1987.

Scheinberg, Labe C., and Nancy J. Holland. *Multiple Sclerosis: A Guide for Patients and Their Families.* New York: Raven Press, 1984.

RELATED ARTICLES

Erickson, Rolland P., Margaret R. Lie, and others. "Rehabilitation in Multiple Sclerosis." *Mayo Clinic Proceedings* 64 (July 1989): 818–828.

Gorelick, P. B. "Clues to the Mystery of Multiple Sclerosis." *Postgraduate Medicine* 85, no. 4 (March 1989): 125–128, 131–134.

Rudick, Richard A. "Helping Patients Live With Multiple Sclerosis: What Primary Care Physicians Can Do." *Postgraduate Medicine* 88, no. 2 (August 1990): 197–200, 203–204, 207.

MUSCULAR DYSTROPHY

OVERVIEW

Muscular dystrophies are a diverse group of disorders in which there is muscular deterioration. It is estimated that about 250,000 to 300,000 persons in this country suffer from one or another of the muscular dystrophies. About two-thirds are children between the ages of three and eighteen years.

These disorders are usually genetically determined, but the nature of the specific defects is unknown. It is hoped that when the defects have been identified, it will be possible to treat these diseases—perhaps by altering genes or by replacing missing substances, in much the same way that insulin injections are used to treat diabetes. Until that research goal is achieved, physical and occupational therapy are advised to try to slow the deterioration that occurs among those with muscular dystrophies. Genetic counseling is important in preventing cases of muscular dystrophies. Patients whose families are at risk should seek this counseling.

The most common types of muscular dystrophies are:

Duchenne's Dystrophy. This is the most common and severe type of muscular dystrophy and is usually first noticed in boys between the ages of two and six years. It is usually transmitted to sons by clinically unaffected mothers. Parents may first suspect that the child is afflicted when he develops a waddling gait and has difficulty rising from the floor and climbing stairs. Laboratory studies and muscle biopsy can confirm the suspected diagnosis. Although the child's pelvic muscles are first involved, weakness spreads to the shoulder and back muscles and then to all the muscles. The disease progresses rapidly, and the patient is not expected to live more than fifteen years after its onset.

Facio-Scapulo-Humeral. This is transmitted as a dominant trait by either parent, and affects males and females equally, appearing in early adolescence or in the twenties. Its most recognizable symptoms are loss of facial expression and difficulty in raising the arms over the head. This is the least threatening form of muscular dystrophy because it progresses slowly and rarely causes an early death, although the patient may eventually have considerable disability.

Limb-Girdle. This is transmitted either as a dominant or recessive trait, or occurs sporadically. A physician or medical geneticist should review each case to see if an inheritance pattern can be determined. Limb-Girdle muscular dystrophy can start anytime from the first to the third decade of life, and occurs in both males and females. The muscles of the pelvis and the shoulder are involved, and the rate of deterioration varies—sometimes being quite slow, and sometimes rapid. The amount of disability also varies, and, in most cases, patients are not threatened with an early death. Other diseases can mimic limb-girdle dystrophy, so it is important to have a thorough evaluation, including "electromyography," which measures the electrical activity of the muscle, and muscle biopsy.

Myotonic Dystrophy. This form of the disease is transmitted as a dominant trait by either parent, and affects males and females equally. It may appear as early as puberty, but it commonly does not show up until young adulthood. Among the early signs of the disease are stiffness in the limbs, especially after exposure to cold; inability to relax the grip after shaking hands; a tendency to trip and fall forward; and loss of facial expression. The disability becomes severe within a 15- to 20-year period after onset, and patients rarely live out a normal life span. Genetic counseling is extremely important in this disorder since children can be severely affected by myotonic dystrophy even when born to mothers who barely show any symptoms.

SOURCE:
California Medical Association. "Muscular Dystrophies." *HealthTips* index 362 (June 1989): 1-2.

GENETIC TRANSMISSION

All forms of muscular dystrophy are caused by gene defects. What has eluded scientists for decades is the identity of the genes and the proteins they produce, as well as the ways in which those proteins are abnormal in the disease. Many questioned the possibility of investigators ever finding the causes of muscular dystrophy.

In 1986, MDA [Muscular Dystrophy Association]-funded researchers made medical history. A Boston-based team of scientists discovered the gene that, when defective, is responsible for Duchenne and Becker muscular dystrophies. One year later, the same research team identified the crucial protein—dystrophin—which in absence or abnormality causes both diseases. Both of these breakthroughs were the culmination of many years of painstaking research by MDA grantees worldwide.

A new and more hopeful era has emerged with these milestone achievements. MDA-backed scientists are using the same state-of-the-art research techniques that led to the Duchenne muscular dystrophy gene and dystrophin breakthroughs in their search for the causes of all types of muscular dystrophy, as well as other inherited neuromuscular diseases.

SOURCE:
Muscular Dystrophy Association. *Facts about Muscular Dystrophy*. May 1990. p. 10.

TREATMENT

There is no successful treatment of the disease. Orthopedic appliances, exercise, physical therapy, and surgery to correct contractures can help preserve mobility. Doctors and nurses often caution family members who are carriers about the risk of transmitting this disease. No form of muscular dystrophy can be detected by amniocentesis, but this procedure can determine the sex of the fetus and is often recommended for carriers who are pregnant.

Nursing care involves the psychologic support of the patient and the family and the encouragement of the patient to avoid long periods of bed rest and inactivity to assure maximum physical activity. Splints, braces, grab bars, and overhead slings help the patient exercise. A wheelchair helps preserve mobility. Other devices that can increase comfort and help prevent footdrop include footboards, high-topped sneakers, and foot cradles. Nurses encourage the patient to maintain peer relationships and often encourage the parents to keep the child in school as long as possible. Nurses provide emotional support for the parents and the patient in coping with continuing changes in the patient's body, and they commonly refer patients to the Muscular Dystrophy Association for further support and assistance.

SOURCE:
"Duchenne's Muscular Dystrophy." In *Mosby's Medical, Nursing, & Allied Health Dictionary*. 3d ed. St. Louis: C. V. Mosby, 1990. p. 393.

RESOURCES

ORGANIZATIONS

Muscular Dystrophy Association. 810 Seventh Ave, New York, NY 10019.

RELATED ARTICLES

Kolata, Gina. "Amid Debate, Scientist Seeks to Treat Muscular Dystrophy." *The New York Times* (May 2, 1991): A1.

Meyer, Charles. "First Human Tests of Myoblast Transfer." *MDA Newsmagazine* 7, no. 2 (Summer 1990): 20-21, 26-27.

Meyer, Charles. "MDA Researchers Uncover the First Clues to the Genetic Cause of Spinal Muscular Dystrophy." *MDA Newsmagazine* 7, no. 2 (Summer 1990): 8-11, 24.

NURSING HOMES

NURSING HOMES—BASIC TYPES

In the first place, the term nursing home is actually a very general name for several different types of medical-care facilities. It has the connotation of a "last stop" for the elderly, but it can actually be a place for people of all ages to convalesce following an accident or serious illness. (It can be a home for mentally retarded persons or for people of any age suffering from chronic illnesses that need constant medical attention.) A nursing home can even be a temporary placement for an elderly person while a family shops around and lines up alternative modes of care.

A nursing home is not for someone who is extremely sick—a hospital is. It is also not a prison where people are segregated from society. It is not a drawn-out hospice program where people are waiting for inevitable deterioration and death. It is, rather, a home for people who have difficulty caring for themselves where rehabilitation on all levels is undertaken. As such, nursing homes provide three basic types of services:

1. **Nursing/medical care**—for example, injections of medication, catheterizations, physical therapy, and other forms of rehabilitative services.

2. **Personal care**—for example, assistance in eating, dressing, bathing, getting in and out of bed, and even making telephone calls.

3. **Residential services**—for example, providing a clean room, good food, and a pleasant atmosphere with appropriate social activities.

Nursing homes can be classified in many different ways. Generally speaking, the most common classifications are by (1) level of care they provide, (2) type of ownership, and (3) type of licensure/accreditation they possess.

Levels of Care

The care provided by nursing homes is generally categorized in one of three ways: skilled, intermediate, and sheltered (custodial). Many facilities provide for both skilled and intermediate care, while some provide for three types on the same campus.

Skilled Nursing Facilities. In these facilities, care is delivered by registered and licensed practical nurses on the orders of an attending physician. . . . The person who requires skilled nursing is often bedridden and not able to help him/herself. An individual may be placed in a skilled nursing facility for either a short or an extended period of time, depending upon the prognosis.

Intermediate Care Facilities. The intermediate care facility provides less intensive care than the skilled facility. The cost is usually less. The patient has a greater degree of mobility and normally is not confined to a bed. Care is also delivered by registered and licensed practical nurses (as well as by an array of therapists). Intermediate care facilities stress rehabilitation therapy, which enables the patient either to return to a normal home setting or at least to regain and/or retain as many functions of daily living as possible. For those patients with chronic conditions, incapable of independent living, these facilities offer a full range of medical, social, recreational, and support services. Intermediate Care Facilities for the Mentally Retarded is a relatively new type of community-based living arrangement, which allows formerly institutionalized and other mentally retarded individuals to be placed in a less restrictive setting. The entire concept is to provide a normal living arrangement for those persons not capable of complete independent living. Some of these facilities are quite small, having fewer than 15 beds.

Sheltered, or Custodial, Care. This level of care is nonmedical in that residents do not require constant attention from nurses or aides. It is designed for those persons who are quite capable of independent living, but who may require some assistance with personal care and homemaking services. A typical sheltered care resident is someone who can no longer (or doesn't wish to) maintain the upkeep of a house or be bothered by everyday activities such as shopping, paying bills, and so forth. A good sheltered care facility emphasizes the social needs of residents while providing a safe secure living arrangement, free from as many anxieties as possible. (Sheltered care facilities are also called "domiciliary care facilities" or "group homes.") Many are affiliated (or have special arrangements) with intermediate care and skilled nursing care facilities as well.

SOURCE:
Bausell, R. Barker, Michael A. Rooney, and Charles B. Inlander. *How to Evaluate and Select a Nursing Home.* Reading, MA: Addison-Wesley, 1988. pp. 1–3.

CHOOSING THE RIGHT NURSING HOME

The first step in the search itself is to compile a list of a half-dozen or so nursing homes that meet such basic criteria as location, the ability to provide key services (e.g., physical therapy), and acceptance of the payment sources you plan on using. Sources for the compilation of this list can include the yellow pages, recommendations from friends and professionals, and lists available from your state or local agency on aging or Nursing Home Ombudsman Program.

The next step is to visit your candidate homes. There are many books on nursing home selection and most have checklists of what to look for. One of the best is *The Nursing Home Handbook,* by Jo Horne (American Association of Retired Persons, 1989, $9.95). Nursing home ombudsmen and state or local nursing home licensing and certification offices can also often provide information on whether the homes you are interested in have a history of meeting regulatory requirements.

Information from checklists and regulatory agencies should, however, be used with caution. As Rosalie Kane [professor of social work and public health at the University of Minnesota] points out, nursing home regulations are "geared more toward ensuring that facilities have the capacity to provide adequate care than that they actually provide it." Most regulations, and many of the items in formal checklists, are also biased towards the view that nursing homes are primarily medical facilities, or "mini-hospitals," instead of homes—places where people may live for many years. This view, says Dr. Kane, emphasizes "physical well-being and safety at the expense of psychological and social well-being and resident satisfaction."

As to the characteristics of a nursing home that do increase "psychological and social well-being and resident satisfaction," a recent study by Dr. Kane offers some clues. Feelings of independence and control are central to the quality of life in a nursing home and Kane's work suggests these can be increased through policies that promote privacy, that allow residents to choose their roommates, to decide on their own wake-up times and to make use of off-premise passes.

Dr. Tellis-Nayak [a sociologist at Chicago's St. Xavier College] also believes that the better nursing homes are those that are less "medicalized." In such homes, he says, the residents do not line the halls restrained or slumped over in wheelchairs. The residents seem well groomed and are encouraged to make choices in matters such as food and scheduling. There is ample opportunity and space for families and friends to visit and volunteers are ever present.

He offers no checklist for identifying such a home, but he does recount the advice given him by the administrator of an "exemplary" nursing home: "Go and ask the residents. Find out how happy they are with the care they receive. Ask their families. And you will know."

SOURCE:
Shepherd, Steven. "Evaluating Nursing Homes: Caregiving with Compassion." *Executive Health Report* 26 (June 1990): 3.

COMPLIANCE WITH GOVERNMENT STANDARDS

Conditions in the nation's skilled nursing facilities improved somewhat last year. But almost one-quarter of all homes did not meet the government's standards for drug administration, and about a third did not meet food-handling standards.

Those are the findings of the Health Care Financing Administration's second annual Nursing Home Information guide, released in late May. The 93-volume guide includes individual reports on each of the 15,600 nursing homes that participate in Medicare and Medicaid. Based on annual inspections by state surveyors, it focuses on 32 of the 500 elements covered in the inspections and gives the home a pass or fail on each.

As such, it represents a broad snapshot of care in the home at a particular point in time and has been criticized by both nursing home officials and patient advocates for lacking specificity. HCFA head Gail Wilensky, PhD, defended the guides, however, saying they are intended only as a starting point to help patients and families evaluate a home, rather than as a "complete measure of quality of care."

Overall, the surveys found that 24% of homes did not meet the standard requiring that nursing home staff follow written orders of the attending physician in administering drugs. Some 36% failed the standard for food storage and preparation; 25% did not meet the standards for resident hygiene; and about 20% failed the standards for rehabilitative care, care of catheterized patients, and skin treatment to prevent bedsores.

Nursing home officials countered that the guides have several problems. American Health Care Assn. Executive Vice President Paul Willging labeled the guides "unreliable" because they provide information only on what was happening on a given day. . . .

In an attempt to make the guide more useful to consumers, several changes were made this year. To give some indication as to whether the home has a continuing problem, for example, this year's guide gives data on compliance with the 32 standards used as performance indicators in both of the last two years. It also notes whether any action was taken against the home for failing to take corrective action.

As an additional gauge of the breadth of a home's problems, the guide also lists any of the 500 standards failed by the home. But these are described only with a number, and readers must look up the corresponding definition in the back of the book. . . .

The guides have been sent to various state agencies and advocacy groups. They are arranged by state, with some states having more than one volume. Copies of single volumes or full sets of the report may be purchased by writing to the Superintendent of Documents, U.S. Government Printing Office, Washington, D.C., 20402.

SOURCE:

McIlrath, Sharon. "HCFA Nursing Home Guide Reports Deficiencies." *American Medical News* 33 (June 8, 1990): 5.

NURSING HOME PATIENT BILL OF RIGHTS

[As suggested by the Health Care Financing Administration, U.S. Department of Health and Human Services, Washington, D.C.]

A patient:

1. is fully informed as evidenced by the resident's written acknowledgement of these rights and of all rules and regulations governing the exercise of these rights.

2. is fully informed of services available in the facility and of related charges for services not covered under Medicare/Medicaid, or not covered by the facility's basic daily rate.

3. is fully informed of his/her medical condition unless the physician notes in the medical record that it is not in the patient's interest to be told, and is afforded the opportunity to participate in the planning of his/her medical treatment and to refuse to participate in experimental research.

4. is transferred or discharged only for medical reasons, or for his/her welfare or that of other residents, and is given reasonable advance notice to ensure orderly transfer or discharge.

5. is encouraged and assisted, through his/her period of stay to exercise his/her rights as a resident and as a free citizen. To this end he/she may voice grievances and recommend changes in policies and services to facility staff and/or outside representatives of his/her choice without fear of coercion, discrimination, or reprisal.

6. may manage his/her personal financial affairs, or is given at least a quarterly accounting of financial transactions made on his/her behalf if the facility accepts the responsibility to safeguard the funds.

7. is free from mental and physical abuse, and free from chemical and physical restraints except as authorized in writing by a physician for a specified and limited period of time or when necessary to protect patients from injury to themselves or others.

8. is assured confidential treatment of his/her personal and medical records and may approve or refuse their release to any individual outside facility.

9. is treated with consideration, respect, and full recognition of his/her dignity and individuality, including privacy in treatment and in care of his/her personal needs.

10. is not required to perform services for the facility that are not included for therapeutic purposes in this plan of care.

11. may associate and communicate privately with persons of his/her choice, and send and receive his/her personal mail unopened.

12. may meet with, and participate in activities of social, religious, and community groups at his/her discretion.

13. may retain and use his/her personal clothing and possessions as space permits, unless to do so would infringe upon rights of other patients, or constitute a hazard of safety.

14. is assured privacy for visits by his/her spouse; if both are inpatients in the facility, they are permitted to share a room.

SOURCE:

Bausell, R. Barker, Michael A. Rooney, and Charles B. Inlander. *How to Evaluate and Select a Nursing Home*. Reading, MA: Addison-Wesley, 1988. 78–79.

RESOURCES

ORGANIZATIONS

American Association of Homes for the Aging. 1129 20th St. NW, Washington, DC 20036.

American Association of Retired Persons. 1909 K St. NW, Washington, DC 20049.

American Health Care Association. 1201 L St. NW, Washington, DC 20005.

PAMPHLETS

American Association of Homes for the Aging:

The Continuing Care Retirement Community.

Living Independently.

Nonprofit Housing and Care Options for Older People.

The Nursing Home.

American Health Care Association:

Here's Help.

Thinking about a Nursing Home?

Welcome to our Nursing Home: A Family Guide.

RELATED ARTICLES

Dawning, Joy. "Making the Nursing Home Decision." *Weight Watchers Women's Health and Fitness News* (January 1991): 4.

"Nursing Homes that Work." *Health After 50* 3, no. 4 (June 1991): 1–2.

Powers, J. S. "Helping Family and Patients Decide Between Home Care and Nursing Home Care." *Southern Medical Journal* 82, no. 6 (June 1989): 723–726.

Sloane, Leonard. "Coping with Selecting a Nursing Home: A Huge Government Report Provides Guidance, but Experts Warn that It Can't Be Used Alone." *New York Times* (June 16, 1990): 16A.

Witchel, Dinah B. "The No-Guilt Guide to Elder Care." *Family Circle* (March 12, 1991): 40, 42, 46–47.

OBESITY

(*See also:* EATING DISORDERS; LIPOSUCTION; WEIGHT CONTROL DIETS)

OVERVIEW

Morbid obesity is a disease. It is a chronic disease with a complex etiology, involving both the patient's genetic background and environment. Studies of twins—particularly adopted twins—suggest that genetic and environmental factors are responsible for 70% of morbid obesity in Americans today. In addition, epidemiological data indicate that if the patient has one parent with a weight problem, then the chance of the patient developing morbid obesity is 60%; if both parents have weight problems, the probability rises to 90%.

With regard to the patient's environment, the American diet looms as a major cause of obesity. High in fat—especially animal fats—and low in fiber, such an unhealthy and calorically dense diet is responsible for a number of health problems in addition to excess weight. These diet-related problems are only compounded by an increasingly sedentary lifestyle that does not exercise the cardiopulmonary system sufficiently. The consumption of a high-fat, calorie-dense diet and the low level of activity among many Americans today certainly helps explain the prevalence of morbid obesity.

There are, however, other factors that require further research before they can be worked into obesity treatment planning. Obesity is also influenced by the patient's metabolism and the interactions between appetite, metabolic rate, adipose tissue and specific neurochemicals. With a greater understanding of these physiological variables, more sophisticated pharmacological and behavioral therapies may be developed, but not in the immediate future.

As with other diseases, whatever the underlying cause, obesity can be diagnosed and classified according to severity. In 1985, the National Institutes of Health Consensus Conference defined obesity as "an excess of body fat frequently resulting in a significant impairment of health." While percent above ideal body weight is commonly used to identify an individual's level of overweight, the body mass index (BMI), defined as weight in kilograms per height in meters squared, is a more direct measurement of fatness. Use of the BMI more clearly distinguishes between groups of obese patients and avoids reference to standard weight-for-height tables developed for normal-weight populations. For example a 5 foot 10 inch male weighing 300 pounds or more or a 5 foot 6 inch female weighing 270 pounds or more would be considered morbidly obese.

From various population surveys, an estimated 1 to 2 million Americans are morbidly or super obese, with an additional 1.24 million persons falling into the category of medically significant obesity. In America, as in other Western societies, the obese population is growing despite the increased awareness of the importance of proper nutrition and exercise. In fact, the 1988 Surgeon General's Report on Nutrition and Health ranks obesity as the number one nutritional problem in the United States. The National Research Council's recent report on Diet and Health further indicates that diet does influence the risk of several major chronic diseases.

SOURCE:

Forse, Armour, Peter N. Benotti, and George Blackburn. "Morbid Obesity: Weighing the Treatment Options." *Nutrition Today* 24 (September-October 1989): 10–11.

HEALTH RISKS

In 1985 a National Institutes of Health panel reviewed the data about overweight and health. The panel strongly advised weight loss for the roughly one in five Americans who are "obese"—20 percent or more above their desirable weight, as defined by the standard weight tables developed by the Metropolitan Life Insurance Co. People who are less overweight may still benefit from slimming down, but the health risks are greatest for those who are most overweight.

"Desirable weight" is a rather arbitrary range that varies with the weight table you choose. Since the Metropolitan tables don't take into account the normal gain in weight as people age, some researchers believe those tables are too strict for older people. Consumers Union's medical consultants prefer the table created in 1985 by the National Institute of Aging's Gerontology Research Center; it's more restrictive for younger people but allows for weight gain with age.

Overweight is associated with an increased incidence of diabetes, heart disease, and hypertension. For obese men, there's a higher rate of cancer of the colon, prostate, and rectum. For women, obesity is linked to cancer of the breast, gallbladder, ovaries, and uterus. Obese people also have a higher incidence of arthritis, gallstones, and gout. Extreme obesity—100 pounds or more overweight—has been linked to early death.

Where you carry your excess weight affects your medical risk. Fat around the waist, particularly the "beer belly" more common among men, seems to pose more of a threat than fat around the hips and buttocks, more common among women. Bulging bellies are associated with an increased risk of cardiovascular disease and diabetes. And studies suggest that abdominal fat increases the risk of coronary heart disease, independent of total body fat.

SOURCE:

"Health Risks of Overweight." *Consumer Reports Health Letter* (February 1990): 11.

CURRENT THERAPIES

Weight control is important in the treatment of hypertension, diabetes mellitus, heart disease and degenerative joint disease. However, substantial, prolonged weight loss is difficult to achieve. Health professionals often have difficulty advising patients about the best method to lose weight. Holmes and associates have analyzed the most popular, available weight-loss methods and provide recommendations for various categories of obese adult patients.

Nutrition counseling, very-low-calorie diets, behavior modification therapy, exercise programs, placement of an intragrastric balloon and gastric restriction are interventions that physicians may recommend for obese patients. Attrition rates, maximal weight loss, long-term weight loss maintenance and morbidity rates should be considered in the evaluation of these interventions.

A low-calorie diet (800 to 1,500 kcal per day) is the first and, for many patients, the only intervention prescribed by physicians. No formal studies have been performed on the impact of diet counseling in the physician's office. Considering the poor record of diet counseling by nutritionists, physicians should not expect much success. Properly supervised, very-low-calorie diets (800 kcal per day) appear safe, but have attrition rates of up to 50 percent. Maintenance of weight loss has also been disappointing.

Behavior modification therapy has become a popular therapeutic approach to weight control. Weight loss has been only moderately successful, and even in the best programs, attrition rates are approximately 15 percent. Courses that combine behavior modification and nutrition education are increasingly available in the community, and physicians should become aware of these resources.

Exercise programs can lead to selective loss of adipose tissue, with preservation (or even an increase) of lean body mass. However, weight loss is slow, and success requires diligence.

The administration of drugs for weight loss is not recommended. Various types of surgery, including jaw wiring and intragastric balloons, have proven successful in certain groups of obese patients. Surgical interventions have significant side effects and risks that should be carefully considered. Risk factors for obesity, such as stress, depression, poverty, poor understanding of nutrition and a strong family history of obesity, should be warning signs for the patient and physician. Preventive education and simple warnings of the risks of obesity before obesity occurs may prove to be the best intervention.

SOURCE:

Holmes, Michelle D., Bernice Zysow, and Thomas L. Delbanco. "An Analytic Review of Current Therapies for Obesity." *Journal of Family Practice* 28, no. 1 (May 1989): 610–616. Cited in "Current Therapies for Obesity." *American Family Physician* 41, no. 1 (January 1990): 317.

BEHAVIORAL TREATMENT

Behavioral programs are among the most widely used approaches for weight loss. There are books and manuals on this approach and the major commercial weight loss centers such as Weight Watchers, Diet Center, and NutriSystem have integrated behavior modification into their programs. Even fad diets and crazy schemes advertised in tabloid newspapers may come with pamphlets or brochures that discuss the importance of behavior change.

There are several reasons for this wide-scale adoption of behavioral techniques and principles. Well over 100 controlled studies testing behavioral approaches have been published, a number far greater than can be claimed by any other approach. This considerable literature is known to researchers, the press, and individuals in policy-making positions, therefore explaining the wide dissemination. In addition, behavioral techniques are particularly helpful in efforts aimed at "life-style change," a philosophy that has captured the public fancy. . . .

Much progress has been made in the development of behavioral programs in recent years. As a consequence, the behavioral approach now is integrated into most programs for weight loss.

Because "behavior modification" is practiced so widely, there is a tendency to believe that it consists of little more than a series of techniques or tricks such as record keeping and slowing eating, and that programs do not vary much in how it is employed. This is mistaken. A modern day, comprehensive program is sophisticated and involves systematic work, not only on eating behavior, but on exercise, attitudes, social relationships, nutrition, and other factors.

The better behavioral programs now are producing weight losses in the range of 25 to 30 lb. The greatest strength of the behavioral approach, however, lies in the maintenance of weight loss. This is an area where exciting developments are occurring. These developments are important, not only to clinicians and programs using behavior modification per se, but to professionals using nearly any approach to weight loss where the maintenance of loss is an issue. The horizon holds much promise for the potential of behavioral approaches, used alone or in combination with other treatments for obesity.

SOURCE:
Brownell, Kelly D., and F. Matthew Kramer. "Behavioral Management of Obesity." *Medical Clinics of North America* 73, no. 1 (January 1989): 185, 199.

SURGICAL INTERVENTION

Intractable morbid obesity is diagnosed if the patient fails to respond to medically supervised conservative treatment. These patients have been unable to reduce their body weight by one-third or their body fat by one-half, and they may not be able to maintain any weight loss that has been achieved. It is inappropriate for the nutritional team to allow the patient to fall into the pattern of weight cycling, and such patients should be considered for surgery. A safe surgical procedure with low morbidity and mortality now exists for these patients, but a careful assessment must still be completed.

Patients with intractable morbid obesity, with few exceptions, are candidates for surgery. The issue of age is important in patient selection. These patients are usually in their thirties and have attempted conservative therapy over 5 to 10 years. Older patients are usually considered for surgery, particularly to reduce the comorbidity of the disease. The strongest indication is in patients older than 50 years of age who suffer degenerative arthritis; often the weight loss after surgery is sufficient to permit these patients to be candidates for joint prostheses, and experienced teams have operated on patients up to age 64 primarily for this reason. . . .

The surgery itself is designed to alter the gastrointestinal tract mechanically in a reversible manner and in such a way that the morbidly obese patient will lose weight and maintain the weight loss. Presently, gastric restrictive operations are the only well-accepted operations for the control of obesity. These operations produce a small pouch with a limited outlet, which results in early pouch filling after eating and, hence, early satiety.

In this operation [gastric bypass procedure], the stomach is reduced in size by applying four rows of stainless steel staples across the top of the stomach. An opening is made in the upper pouch of the stomach, and a portion of the small intestine is attached to this opening. Since food passes through the entire bowel, which allows complete digestion of nutrients, diarrhea should not occur.

An alternative procedure [is] vertical banded gastroplasty. As with the gastric bypass, the stomach is reduced in size by use of four rows of staples. The outlet of the upper pouch is made in such a manner that it empties into the rest of the stomach; the small intestine is not used in the surgical procedure at all. The stomach opening is then banded by a piece of mesh to prevent it from enlarging during the years after surgery.

Patients will often test their new stomach by experimenting with excessive eating; this should be prevented by a careful postoperative feeding regimen. Excessive eating following the gastroplasty leads to bloating of the pouch and nausea and vomiting. If the wrong foods are eaten, the pouch can become blocked and produce the same symptoms. In gastric bypass patients, these problems may be accompanied by a "dumping syndrome" as well. In this situation, excessive food or the wrong types of food, such as those rich in carbohydrates, produces an osmotic distension of the intestine attached to the pouch. The resultant symptoms include a fast heart rate, sweating and abdominal pain. Because these negative experiences enhance motivation of the patient to make the right behavioral changes, gastric bypass patients often achieve an additional 20-pound weight loss.

Obesity treatment does not end with the completion of the surgery. Major alterations in eating behavior are required, and the medical team must continue to support each patient throughout the postoperative period.

SOURCE:
Forse, Armour, Peter N. Benotti, and George Blackburn. "Morbid Obesity: Weighing the Treatment Options." *Nutrition Today* 24 (September-October 1989): 14, 15.

RESOURCES

ORGANIZATIONS

American Dietetic Association. 208 S. LaSalle St., Suite 1100, Chicago, IL 60604.

American Society of Bariatric Physicians. 5600 S. Quebec, Suite 310B, Englewood, CO 80111.

Overeaters Anonymous. P.O. Box 92870, Los Angeles, CA 90009.

RELATED ARTICLES

Holmes, Michelle D., Bernice Zysow, and Thomas L. Delbanco. "An Analytic Review of Current Therapies for Obesity." *The Journal of Family Practice* 28, no. 5 (May 1989): 610–616.

Keesey, Richard E. "The Body-Weight Set Point: What Can You Tell Your Patients?" *Postgraduate Medicine* 83, no. 6 (May 1, 1988): 114–118, 121–122, 127.

Leary, Warren E. "U.S. Panel Endorses Bypass Surgery for Obesity." *The New York Times* (March 28, 1991): B7.

Shepherd, Steven. "Bariatric Surgery . . . The Best Treatment Today for Extreme Obesity." *Executive Health Report* 24 (April 1988): 7.

OBSESSIVE-COMPULSIVE DISORDER

OVERVIEW

In the mental illness called obsessive-compulsive disorder (OCD), a person becomes trapped in a pattern of repetitive thoughts and behaviors that are senseless and distressing but extremely difficult to overcome. The following are typical examples of OCD:

Troubled by repeated thoughts that she may have contaminated herself by touching doorknobs and other "dirty" objects, a teenage girl spends hours every day washing her hands. Her hands are red and raw, and she has little time for social activities.

A middle-aged man is tormented by the notion that he may injure others through carelessness. He has difficulty leaving his home because he must first go through a lengthy ritual of checking and rechecking the gas jets and water faucets to make certain that they are turned off.

Several times a day, a young mother is seized by the fearful thought that she is going to harm her child. However hard she tries, she cannot get rid of this painful and worrisome idea. She even refuses to touch the kitchen knives and other sharp objects because she is afraid that she may use them as weapons.

If OCD becomes severe enough, it can destroy a person's capacity to function in the home, at work, or at school. That is why it is important to learn about the disorder and the treatments that are now available.

SOURCE:
National Institute of Mental Health. *Obsessive-Compulsive Disorder.* DHHS Pub. No. (ADM) 91-1597. 1991, 2.

KEY FEATURES OF OCD

Obsessions

These are unwanted ideas or impulses that repeatedly well up in the mind of the person with OCD. Again and again, the individual experiences a disturbing thought, such as, "My hands may be contaminated—I must wash them"; "I may have left the gas on"; or "I am going to injure my child." These thoughts are felt to be intrusive and unpleasant. They produce anxiety.

Compulsions

To deal with their anxiety, most people with OCD resort to repetitive behaviors called compulsions. The most common of these are washing and checking, as in the first two previous examples. Other compulsive behaviors include counting (often while performing another compulsive action such as hand washing) and endlessly rearranging objects in an effort to keep them in perfect alignment or symmetry with each other. These behaviors generally are intended to ward off harm to the person with OCD or others. They are usually quite stereotyped, with little variation from one time to the next, and are often referred to as rituals. Performing these rituals may give the person with OCD some relief from anxiety, but it is only temporary.

Insight

People with OCD generally have considerable insight into their own problems. Most of the time, they know that their obsessive thoughts are senseless or exaggerated, and that their compulsive behaviors are not really necessary. however, this knowledge is not sufficient to enable them to break free from their illness.

Resistance

Most people with OCD struggle to banish their unwanted, obsessive thoughts and to prevent themselves from engaging in compulsive behaviors. Many are able to keep their obsessive-compulsive symptoms under control during the hours when they are at work or attending school. But over the months or years, resistance may weaken, and when this happens, OCD may become so severe that time-consuming rituals take over the person's life and make it impossible for him or her to continue activities outside the home.

Shame and Secrecy

People with OCD generally attempt to hide their problem rather than seek help. Often they are remarkably successful in concealing their obsessive-compulsive symptoms from friends and coworkers. An unfortunate consequence of this secrecy is that people with OCD usually do not receive professional help until years after the onset of their disease. By that time, obsessive-compulsive habits may be deeply ingrained and very difficult to change.

Interference

A person is not considered to have OCD unless the obsessive and compulsive behaviors are extreme enough to interfere with everyday life. People with OCD should not be confused with a much larger group of individuals who are sometimes called "compulsive" because they hold themselves to a high standard of performance in their work and even in recreational activities. This type of "compulsiveness" often serves a valuable purpose, contributing to a person's self-esteem and success on the job. In that respect, it differs from the life-wrecking obsessions and rituals of the person with OCD.

Long-Lasting Symptoms

OCD tends to last for years, even decades. The symptoms may become less severe from time to time, and there may be long intervals when the symptoms are mild, but generally OCD is a chronic disease.

SOURCE:

National Institute of Mental Health. *Obsessive-Compulsive Disorder.* DHHS Pub. No. (ADM) 91-1597. 1991. pp. 3-5.

BEHAVIOR THERAPY

There is little evidence that psychodynamic psychotherapy is effective in patients with obsessive-compulsive disorder. On the contrary, the symptoms of many patients with the disorder fail to resolve with insight-oriented psychotherapy. While psychotherapy may be useful for other problems in patients with obsessive-compulsive disorder, it cannot be recommended as a primary treatment for obsessive-compulsive disorder itself.

Behavior therapy, on the other hand, is of proven benefit in obsessive-compulsive disorder. Improvement of symptoms has been shown to persist over time, with a parallel improvement in depressive symptoms and overall functioning in family and work settings. Treatment consists of exposure and response prevention, directed primarily toward the patient's compulsions, since it is more difficult to gain access to a patient's obsessions. . . .

Behavior therapy is generally considered the treatment of first choice, because it has been shown to be at least as effective as psychopharmacologic interventions in reducing the symptoms of obsessive-compulsive disorder. However, as many as 15 percent of patients refuse behavior therapy, and another 10 percent are unable to comply with the suggested regimen for exposure and response prevention. A number of patients simply do not improve, despite a high level of compliance. A few patients also have severe depressive symptoms that warrant drug therapy. These facts, as well as the occasional unavailability of behavior therapy and its time-consuming nature, make drug therapy an attractive option for many patients.

SOURCE:

March, John S., Hugh Johnston, and others. "Obsessive-Compulsive Disorder." *American Family Physician* 39, no. 5 (May 1989): 179-180.

DRUG THERAPY

FDA has approved the prescription drug clomipramine for the treatment of severe obsessive-compulsive disorder.

People with this disorder have recurrent ideas, thoughts, images, or impulses that they know are irrational but cannot control. They also engage in repetitive actions such as excessive hand-washing, which they also recognize as irrational.

Psychotherapy, behavior therapy, and various drugs have been used to treat obsessive-compulsive disorder without much success. Clomipramine is the first substantially effective drug treatment.

The drug's most serious side effect is seizure, which may occur in about 1.5 percent of treated patients each year. Other possible side effects include dry mouth, constipation, increased appetite, decreased sex drive, ejaculation failure, and impotence.

The drug is manufactured by Ciba-Geigy Pharmaceuticals of Summit, NJ, and will be marketed under the trade name Anafranil.

SOURCE:

"Drug Approved for Psychiatric Disorder." *FDA Consumer* (March 1990): 5.

OBSESSIVE-COMPULSIVE DISORDER IN CHILDREN

Over the years it has become apparent that children suffer from many of the same psychological disorders as adults. And now, obsessive-compulsive behavior disorders will have to be added to an already long list.

Dr. Henrietta Leonard discussed this disorder at a recent pediatric symposium. Obsessive-compulsive behavior is more distressing because it can significantly interfere with children's lives. The most commonly encountered symptoms include excessive hand washing, grooming and bathing. Some children are compelled to enter and exit a doorway the same number of times. This may not seem a problem if it is only once or twice, but what happens if it's 15–20 times? Other children will always do tasks in groups of five, ten or fifteen. Others become hoarders, collecting nothing but garbage.

This is the type of behavior that might be picked up by a daycare provider who has the opportunity to observe the child over a long period of time in a variety of both normal, everyday situations, and socially stressful ones as well. This type of stress might even help elicit some of this unusual behavior. Observations like this made by someone who knows the child well is invaluable.

The disorder tends to run in families and can become debilitating. Recurrent non-functional behavior can overwhelm a child's ability to lead a normal life. Fortunately most of these youngsters can be successfully treated with either behavior modification or medication.

SOURCE:
"Obsessive-Compulsive Children." *Parents' Pediatric Report* 7, no. 5 (June 1990): 36.

RESOURCES

ORGANIZATION
OCD Foundation Inc. P.O. Box 9573, New Haven, CT 06535.

BOOKS
Barlow, D. H. *Anxiety and Its Disorders*. New York: Guilford Press, 1988.

Insel, T. R. (ed.). *New Findings in Obsessive Compulsive Disorders*. Washington: American Psychiatric Press, 1984.

Rapoport, J. L. *The Boy Who Couldn't Stop Washing*. New York: Dutton, 1989.

RELATED ARTICLES
Greist, John H., Rapoport, Judith L., and others. "Spotting the Obsessive-Compulsive." *Patient Care* 24 (May 15, 1990): 47–61.

Greist, John H. "Treatment of Obsessive Compulsive Disorder: Psychotherapies, Drugs, and Other Somatic Treatment." *Journal of Clinical Psychiatry* 51 (8 suppl.) (August 1990): 44–50.

Jenike, Michael A. "Approaches to the Patient with Treatment-Refractory Obsessive Compulsive Disorder." *Journal of Clinical Psychiatry* 51 (2 suppl.) (February 1990): 15–21.

Jenike, Michael. "Obsessive-Compulsive Disorder." *Harvard Medical School Health Letter* 15, no. 6 (April 1990): 4–7.

Leonard, Henrietta L., and others. "Childhood Rituals: Normal Development or Obsessive-Compulsive Symptoms?" *Journal of the American Academy of Child and Adolescent Psychiatry* 29 (January 1990): 17–23.

Thoren, Peter, Marie Asberg, and others. "Clomipramine Treatment of Obsessive-Compulsive Disorder." *Archives of General Psychiatry* 37 (November 1980): 1281–1285.

Zohar, Joseph and Thomas R. Insel. "Diagnosis and Treatment of Obsessive-Compulsive Disorder." *Psychiatric Annals* 18, no. 3 (March 1988): 168–171.

ORGAN TRANSPLANTS

OVERVIEW

The first successful human transplant operation, of a single kidney, was performed between identical twins in Boston in 1953. It was followed by several failures, notably a wave of human heart transplants in the late 1960's. But subsequent improvement in understanding the immune system and development of new drugs to ward off rejection of donated tissues have made organ transplantation one of the most spectacular medical advances in decades. Now more than 250 teams transplant single organs in the United States with overall one-year success rates for grafts that range from about 85 percent for hearts to 77 percent for kidneys to about 60 percent for pancreases and livers, according to the United Network for Organ Sharing, which keeps a registry. But the rates for each type of organ transplant vary widely among medical centers.

The first multiple organ transplant operations—pancreas-kidney and heart-lung combinations—were done in the mid-1960s. They failed, and a moratorium was declared. But multiple-organ transplants have made an astonishing comeback this decade after the introduction of the drug cyclosporine, which prevents the body from rejecting the new organs.

The number of multiple-organ transplant operations is just a thin fraction of the estimated 13,000 transplant operations to be done in the United States this year.

The survival rates for multiple-organ transplants are generally a few percentage points lower than for a single organ, but the figures depend on the surgical team. Only a small fraction of the 250 teams are qualified to do multiple-organ transplants.

The earliest and still most common multiple-organ transplants are those given to patients with kidney failure from type 1 or juvenile diabetes. More than 1,800 operations involving pancreas-kidney-duodenum combinations have been done since the first one in 1966.

SOURCE:

Altman, Lawrence K. "With New Boldness, Surgeons Create Patchwork Patients." *New York Times* (December 12, 1989): 21.

ORGAN TRANSPLANTS AND THE IMMUNE SYSTEM

The major challenge to organ transplantation is rejection by the body's immune system. Programmed to defend your body against disease-causing bacteria, viruses and fungi, your immune system also regards the cells of transplanted tissue as foreign.

If you were to have a transplant and preventive steps were not taken, your immune system immediately would set out to destroy the new tissue by activating release of white blood cells called T lymphocytes. If unchecked, T cells would attack and eventually destroy the transplanted organ. For this reason, preventive measures are routinely administered.

Kidney, heart, lung, liver, pancreas and allogenic skin transplants are particularly vulnerable to rejection. The cornea and bone usually are less susceptible to rejection. Because bone marrow contains its own T cells, it is unique in its ability to identify the recipient's tissues as "foreign," leading to what specialists in blood disorders call a graft vs. host disease (GVHD).

To minimize rejection and the eventual destruction of transplanted tissue, doctors use these techniques:

- **Cross-matching blood**—Your immune system regards proteins in your blood as foreign only if they differ from your own proteins. By matching the recipient's and donor's ABO blood types, doctors greatly increase chances for acceptance of the organ.

- **Tissue typing**—If you need an organ transplant, the ideal donor is your identical twin. That's because identical twins have identical blood proteins. To further enhance compatibility, doctors match another protein in the blood. This protein is called the human leukocyte antigen (HLA) system.

Because most transplant candidates don't have an identical twin, doctors use the HLA system to judge whether there's a good match between donor and recipient. The more compatible HLA antigens are between donor and recipient, the less chance for rejection.

Among brothers and sisters, about one in four inherit identical HLA proteins, making a brother or sister the next best match if there's no identical twin. Two out of four brothers and sisters share half their HLA antigens; one in four are completely mismatched.

- **Immune-suppressing therapy**—Before operating, physicians use a variety of drugs and techniques to suppress the immune response and thus prepare the individual for surgery. Because every approach weakens the body's normal defense against illness, doctors must strike a delicate balance between preventing rejection and allowing a fatal infection.

During the past decade, an anti-rejection drug called cyclosporine has gained wide acceptance. Unlike other drugs, it has a more focused impact on the immune system.

Another family of drugs, called corticosteroids, also helps prevent rejection. Prednisone, for example, is widely prescribed for this purpose. These drugs are most commonly used to treat episodes of acute rejection.

SOURCE:

"Organ Transplantation: The Gift of New Life. Part I." *Mayo Clinic Health Letter: Medical Essay.* (November 1990): 3-4.

HEART TRANSPLANTATION

Heart transplantation has been performed for more than 20 years with increasing success. It is now performed in many hospitals all over the world.

Heart transplantation is not a solution to all heart problems. In fact, it is suitable for only a few persons with only certain kinds of heart disease. The usual profile for a candidate for heart transplantation is age under 55 to 60 years, psychologically stable, and surrounded by a supportive family. All of the other vital organs must be in excellent health, particularly the kidneys, liver, and lungs. Transplantation may be appropriate for people with heart failure and certain diseases of the heart that are serious enough that life expectancy is decreased to less than 2 to 3 years.

Before the operation, a donor heart must be found. Most often, this heart comes from the body of a healthy person who died in an accident but did not sustain heart injuries.

The donated heart generally is brought to the recipient, transported in a special solution. The recipient's chest cavity is opened and the diseased heart is removed; then, the new organ is put in place. During this portion of the procedure, the pumping of oxygenated blood to the body is taken over by a heart-lung machine, as is done routinely in many kinds of heart surgery.

All transplanted organs are susceptible to rejection. The body's immune system recognizes the transplanted tissue as foreign and produces antibodies to attack the "intruder."

In order to minimize the risk of rejection of a transplanted heart, you will be given drugs that suppress your body's normal immune response. Some of these "immunosuppressive drugs" will be used for a short term and will be discontinued shortly after the operation. You must take others for the rest of your life. These drugs have side effects; they decrease your body's ability to recognize and resist infectious disease. Therefore, dosages must be adjusted carefully.

Most successful recipients of heart transplants seem to recover and to carry on relatively normal lives. Approximately 80 percent of those who have received heart transplants are alive and active 1 year after the operation; some have lived for more than a decade.

Heart transplantation remains a complicated procedure. For success, this procedure requires a well-organized team of experienced transplantation specialists and a motivated recipient. If you have a transplant, you will continue to see members of the transplantation team for the rest of your life. They will carefully adjust medications and perform periodic heart biopsies to monitor rejection, and they will treat any complications.

Transplantation is most appropriate in those cases in which it is the only hope for survival and the possibility of success is high.

SOURCE:

Larson, David E. (ed.). *Mayo Clinic Family Health Book.* New York: William Morrow and Company, 1990. p. 833.

NEED FOR ORGAN DONORS

While technological advances have propelled transplantation forward at an impressive clip, the number of organ donors has remained static. In fact, the ever-increasing shortfall of donated organs has become the major limitation in organ transplantation.

Hospitals are required to request organ donation from the next-of-kin when someone dies. Even if the potential donor carried a donor card, the law requires that a family member must consent to the donation. Failure of many families to consent—and, in some cases, failure of hospital personnel to ask—contributes to the organ shortage.

Though highly controversial, a possible scenario in the not-too-distant future is establishment of financial incentives for family consent. One proposal suggests that the next-of-kin who consents to organ donation be paid in the form of a federally funded life insurance policy. Other proposals involve federal grants for free burial and breaks on estate taxes.

While government officials study various strategies to increase the number of donated organs, a national computer registry ensures the best use of those that are available. Everyone awaiting a transplant is registered in the system, which is operated by the United Network for Organ Sharing (UNOS). When a donor is identified, hospital staff immediately communicate specific information about the donor to the UNOS Organ Center. Using the computer registry, the center identifies potential recipients.

The most important criterion in selecting a recipient is match. The tissue of the donor and recipient must be as similar as possible. Medical urgency, genetic compatibility, logistics and time on the waiting list are other factors that are considered.

SOURCE:

"Organ Transplants: From Science Fiction to Mainstream Medicine." *The University of Texas Lifetime Health Letter* 3, no. 7 (July 1991): 6.

RESOURCES

ORGANIZATIONS

National Bone Marrow Donor Registry. St. Paul Red Cross, 100 S. Robert Street, St. Paul, MN 55107.

Pittsburgh Transplant Foundation. 5743 Center Ave., Pittsburgh, PA 15206.

United Network for Organ Sharing. 3001 Hungary Spring Rd., P.O. Box 20810, Richmond, VA 23228.

PAMPHLETS

American Liver Foundation:

Facts on Liver Transplantation. n.d. 6 pp.

Leukemia Society of America:

Bone Marrow Transplantation: Questions & Answers. 1987. 12 pp.

National Cancer Institute:

Bone Marrow Transplantation: Research Report. NIH Pub. No. 90-1178. August 1989. 27 pp.

RELATED ARTICLES

Kirkpatrick, Charles H. "Transplantation Immunology." *JAMA* 258, no. 20 (November 27, 1987): 2993-3000.

"Organ Transplantation: The Gift of New Life. Part II." *Mayo Clinic Health Letter: Medical Essay* (January 1991): 1-7.

Salvatierra, Oscar, Jr. "Optimal Use of Organs for Transplantation." *New England Journal of Medicine* 318, no. 20 (May 19, 1988): 1329-1331.

Starzl, Thomas E., and John J. Fung. "Transplantation." *JAMA* 263 (May 16, 1990): 2686-2687.

OSTEOPOROSIS

(*See also:* ESTROGEN REPLACEMENT THERAPY; MENOPAUSE)

OVERVIEW

Osteoporosis literally means "porous bone." While the outer form of the bones does not change (unless there is a fracture), the bones have less substance and so are less dense. Osteoporosis is a common condition, affecting as many as 15 to 20 million individuals in the United States. It has been estimated to lead to 1.3 million bone fractures a year in people over 45 years of age, which is about 70 percent of all fractures occurring in this age group. Looked at in another way, each year about 1.7 percent of Americans between 45 and 64 years old and 2 percent of those age 65 and older break a bone because of osteoporosis.

In osteoporosis bone mass decreases, causing bones to be more susceptible to fracture. A fall, blow, or lifting action that would not normally bruise or strain the average person can easily break one or more bones in someone with severe osteoporosis.

The spine, wrist, and hip are the most common sites of osteoporosis-related fractures, although the disease is generalized, that is, it can affect any bone of the body.

When the bones of the spinal column (the vertebrae) are weakened, a simple action like bending forward to make a bed or lifting a heavy roast pan out of the oven can be enough to cause a "crush fracture," or "spinal compression fracture." These vertebral crush fractures often cause back pain, decreased height, and a humped back or a "dowager's hump."

The occurrence of osteoporosis of the spine increases with age. One recent study of a group of about 2,000 women showed x-ray evidence of osteoporosis in the spine in about 29 percent of those age 45 and 54 years, 61 percent of those age 55 to 64, and 79 percent of those age 65 and older. Vertebral crush fractures are more common in women than men and generally occur in women between 55 and 75 years of age.

Wrist fractures also occur commonly among people with this disorder. For example, an otherwise healthy, vigorous woman in her fifties or sixties slips on ice, falls, reaches out to catch herself, and is taken to the emergency room with a broken wrist.

Osteoporosis is often the underlying cause of the broken hips suffered by more than 200,000 Americans over age 45 each year. A fall from a standing position can fracture a hip weakened by osteoporosis. In cases of severe osteoporosis, a change of posture or weight distribution alone can actually break the hip, and the fracture then causes a fall.

People who have hip fractures due to osteoporosis are generally older than people who suffer spinal fractures. There is more even distribution between women and men than with vertebral fractures, the rates for hip fractures being two to three times higher in women than in men.

A number of risk factors for osteoporosis have been identified. These include:

- **Being a woman.** Osteoporosis—as evidenced by vertebral fractures—is estimated to be six to eight times more common in women than in men, partly because women have less bone mass to begin with. Furthermore, for several years after menopause, women also lose bone much more rapidly than men do, due to a fall in their bodies' production of estrogen.
- **Early menopause.** This is one of the strong predictors for the development of osteoporosis, especially if menopause is induced by surgery or other means that remove both ovaries or cause a sufficient drop in estrogen. Many experts define "early" menopause as menopause occurring before the age of 45.

- **Being white, that is, Caucasian.** White women are at higher risk than black women, and white men are at higher risk than black men. Some experts estimate that by age 65 a quarter of all white women have had one or more fractures related to osteoporosis. Oriental women are also thought to be at greater risk for the disease, but there are not enough data to confirm this.
- **A chronically low calcium intake.**
- **Lack of physical activity.** However, exercising at an extreme level that halts menstruation in a young woman also may lead to bone loss.
- **Being underweight.** (This is not to suggest that being overweight is a good idea. Both overweight and underweight people are better off trying to attain their desirable weight.)

SOURCE:
National Institute of Arthritis and Musculoskeletal and Skin Diseases. *Osteoporosis: Cause, Treatment, Prevention.* NIH Pub. No. 86-2226. 1986. pp. 4-7.

PREVENTION AND TREATMENT

The FDA Working Group on Osteoporosis identified nutrition and exercise as two of the key areas related to osteoporosis prevention. Osteoporosis is a multi-factorial disorder. Important non-dietary factors influence the risk for osteoporosis, including a person's age, sex, race, physical activity, stature, & hormonal status; but, nutrition and exercise are the only factors that can be controlled by the individual. More than any of the other measures that can be taken to reduce the risk of osteoporosis, nutrition and exercise have received considerable media and consumer attention, and have been touted too often as singular and simplistic solutions to prevent fractures by building bone mass and stopping bone loss.

The prevention of osteoporosis in women at risk for this condition is a lifetime process. At different phases of her life, a woman will use different strategies to build bone mass and stop bone loss. Women and their physicians should work together to decide whether a woman is at risk for osteoporosis, what strategies are needed to reduce the risk of osteoporosis and the appropriate ages for using these strategies, and what types of monitoring and follow-up are needed to judge the effectiveness of prevention strategies. Nutrition and exercise are two factors that women can control as they attempt to prevent osteoporosis.

Nutrition as a strategy for preventing osteoporosis is primarily related to adequate calcium intake during active bone-forming years (approximately 10 to 35 years of age). Evaluating the calcium adequacy of the diet requires women to take an active role in becoming informed about sources of calcium, and ultimately in changing their diet to increase the level of calcium intake. It also requires women to become knowledgeable about the interaction between other nutrients and calcium (i.e., the "calcium depleters") and the limits of preventing osteoporosis through calcium intake. Women do have an active role to play in controlling the nutrition factor related to osteoporosis prevention. The most effective role will be played by women who work with their health care provider to develop a strategy that will work within the context of their individual lifestyles.

Exercise is another factor related to osteoporosis prevention that women should know about, particularly the role exercise can play in the prevention of osteoporosis, and the types of exercises women at risk for osteoporosis should pursue. . . .

- Surveys indicate that a majority of women in the United States do not achieve a dietary intake of even 800 mg of calcium per day from food sources.
- Adults normally adapt to low calcium intake mainly by increasing the fraction of dietary calcium absorbed, but adaptation is impaired by menopause and by the aging process.
- A daily intake of 1,000 mg of calcium per day is considered a desirable goal. This level of calcium intake can be achieved by dietary means alone, preferably from a diet that includes three servings of dairy products (preferably low-fat).
- Children, adolescents, pregnant women, and individuals with osteoporosis or judged to be at increased risk of osteoporosis should consume from 1,200 to 1,500 mg of calcium per day.
- Calcium supplements may be useful for individuals who cannot tolerate milk products, but education is needed on appropriate use of calcium supplements, side effects, forms in which they are best absorbed, and interactions with other medications. . . .

The following are the primary health messages related to drug therapy for the prevention and treatment of postmenopausal osteoporosis:

- Women and their physicians are faced with the dilemma of using estrogen alone to prevent osteoporosis but increasing the risk of endometrial cancer, or combining estrogen and progestin to reduce this risk, but in turn, possibly blunting the protective effect of estrogens on heart disease. These benefits and risks need to be further evaluated before arriving at definitive recommendations for treating women with hormone replacement therapy.
- Under certain conditions, estrogen replacement therapy is of established benefit in preventing postmenopausal bone loss.
- Soon after menopause, estrogen deficiency induces a transient phase of accelerated bone loss that calcium cannot be expected to correct.
- Effectiveness of estrogen therapy is greatest when started near menopause, but continues up to 65 or 70 years of age.
- Estrogen replacement therapy may be associated with an increased risk of endometrial cancer.

- The majority of available studies do not suggest an association of estrogen therapy and breast cancer at any time. The evidence of this association is less clear after 20 years of estrogen use.
- Combining progestin with estrogen replacement therapy reduces the risk of endometrial cancer.
- The majority of evidence suggests that estrogen use has a protective effect against cardiovascular disease, but this is probably blunted by the concomitant use of progestin.
- Because of this effect on cardiovascular disease, overall mortality is decreased in women on estrogen therapy, even though the incidence of endometrial cancer is increased.
- Patient compliance is an important factor in long-term estrogen therapy. Educating women on the benefits of hormonal therapy on bone mass content, and documenting these changes, along with changes in life-style and exercise regimens, may make a positive impact on the health of climacteric women and their environment.

SOURCE:
"Proceedings of the National Conference on Women's Health. Series: Special Topic Conference on Osteoporosis. Oct 30, 1987." *Public Health Reports* (September-October 1989): supp.: 2-4.

TREATMENT

The most successful therapies for preventing osteoporosis have been those that are anti-resorptive. Hormone replacement prevents bone loss, and hence osteoporotic fracture, in the long-term. There are many other benefits of this therapy and it is suitable for most women. However, the addition of a progestagen (given for a minimum of 12 days each month) to the continuous oestrogen treatment is mandatory in women who have not had a hysterectomy to prevent endometrial hyperplasia. This treatment usually results in a regular withdrawal bleed, which becomes less well tolerated with increasing age. Some women—e.g., those with hormone-sensitive tumours—are unable to receive hormone replacement.

Prevention of bone loss is most effective in the earliest stages of osteoporosis, before perforation and removal of trabecular elements lead to irreversible destruction of bone microstructure, but it is still important to arrest further loss even in patients with established osteoporosis to reduce the risk of further fractures. Calcitonin is effective in the prevention and treatment of osteoporosis but has to be administered by subcutaneous injection, which makes its widespread use impractical. When nasal spray preparations become generally available they will form a realistic treatment strategy.

Bisphosphonates are another class of antiresorptive agents. They are widely used in the treatment of Paget's disease, and are very successful in the management of malignant hypercalcaemia. These drugs, which can be administered orally, are now being tried for the prevention and treatment of osteoporosis and appear to be effective. Endronate disodium, a widely available bisphosphonate, has now been studied in a double-blind, placebo-controlled trial in women with postmenopausal osteoporosis. Cyclical etidronate was given orally in a dose of 400 mg daily—two weeks' treatment was repeated every 3 months over 3 years. Therapy resulted in a modest increase in vertebral bone density which, most importantly, led to a significant reduction in new fractures compared with the control group.

Another approach is to stimulate new bone formation. Sodium fluoride is the best established agent in this respect, and preliminary trials with this drug have been encouraging. Fluoride causes a sustained increase in bone density, but there are some important drawbacks to this therapy. Significant proportions of patients either do not respond to the treatment or get side-effects, including gastrointestinal bleeding, lower limb pain, and the suggestion of an increase in the incidence of femoral neck fracture.

SOURCE:
"New Treatments for Osteoporosis." *The Lancet* 335, no. 8697 (May 5, 1990): 1065–1066.

OTHER POSSIBLE THERAPIES

In clinical studies, calcitonin, a thyroid hormone that inhibits the breakdown of bone, has been reported to reduce back pain from compression fractures; however, the hormone has not yet been proven to prevent fractures. With long-term use, some women develop antibodies to calcitonin, rendering the drug ineffective. FDA has approved an injectable form of calcitonin for treating osteoporosis. The effectiveness of a nasal spray version is being studied.

Researchers are also investigating several non-hormonal therapies. Currently, the most promising is etidronate, a drug used in treating Paget's disease of bone (a condition characterized by an excessive bone turnover that results in new bone being dense but fragile).

In a study by the Emory University School of Medicine in Atlanta, and reported in the July 1990 issue of *The New England Journal of Medicine,* 429 post-menopausal women who had suffered one to four spinal fractures took either a placebo or etidronate for 14 days, followed by calcium supplementation for 76 days (to match the body's 90-day bone turnover cycle). Etidronate slowed the loss of bone resorption while the calcium helped build bone mass, resulting in a 4 to 5 percent increase in spinal bone density. The women on the drug-and-supplement regimen also suffered less than half the vertebral fractures as the group receiving the placebo. On the minus side, the study found neither evidence of improved bone mass in the wrist and hip, nor any indication that fractures at those sites could be prevented.

Sodium fluoride, another experimental treatment for osteoporosis-related spinal fractures, increased bone mass but did not prevent fractures in a Mayo Clinic study of 202 women 50 to 75 years old, reported in *The New England Journal of Medicine* in March 1990. The group treated with a combination of sodium fluoride and calcium had a 35 percent increase in spinal bone density. The new bone was structurally abnormal and weak, however. The number of spinal fractures was not significantly different between the treated and placebo groups. Furthermore, the treated group sustained more broken hips.

SOURCE:

Papazian, Ruth. "Osteoporosis Treatment Advances." *FDA Consumer* 25, no. 3 (April 1991): 32.

RESOURCES

ORGANIZATIONS

FDA Women's Health Initiative. Office of Consumer Affairs, Food and Drug Administration, Rockville, Maryland 20857.

National Institute of Arthritis and Musculoskeletal and Skin Diseases. National Institutes of Health, Bethesda, Maryland 20205.

National Institute of Diabetes and Digestive and Kidney Diseases. National Institutes of Health, Bethesda, Maryland 20205.

National Institute on Aging. National Institutes of Health, Bethesda, Maryland 20205.

National Osteoporosis Foundation. 1625 Eye Street NW, Washington, DC 20006.

Office of Disease Prevention and Health Promotion. U.S. Public Health Service, Washington, DC 20201.

PAMPHLETS

American Academy of Orthopaedic Surgeons:

Osteoporosis.

American College of Obstetricians and Gynecologists:

Preventing Osteoporosis.

Food and Drug Administration, Office of Consumer Affairs:

Here are Some Things You Should Know about Prescription Drugs.

Osteoporosis, Calcium and Estrogens.

Please Pass that Woman Some More Calcium and Iron.

National Institute of Aging:

The Menopause Time of Life.

Osteporosis: The Bone Thinner.

National Institute of Arthritis and Musculoskeletal and Skin Diseases, National Institutes of Health:

Osteoporosis: Cause, Treatment, Prevention.

Weldon, Barbara. *Osteoporosis: A Growing National Problem.*

National Institutes of Health, Office of Medical Applications of Research:

Osteoporosis. 1984.

National Osteoporosis Foundation:

Osteoporosis: A Woman's Guide.

BOOKS

McIlwain, Harris H., and others. *Osteoporosis: Prevention, Management, Treatment.* New York: Wiley, 1988.

Peck, William A., and Louis V. Avidi. *Osteoporosis: The Silent Thief.* Glenview, IL: Scott, Foresman, 1988.

RELATED ARTICLES

"Better Prognosis for Osteoporosis." *Johns Hopkins Medical Letter* 2, no. 7 (September 1990): 1–2.

"Consensus Development Conference: Prophylaxis and Treatment of Osteoporosis." *The American Journal of Medicine* 90 (January 1991): 107–110.

"Important New Advance in Osteoporosis Treatment." *Medical Update* 14, no. 4 (October 1990): 1–2.

Lindsay R. "Osteoporosis: An Updated Approach to Prevention and Management." *Geriatrics* 44, no. 1 (January 1989): 45–54.

"Osteoporosis." *Mayo Clinic Health Letter* 8 (May 1990): 5–6.

Papazian, Ruth. "Osteoporosis Treatment Advances." *FDA Consumer* (April 1991): 29–32.

Thorneycroft, I. H. "The Role of Estrogen Replacement Therapy in the Prevention of Osteoporosis." *American Journal of Obstetrics and Gynecology* 160, no. 3, part 2 (May 1989): 1306–1310.

Walden, O. "The Relationship of Dietary and Supplemental Calcium Intake to Bone Loss and Osteoporosis." *New England Journal of Medicine* 89, no. 3 (March 1989): 397–400.

Watts, N. B. "Osteoporosis." *American Family Physician* 38, no. 5 (November 1988): 193–207.

Watts, N. B., S. T. Harris, and others. "Intermittent Cyclical Etidronate Treatment of Postmenopausal Osteoporosis." *New England Journal of Medicine* 323, no. 2 (July 12, 1990): 73–79.

Weinerman, S. A., and R. S. Bockman. "Medical Therapy of Osteoporosis." *Orthopedic Clinics of North America* 21, no. 1 (January 1990): 109–124.

OVARIAN CANCER

OVERVIEW

Ovarian cancer is on the minds of a lot of women these days. It's the cancer that killed comedienne Gilda Radner at age 42, and in the ABC-TV series *thirtysomething*, one of the lead characters (Nancy Weston) battled the disease.

Though cancer specialists have made encouraging strides against many types of cancer, ovarian cancer remains a stubborn and worrisome affliction. Ovarian cancer strikes 20,500 American women each year—about one woman in 70 will develop the disease.

Progress against this deadly disease has been slow but not without a few bright spots. In the last decade, new chemotherapy regimens have improved the survival rates. And researchers are exploring the use of ultrasound as a means of detecting ovarian cancers early.

For now, awareness of risk factors and familiarity with some of the subtle symptoms that occasionally accompany ovarian cancer are a woman's best protection against the disease.

Most cases of ovarian cancer develop in postmenopausal women. Some research suggests that women who have not had children or those who have had only one pregnancy may be at somewhat higher risk.

A family history of ovarian cancer—specifically two or more blood relatives with the disease—also appears to increase the risk. According to the American Cancer Society, nuns, Jewish women and women who have never been married are more likely to develop ovarian cancer.

A personal history of breast, endometrial or colon cancer also increases the risk. However, prior use of oral contraceptives may offer some protection against the disease.

Unfortunately, ovarian cancer typically is symptom-free in its early stages. The abnormal cell growth occurs quietly and usually isn't detected until it has spread to other parts of the abdomen.

Nonetheless, some women with ovarian cancer recall experiencing vague digestive disturbances, such as abdominal discomfort, indigestion, bloating or gas, before their disease was diagnosed.

Although these aren't symptoms that would normally lead a woman to rush to the doctor's office, persistent, unexplained abdominal discomfort calls for a thorough gynecologic evaluation.

A reliable means of detecting ovarian cancer in its early stages has continued to elude cancer researchers.

"As yet, there really isn't a good diagnostic tool for ovarian cancer," says David Gershenson, M.D., professor and deputy chairman of gynecology at The University of Texas M.D. Anderson Cancer Center in Houston. "About 75% of ovarian cancers are diagnosed only after they've already spread well outside the ovary into the upper abdomen."

Finding a reliable diagnostic test is critical: Today, only one in three women with ovarian cancer survives five years or more. But the five-year survival rate jumps to 90% for women whose cancer is found early.

Some cancer researchers are optimistic about two potential screening methods: pelvic ultrasonography and a blood test that can detect the cancer-related protein CA 125.

Neither approach is currently recommended as a screening method for the general population. But the two techniques may one day be useful in monitoring women at high risk of developing the disease.

A British study published in late 1989 first indicated that abdominal ultrasound could detect cancerous tumors in their early stages. And a newer "transvaginal" technique, which uses a vaginal probe to create an image of the ovaries, may turn out to be even better. Studies examining the usefulness of transvaginal ultrasound as a screening device are now under way.

Measurement of the "tumor marker" CA 125 also has shown some promise. CA 125 has been used for years to monitor ovarian cancer patients' responses to treatment and as a means of detecting treatment relapses.

In recent studies, women without known disease have been tested for CA 125. Researchers are trying to determine whether a blood test for the tumor marker might be able to detect early cancers.

Thus far, study results indicate that CA 125 is not useful as a general screening method because unrelated gynecologic conditions also can cause CA 125 levels to rise. But some research suggests that for certain high-risk women, very high levels of the protein or a sudden upsurge in CA 125 can predict the presence of an ovarian cancer.

Patients with ovarian cancer typically undergo surgery to remove one or both ovaries. (In pre-menopausal women, a normal ovary may be spared). When the cancer has spread beyond the ovaries, the surgeon will attempt to remove as much of the tumor as possible from other areas of the body.

Surgery is followed by chemotherapy, most often with one of two potent drugs—cisplatin or carboplatin—and usually in tandem with a third drug, cyclophosphamide. Most doctors credit this combination drug therapy with improvements in survival rates during the last decade.

Researchers are experimenting with other new drugs, including a promising chemotherapeutic medication called Taxol. Some cancer specialists also are optimistic about the possible advantages of an alternative way of delivering drugs: filling the abdominal cavity with the medications rather than administering them intravenously. This technique may be particularly effective for patients who have only microscopic remnants of the disease after surgery.

As cancer researchers and patients continue to grapple with this difficult disease, women at risk of developing ovarian cancer can take a few precautions. All women over age 50 should have annual pelvic exams; more frequent exams may be in order for women with a mother or sisters with the disease.

Some doctors recommend even stronger action for women with a strong family history of ovarian cancer. These women, they advise, should consider having their ovaries removed if they have finished having children.

SOURCE:
"The Difficult Battle Against Ovarian Cancer." *The University of Texas Lifetime Health Letter* 3, no. 1 (January 1991): 3, 6.

TYPES OF OVARIAN CANCER

The most common form of ovarian cancer arises from the cells covering the surface of the ovary and is known as epithelial carcinoma. There are five major types of this carcinoma—serous, mucinous, endometrioid, clear cell and undifferentiated. Epithelial carcinomas are further divided into grades, according to how virulent they appear on microscopic examination.

Tumors of low malignant potential, also known as borderline tumors, are the most well-differentiated malignancy (Grade 0) and account for 15 percent of all epithelial carcinomas of the ovary. The other three grades are well-differentiated (Grade 1), moderately differentiated (Grade 2) and poorly differentiated (Grade 3). Well-differentiated tumors have a better prognosis than poorly differentiated tumors. Clear cell carcinoma and especially undifferentiated carcinoma have a poorer prognosis than the other cell types.

The two other major kinds of ovarian cancer—germ cell tumors, which arise from the eggs, and ovarian stromal tumors, which arise from supportive tissue—are relatively uncommon and account for less than 10 percent of all ovarian malignancies.

SOURCE:
Stern, Jeffrey L. "Ovary." In *Everyone's Guide to Cancer Therapy*. Kansas City: Andrews and McMeel, 1991. p. 456.

STAGING

Once ovarian cancer has been diagnosed, it is important to determine the extent (stage) of the disease. Staging is essential in selecting appropriate treatment and in determining prognosis. Accurate staging depends on the findings of the laparotomy, lymphangiography, IVP, barium enema, and other diagnostic procedures.

The most common staging system used in the United States was developed by the International Federation of Gynecology and Obstetrics. In this system, epithelial ovarian cancers, stromal tumors, and germ cell ovarian cancers are divided into four stages.

- **Stage I:** Cancer is limited to the ovaries. Stage IA: Cancer is limited to one ovary. There is no fluid in the abdomen, cancer is not found on the outer surface of the ovary, and the ovarian capsule is intact. Stage IB: Cancer is found in both ovaries. There is no fluid in the abdomen, no cancer is found on the outer surfaces of the ovaries, and the ovarian capsules are intact. Stage IC: The tumor involves one or both ovaries and displays one of the following characteristics: There is cancer on the outer surface of one or both ovaries, the capsule is ruptured, abdominal fluid is present, or the pelvic and abdominal washings contain cancer cells.
- **Stage II:** The cancer is found in one or both ovaries and has spread to the uterus, fallopian tubes, or other tissues in the pelvis. Stage IIA: Cancer has spread to the uterus and/or fallopian tubes. Stage IIB: Cancer

has spread to other pelvic tissues. Stage IIC: Cancer has spread to the pelvis and includes one of the following characteristics: There is cancer on the outer surface of one or both ovaries, the capsule has ruptured, abdominal fluid is present, or the abdominal washings contain cancer cells.

- **Stage III:** The cancer involves one or both ovaries and has spread to the lymph nodes in the abdomen or to the outer surface of other organs in the abdomen, such as the liver or intestine. Stage IIIA: Cancer is limited to the pelvis, and the lymph nodes are not involved, but there are microscopic deposits of cells on the outer surfaces of abdominal organs. Stage IIIB: Cancer is limited to the pelvis, and the lymph nodes are negative, but there is cancer on abdominal organs that is not larger than 2 centimeters (about 3/4 of an inch). Stage IIIC: The cancer that affects the abdomen is larger than 2 centimeters, and/or there are positive lymph nodes.
- **Stage IV:** The cancer involves one or both ovaries and has spread to the inside of the liver or other abdominal organs or to other organs outside the abdomen.

SOURCE:
National Cancer Institute. *Cancer of the Ovary: Research Report.* NIH Pub. No. 89-3014. 1989. pp. 8-9.

TREATMENT

Stage I. Surgical removal of the ovaries, fallopian tubes, and uterus is the usual treatment for patients with ovarian cancer in stages IA and IB. In some patients with stage IA ovarian cancer who still wish to have children, only the involved ovary and accompanying fallopian tube are removed. In patients with stage IC ovarian cancer, surgery may be followed by chemotherapy (usually a combination of cisplatin and cyclophosphamide) or intraperitoneal P32 radiation therapy.

Stage II. Treatment for stage II ovarian cancer involves total hysterectomy (removal of the uterus and cervix) with removal of both ovaries and fallopian tubes. Cancer that cannot be removed completely by surgery is called residual disease. Patients with a residual cancer less than 3/4 inch in diameter may also receive intraperitoneal P32 radiotherapy or external beam radiation to the pelvis and abdomen. Patients with residual disease larger than 3/4 inch are usually treated with chemotherapy. The most widely tested combination of drugs is CP (cyclophosphamide and cisplatin). Other combinations include:

- CAP: cyclophosphamide, doxorubicin, and cisplatin;
- CHAD: cyclophosphamide, hexamethylmelamine, doxorubicin, and cisplatin; and
- AP: doxorubicin and cisplatin.

Patients with stage II ovarian cancer are encouraged to participate in clinical trials of promising new treatments. For example, researchers are comparing the benefits of intraperitoneal radiotherapy to combination chemotherapy used in addition to surgery in patients with minimal residual disease. Studies also are under way to examine the effectiveness of intraperitoneal chemotherapy (drugs are placed directly into the abdominal cavity rather than injected into a vein).

SOURCE:
National Cancer Institute. *Cancer of the Ovary: Research Report.* NIH Pub. No. 89-3014. 1989. p. 11.

OVARIAN CANCER LINKED TO DAIRY PRODUCTS

A study suggests that some women eating yogurt and other dairy products may face an increased risk of ovarian cancer, adding another link between diet and malignancies. The surprising findings show elevated risk in women who may have inherited a flawed enzyme that poorly metabolizes a certain dairy sugar—a risk that grows with the amount of dairy products consumed. Researchers say the report is the first to associate dairy products with human ovarian cancer, which will strike an estimated 20,000 U.S. women in 1989.

"We hesitate to make broad public health recommendations on the basis of the first and only finding related to dairy products," says lead author Daniel W. Cramer of Brigham and Women's Hospital and Harvard Medical School in Boston. Cramer adds that if others confirm these results, avoiding dairy products may help prevent ovarian cancer, especially in women who inherit the flawed enzyme.

In the meantime, cancer experts say people should interpret the study with caution. "These results have to be validated by other studies before you can decide whether public health action should be taken," comments Lawrence Garfinkel of the American Cancer Society in New York City. "I don't think people should stop eating yogurt or cottage cheese because of this one study."

SOURCE:
Fackelmann, K. A. "Dairy Sugar Linked to Ovarian Cancer." *Science News* 136 (July 22, 1989): 52.

RESOURCES

PAMPHLETS
American Cancer Society:

Facts on Ovarian Cancer. 1988. 9 pp.

National Cancer Institute:

What You Need to Know about Ovarian Cancer. NIH Pub. No. 91-1561. May 1990. 24 pp.

RELATED ARTICLES
Berek, Jonathan S. "Adjuvant Therapy for Early-Stage Ovarian Cancer." *New England Journal of Medicine* 322 (April 12, 1990): 1076-1078.

Cramer, Daniel W., and others. "Galactose Consumption and Metabolism in Relation to the Risk of Ovarian Cancer. *The Lancet* 2 (July 8, 1989): 66–71.

"Ovarian Cancer, the Silent Stalker, Is Striking More Women." *Scripps Clinic Personal Health Letter* (January 1991): 5–7.

"Should You Be Screened for Ovarian Cancer?" *The Johns Hopkins Medical Letter, Health After 50* (November 1990): 7.

PACEMAKERS

OVERVIEW

Basically, your heart is a pump made of special muscle that pumps blood carrying oxygen and nourishment to all the cells of your body. This function is vital, because without a constant supply of oxygen and nourishment your cells will die.

The heart beats or pumps blood because special cells in your heart (the heart's natural pacemaker) produce electrical impulses that cause the heart to contract and pump blood. These impulses travel from the pacemaker down certain muscle paths in the muscle walls, producing a contraction.

As long as these electrical impulses flow down the heart's walls at regular intervals, your heart pumps at a rhythmic pace. Sometimes, however, something happens to interfere with the electrical impulses of your heart's natural pacemaker. When that happens, the natural pacemaker can't do its job as well as it needs to.

Problems that involve your heart's natural pacemaker include 1) a complete block of the heart's electrical pathways, 2) a slow beat, or 3) an irregular rhythm. If you have a slow and often irregular heartbeat, or if your heartbeat is sometimes normal and sometimes too fast or too slow, your doctor may recommend an artificial pacemaker.

The reason a pacemaker is necessary in such cases is that when your heart pumps too quickly or too slowly, or irregularly, it can't send as much blood to the various parts of the body as it could if it was working properly. The result is that not enough food and oxygen gets to the cells.

An artificial pacemaker works in about the same way as your heart's natural pacemaker. It's a small unit that uses batteries to produce the electrical impulses that make your heart pump. The impulses flow through tiny wires to your heart, and are timed to flow at regular intervals just as impulses from your heart's natural pacemaker would normally do. With the help of an artificial pacemaker your heart should pump almost as well as it did before problems developed.

Significant technological advances have taken place in recent years in pacemakers. Modern pacemakers last much longer than earlier models; some, in fact, are nuclear-powered. As with any electronic device, your artificial pacemaker will require some care. The batteries, for example, will wear down over time and will need to be replaced. As the batteries wear down, your pacemaker will slow down, but it won't stop. The first warning that the batteries are wearing out will be a change in your pulse rate. If your pulse suddenly drops to 40 or 50 beats per minute, tell your doctor.

If your pacemaker or its batteries need replacement, a minor surgical procedure is necessary. Your doctor can explain it to you.

SOURCE:
American Heart Association. *Living with Your Pacemaker.* 1986. pp. 2–3.

TYPES OF PACEMAKERS

Although it is a simplification, we can think of pacemakers as one of three kinds: a) the single-chamber unit, b) the dual-chambered unit, and c) the AICD or pacemaker-defibrillator.

The single-chamber unit is the most commonly used, the smallest in size, the most reliable, and the least expensive. It is nearly always composed of a power source which is placed in a small pocket created surgically in the chest wall, in the region of the upper portion of the breast. A covered wire electrode is inserted into a certain vein and introduced into the tip of the right ventricle, the chamber of the heart that delivers the blood to the lungs. The surgery is nearly always done under simple local anesthesia; it is safe and essentially without complication. These single-chamber units have the capacity to recognize a normal heartbeat and when this occurs, they are suppressed and no electrical discharge occurs. When the heart pauses beyond a set period of time, the pacemaker activates; an electrical impulse is sent through the electrode to the heart, and the heart dutifully contracts.

Dual-chamber units are used less frequently but add an important component of efficiency to the contraction of the heart. The dual electrodes allow the pacemaker to mimic the normal contraction sequence of the beating heart, i.e., contraction of the upper chambers, a brief period to allow the mitral and tricuspid valves to open so that blood can be pumped into the lower chambers, following which there is contraction of these heavy muscular pumps with opening of the aortic and pulmonary valves, and the cardiac cycle is completed.

As with the single-chamber unit, these more complex electronic devices are programmed to function only when need is demonstrated. This occurs where there is a failure in generation of the normal electrical impulse and correct tracking along appropriate pathways through the heart muscle. Dual-chamber pacemakers are also usually located in the tissues of the upper chest, with covered wires passing through veins into the heart muscle. In this case, however, one wire is lodged in the upper chamber (the atrium) and the other in the lower chamber (the ventricle) as with the single-chamber unit. This surgery is also done under local anesthesia and differs little from the single-chamber procedure. Because they are more complex electronically, dual-chamber units are slightly larger, more expensive, and have expanded programmable functions that allow for a wide variety of heart rates.

A new variation of pacemaker has recently shown great success. It is an activity-driven unit, and the rate will change dependent upon the movement of the patient. In sleep, the rate is slow. As the patient becomes more active, delicate sensors "tell" the pacemaker to increase the rate of electrical discharge, and the heart rate speeds up to meet the demands of greater physical activity. These newer units have restrictions built into the circuitry so that the rate will not drop to dangerously low levels or accelerate beyond the ability of the heart to handle the new rate.

Another variety of pacemaker reflects a new generation of electronics for a somewhat different problem. It is calculated that approximately 400,000 Americans die yearly as a result of a sudden malignant heart rhythm abnormality. This is usually what is termed ventricular fibrillation, but may rarely be due to a sudden arrest of all electrical and mechanical activity of the heart. Fortunately, this catastrophe seldom comes without warning. When the warning is heeded, the patient may benefit from what is now termed an AICD (Automatic Implantable Cardioverter Defibrillator). Invented by Dr. Michael Miroski, the AICD has united the skills of the engineer, metallurgist, chemist, physician, mathematician, electronic technician and nurse with the result being an instrument that stretches the limits of one's imagination. The AICD monitors every beat of the heart, recognizes and identifies major rate and rhythm changes, and when appropriate criteria are met, will deliver an electrical shock to the heart. This shock suspends all electrical and mechanical activity for a split-second. In the vast majority of instances, that is all that is needed, and the normal sequence of automatic heart rhythm is restored.

SOURCE:

Carmichael, David P. "Pacemakers: Cardiac Sparkplugs." *HeartCorps* 2 (July/August 1989): 36-37.

UNJUSTIFIED AND INAPPROPRIATE USE

Because of allegations that the implantation of many permanent cardiac pacemakers has been unjustified, we reviewed the indications for all new pacemakers implanted at 30 hospitals in Philadelphia County between January 1 and June 30, 1983, and paid for by Medicare.

Complete chart data were evaluated for 382 implants. We determined whether the indications for implantation were appropriate and adequately documented on the basis of standard clinical practice. Implants were classified as possibly indicated primarily because of inadequate diagnostic evaluation (63 percent) or inadequate documentation (36 percent). Implants were classified as not indicated primarily because a rhythm abnormality was incorrectly identified as a justifiable indication (84 percent).

We found that 168 implants (44 percent) were definitely indicated, 137 (36 percent) possibly indicated, and 77 (20 percent) not indicated. Unwarranted implantation was both prevalent (73 percent of hospitals had an incidence of 10 percent or more) and independent of the type of hospital (university teaching, university-affiliated, and community hospitals). The additional tests most often required to clarify the need for a pacemaker in inadequately evaluated cases included electrophysiologic studies (37 percent) and ambulatory monitoring (31 percent).

We conclude that in a large medical population in 1983, the indications for a considerable number of permanent pacemakers were inadequate or incompletely documented.

SOURCE:

Greenspan, Allan M., and others. "Incidence of Unwarranted Implantation of Permanent Cardiac Pacemakers in a Large Medical Population." *The New England Journal of Medicine* 318, no. 3 (January 21, 1988): 158.

INTERFERENCE BY MICROWAVE OVENS

Probably the most publicized source of pacemaker interference has been the microwave oven. Although today's pacemakers are safe and can overcome some electromagnetic interference, your patient still needs to be aware of some potential hazards.

Electromagnetic interference (EMI) refers to any exogenous (electrical, magnetic, or galvanic) or endogenous (from muscular activity, also called myopotential) signal that alters the function of a pacemaker. Unlike earlier, more vulnerable models, pacemakers are now encased in heavy metal to protect the circuitry from outside signals. Interference from myopotentials has been further limited by the use of the bipolar lead wire, which reduced the distance to be traveled by electric current. In addition, an interference protection signal switches the pacemaker to an interference mode until the disruptive signal vanishes. The interference mode is a fixed rate that ignores the patient's intrinsic rhythm until the interference vanishes. However, there are still a number of potential hazards to the pacemaker patient that require certain safeguards. . . .

At home, the pacemaker patient can safely turn on light switches, televisions, and radios and sleep under an electric blanket. He can use hand drills, battery-operated toothbrushes, and blow dryers, but advise him to avoid holding such devices right next to his pacemaker. Any of these appliances, held right over the insertion site, could emit interfering signals—as happens when you turn on an electric mixer while watching television. The interference mode will temporarily place the pacemaker in a fixed mode. If due to malfunction this does not happen, the patient will have symptoms of a malfunctioning pacemaker, such as dizziness, faintness, and a slow pulse. The demand pacemaker, which may sense EMI as intrinsic beeps, will shut itself off. Advise all patients to have all battery-operated and electrical appliances checked to be sure they are properly grounded and well-maintained.

Microwave ovens manufactured more than ten years ago can leak current and, theoretically, can interfere with pacemaker function. If the patient is in doubt about the safety of a microwave oven, suggest that he protect himself by staying at least six feet away from the oven while it is in use.

People with pacemakers can safely drive, use burglar alarm systems, and pass through metal detectors in airports. However, as pacemakers will trigger alarms in metal detectors, advise the patient to show his pacemaker identification card (available from his physician or clinic) to airport security personnel before passing through the detector.

Patients who work near electric welders, electric steel furnaces, or radio or television transmitters should discuss possible hazards with their cardiologists, who may advise a change of occupation. High-frequency emitting devices can switch a pacemaker to an interference mode.

SOURCE:
Barredo, Josephine. "What Really Interferes with Pacemakers?" *American Journal of Nursing* (December 1990): 24, 25.

RESOURCES

RELATED ARTICLES

Brinker, Jeffrey A. "Pursuing the Perfect Pacemaker." *Mayo Clinic Proceedings* 64 (May 1989): 587–591.

Dugan, Lois. "What You Need to Know about Permanent Pacemakers." *Nursing* 21 (June 1991): 46–52.

Franklin, Jay Olen, and Jerry C. Griffin. "Implantable Devices and Electrotherapy for Arrhythmias." *Hospital Practice* (December 15, 1988): 135–150.

Kastor, John A. "Pacemaker Mania." *The New England Journal of Medicine* 318, no. 3 (January 21, 1988): 182-183.

Lagergren, Hans. "25 Years of Implanted Intracardiac Pacers." *The Lancet* (March 19, 1988): 636–638.

PAP SMEARS

(*See also:* CERVICAL CANCER)

AN EARLY WARNING OF CANCER

Studies show that women who become sexually active early in their teen years, who have multiple sex partners, who have their first child before the age of 20, and who have many pregnancies are at higher than average risk. Also at higher risk are women whose sex partners have other partners.

The risk of cervical cancer is much lower in women in monogamous relationships, and studies indicate that the disease occurs much less often in celibate women. But recent studies show that half of all married women and from 70 to 80 percent of married men have had multiple sex partners. About half of all teenagers have had more than one sexual partner by the time they reach 15, according to ACOG [American College of Obstetricians and Gynecologists]. In effect, then, the consortium of medical groups recommends that nearly all women who are sexually active have annual Pap tests regardless of age, according to William Creasman [professor and head of the Department of Obstetrics and Gynecology at the University of South Carolina].

"If a woman is in any of these high-risk groups she should have annual Pap tests and cervical exams," says George Morley, M.D., the president of ACOG. "To do any less is to play Russian roulette with her life. The annual Pap test will be her early warning system to protect her health and perhaps her life."

SOURCE:
Hale, Ellen. *The Controversial Pap Test: It Could Save Your Life*. DHHS Publication No. (FDA) 90-1159. September 1989, p. 3.

SUCCESS AS A SCREENING METHOD

A Pap test is the first line of defense in diagnosing cervical cancer, which can be treated successfully if it is caught early. Since the introduction of the Pap test, the number of deaths from cancer of the cervix has dropped by 70%.

The Pap test is the procedure in which a sample of cells, called a smear, is gently scraped off the cervix. This sample is looked at under a microscope in a lab to detect any changes or abnormalities in the cells. The results are classified according to the appearance of the cells. About 5 of every 100 women are told that their Pap test shows abnormal cells. An abnormal Pap test does not always mean that there is cancer; a number of things can cause an abnormal smear.

A change in the cells on the surface of the cervix which can lead to cancer is known as cervical intraepithelial neoplasia (CIN). At one time, these changes were called dysplasia. CIN is not cancer; it is, however, a condition where normal cells show some change. This change does not produce any symptoms. In some women, untreated CIN may progress to cervical cancer. Women are at high risk of getting CIN and cancer of the cervix if they started sexual activity before age 18, have had multiple sex partners or their partners have had multiple partners. Women who have had viral infections transmitted through sexual intercourse are also at high risk. Since CIN does not produce any noticeable symptoms, the annual Pap test, especially for women in a high-risk group, serves as the early warning system for catching the condition before it becomes cancer.

If the Pap smear is abnormal the physician should follow up with a colposcopy—a direct examination of the cervix with a special microscope called a colposcope. During the colposcopy, several sites on the cervix may be selected for a biopsy, which involves the removal of a sample of tissue for examination. Treatment for CIN depends on the severity and extent of the condition and the woman's medical history. It could include removing the abnormal part of the cervix by either heating (electrocoagulation) or freezing (cryosurgery), using laser therapy or removing a cone-shaped portion of the cervix (conization) which can define the physical limits of CIN and determine the degree of abnormality.

Cervical cancer is a slow-growing disease which begins as a small group of cells. In its mildest form, which is not yet a true cancer, it is called CIN III, carcinoma in situ (CIS) or Stage 0 Cervical cancer. This means that the cancer has not penetrated the supporting tissue of the cervix and is "noninvasive." At this stage, it can always be treated successfully.

Cervical cancer becomes more serious when it begins to invade the cervix. At this point, the cancer has penetrated deeper into the tissues of the cervix and may have spread to other organs. Treatment depends on the extent of the disease, the woman's age, general health, medical history and other factors. Most often cancers of the cervix are treated with surgery or radiation.

It is important to remember that almost all women with cervical cancer can be cured if the disease is diagnosed in its early stages. An annual Pap test is recommended for women who are sexually active or who have reached age 18. After three or more consecutive annual examinations with normal findings, a woman may have the test less frequently at the discretion of her physician. One study has shown that women who have Pap tests at intervals of more than two years appear to have a higher risk of cervical cancer than women who have the tests every one to two years. The Pap smear and regular pelvic examinations are the best ways to catch problems and can help make an early life-saving diagnosis.

SOURCE:
"Understanding Cervical Cancer." *HealthTips* (March 1990): 1–2.

RECOMMENDED FREQUENCY OF TESTING

Regular Pap smears are recommended for all women who are or have been sexually active. Testing should begin when the woman first engages in sexual intercourse. Adolescents whose sexual history is thought to be unreliable should be presumed to be sexually active at age 18. Pap tests are appropriately performed at an interval of one to three years, to be recommended by the physician on the basis of risk factors (e.g., early onset of sexual intercourse, history of multiple sexual partners, low socioeconomic status). Pap smears may be discontinued at age 65, but only if the physician can document previous Pap screening in which smears have been consistently normal.

The effectiveness of cervical cancer screening is more likely to be improved by extending testing to women who are not currently being screened and by improving the accuracy of Pap smears than by increasing the frequency of testing. Studies suggest that those at greatest risk for cervical cancer are the very women least likely to have access to testing. Inadequate Pap testing is most common among blacks, the poor and the uninsured, the elderly and those living in rural areas. In addition, many women who are tested receive inaccurate results because of interpretive or reporting errors made by cytopathology laboratories or specimen collection errors made by clinicians. The failure of some physicians to provide adequate follow-up for abnormal Pap smears is another source of delay in the management of cervical dysplasia.

SOURCE:
U.S. Preventative Services Task Force. "Screening for Cervical Cancer." *American Family Physician* 41, no. 3 (March 1990): 856.

TEST ACCURACY

The American College of Obstetricians and Gynecologists believes that up to 40 percent of Pap smears may fail to disclose cancer or the cellular abnormalities that can lead to it. As many as half of those errors may result from inadequate sampling; the rest are apparently caused by shortcomings in the laboratories.

Currently, the Federal Centers for Disease Control requires that cytology laboratories engaged in interstate commerce (and thus subject to federal regulation) must rescreen 10 percent of negative Pap smears as a means of quality control. New York state licenses laboratories only after a mandatory examination of the cytotechnologists. A California law forbids that state's cytotechnologists from screening more than 75 slides a day.

And Congress last year (1988) amended the 20-year-old Clinical Laboratory Improvement Act to require quality standards for the estimated 12,000 labs receiving Medicare and Medicaid funding or engaging in interstate commerce. Congress also ordered the Health Care Financing Administration (HCFA) to regulate doctors' office laboratories that examine Pap smears.

SOURCE:
Hale, Ellen. *The Controversial Pap Test: It Could Save Your Life.* DHHS Publication No. (FDA) 90–1159. September 1989. p. 3.

CLASSIFICATION OF TEST RESULTS

Last year, the National Cancer Institute announced a new system for reporting the results of cervical smears, which is intended to encourage long overdue uniformity and quality control. Under the old system, results were given according to one of five different classifications. Class 1 was normal and class 5 was cancer. But laboratories differed in their interpretation of the meanings of classes 2, 3, and 4 (which included everything from abnormal cells to precancers). Furthermore, the classification system didn't allow for the diagnosis of noncancerous conditions, such as infections.

The new system of reporting the results of a Pap smear, called the Bethesda System, involves the use of uniform terminology, a report on the adequacy of the smear and the use of clear diagnostic terms to describe findings that include infections, precancers, and cancerous cell changes. Whether a lab chooses to use the new system is purely voluntary.

"What's important about the Bethesda System is the uniformity," explained Diane Solomon, M.D., chief of the National Cancer Institute's cytopathology section, in a telephone interview. Under the old Pap classification system, what was a Class 2 in one lab could be Class 3 in another. "Each lab may have developed its own kind of descriptive terminology to supplement the Pap class system so what you ended up with was a hodgepodge of different diagnostic terminology that physicians didn't always understand."

SOURCE:
Screening for Cervical Cancer: Room for Improvement. *HealthFacts* 15, no. 136 (September 1990): 3-4.

RESOURCES

ORGANIZATIONS

American Cancer Society. National Office, 4 East 35th St., New York, NY 10001.

American College of Obstetricians and Gynecologists. 600 Maryland Avenue SW, Suite 300 East, Washington, DC 20024.

National Cancer Institute. Office of Cancer Communications, NIH Building 31, 9000 Rockville Pike, Bethesda, MD 20205.

RELATED ARTICLES

Eddy, David E. "Screening for Cervical Cancer." *Annals of Internal Medicine* 113, no. 3 (August 1990): 214-226.

Gall, Stanley A. "Pap Smears: Do Them Right and Every Year—Forever!" *Postgraduate Medicine* 85, no. 6 (May 1, 1989): 235-239.

Koss, Leopold G. "The Papanicolaou Test for Cervical Cancer Detection: A Triumph and a Tragedy." *JAMA* 251, no. 5 (February 3, 1989): 737-743.

Lundberg, George D. "The 1988 Bethesda System for Reporting Cervical/Vaginal Cytological Diagnoses." *JAMA* 262, no. 7 (August 18, 1989): 931-934.

Pomidor, William J. "Pap Tests: What Every Woman Must Know Now." *Medical Selfcare.* (March/April 1989): 37-41.

PARKINSON'S DISEASE

OVERVIEW

Before 1817, what we now know as Parkinson's disease was just one of a number of similar disorders of movement. Then a British doctor, James Parkinson, published a paper on what he called "shaking palsy." In it, he described the major symptoms of the disease that would later bear his name.

Dr. Parkinson's observations allowed the disease to be studied as a special illness for the first time. During the next century, scientists defined its distribution, symptoms and onset, and the prospects for recovery. But most important, in the early 1960's they identified the fundamental brain defect that is the hallmark of the disease. This information led to the first effective treatment for parkinsonism and suggested ways of devising new and more effective therapies.

Very few persons with Parkinson's disease develop serious symptoms before age 40. The great majority of cases are diagnosed between ages 60 and 70, so that the average age of parkinsonian patients is 65 years. In one community studied, the frequency of the disease in those above 50 increased markedly with age. The increasing number of older persons in the U.S., therefore, would seem to foreshadow an increase in the number of people who will develop parkinsonism.

Both men and women appear to be equally affected. There are now perhaps 500,000 people with the disease in the United States, but this number is not exact since many cases are not severe enough to need treatment.

Among many populations in the world, there is wide variation in the occurrence of Parkinson's disease. Some scientists believe that high disease rates in certain populations might be due to an increased genetic susceptibility; but other research findings suggest that heredity may not play a major role in determining who gets the disease. An NINCDS [National Institute of Neurological and Communicative Disorders and Stroke] study of over 40 Parkinson's disease patients who had an identical twin uncovered only one case in which the twin also had the disease. This and other findings lend support to the likelihood that an environmental factor, rather than heredity, causes parkinsonism—an idea that is now being investigated.

The first signs of Parkinson's disease may appear to be simply part of the normal aging process: a little shakiness, some difficulty in rising from a deep, comfortable chair. This is especially true since most symptoms of Parkinson's are first noticed when persons are in their sixties.

But the signs very gradually become more pronounced and extensive. The shaking or tremor that affects about two-thirds of parkinsonian patients begins to interfere with daily activities. It may be more difficult to hold utensils steady when eating. A newspaper may shake enough to make it hard to read.

The shaking may become worse when the patient is relaxed. This is characteristic of Parkinson's. A few seconds after the hands are rested on a table, for instance, the shaking is most pronounced.

Although tremor is usually the most obvious early sign of Parkinson's disease, a more distressing problem to the patient is the symptom known as bradykinesia—the gradual loss of spontaneous movement. A person with Parkinson's may sit in one position for a long time without moving. Or the patient may find it difficult to start walking.

Bradykinesia may lead to the loss of facial expression. This is not a sign of an emotional problem, but a loss of activity in the nerves that control the facial muscles. The link between emotions and facial expressions is instinctive: expressions don't require conscious thought. In Parkinson's, a patient may have natural emotional responses, and not be aware that his or her face is not showing those feelings.

A parkinsonian patient may also have flat, expressionless speech. About half of Parkinson's disease patients experience such problems as loss of volume, difficulty beginning to speak, or inability to speak clearly. Again, these are not emotional problems, but a loss of normally spontaneous activity of the nerves and muscles.

A third characteristic of Parkinson's disease is rigidity. This symptom may not be as obvious to patients as is tremor. They may be aware only of a certain amount of stiffness when they move their arms or legs. But if another person tells a patient to relax and then tries to move the patient's arm, the movements will be ratchetlike: resistance, followed by a quick short movement, then rigidity again. The result is a series of short, jerky motions, as though the arm is being moved by a gear.

A major principle in the body is that all muscles have an opposing muscle. Movement is possible not just because one muscle becomes more active, but because the opposing muscle relaxes. It may be a disturbance of this dynamic balance that causes rigidity.

Parkinsonian patients may also experience other motor problems. For instance, the posture may become stooped with the shoulders bent forward. When the person is standing at rest, the arms may not hang down in the normal way, but may bend upward from the elbow. . . .

Without treatment, Parkinson's disease becomes progressively more severe and disabling. But different patients experience different rates of disease progression. It is generally agreed, however, that with current treatments, many parkinsonian patients enjoy a normal life span.

The course of the disease is variable. With time, patients whose symptoms appeared only on one side of the body may have movement problems on the other side as well. On the other hand, cases of one-sided parkinsonism with no further development of movement problems are well known.

The patient may also begin to experience certain annoying problems, such as drooling. This comes from the difficulty in swallowing due to decreased function of the throat muscles. This swallowing problem can also make eating difficult, and can lead to choking if the patient is not careful. To some extent the patient can control this problem by eating slowly and swallowing often.

There may also be overproduction of the normal oily coating of the skin, a condition called seborrhea. Its cause is poorly understood. The condition is not dangerous, but does require extra care.

The more serious symptoms of advanced Parkinson's disease are aggravations of the movement problems, such as a severe loss of the sense of balance, sometimes compounded by loss of the normal armswing that we all use to maintain our walking rhythm. The short steps characteristic of a parkinsonian patient's walk are an attempt to compensate for lost stability.

SOURCE:

National Institute of Neurological Disorders and Stroke. *Parkinson's Disease: Hope Through Research.* NIH Pub. No. 83-139. June 1983. pp. 3-6, 7.

TREATMENT WITH DRUGS

Carbidopa/levodopa remains the most potent drug for the treatment of Parkinson's disease. Several newer medications may help stabilize and improve such problems as fluctuating responses to the medication, drug-induced dyskinesias and refractory symptoms. Patients with fluctuating responses that do not respond to adjustments in the carbidopa/levodopa dose may benefit from the addition of a direct-acting dopamine agonist, such as pergolide or bromocriptine. While carbidopa/levodopa and the direct-acting dopamine agonists have a proven track record as symptomatic treatment, they probably do not alter the pathologic process underlying this progressive condition. On the other hand, two studies have shown that selegiline might slow the progression of Parkinson's disease, independent of any direct effects on symptoms.

Medical treatment of Parkinson's disease can be very gratifying to both the physician and the patient. Symptomatic treatment often produces dramatic results and can return patients who were once disabled by the disease to the mainstream of life. However, Parkinson's disease is a progressive condition and medical control may wane with time; fluctuating responses, medication-induced dyskinesia and refractory symptoms may develop. Fortunately, some of these problems can be countered by medication adjustments, including the use of some of the newer antiparkinson drugs. The complexities of the therapeutic responses and the availability of new medications require a strategy to optimize the patient's functional status.

SOURCE:

Ahlskog, J. Eric, and John M. Wilkinson. "New Concepts in the Treatment of Parkinson's Disease." *American Family Physician* (February 1990): 574-584.

FETAL CELL TRANSPLANTS

After 10 years of experiments with animals, and just three years with humans, scientists say they are tremendously encouraged by fetal cell transplants as a treatment for Parkinson's disease, a devastating condition that has no cure.

Of the estimated 100 patients worldwide who have been implanted with fetal brain cells over the last three years, they said, nearly all have shown at least minor improvement in their symptoms and many have gotten dramatically better. Although no one has been cured of

Parkinson's disease and scientists do not yet understand how fetal cells exert a therapeutic effect, those conducting the transplant experiments should forge ahead, according to researchers who are presenting their latest findings here this week at the annual meeting of the Society for Neuroscience. . . .

Ideas Behind Therapy

The transplant therapy is based on theories about the differences in the brain before birth and in old age. In old age, the brain has a limited capacity to make new connections and to repair itself, researchers say. And when the brain is diseased, this capacity is severely hampered or disappears. A fetal brain, on the other hand, is designed to make new connections and complicated circuits. As such, fetal brain cells are endowed with special chemicals that could—if implanted in an old brain—restore lost substances or induce the regrowth of lost connections.

Parkinson's disease occurs when cells die inexplicably in a region of the brain called the substantia nigra. In a healthy brain, nerve cells in this region communicate with nerve cells in the nearby striatum, made up of the caudate and putamen, using the chemical transmitter dopamine. When dopamine fails to reach the striatum, patients develop the classic symptoms of Parkinson's disease—tremor, a slowing of movement and rigidity. The disease affects 500,000 Americans, mostly over age 50. Drugs can slow this disease process but eventually stop working.

The goal of fetal cell therapy in Parkinson's disease, researchers said, is to replace dopamine-releasing cells exactly where they are needed, in the striatum. The cells are obtained from 6- to 11-week-old fetuses in a brain region destined to develop into the substantia nigra. The cells are typically placed in a liquid suspension and injected into the adult brain with special needles. Many patients are given drugs to prevent rejection of foreign tissue.

SOURCE:
Blakeslee, Sandra. "Fetal Cell Transplants Show Early Promise in Parkinson Patients." *The New York Times* (November 12, 1991): B6.

SURGICAL TREATMENT

None of the available drugs is viewed as a cure-all for Parkinson's disease. And the same can be said for a new surgical technique—transplanting dopamine-secreting cells from the patient's own adrenal glands to the brain.

Nonetheless, even skeptics admit that the adrenal transplants seem to have dramatically reversed the course of Parkinson's disease in some patients.

The surgery was first successfully performed in Mexico City in 1987 and has spread to several medical centers in the U.S., including The University of Texas Medical School at Houston.

Only a few hundred patients worldwide have undergone the procedure, and some have fared quite well. These patients have experienced significant improvements, including improved mobility, reduced rigidity and less need for medication. But for other patients, the surgery hasn't had much effect, and medical opinion remains divided on the value of this relatively new operation.

SOURCE:
"Parkinson's Disease: New Hope on the Horizon." *The University of Texas Lifetime Health Letter* 2, no. 9 (September 1990): 1.

COPING

Whether diagnosis is made early in the case of those who attend to minor physical problems immediately, or very late in the case of those who ignore even serious symptoms, it becomes necessary for everyone with the illness to adapt to it.

Those who accept the condition and seek helpful information, are better able to plan their existence with it intelligently.

Those who try to hide it from people around them and even from themselves, face a long series of mentally painful episodes.

In such instances, the battle to deny what is actually taking place may produce years of tension and anxiety.

The way an individual reacts to a diagnosis of Parkinson's disease depends in large measure upon what his or her thinking and outlook on life was before the illness.

It's important to recognize, however, that Parkinson's disease is a unique experience. It cannot be reacted to as if it were a minor problem. It does not disappear and is likely to get worse with time.

While some cases progress extremely slowly, others become severe very rapidly. No case can be predicted in advance. Whatever happens, the patient with Parkinson's disease needs to accept it as part of his or her life.

Focusing on the disaster element of Parkinson's may be hard to avoid doing at times. But this causes added emotional pain and may intensify the symptoms themselves.

As much as possible, it will help the patient to concentrate on the positives in life, to adopt the attitude, "I will do the best I can."

Many Parkinson patients find that their lives are still enjoyable even though the illness prevents them from acting in ways they previously did.

It is very important for close relatives to understand this, because their attitudes and reactions often influence the one who has the disease.

A positive and accepting attitude in the patient's spouse or other family members and friends can do much to maintain a spirit of well-being and relieve many of the fears and anxieties that may overtake the Parkinson patient.

SOURCE:
National Parkinson Foundation. *The Parkinson Handbook: A Guide for Parkinson Patients and Their Families*. n.d. p. 16.

RESOURCES

ORGANIZATIONS
American Parkinson Disease Association. 60 Bay Street, Suite 401, Staten Island, NY 10301.

National Parkinson Foundation, Inc. 1501 NW Ninth Avenue / Bob Hope Road, Miami, FL 33136.

Parkinson's Disease Foundation. William Black Medical Research Building, Columbia-Presbyterian Medical Center, 650 West 168th Street, New York, NY 10032.

PAMPHLETS
Parkinson's Disease Foundation:

The Parkinson Patient at Home: For the Patient Who Is Not Responding Well to Levodopa Therapy. 1980.

Parkinson's Disease, Progress, Promise and Hope. n.d.

BOOKS
Goodwin-Austin, Richard. *The Parkinson's Disease Handbook*. Baltimore, MD: International Health. 1990.

Pierce, Jon Robert. *Living with Parkinson's Disease: Or Don't Rush Me! I'm Coping as Fast as I Can*. Knoxville, TN: Spectrum Communications, 1990.

RELATED ARTICLES
Calesnick, Benjamin. "Selegiline for Parkinson's Disease." *American Family Physician* 41 (February 1990): 589–591.

Marsden, C. D. "Parkinson's Disease." *The Lancet* 335 (April 21, 1990): 948–952.

Parkinson Study Group. "Effect of Deprenyl on the Progression of Disability in Early Parkinson's Disease." *The New England Journal of Medicine* 321, no. 20 (November 16, 1989): 1364–1371.

Pearce, J. M. S. "Progression of Parkinson's Disease: Drug Treatment May Slow the Disease Process." *British Medical Journal* 301, no. 6749 (September 1, 1990): 396.

PELVIC INFLAMMATORY DISEASE (PID)

(*See also:* CHLAMYDIA; GONORRHEA;
SEXUALLY TRANSMITTED DISEASES; SYPHILIS)

OVERVIEW

The most serious and common complication of sexually transmitted diseases (STD's) among women is pelvic inflammatory disease (PID), an infection of the upper genital tract. PID can affect the uterus, ovaries, fallopian tubes, or other related structures; it can be acute (short-term) or chronic (long-lasting). PID can lead to infertility, tubal pregnancy, chronic pelvic pain, and other serious consequences.

Each year in the United States, an estimated 1 million women experience an episode of PID, and nearly one-fifth of these are teenagers. More than 100,000 women become infertile (cannot become pregnant) each year as a result of PID, and a large proportion of the 70,000 ectopic (tubal) pregnancies occurring every year are due to the consequences of PID.

PID occurs when disease-causing organisms migrate upwards from the vagina and cervix into the reproductive organs. Many different organisms can cause PID, but most cases are associated with gonorrhea and chlamydial infections. Scientists have also found that bacteria normally present in the vagina and cervix may also play a role.

Investigators are learning more about how these organisms cause PID. The gonococcus probably travels to the fallopian tubes, where it penetrates the cells of the tube's lining and destroys them, producing a pus-like substance. The pus can carry the infection to other organs, resulting in more inflammation, pus, and scarring. Chlamydiae and other bacteria may behave in a similar manner and may attach to sperm, which then can carry the organisms into the upper genital tract. It is not known how other bacteria that normally inhabit the vagina (e.g., organisms such as *Gardnerella vaginalis* and *Bacteroides*), enter the upper organs, but it appears likely that the normal cervical defenses break down and allow access to the uterus and tubes. The organisms may gain access more easily during menstruation.

The major symptoms of PID are lower abdominal pain, discharge from the cervix or vagina, and fever. Often only some of these symptoms appear, and other symptoms such as pain in the right upper abdomen can occur as well. PID, particularly when caused by chlamydia, may produce only minor symptoms, even though it can seriously damage the pelvic organs.

A patient's symptoms alone are not enough to confirm a diagnosis of PID. Laboratory tests can aid in establishing the diagnosis, but the diagnosis can only be confirmed by a procedure called laparoscopy. In this procedure, a small incision is made just below the woman's navel. A tiny tube with a lighted end is inserted to allow the doctor to view the internal organs as well as take a sample of tissue if necessary.

SOURCE:
National Institute of Allergy and Infectious Diseases. *Pelvic Inflammatory Disease.* NIH Pub. No. 87–909F. August 1987. pp. 1–2.

* * *

Pelvic infection and pelvic inflammatory disease (PID) are general terms for infection anywhere in a woman's pelvic organs. Your clinician may also use more precise terms to indicate which specific areas are infected:

- Endometritis: infection of the endometrium or lining of the uterus
- Myometritis: infection of the muscular layers of the uterus
- Salpingitis: infection of the fallopian tubes
- Oophoritis: infection of the ovaries

- Unilateral: affects one side of paired structures such as the tubes or ovaries
- Bilateral: affects both sides of paired structures such as the tubes or ovaries
- Pelvic abscess: walled-off pocket of infection in the pelvic cavity
- Peritonitis: infection of the peritoneum, a thin, strong membrane that lines the abdominal cavity
- Pelvic inflammatory disease (PID): generic term for infections in the uterus, tubes, ovaries, and/or pelvis

PID attacks more than 1 million women a year in the United States, and some 300,000 of them are hospitalized for treatment. Most cases of PID are thought to be polymicrobial in nature; that is, two or more types of pathogens are present at the same time. Chlamydia or gonorrhea is a culprit in over half of all PID.

SOURCE:
Stewart, Felicia H., and others. *Understanding Your Body: Every Woman's Guide to a Lifetime of Health.* New York: Bantam, 1987. pp. 489–490.

EFFECT OF IUDs

We found no consistent differences in the risk of pelvic inflammatory disease associated with IUD use among women in different categories of gonorrhea history, frequency of intercourse, or number of recent sexual partners. However, among women with only one sexual partner, married and cohabiting women had little appreciable increased pelvic inflammatory disease risk associated with IUD use compared with those using no contraception, whereas previously and never-married women using IUDs had relative risk estimates of 1.8 and 2.6, respectively. These results suggest that women at low risk of acquiring sexually transmitted infections have little increase in the risk of pelvic inflammatory disease from use of an IUD.

SOURCE:
Lee, Nancy C., George L. Rubin, and Robert Borucki. "The Intrauterine Device and Pelvic Inflammatory Disease Revisited: New Results from the Women's Health Study." *Obstetrics and Gynecology* 72, no. 1 (July 1988): 1.

EFFECT OF DOUCHING

Several studies have shown that women with P.I.D. are much more likely to have used douches than women who do not get the disease.

More research is needed to determine whether douches cause P.I.D. or whether women use douches because they mistakenly think it will help with the symptoms of P.I.D., said Dr. King Holmes, an expert in sexually transmitted diseases at the University of Washington in Seattle.

"It is not absolutely certain that douching causes complications leading to P.I.D., but all the good studies point in that direction," he said.

Dr. Holmes added: "There is no known benefit of douching. It has no purpose. And there is some risk. So my personal advice is that women should not use douches."

Douche manufacturers referred questions to Dr. Suzanne Trupin of the University of Illinois, who acknowledged that douching is "for the most part a cosmetic thing."

She continued: "Women state that they feel clean and fresh after they douche. So if it isn't harmful, women who wish to douche should be able to. There is no medical evidence yet that douching causes P.I.D."

SOURCE:
Hilts, Philip J. "Growing Concern Over Pelvic Infection in Women." *The New York Times* (October 11, 1990): B7.

TREATMENT

Drug therapy for PID must be prompt and appropriate, and last long enough to eradicate the infective organisms. Ideally, treatment should be instituted within 48 hours of the onset of symptoms. Inadequate therapy may lead to infertility, recurrent disease, or a tubo-ovarian abscess. The patient must understand the possible consequences of failing to comply with treatment; a chlamydial infection, for example, may simply fade away without therapy, but leave tubal adhesions. The physician should initiate empiric therapy while awaiting the results of cultures.

In general, a woman who understands the importance of complying exactly with the treatment regimen may be an appropriate candidate for outpatient treatment. In addition, she must agree to return for follow-up in 36–48 hours. It is important to recognize, however, that a woman with mild symptoms may have significant tubal disease, and IV [intravenous] treatment may be more appropriate.

The Centers for Disease Control (CDC), Atlanta, currently recommend the following regimen for outpatients with PID: ceftriaxone sodium (Rocephin) 250 mg IM [intramuscular] in one dose, plus doxycycline hyclate (Doryx, Vibramycin, Vibra-Tabs, etc.) 100 mg bid po [by mouth] for 10–14 days. (Ceftriaxone is now available in 250-mg vials, thus reducing waste.) Other third-generation cephalosporins that are active against *N. gonorrhoeae* may be used in place of ceftriaxone. Another alternative to doxycycline is clindamycin HCl (Cleocin HCl) 450 mg q6h [every 6 hours] po.

Experts in the treatment of PID, as well as personnel at the CDC, advise that a patient with PID be hospitalized if any of the following criteria apply:

- The diagnosis of PID is uncertain.

- Follow-up within 36–48 hours is possible only if she is hospitalized.
- She has a high fever (38.3-40.0°C [101-104°F]).
- It has been impossible to rule out surgical emergencies such as appendicitis and ectopic pregnancy.
- She has another severe illness that could complicate the course of PID or have an adverse effect on treatment.
- She is prepubertal.
- Outpatient therapy has been ineffective.
- She has a pelvic abscess.
- The pregnancy test is positive.

In addition, admission should be considered for a woman with a poor nutritional state or low resistance to infection (alcoholic, for example). Another candidate for inpatient treatment is someone who seems unlikely to comply with the outpatient regimen.

SOURCE:
Gall, Stanley A., Bente Hoegsberg, and Philip B. Mead. "PID: Often Subtle, Always Dangerous." *Patient Care* (August 15, 1988): 230.

RESOURCES

RELATED ARTICLES

Dranov, Paula. "PID: The Silent Threat." *Glamour* (March 1991): 82, 86.

Marchbanks, Polly A., Nancy C. Lee, and Herbert B. Peterson. "Cigarette Smoking as a Risk Factor for Pelvic Inflammatory Disease." *American Journal of Obstetrics and Gynecology* 162 (March 1990): 639–644.

Shafer, Mary-Ann, and Richard L. Sweet. "Pelvic Inflammatory Disease in Adolescent Females: Epidemiology, Pathogenesis, Diagnosis, Treatment, and Sequelae." *Pediatric Clinics of North America* 36, no. 3 (June 1989): 513–532.

Wolner-Hanssen, Pal, and others. "Decreased Risk of Symptomatic Chlamydial Pelvic Inflammatory Disease Associated with Oral Contraceptive Use." *JAMA* 263, no. 1 (January 5, 1990): 54–59.

PESTICIDE RESIDUES IN FOOD

OVERVIEW

Despite the fact that bacterial contamination is much more of an immediate threat to health than contamination from pesticides, the word pesticide continues to instill greater fear in many consumers than the word bacteria. Perhaps that's because control over pesticides is largely out of consumer's hands. These chemicals cannot be completely eradicated simply by paying careful attention to preparation and cooking methods.

Two supermarket chains in California have responded to consumers' anxiety over not being able to do something about pesticides in foods by subjecting many of the fruits and vegetables they sell—including tomatoes, potatoes, oranges, lettuce, apples, and corn—to laboratory tests for residues of certain pesticides. If the pesticide levels are higher than the limit set by the federal government, the produce is not put on the market.

On the surface, such testing programs seem to be just what's needed because they give consumers a choice they lacked previously. That is, those who do the grocery shopping can shop where they are assured the pesticide levels are safe, or they can take their chances elsewhere. But as was discovered soon after the testing procedures went into effect, it's not simple. For one thing, the findings on levels of pesticide residues vary depending on the lab doing the testing and the method of analysis used. One supermarket, for example, offered apples that contained no detectable pesticide residues according to a report from a laboratory that was able to check for chemicals at levels as low as 200 parts per billion. But a second lab, one that used more advanced testing methods and could detect pesticides in even lower concentrations, did find residues in the apples.

Such a discrepancy raises a larger question than whether those particular apples were safe to eat: Does the detection of pesticide residues in food necessarily mean the food is harmful? Twenty-five years ago scientists could detect pesticide levels in foods in concentrations of something on the order of one part per million. Now, as a result of advanced laboratory methodologies, they can detect as little as one part per trillion in some cases. But we have no definitive evidence that such minute traces are biologically significant. Indeed, scientists now know that arsenic in tiny amounts is an essential nutrient, whereas it was once detectable only at poisonous levels.

Even with these advances, the fact is that certain pesticides have been found to be capable of causing serious health problems. (That is why, for instance, the potentially cancer-causing agent EDB was taken off the market in 1984.) Furthermore, even though about 25 percent of our fresh fruits and substantial amounts of our winter vegetables are imported from countries that do not share the comparatively strict pesticide regulations the United States has set, hardly any imported produce is tested for pesticide levels before it is allowed into the country. Indeed, summoned before Congress to answer charges that his agency was not doing an adequate job of screening imported fruits and vegetables, FDA commissioner Dr. Young admitted there were unacceptable lapses in surveillance of imported produce.

Still, the federal government is stepping up its efforts to control the levels of harmful pesticides in food and tests new pesticides so carefully for safety that years elapse between the time they are developed and the time they are used on farms. Then, too, violations of pesticide limits set by the Environmental Protection Agency for produce grown in the U.S. are estimated to be quite rare—on the order of one percent or less. And despite the widespread fear of pesticides as potent carcinogens, the death rate from cancer in the 1950s, 60s, and 70s—

the decades when pesticide usage increased most dramatically—rose only slightly. Hundreds of thousands more cases of cancer could be averted by a decline in cigarette smoking, in fact, than by avoiding fresh fruits and vegetables.

SOURCE:
"Is There Anything That Is Still Safe to Eat?" *Tufts University Diet and Nutrition Letter* 6 (August 1988): 4-5.

FEDERAL REGULATION

Data from FDA's pesticide monitoring programs indicate there is no factual basis for widespread public concern that pesticides present a health hazard in the American diet.

Three federal agencies share the responsibility for monitoring pesticide levels in foods. The Environmental Protection Agency registers or approves the use of pesticides and establishes tolerances for those whose use may lead to residues in foods. The FDA is responsible for enforcing these tolerances for foods shipped in interstate commerce, except for meat and poultry, which are the responsibility of the U.S. Department of Agriculture. A tolerance is the maximum amount of residue expected in a food when a pesticide chemical is used according to the label directions, provided that the level does not present an unacceptable health risk. In 1987, there were 320 pesticide chemicals with established food and/or feed tolerances in the United States.

According to the latest FDA report—published in November 1988—data from over 25 years of monitoring show that above-tolerance levels are rarely found and indicate that pesticide chemicals are generally used according to label directions. Some violations result from misuse, unusual weather conditions, or poor agricultural practices. However, most violations involve foods that contain small amounts of pesticides for which no tolerance has been set. For example, if a pesticide registered for use in lettuce but not cabbage is found in cabbage, any amount is illegal even though it may not present a health risk.

Under its regulatory monitoring program, the FDA collects samples from individual lots of both domestically grown and imported food and analyzes them for pesticide residues. When violative residues are found, the agency can stop the food from being marketed.

The FDA also does a Total Diet Study (also called a Market Basket Study) designed to estimate the dietary intakes of pesticide residues for eight age/sex groups from infants to senior citizens. Industrial chemicals, heavy metals, radionuclides and essential minerals are also measured. To obtain the samples, FDA personnel purchase foods from local supermarkets or grocery stores four times a year throughout the United States. Each market basket contains 234 individual items judged through nationwide dietary surveys to represent what Americans eat. The foods are prepared for eating and then analyzed for pesticide residues. The results of these analyses are combined with data on food consumption to estimate the actual amounts of pesticide residues in foods as they are usually eaten.

During Fiscal Year 1987, the FDA's regulatory monitoring program analyzed 14,992 samples, 6,503 produced in this country and 7,989 imported from 79 countries. Residues were found in 42% of domestic samples and 44% of imported samples, but the levels involved were usually insignificant. Fewer than 1% of the samples contained residues that exceeded regulatory limits, but 81% of these were cases in which no tolerance had been established for a specific pesticide/commodity combination. These findings were supported by the Total Diet Study data, which showed that the dietary intake of pesticide residues was only a small fraction of acceptable limits.

SOURCE:
"New FDA Report on Pesticide Levels in Foods." *Nutrition Forum* 6 (January/February 1989): 6.

MINIMAL HEALTH RISKS CLAIMED

There are no all-purpose definitions of what a safe food supply really means. For example, different government agencies use different cancer risk standards. And, what a toxicologist considers safe and what a consumer thinks is safe may vary dramatically, based on a variety of factors including knowledge, opinion and confidence in the regulatory system. Consequently, the questions about the safety of the food supply must switch from "Is it safe?" to "Is it safe compared to what?" and "Is it safe enough?" . . .

ACSH [American Council on Science and Health] takes the position that:

- There is no scientific evidence that residues in food from the regulated and approved use of pesticides has ever been the cause of illness or death in either adults or children.
- There are valid reasons to use man-made chemicals to produce an adequate, wholesome and economical food supply. In 1989, less than two percent of the population is engaged in food production for a nation of 248 million Americans.
- A chemical's presence alone, at levels currently detected and detectable in the consumer's diet, does not necessarily suggest that a hazard is present.
- Prevention of excess levels of pesticides in the diet results from the very large safety margins factored into allowable residues in food, from the breakdown characteristics of the chemicals themselves, and from the rigorous regulatory system which licenses and monitors pesticides in food production, transportation and storage.
- The advantages to health of maintaining a varied diet, particularly eating more fruits and vegetables, far outweigh the insignificant risks from pesticide residues, if present at all.

SOURCE:
American Council on Science and Health. *Pesticides and Food Safety.* June 1989. pp. 3-4.

CONCERNS ABOUT ADVERSE HEALTH EFFECTS

Although the American food supply is regarded by many as the safest in the world, recent events have increased consumer concerns about pesticides (fungicides, herbicides, insecticides and rodenticides) in foods. First it was concern about alar in apples, followed by cyanide in grapes and most recently, aldicarb in bananas.

There's good reason to question these chemicals. In laboratory animals, some have been linked to birth defects, sterility, tumors, organ damage and injury to the central nervous system. And it's hard to escape their detrimental influence, since some persist indefinitely in the environment.

What's more, questions are being raised about the effectiveness of many of these chemicals in improving crop yields in the first place. Between 1969 and 1980, for example, the number of insects resistant to insecticides nearly doubled, leading to still greater use. Since the 1940's pesticide use has increased tenfold.

Consumer groups say that governmental attempts to regulate pesticide levels in foods are in shambles. Their concerns center around two issues: the safety of pesticides currently in use, and the amounts of pesticide residues found in our foods. . . .

Once a pesticide is approved for use, as in crop spraying, the Food and Drug Administration (FDA) monitors its levels in foods. Critics, however, contend that the FDA does a poor job. The National Resources Defense Council (NRDC) issued a report in February of this year entitled "Intolerable Risk: Pesticides in Our Children's Food." In it, the NRDC says, "Routine FDA monitoring methods cannot detect approximately 60 percent of pesticides likely to leave residues on food."

In addition to chemical residues left from accepted use of pesticides, there is also the problem of chemical misuse. The most dramatic demonstration of what can happen when pesticides are used improperly occurred in California in 1985 when 1,000 people became ill after eating watermelon contaminated with aldicarb. The chemical had been illegally applied to watermelons during the growing process.

The bottom line is that gaps exist in our knowledge of the safety of currently used pesticides. And while the EPA is trying to close the gap through stricter standards, present monitoring cannot dependably detect unsafe levels or misuse of pesticides. "You're talking about several hundred pesticides and hundreds of different commodities," says Pat Lombardo, Manager of the Food and Drug Administration's Pesticides and Chemical Contaminants Program, "To test all commodities from all areas on an ongoing basis is just impossible."

California consumers recently sent a clear message to the food industry that they are concerned. The "Safe Drinking Water and Toxic Enforcement Act of 1986," more commonly known as Proposition 65, requires that Californians be given a "clear and reasonable warning" of the presence of significant levels of substances in consumer products or those discharged into the environment that are known to cause cancer or reproductive toxicity. In California supermarkets, warnings are now posted about foods deemed by the state of California to be potentially harmful.

SOURCE:
Hudnall, Marsha. "Pesticides in Foods: Putting the Problem in Perspective." *Environmental Nutrition* 12 (May 1989): 1, 2.

AMERICAN CANCER SOCIETY POSITION STATEMENT

Whereas: The Society [American Cancer Society] recognizes that estimation of safe exposure levels involves difficult risk assessment calculations and that the process of translating such calculations into acceptable food tolerance levels is complex. More research is needed so that this risk assessment process can be as accurate as possible, especially with respect to exposures during early childhood development. By understanding such risks more fully we can improve our ability to make national cost-benefit judgements between potential adverse biologic effects of pesticides and the beneficial aspects of their use in food production.

Therefore, Be It Resolved: The American Cancer Society recognizes that many pesticides possess cancer-producing potential for humans. It is essential, therefore, that we do everything possible to assure that the pesticide residues in foods be kept at safe levels.

SOURCE:
"Pesticides: American Cancer Society Position Statement." *CA: A Cancer Journal for Clinicians* 39 (July-August 1989): 226.

RISKS IN CHILDREN

In a recently completed survey of residential pesticide use, the Environmental Protection Agency (EPA) found traces of up to 10 different pesticides in the air of randomly sampled homes. In the majority of homes more than three pesticides were detected.

This widespread residential use of pesticides is a particularly important problem because people are potentially being exposed for a lifetime. Young children are more sensitive to the adverse effects of pesticides than adults because important organ systems are not fully developed at birth. The infant's liver and kidneys are both less able to remove poisons from the blood stream and excrete them. This means that any given dose to a child persists and/or builds up faster than it would in an adult. In addition, the barrier between blood and brain is immature in young children and allows more toxic material to get to the brain than would occur in an adult. If a toxin blocks the development of the central nervous system at an early stage, mental abnormalities may be permanent, as can be seen after exposure to small amounts of lead.

In addition to skin and inhalation exposure, children have a relatively high oral intake of pesticides. The high incidence of accidental poisonings is well known. In 1988, 60 percent of the 63,345 pesticide exposures reported to the Poison Control Center were seen in children under six years old. What may be more important, however, is children's relatively high intake of what most people consider healthy food. The FDA has set the level of pesticides allowed in food on the basis of the amount an adult would take in if he ate a normal balanced diet. Children, however, eat much more fruit and drink much more fruit juice than adults. In addition, because they are growing, they have high metabolic rates and they eat more per pound of body weight than do adults. Therefore the amount of pesticides children eat relative to their size may exceed the acceptable daily intake by several thousandfold.

SOURCE:
"Pesticides Are Even More Harmful to Children than Adults." *Public Citizen Health Research Group Health Letter* (February 1991): 10–11.

EPA (ENVIRONMENTAL PROTECTION AGENCY) PESTICIDES INFORMATION HOTLINE

"What are the health risks associated with eating apples sprayed with Alar?" "Can I plant tomatoes next to my house after it's been treated for termites?" "If I spray my garden with pyrethrin to keep pests away, can I eat the vegetables I harvest during the following week?" These and related questions can be answered by dialing the National Pesticide Telecommunications Network Hotline. Funded by the Environmental Protection Agency and operated at Texas Tech University, the hotline provides consumers with health and environmental information regarding specific pesticides used around the house and garden as well as on supermarket produce. Operators are reachable 24 hours a day, 365 days a year at 1-800-858-PEST.

SOURCE:
"Pesticide Watch." *Tufts University Diet and Nutrition Letter* 8 (April 1990): 1.

RESOURCES

ORGANIZATIONS

American Council on Science and Health. 1995 Broadway, New York, NY 10023.

Center for Science in the Public Interest. 1501 16th St. NW, Washington, DC 20036.

Environmental Protection Agency. 401 M St. SW, Washington, DC 20460.

Food and Drug Administration. 5600 Fishers Lane, Rockville, MD 20857.

National Pesticide Telecommunications Network. Texas Tech University and Environmental Protection Agency, Thompson Hall, Room S-129, Lubbock, TX 79409.

Natural Resources Defense Council. 122 East 42nd St., New York, NY 10168.

RELATED ARTICLES

"A Guide to Choosing a Low-Pesticide Diet?" *Tufts University Diet and Nutrition Letter* 8 (February 1991): 2.

Lefferts, Lisa Y. "Carcinogens Au Naturel?" *Nutrition Action Health Letter* 17, no. 6 (July/August 1990): 1, 5–7.

Stone, Pat. "Is It Really Organic? The Label Implies It but It Ain't Necessarily So." *American Health* (July/August 1990): 37–41.

Young, Frank E. "Weighing Food Safety Risks." *FDA Consumer* 23 (September 1989): 8–13.

PHOBIAS AND PANIC DISORDERS

OVERVIEW

Mental health professionals now recognize three types of phobia—simple phobia, social phobia, and agoraphobia (with and without panic attacks)—and a separate diagnosis for people who repeatedly experience severe attacks of panic.

The most common of the various phobias is simple phobia, the unreasonable fear of some object or situation. Bees, germs, heights, odors, illness, and storms are examples of the things commonly feared in simple phobias.

If you have a simple phobia, it might have begun when you actually did face a risk that realistically provoked anxiety. Perhaps, for example, you found yourself in deep water before you learned to swim. Extreme fear was appropriate in such a situation. But if you continue to avoid even the shallow end of a pool, your anxiety is excessive and may be of phobic proportions.

Simple phobias, especially animal phobias, are common in children, but they occur at all ages. The best evidence to date suggests that between 5 and 12 percent of the population have phobic disorders in any 6-month period.

The recognition by most phobics that their fears are unreasonable doesn't make them feel any less anxious. Simple phobias do not often interfere with daily life or cause as much subjective distress as most other anxiety disorders.

The person with a social phobia is intensely afraid of being judged by others. Even at a gathering of many people, the social phobic expects to be singled out, scrutinized, and found wanting. Thus, the person with a social phobia feels compelled to avoid social situations associated with such apprehensions.

If you have a social phobia, you might be afraid to go to a party because you fear that other people will laugh at your clothing or think you are hopelessly stupid because you won't be able to think of anything to say. Like people with simple phobias, you work hard to avoid these anxiety-provoking situations.

People with social phobias are usually most anxious over feeling humiliated or embarrassed by showing fear in front of others. Ironically, they are often so crippled by the inhibitions resulting from such fears that they, in fact, may have difficulty thinking clearly, remembering facts, or expressing themselves in words. Even success in social situations fails to make them feel more confident. They are likely to think something like, "Next time I'll fall on my face."

Although studies of the incidence of social phobias are so far only preliminary, most experts believe social phobias are not as common as simple phobias. But because they result in considerable distress, people who suffer from them are more likely to seek treatment than are people with simple phobias. Social phobias tend to begin between the ages of 15 and 20 and, if left untreated, continue through much of the person's life. Often, social phobics suffer from symptoms of depression, and many also become dependent on alcohol.

Another group of anxious people are subject to devastating episodes of panic that are unexpected and seemingly without cause. Such unpredictable panic attacks are marked by an overwhelming sense of impending doom and a host of bodily symptoms. The person's heart races and breathing quickens, as he gasps for air. Sweating, weakness, dizziness, and feelings of unreality are also common. The person having a panic attack fears he is going to die, go crazy, or at least lose control.

Panic disorder is diagnosed when patients experience repeated episodes of such panic. Although people with simple or social phobias may sometimes experience panic, they are clearly responding to an encounter—or an anticipated encounter—with the object or situation they fear. Such is not the case with panic disorder, when the fear strikes from nowhere, seemingly "out of the blue."

People with simple and social phobias can also predict that they will feel fear every time they come close to a cat, climb to the roof of a tall building, or encounter whatever else they fear. People with panic disorder, by contrast, never can predict when they will suddenly be struck by panic. Some situations may seem more "dangerous," especially those that make escape difficult, but an attack does not invariably occur in those situations.

Panic disorder, which runs in families, afflicts some 1.2 million Americans. For most, panic attacks begin sometime between the ages of 15 and 19.

Many people who suffer from panic attacks go on to develop agoraphobia, a severely handicapping disorder that often prevents its victims from leaving their homes unless accompanied by a friend or relative—a "safe" person. The first panic attack may follow some stressful event, such as a serious illness or the death of a loved one. (The agoraphobic often doesn't make this connection, though.) Fearing more attacks, the person develops a more-or-less continual state of anxiety, anticipating the next attack, avoiding situations where he would be helpless if a panic attack occurred. It is this avoidance behavior that distinguishes agoraphobia from panic disorder. Two different types of anxiety appear to afflict the person with agoraphobia—panic and the "anticipatory anxiety" engendered by expectations of future panic attacks.

If you have agoraphobia, chances are it developed something like this: One ordinary day, while tending to some chore, taking a walk, driving to work—in other words, just going about your usual business—you were suddenly struck by a wave of awful terror. Your heart started pounding, you trembled, you perspired profusely, and you had difficulty catching your breath. You became convinced that something terrible was happening to you, maybe you were going crazy, maybe you were having a heart attack, maybe you were about to die. You desperately sought safety, reassurance from your family, treatment at a clinic or emergency room. Your doctor could find nothing wrong with you, so you went about your business, until a panic attack struck you again. As the attacks became more frequent, you spent more and more time thinking about them. You worried, watched for danger, and waited with fear for the next one to hit.

You began to avoid situations where you had experienced an attack, then others where you would find it particularly difficult to cope with one—to escape and get help. You started by making minor adjustments in your habits—going to a supermarket at midnight, for example, rather than on the way home from work when the store tends to be crowded.

Gradually, you got to the point where you couldn't venture outside your immediate neighborhood, couldn't leave the house without your spouse, or maybe couldn't leave at all. What started out as an inconvenience turned into a nightmare. Like a creature in a horror movie, fear expanded until it covered the entire screen of your life.

To the outside observer, a person with agoraphobia may look no different from one with a social phobia. Both may stay home from a party. But their reasons for doing so are different. While the social phobic is afraid of the scrutiny of other people, many investigators believe that the agoraphobic is afraid of his or her own internal cues. The agoraphobic is afraid of feeling the dreadful anxiety of a panic attack, afraid of losing control in a crowd. Minor physical sensations may be interpreted as the prelude to some catastrophic threat to life.

Agoraphobics may abuse alcohol in an effort to keep the anticipatory anxiety in check. Their pattern of abuse appears to be different from the binging characteristic of alcoholism, however. The agoraphobic usually takes small amounts of alcohol, avoiding loss of control. Other drugs may also be abused.

Agoraphobia typically begins during the late teens or twenties. The best surveys done to date show that between 2.7 percent and 5.8 percent of the U.S. adult population suffer from agoraphobia. Women are affected two to four times more often than men. The condition tends to run in families.

Recent surveys have found that many people are afraid to leave their homes. Most likely, they are not all suffering from agoraphobia. Some people may stay confined because of depression, fear of street crime, or other reasons. These surveys also show, however, that many agoraphobics may have never suffered a panic attack. This finding suggests that their agoraphobia may have developed in ways different from that outlined above.

Panic and agoraphobia have received a great deal of attention from clinical investigators in recent years. Some believe that panic attacks are a severe expression of general anxiety, while others think that they constitute a biologically distinct disorder, possibly related to depression, possibly indistinguishable from agoraphobia. This controversy will probably be resolved through more research in the coming years.

SOURCE:

National Institute of Mental Health. *Useful Information on Phobias and Panic.* DHHS Pub. No. (ADM) 89-1472. 1989. pp. 5-11.

PANIC DISORDER

Two to five percent of Americans are thought to suffer panic disorder, so you are not alone if you experience these symptoms. Most often, panic disorder first strikes people in their early twenties. A severe life stress, such as the death of a loved one, can precipitate panic attacks.

A 1986 study by the National Institute of Mental Health showed that 5.1% to 12.5% of people surveyed had experienced phobias in the past 6 months. The study estimated that 24 million Americans will experience some phobias in their lifetimes.

Phobias are the leading psychiatric disorders among women of all ages. One survey showed that 4.9% of women and 1.8% of men have panic disorder, agoraphobia, or other phobias.

No one really knows what causes panic disorder, but several theories are being researched. Panic disorder seems to run in families, and this suggests the disorder has some genetic inheritability or predisposition.

Some theories suggest that panic disorder is part of a more generalized anxiety in the people who experience panic attacks or that severe separation anxiety can develop into panic disorder or phobias, most often agoraphobia. Cognitive theorists believe that one's "wrong thinking" maintains an anxiety level that can trigger panic attacks.

Biological theories point to possible physical defects in a person's autonomic (or automatic) nervous system. General hypersensitivity in the nervous system, increased arousal, or a sudden chemical imbalance can trigger panic attacks. Caffeine, alcohol, and several other agents can also trigger these symptoms.

Researchers have found that sodium lactate, when injected into the bloodstream of some people who are predisposed to panic attacks, will induce such attacks. This suggests that people who experience panic attacks may have trouble metabolizing lactate, a substance usually produced by muscles during exercise.

Recovery from panic disorder appears to be most successful when a combination of treatments is used in fighting the disorder. Most often, medication is used to block panic attacks, and when it is used in combination with cognitive or behavioral therapy, it allows people to overcome their fears and return to normal, functional living.

Sadly, although treatments can be quite successful—75% to 90% of those treated show significant improvement—only about one quarter of those who suffer this disorder ever seek appropriate treatment.

Cognitive therapy is used to help people think and behave appropriately, thus making the feared object or situation less threatening through supported exposure and hierarchical desensitization (being exposed to, and slowly getting used to, the thing that is so frightening). Family members and friends play an important role in this process as they provide support, assistance, and encouragement.

Medication is most effective when used as part of a more comprehensive treatment plan that involves supportive therapy. Antidepressants, such as imipramine and phenelzine, and antianxiety agents, such as alprazolam, are most successful. Beta blockers, which limit neuron activity in the brain, are helpful with social phobias. If you are seeking medical treatment, ask your doctor about these medications or others that may help you.

Psychotherapy and healthy living habits are also believed to help people overcome the burdens placed on them by panic disorder. Exercise, a proper and balanced diet, moderate use of caffeine or alcohol, and reduced stress can help tremendously.

Peer support is a vital part of overcoming panic disorder. Family and friends can play a significant role in the treatment process and should be informed of the treatment plan and of the ways they can be most helpful.

SOURCE:
National Alliance for the Mentally Ill. *Panic Disorder*. n.d. pp. 3–4.

TREATMENT

Phobia treatment programs now exist in many parts of the United States. These programs use a variety of behavioral therapy techniques to help clients confront and overcome their fears. In addition, through these programs drugs may be recommended and prescribed for individuals likely to benefit from them.

In a typical program, phobic individuals work together in groups with a trained group leader. In some programs, family members and friends are also invited to attend the weekly meetings. Group sessions are used to teach attitudes and skills that are helpful in overcoming phobias. The client also has weekly practice sessions, either alone or in a group, with a therapist who is a mental health professional or a recovered phobic. During these sessions, the client uses his new coping skills in situations he would previously have avoided. With the therapist at his side, he gradually takes progressively more difficult steps toward his final goal. Setbacks are expected and viewed as opportunities for further practice and gain. Agoraphobic clients who are housebound sometimes begin their treatment in their own homes.

Although organized phobia treatment programs offer many advantages, they do not exist in all areas. Many individual therapists are experienced at working with phobic patients, and some will accompany their patients in fear-producing situations.

Referrals to treatment programs and therapists can be obtained by calling or writing to the local, regional, or State chapters of the American Psychological Association, the American Psychiatric Association, the National Association of Social Workers, the American Nurses Association, the National Mental Health Association, the American Association for Counseling and Development, and the Phobia Society of America. In addition, several books and tape cassettes offer self-treatment programs. Since the effectiveness of these programs has not been evaluated, referral to them in this pamphlet does not imply an endorsement by the National Institute of Mental Health.

A word of caution: Not every form of treatment is appropriate for every patient or client. Nor does every therapist or phobia program offer all forms of treatment—psychotherapy, behavior therapy, and medications. Often, a combination of these treatments is necessary. If you feel that you are not being helped by one clinic, program, or therapist, you may wish to seek help elsewhere.

SOURCE:
National Institute of Mental Health. *Useful Information on Phobias and Panic.* DHHS Pub. No. (ADM) 89-1472. 1989. pp. 35-37.

RESOURCES

ORGANIZATIONS

American Psychiatric Association. 1400 K Street NW, Washington, DC 20005.

National Institute of Mental Health. 5600 Fishers Lane, Rockville, MD 20857.

Phobia Society of America. P.O. Box 2066, Rockville, MD 20852-2066.

PAMPHLET

American Psychiatric Association:

Let's Talk Facts About Panic Disorder. 1989. 9 pp.

BOOKS

Greist, John H., James W. Jefferson, and Isaac M. Marks. *Anxiety and Its Treatment: Help Is Available.* Washington, DC: American Psychiatric Press, 1986.

Sheehan, David V. *Anxiety Disease and How to Overcome It.* New York: Scribner, 1984.

Wilson, R. Reid. *Don't Panic: Taking Control of Anxiety Attacks.* New York: Harper & Row, 1987.

RELATED ARTICLES

Brown, Harriet. "Help, I'm Having a Panic Attack!" *American Health* (March 1991): 44-48.

Christenson, Gary A., and Thomas B. Mackenzie. "Social Phobia: Recognizing the Distress Signals." *Postgraduate Medicine* 86, no. 6 (November 1, 1989): 197-202.

McCann, Daniel. "Dental Phobia: Conquering Fear with Trust." *Journal of the American Dental Association* 119 (November 1989): 593-598.

"Panic Attacks: They're Sudden and Terrifying but Respond Well to Treatment." *Mayo Clinic Health Letter* (October 1988): 2.

"What Precipitates Agoraphobia?" *The Lancet* 335 (June 2, 1990): 1314-1315.

PNEUMONIA

OVERVIEW

Inflammation of the lungs due to infection. Pneumonia is the sixth most common cause of death in the US, primarily because it is a common complication of any serious illness. It is more common in males, during infancy and old age, and in those who have reduced immunity to infection (such as alcoholics).

There are two main types of pneumonia: lobar pneumonia and bronchopneumonia. In lobar pneumonia one lobe of one lung initially is infected. In bronchopneumonia, inflammation starts in the bronchi and bronchioles (airways) and then spreads to affect patches of tissue in one or both lungs.

Most cases of pneumonia are caused by viruses or bacteria. Causes of viral pneumonia include adenovirus, respiratory syncytial virus, or a coxsackievirus. The most common bacterial pneumonia is caused by *Streptococcus pneumoniae.* Other causes of bacterial pneumonia include *Hemophilus influenzae, Legionella pneumophilia* [Legionnaire's disease], and *Staphylococcus aureus.* Pneumonia may also be caused by a *mycoplasma* (an organism that is intermediate between a bacterium and a virus) or by a *chlamydial infection*; Q fever is a type of pneumonia caused by a *rickettsia.*

Rarely, pneumonia may be due to a different type of organism, such as fungi, yeasts, or protozoa. These types usually occur only in people with immunodeficiency disorders (e.g., pneumocystis pneumonia, caused by a protozoon, commonly occurs in people with AIDS).

Symptoms and signs typically include fever, chills, shortness of breath, and a cough that produces yellow-green sputum and occasionally blood. Chest pain that is worse when breathing in may occur because of pleurisy (inflammation of the membrane lining the lungs and chest cavity).

Potential complications include pleural effusion (fluid around the lung), empyema (pus in the pleural cavity), and, rarely, an abscess in the lung.

The physician gives the patient a physical examination, listening to chest sounds through a stethoscope. The diagnosis may be confirmed by a chest X ray and by examination of sputum and, occasionally, of blood for microorganisms.

Patients with mild pneumonia can usually be treated at home, but hospitalization is necessary in severe cases. The drugs prescribed depend on the causative microorganism; they may include antibiotic drugs or antifungal drugs. Aspirin or acetaminophen may be given to reduce fever. In severe cases, oxygen therapy and artificial ventilation may be required.

The majority of sufferers recover completely within two weeks. However, some elderly or debilitated people fail to respond to treatment; progressively more lung tissue is affected and death occurs as a result of respiratory failure.

SOURCE:

Clayman, Charles B. (ed.). "Pneumonia." In *The American Medical Association Encyclopedia of Medicine.* New York: Random House, 1989. pp. 803–804.

PREVENTIVE INOCULATION

Pneumonia used to be called "the friend of the aged" in the days before antibiotics, because it was that which finally and quietly terminated life for many in the end stages of other diseases. In this antibiotic era, however, we are inclined not to give it the attention it still deserves.

Pneumococcal pneumonia accounts for 500,000 cases of the bacterial pneumonias seen in this country each year, and although it usually responds to antibiotics, it can be at worst fatal and at best a debilitating disease. Yet only 10-to-20 percent of those at greatest risk for developing the disease are given the vaccine, which is 90 percent effective and whose protection lasts 5-to-10 years. This high-risk group includes persons older than 65; those with such chronic health problems as diabetes, heart disease, and kidney disease, to name just three; health care workers or family members caring for the chronically ill; and children with such chronic pulmonary problems as asthma.

Reactions to the vaccine are minimal or, for many, non-occurring. If you are in any of the above groups, ask your doctor for the vaccine if he has not already offered it.

SOURCE:
"Pneumococcal Vaccine." *Medical Update* 14 (March 1991): 6.

EFFECTIVENESS OF PNEUMOCOCCAL VACCINES

Pneumococcal infections are no less important today than they were in the pre-antibiotic era. Serious pneumococcal infections are common and an excessive number of deaths still occur despite effective antimicrobial agents. Pneumonia mortality and hospitalization rates have increased among older Americans in the past decade, with pneumonia and influenza becoming the fifth leading cause of death. This increase is particularly troublesome because it has occurred during a national commitment by the Surgeon General to reduce premature deaths from pneumonia. Pneumococcal pneumonia is the most common community-acquired bacterial pneumonia. Its highest incidence is in middle-aged men during the months of April and October, but it affects persons of any age, anytime. Consequently, a polyvalent pneumococcal polysaccharide vaccine was developed for the prevention of serious pneumococcal infections. Its widespread use in adults "at risk" for pneumonia—immunocompromised, with chronic diseases, or over 65 years of age—can be expected to reduce mortality, morbidity, and associated health care costs.

Pneumococcal vaccines (23-valent) have been shown to be efficacious and safe in the prevention of pneumococcal infections, especially pneumonias.

SOURCE:
Gable, Carol Brignoli. "Pneumococcal Vaccine: Efficacy and Associated Cost Savings." *JAMA* 264 (December 12, 1990): 2910-2915.

PNEUMOCYSTIS CARINII PNEUMONIA

Pneumocystis carinii is an opportunistic pathogen [microorganism producing disease] whose natural habitat is the lung. The organism is an important cause of pneumonia in the compromised host. . . .

P. carinii pneumonia occurs in the following hosts: premature, malnourished infants; children with primary immunodeficiency diseases; patients receiving immunosuppressive therapy (particularly corticosteroids) for cancer, organ transplantation, and other disorders; and patients with the acquired immunodeficiency syndrome. AIDS is by far the most common underlying disease for *P. carinii*; conversely, *P. carinii* is the most common opportunistic infection in AIDS, occurring in at least 60 percent and perhaps up to 80 to 90 percent of patients during their lifetime.

Available data suggest that impaired cellular immunity is the major host predisposing factor in the development of pneumocystosis [infection with *Pneumocystis carinii*]. Antibodies are produced locally and systemically in response to exposure to *P. carinii*, but do not appear to have a protective role. *P. carinii* pneumonia which develops with the use of immunosuppressive drugs probably represents reactivation of latent infection. In some reports the incidence of the disease has been related to the intensity of the immunosuppression. . . .

The two major drugs used in the treatment of *P. carinii* pneumonia have been trimethoprim-sulfamethoxazole (TMP-SMX) and pentamidine isethionate.

SOURCE:
Wilson, Jean D., and others (eds.). "*Pneumocystis Carinii* Pneumonia." In *Harrison's Principles of Internal Medicine.* Twelfth edition. New York: McGraw-Hill, 1991. pp. 799–800.

PREVENTION OF PNEUMONIA IN AIDS PATIENTS

FDA has approved expanded distribution of an experimental drug to help prevent pneumonia in AIDS patients. The drug, aerosolized pentamidine, can now be used in persons infected with the AIDS virus who have had at least one episode of *Pneumocystis carinii* pneumonia—a life-threatening infection that often afflicts AIDS patients—or who have T helper (T4) cell counts of 200 or less per cubic millimeter of blood. (T helper cells, white blood cells that are critical parts of the body's immune system, are destroyed by the AIDS virus. Healthy people normally have T helper cell counts of 1,000 or more.) A study supported by the National Institute of Allergy and Infectious Diseases found that a significant percentage of AIDS-infected individuals with such low T4 cell counts are at risk of developing *Pneumocystis* pneumonia even if they have no symptoms of AIDS.

As many as 50,000 AIDS patients may benefit from the broadened use of aerosolized pentamidine. According to the approval, the drug should be given through a special nebulizer—a device to reduce a liquid to a fine spray so it can be inhaled—at a dosage of 300 milligrams every four weeks. The dosage is based on results of a study by the San Francisco Community Consortium, a group of doctors experienced in treating people with AIDS. While the dosage did not provide complete protection, it did significantly reduce the incidence of pneumonia.

SOURCE:
"Wider Use of Pneumonia Drug Approved." *FDA Consumer* 23 (April 1989): 4.

RESOURCES

ORGANIZATION
American Lung Association. 1740 Broadway, New York, NY 10019.

PAMPHLET
American Lung Association:

Facts about Pneumonia. 0029. 1988.

RELATED ARTICLES
Bryan, Charles S. "Preventing Pneumonia and Influenza Deaths: A Strategy for Increasing Vaccination of High-Risk Patients." *Consultant 30* (November 1990): 68–75.

"Just One Shot for Pneumonia?" *Consumer Reports Health Letter* 3, no. 1 (January 1991): 6.

Mostow, S. R., T. R. Cate, and F. L. Ruben. "Prevention of Influenza and Pneumonia." *American Review of Respiratory Disease* 142, no. 2 (August 1990): 87–88.

"Pneumonia: Renewed Respect for an Old Killer." *University of Texas Lifetime Health Letter* 3, no. 1 (January 1991): 1, 5.

"TB and Pneumonia Alert." *Woman's Day* 53, no. 4 (February 6, 1990): 21.

"An Untimely—And Unnecessary—Death." *Medical Update* 14, no. 2 (August 1990): 6.

Wasco, James. "Can What Killed the Muppet Man Kill You?" *Woman's Day* 53, no. 13 (September 4, 1990): 14.

POISON IVY

OVERVIEW

This ubiquitous weed—ivy in the East, oak in the West and sumac and ivy in the South—grows practically everywhere in the United States, except Hawaii, Alaska, and some desert areas of Nevada. It is the single most common cause of allergic reactions in the United States and will affect ten to 50 million Americans every year.

Poison ivy rash is allergic contact dermatitis caused by a substance called urushiol, found in the sap of poison ivy, poison oak and poison sumac. Urushiol (pronounced you-roo-shee-ol) is a colorless, or slightly yellow, oil that oozes from any cut, or crushed, part of the plant, including both stem and leaves. Simply brushing against a plant may not cause a reaction. On the other hand, you may develop dermatitis without ever coming into contact with poison ivy, because the urushiol is so easily spread. Sticky, and virtually invisible, it can be carried on the fur of animals, on garden tools, or golf ball, or on any objects that have come into contact with a broken plant. After exposure to air, urushiol turns a brownish-black, making it easier to spot, and is neutralized to an inactive state by water.

Once it touches the skin, the urushiol begins to penetrate in a matter of minutes. In those sensitive to the chemical, reaction will appear in the form of a linear rash (sometimes resembling insect bites) within 12-48 hours. Redness and swelling will be followed by blisters and severe itching. In a few days, the blisters become crusted and begin to scale and the dermatitis will usually take about ten days to heal, sometimes leaving small pigmented spots, especially in dark skin. The rash can affect almost any part of the body, although areas where the skin is thinner are more sensitive to the ivy sap. The soles of the feet and palms of the hands are thicker and less susceptible.

Sensitivity to poison ivy is not something we are born with. It develops only after several encounters with the plants, and sometimes over many years. Studies have shown that approximately 85 percent of the population will develop an allergic reaction if exposed to poison ivy, but this sensitivity varies with each individual according to circumstance, age, genetics or previous exposure. Although they are not sure why, scientist say that an individual's sensitivity to poison ivy is not a static phenomenon—it changes with time, and tends to decline with age. Typically, an initial bout of dermatitis will occur in children somewhere between the ages of 8 and 16, and can be quite severe. However, if these individuals are not repeatedly exposed to poison ivy, or urushiol, sensitivity will probably be halved by the time they reach their thirties.

Investigators have found that in people who reach adulthood without becoming sensitized, there is only a 50 percent chance of developing an allergy to poison ivy. Similarly, those who were once allergic may lose their sensitivity later in life. However, dermatologists say it's not safe to assume you are one of the few people who are not sensitive—only 10 to 15 percent of the population is believed to be tolerant. Conversely, that same percentage (25-40 million people) is thought to be particularly susceptible to poison ivy. These people will develop a dermatitis characterized by extreme swelling on the face, arms and genitals. In such severe cases, treatment by a dermatologists will be required.

SOURCE:
American Academy of Dermatology. *Poison Ivy*. 1990. pp. 1-3.

TREATMENT

Mild Dermatitis—Local treatment often suffices when there are a limited number of affected areas and the eruption is not frankly vesicular [blister-like] or bullous [eruptions filled with fluid]. A high-potency corticosteroid cream can be used on the most uncomfortably itchy sites: clobetasol propionate (Temovate) cream, betamethasone dipropionate (Diprolene) cream. Medium-strength corticosteroid creams can be used over more extensive areas of involvement: betamethasone dipropionate (Diprosone) cream, betamethasone valerate (Valisone) cream, fluocinonide (Lidex) cream, triamcinolone acetonide 0.5 percent cream (Aristocort HP cream, Kenalog HP cream). All these creams can be applied sparingly two to three times daily without bandages.

Calamine lotion containing menthol 0.25 percent and phenol 0.5 percent can be applied three to six times daily, preferably with a paint brush. It is not necessary to wash off remnants of previous applications of the lotion.

Dexamethasone (Decspray) can be used two to three times daily.

Moderately Severe Dermatitis—In these cases, one can add cool, wet compresses for ten to fifteen minutes four to six times daily. The compress solution can be kept in a bowl standing in a larger bowl containing ice cubes. Ordinary tap water or Burow's solution (one package of Domeboro per pint of water) can be applied, or milk (not skim milk) can be used to avoid excessive drying of the skin. The aforementioned topical steroid preparations can be used; when there is much redness and swelling, it is helpful to apply a dressing with occlusive [air tight] plastic wrap or other impermeable material over the cream during the night. This increases the penetration of the steroid into the skin and augments its anti-inflammatory action. Antihistamines of the H1-blocking variety, for example, hydroxyzine 10 to 25 mg, cyproheptadine 4 mg, promethazine 12.5 mg, diphenhydramine 25 mg, taken one to four times daily, are often helpful to treat the itching.

Severe Dermatitis—Tub baths two to six times daily for fifteen to twenty minutes can be used by patients with widespread, severe eruptions. Plain water or water with the addition of colloidal oatmeal (Aveeno) is recommended. The patient should determine whether cool or fairly hot baths provide the greatest relief. Such baths are particularly useful during itching crises at night.

Barring medical contraindications, severe poison ivy dermatitis is an indication for the systemic administration of glucocorticosteroids, which produce significant involution of the lesions and suppress itching.

SOURCE:
Baer, Rudolf L. "Poison Ivy Dermatitis." *CUTIS* 46 (July 1990): 36.

PREVENTION

The best way to treat poison ivy is not to get it. A small study found that Ivy Shield [TM], an over-the-counter skin cream, helps prevent poison ivy. To test the effectiveness of this cream, volunteers applied it to their forearms. Four hours later, urushiol (the chemical that causes the itches and blisters of poison ivy and oak) was applied to their forearms. The cream was effective in preventing reactions in those who are "moderately sensitive" to poison ivy, but wasn't beneficial for people "extremely sensitive." Although this product isn't a guaranteed way to avoid getting poison ivy or oak, it seems to help.

SOURCE:
"Poison Ivy Protection." *Pediatrics for Parents* 10 (July-August 1989): 7.

* * *

Here are some preventive tips to keep in mind:

- Learn to recognize poison oak, ivy and sumac.
- When hiking in areas that are known to have these plants, wear clothing that will cover the skin.
- Wash all exposed body areas with water and soap or detergent as soon as possible after exposure to the plant. Be sure to clean thoroughly under the nails. The sap takes effect very quickly, so the washing must occur immediately. If this is not possible, it is still recommended to wash at the earliest opportunity.
- Remove all clothing and shoes that may have been in contact with the plants and wash them thoroughly with soap or detergent. Avoid skin contact with them until after the cleansing.
- Bathe the family pet if it was in contact with the plants.

SOURCE:
"Rhus Dermatitis (Poison Oak)." *HealthTips* no. 345 (December 1989-January 1990): 10.

RESOURCES

ORGANIZATION

American Academy of Dermatology. 1567 Maple Ave., Evanston, IL 60201.

RELATED ARTICLES

Epstein, W. L. Topical Prevention of Poison Ivy/Oak Dermatitis. *Archives of Dermatology* 125, no. 4 (April 1989): 499-501.

Guin, Jere D., Albert M. Kligman, and Howard I. Maibach. "Treating Poison Ivy, Oak, and Sumac." *Patient Care* 23 (June 15, 1989): 227-235.

Shepherd, Steven. "The Scourge of the Great Outdoors: Poison Oak and Poison Ivy." *Executive Health Report* (May 1990): 2-3.

PREMENSTRUAL SYNDROME (PMS)

(*See also:* MENSTRUATION)

OVERVIEW

Premenstrual syndrome (PMS) is the term used to describe a group of physical or behavioral changes that some women go through before their menstrual periods begin every month. PMS can produce discomfort in different parts of the body; it can also cause unpleasant emotional feelings. For reasons that remain unclear, these physical discomforts or mood changes begin at various times near the end of the menstrual cycle and usually disappear after a woman has begun her menstrual period. They reappear at about the same time each month.

The degree of discomfort from PMS varies with each individual. Most women with PMS have symptoms that cause a mild or moderate degree of distress. In about 10% of women with PMS, symptoms may be severe.

PMS can have a major impact on a woman's life:

- On the job or at home, a woman may not be able to function as well when symptoms occur.
- Problems caused by PMS may trigger marital and family conflicts.
- A woman may become less outgoing socially and avoid friends when symptoms occur.

Women who have PMS can be helped. Education is the most important step in understanding this condition. Certain treatments can be useful in some women. . . .

A number of changes that cause various degrees of discomfort have been found in women with PMS:

Physical Changes. Bloating, weight gain, breast soreness, abdominal swelling, headache, clumsiness, constipation, swollen hands and feet, and fatigue.

Behavioral Changes. Depression, irritability, anxiety, tension, mood swings, inability to concentrate, and a change in sex drive.

You don't have to have all of these problems to have PMS. Most women with PMS have only certain ones. Some women have more difficulty with changes that affect their bodies; others have more problems with emotional changes. The severity of discomfort felt also varies from woman to woman. Some months may be more stressful than others. Occasionally, PMS disappears temporarily for no reason.

No one knows for certain what causes PMS. It is probably related to the change in hormone levels that occurs in a woman's body before menstruation. Nor do doctors know why some women are more severely affected than others. Some well-publicized "simple answers" to PMS cannot be documented by scientific studies.

True, PMS occurs only when the ovaries are working to make both estrogen and progesterone—it has been detected only in women between puberty and menopause.

But PMS is probably not caused by hormone deficiencies or excesses. Hormone levels appear to be normal in women with PMS. Researchers are now studying the possibility that estrogen and progesterone may act in combination with chemicals made in the brain to cause some of the symptoms of PMS.

The most important aspect of PMS is that it follows a pattern. Changes always occur during the second half of the menstrual cycle and are repeated each month. To be called PMS, symptoms must follow a certain pattern:

- Women with PMS may have discomfort during the last 3–14 days before their menstrual periods.
- They usually gain rapid relief of their symptoms once their menstrual periods start.

This pattern must be repeated for at least two cycles before PMS is considered as a possible reason for the symptoms. If the problem is PMS, a woman should also be free of typical discomfort for at least 2 weeks a month. Any problem that lasts longer than 2 weeks is probably not PMS.

SOURCE:
American College of Obstetricians and Gynecologists. *Premenstrual Syndrome.* 1985. pp. 1, 4–5.

DIAGNOSIS

Premenstrual problems can be divided into four distinct categories with standardized critera:

1. Premenstrual symptoms or changes. Almost all women experience at least one premenstrual symptom or change, but these are typically mild, do not interfere with functioning, and are considered normal.

2. Premenstrual syndrome. This consists of two or three symptoms (e.g. fatigue, irritability) that are also not severe enought to interfere wtih functioning.

3. Premenstrual disorder. A true premenstrual disorder—as defined by the American Psychiatric Association—comprises five or more symptoms, one of which involves mood, that are severe enough to impair daily functioning.

4. Premenstrual exacerbation of a chronic condition. Many chronic medical and emotional problems (such as depression, endometriosis, seizure disorder, asthma, allergy) are exacerbated during the premenstrual phase.

The failure of patients, clinicians, and even researchers to differentiate among these conditions has greatly hampered both diagnosis and research.

SOURCE:
Gise, Leslie Hartley. "Premenstrual Syndrome: Which Treatments Help?" *Medical Aspects of Human Sexuality* (February 1991): 62–63.

* * *

In its broadest context, PMS may be defined as "the cyclic recurrence in the luteal phase [after ovulation] of the menstrual cycle of a combination of distressing physical, psychological, and/or behavioral changes of sufficient severity to result in deterioration of interpersonal relationships and/or interference with normal activities." Such a definition would exclude many women with mild premenstrual changes, such as acne, craving for sweets, bloating, constipation, and breast tenderness, which rarely if ever disrupt lifestyle or interpersonal relationships. It would include those with more severe luteal-phase symptoms, such as depression, mood swings, irritability, anxiety, fatigue, insomnia, and headaches, if these resulted in social withdrawal, deterioration of interpersonal relationships due to increased verbal or physical aggression, suicidal thoughts or actions, or impaired cognition or performance. Daily records confirming the severity, impact, and timing of symptoms are essential to confirm the diagnosis and rule out more chronic disorders of mood or behavior that may worsen during the premenstrual period.

The very diagnosis of PMS has been hotly contested on a number of fronts. Some feminists have presented arguments for and against the recognition of the syndrome as a distinct clinical entity, based on their perceptions of whether its acknowledgment as a disorder would help the afflicted women or serve to undermine the quest for equality for women.

SOURCE:
Reid, Robert L. "Premenstrual Syndrome." *The New England Journal of Medicine* 324, no. 17 (April 25, 1991): 1208.

TREATMENT WITH PROGESTERONE

Use of progesterone in clinical practice indicates that it can be effective in the treatment of severe symptoms associated with PMS, although it has not been shown to help all women. However, numerous testimonials from women who have used progesterone therapy suggest that it can relieve severe physical symptoms such as migraine headaches. Women report that progesterone has minimized erratic, self-destructive and dangerous behaviors. These behaviors include angry outbursts that can lead to quitting a job, rage that can result in child abuse, anger and resentment that can lead to divorce, and the kind of desperate depression that can make a woman feel suicidal.

If you are still suffering from PMS symptoms after trying all the self-help treatments for PMS, you must decide if your symptoms are severe enough that they necessitate progesterone therapy. In making the decision, you need to weigh the risks between possible long-term side effects of progesterone against the consequences of PMS symptoms.

What is the best way for you to go about deciding whether you should use progesterone? If I were counseling you at the PMS Clinic, I would ask you: "Are your symptoms interfering significantly with your personal or professional life?"

If your answer was "yes," then you might benefit from progesterone therapy. If your PMS symptoms are damaging your relationships and your self-esteem, you need to stop the destructive process and stabilize your situation. You need to find a doctor who can assist you in getting effective medical treatment.

SOURCE:
Bender, Stephanie DeGraff, and Kathleen Kelleher. *PMS: A Positive Program to Gain Control.* Tucson, AZ: The Body Press, 1986. pp. 157, 158.

* * *

The value of progesterone, long thought to be the only effective treatment for premenstrual syndrome (PMS), has been disproven in a large study published recently in *JAMA* (18 July 1990). About seven million women are said to experience at least some of the broad array of PMS symptoms—from breast tenderness to irritability—each month before the menstrual period.

The extensive media coverage given PMS in the early 1980s spawned clinics across the country claiming an expertise not found in the ordinary gynecologists's office. Nutritional counseling and short-term psychotherapy were offered but the big draw was the hormone drug progesterone, because PMS was believed to be caused by progesterone deficiency. This was a theory proposed by the British physician and author, Katharina Dalton, who was invariably mentioned in every major article on PMS.

While progesterone drugs were—and still are—not approved by the FDA for the treatment of this disorder, doctors prescribe them anyway. (Progesterone is approved only for the treatment of irregular periods and uterine bleeding.) This is a common practice that is ethical only when the woman is fully informed of the fact that the drug has never been tested and proven safe or effective for the treatment of PMS. In the heyday of PMS clinics, informal surveys indicated that informed consent was relatively uncommon. There is good reason to use this drug with caution since it is associated with blood-clotting and cancer in laboratory animals.

Today, progesterone is the most widely used treatment for PMS, despite the failure of six out of seven studies to find it any more effective than a placebo. Since all these studies were criticized for various reasons, such as a small number of participants (none had more than 35) or too low a dose of progesterone, Ellen Freeman, Ph.D., and colleagues at several Philadelphia medical centers, conducted a new study designed to provide definitive answers.

The 168 participants who had suffered from PMS for about eight years took vaginal suppositories containing either a placebo or progesterone in doses ranging from 400 to 800 mg. Without knowing when they were taking the active treatment, the women alternated each over a four-month period. Progesterone produced no significant improvement in emotional or physical distress.

SOURCE:
"Drug Used to Treat PMS Found Ineffective." *HealthFacts* (August 1990): 5.

RESOURCES

ORGANIZATION
American College of Obstetricians and Gynecologists. 600 Maryland Avenue SW, Suite 300 East, Washington, DC 20024.

BOOKS

Bender, Stephanie DeGraff, and Kathleen Kelleher. *PMS: A Positive Program to Gain Control.* Tucson, AZ: The Body Press, 1986.

Nazzaro, Ann L., and Donald R. Lombard. *The PMS Solution: Premenstrual Syndrome, the Nutritional Approach.* Minneapolis: Winston Press, 1985.

RELATED ARTICLES

Chrisler, Joan C., and Karen B. Levy. "The Media Construct a Menstrual Monster: A Content Analysis of PMS Articles in the Popular Press." *Women & Health* 16 (Summer 1990): 89.

Endicott, Jean, and others. "Helping the Patient with PMS." *Patient Care* 24 (February 15, 1990): 44–61.

Keye, William R., Jr. "Premenstrual Syndrome: Seven Steps in Management." *Postgraduate Medicine* 83, no. 3 (February 15, 1988): 167–173.

"The Latest News on Premenstrual Syndrome." *Good Housekeeping* (February 1991): 116, 118.

Osofsky, Howard J. "Efficacious Treatments of PMS: A Need for Further Research." *JAMA* 264, no. 3 (July 18, 1990): 387.

"PMS Sure Remains Elusive." *Consumer Reports Health Letter* (October 1990): 78.

"Premenstrual Syndrome: Self-Help, New Drugs Can Ease the Monthly Misery." *University of Texas Health Letter* (April 1990): 6.

PRENATAL TESTING

(*See also:* DOWN SYNDROME)

OVERVIEW

As more and more women delay childbirth into their 30s and even 40s—the number of first births among this group has increased fourfold in the past two decades—prenatal testing has taken on increased importance. Most of these women will give birth to healthy, normal infants. Ninety-seven percent of all prenatal tests reveal no abnormality. But it is undeniable that an older woman's risk of having a baby with certain disabilities increases significantly with age. At 35 a woman's chance of giving birth to an infant with a chromosomal abnormality is one in 192, but by the time she's 45, the figure shoots up to one in 21.

The father's age—not just the mother's—may also play a role in a baby's health, says Mark I. Evans, M.D., director of reproductive genetics at Hutzel Hospital in Detroit. In all likelihood the father is older than the mother, and sperm, like eggs, can be altered by time.

Whatever the cause of birth defects, modern technology is now better able to discover them in utero and with greater accuracy than when the first tests were done in the late '60s. In a very few cases, it is possible to treat the infant in the womb—even surgery has been successfully performed on a fetus. More frequently, treatment begins right after birth, and knowing what to expect allows parents and physicians to prepare for the baby's arrival so the best care will be readily available.

While a test may bring peace of mind and improve a child's chances, some procedures carry a slightly increased risk of miscarriage. And results may cause unnecessary worry if they are inconclusive. Finally, if a test does reveal a serious, untreatable defect, parents may grapple with the agonizing decision of whether to terminate the pregnancy. Thus, tests should not be used indiscriminately and most are recommended only when the mother is over 30 or there is a family history of genetic disease. Here's where we are now.

Maternal Serum Alpha-Fetoprotein (MSAFP) test is a simple blood test performed in the 14th to 16th week on nearly all pregnant women. The test measures the maternal blood level of alpha-fetoprotein (AFP), a protein produced by the fetus.

"Between 40 and 50 percent of patients with high AFP readings develop some complication, such as toxemia, premature labor, poor fetal growth or stillbirth, and so the test warns us when a pregnancy should be monitored carefully," says Albert Haverkamp, M.D., director of perinatology at Kaiser-Permanente Hospital in Denver.

A high AFP level can also indicate a neural-tube defect—in which either the brain or spinal cord does not form correctly—or an abdominal wall defect. However, while AFP screening detects about 80 percent of these abnormalities, only 2 to 4 percent of women with elevated levels actually have an abnormal fetus. More often, high readings result from twins or a pregnancy that is further along than originally believed, since AFP levels increase as the pregnancy progresses. Thus its primary use is as a screening tool to determine whether further tests are warranted. AFP is as safe as any other blood test. Cost: about $35.

Ultrasound creates a picture of the fetus using high-frequency sound waves. The test is usually performed in the 18th or 19th week and can detect many physical abnormalities, including neural-tube defects and malformations of the heart.

The test itself is simple and painless. The woman lies on her back and the doctor moves a microphone-like device called a transducer over her abdomen. Sound waves produced by the transducer are bounced off fetal bones and tissues and are then converted into images on a television monitor. These images can be recorded for further study.

The test has been used safely now for 25 years, and 60 to 80 percent of pregnant women in this country have this test done at least once. Cost: $50 to $300.

Amniocentesis can be used to identify genetic abnormalities, hereditary diseases, neural-tube defects and the sex of the fetus. It is usually done in the 16th to 18th week of pregnancy.

Using ultrasound as a guide, the physician inserts a long, thin needle into the abdomen and withdraws a small amount of the amniotic fluid from the sac surrounding the fetus. Fetal cells from the fluid are then grown in the laboratory for two to three weeks, at which time they are analyzed. Unfortunately, this means that results are not available until late in the second trimester. Amniocentesis also raises the risk of miscarriage by about a half of 1 percent, and there is a slight chance of infection. Cost: $800 to $1,500.

Chorionic-villus sampling (CVS) is similar to amniocentesis but allows an earlier diagnosis, as it is performed in the ninth to 12th week of pregnancy with results available in a few days. It too detects genetic abnormalities and hereditary diseases, as well as the baby's sex, but will not pick up neural-tube defects.

Guided by ultrasound, the physician inserts a catheter through the cervix to the uterus to remove a small amount of the chorionic villi (a part of the placenta), which has the same genetic makeup as the fetus. The tissue is then cultivated and examined.

Some doctors believe that CVS is as safe as if not safer than amniocentesis. "Because CVS only goes as far as the placenta, it does not get as close to the fetus," says Joe Leigh Simpson, M.D., chairman of obstetrics and gynecology at the University of Tennessee in Memphis. However, a recent study conducted by the National Institute of Child Health and Human Development suggests that CVS may entail a slightly higher risk of miscarriage. The key seems to be the skill of the doctor. Cost: $800 to $1,100.

SOURCE:

Morrison, Maggie. "Prenatal Testing: Peering Into the Womb." *McCalls* (October 1990): 160, 162.

DETECTION OF GENETIC PROBLEMS

Here are a few of the most common genetic problems prenatal testing can detect:

Cystic fibrosis. A disease which affects the pancreas, respiratory system, and sweat glands, this problem strikes 1 in 2,000 children, mostly whites. Parents from families with histories of cystic fibrosis can be screened before pregnancy to see if they are non-diseased carriers of the abnormal gene. If both parents carry the cystic fibrosis gene, the pregnant woman can be tested with CVS or amniocentesis to see if the baby is affected.

Sickle cell anemia. Common among blacks, this disease causes anemia, infections, and pain requiring frequent hospitalization. Prepregnancy screening can detect carriers. If both parents carry the gene, the pregnant mother can be tested with CVS or amniocentesis to see if the baby has the disease.

Tay-Sachs disease. Common among Jews of Northeastern European descent, this disease causes retardation, blindness, and early death among affected children. Jewish parents should be screened before pregnancy. If both carry the non-symptomatic gene, the fetus can be tested for the disease.

Duchenne's muscular dystrophy. Mothers carry the gene for this X-linked disease which causes paralysis, muscular degeneration, and early death among male children. Women with family histories can be tested before pregnancy. If they carry the gene, prenatal testing can determine if the fetus is affected.

Down's syndrome. Once commonly called "mongolism," this condition is characterized by mental retardation, heart defects, and decreased life expectancy. It may run in families or arise spontaneously, particularly among older mothers. Mothers over age 35 should be tested. After age 40, the risk rises as high as 1 in 50 pregnancies.

Neural tube defects (spina bifida or anencephaly). These abnormalities result from the spinal cord's failure to close during embryonic development. Fetuses with anencephaly are born without brains and generally die within a few days. Spina bifida infants have normal brains but varying degrees of openings in the low back area of the spinal column and may suffer leg paralysis and lack bladder and bowel control.

These serious neural tube defects can usually be detected with a maternal blood test performed at 16 to 18 weeks which measures the amount of a protein called alpha-fetoprotein normally produced by the fetus. Abnormally high levels of the protein may indicate a neural tube defect. It may also indicate twins and help date pregnancy. Women with high levels of alpha-fetoprotein should be tested further with ultrasound and amniocentesis for a more accurate diagnosis.

SOURCE:

Greenwood, Sadja. "Prenatal Testing Update." *Medical SelfCare* (March/April 1989): 19–20.

ALPHA-FETOPROTEIN SCREENING

Many obstetricians now routinely offer their pregnant patients the option of a blood test called the maternal serum alpha-fetoprotein (MSAFP) screening test. This test identifies pregnancies at higher-than-average risk of certain serious birth defects and can provide valuable information about the developing fetus. But an abnormal result can cause a great deal of anxiety for a pregnant woman unless she understands that in most cases abnormal results do not reflect anything wrong with the fetus. The following addresses common questions about the use and limitations of MSAFP testing.

What is alpha-fetoprotein?

Alpha-fetoprotein (AFP) is a substance produced by the fetal liver. The fetus excretes some of this protein into the amniotic fluid. A small amount of AFP passes into the maternal bloodstream, where the concentration rises gradually until late in pregnancy.

AFP levels can be measured during pregnancy in either the mother's blood or amniotic fluid to look for certain birth defects.

What does a low MSAFP reading mean?

A more recent and still unexplained finding is that low MSAFP readings are sometimes associated with chromosomal abnormalities, such as Down syndrome. However, a finding of low MSAFP does not seem to be as predictive in identifying chromosomal abnormalities as high MSAFP is for neural tube defects.

If a woman has a low MSAFP level, her physician may repeat the test, and perform ultrasound to confirm gestational age. Many physicians may then discuss the option of amniocentesis with the pregnant woman to detect or rule out chromosomal abnormalities, especially if she has other risk factors for this kind of birth defect—the usual one being her age.

If a woman has a low MSAFP level, her physician may perform ultrasound to confirm gestational age, or possibly repeat the test. Many physicians may then discuss the option of amniocentesis with the pregnant woman to detect or rule out chromosomal abnormalities. Some women have other risk factors for this kind of birth defect, such as family history or age 35 or above, that add weight to consideration of amniocentesis.

What are the benefits of MSAFP screening?

For the great majority of women, screening provides reassurance that the fetus is not apparently affected by certain serious birth defects. Test results can lead to a more effectively managed pregnancy. For example, finding the correct gestational age helps determine whether the fetus is growing at a normal rate. Detecting a twin pregnancy also allows for the special prenatal care needed in a multiple pregnancy.

When a neural tube defect or other problem is diagnosed, or suspected, specially trained personnel can provide information and support. Delivery may be planned in a center equipped to deal with an affected newborn, possibly improving the outlook for the baby, who may require surgery or treatment soon after birth.

In some cases, abnormal MSAFP test results remain unexplained. Abnormal readings have been linked with pregnancy problems such as abruption (detachment) of the placenta and low birthweight, and the physician can monitor such pregnancies with these possibilities in mind.

March of Dimes-supported researchers are currently investigating whether unexplained abnormal readings can serve as an early warning signal for a number of pregnancy-related problems.

SOURCE:
March of Dimes Birth Defects Foundation. *Alpha-Fetoprotein Screening.* Public Health Education Information Sheet. January 1991. p. 1.

CHORIONIC VILLUS SAMPLING (CVS)

The chorion is a membrane that surrounds the fetal gestational sac. It develops from the same cells from which the fetus develops and is located just outside of the amniotic membrane. The chorion's surface is covered with fingerlike projections (villi) in early pregnancy. As the pregnancy progresses, the villi on one surface of the chorion grow to attach the gestational sac to the uterine lining. The villi eventually form a part of the placenta with a large surface area that allows for the exchange of oxygen and nutrients from mother to fetus. Since the chorion begins from the same cells as the fetus, a sample of the chorion will be identical in genetic makeup to that of the fetus.

CVS is usually performed at nine to twelve weeks from the first day of the last menstrual period. Amniocentesis, on the other hand, has traditionally been performed later in pregnancy, around sixteen weeks after the last menstrual period. Unlike CVS, which involves taking a sample of the chorionic villi, amniocentesis involves drawing amniotic fluid from the sac surrounding the fetus.

In addition to the difference in gestational age at the time the tests are performed, the techniques for examining the chorionic villi tissue differ from those used to examine the amniotic-fluid cells. Also, the waiting time for obtaining the results is usually much shorter with CVS than with amniocentesis; the results of CVS are usually available within one week, while amniocentesis results are available within two to four weeks. . . .

Chorionic villus sampling, while no longer considered to be an experimental procedure, is still somewhat new compared with amniocentesis. The potential risks associated with amniocentesis are well known: serious complications are rare, with pregnancy loss occurring in about .5 percent of procedures. The risks associated with CVS are also small, with miscarriages occurring in 1 percent of procedures. It is difficult to determine which of these pregnancies might have resulted in a miscarriage even if CVS had not been performed. Another problem with CVS is that obtaining a sample of tissue may be unsuccessful. This may be due to anatomical problems, such as uterine fibroids (benign tumors).

Both CVS and amniocentesis are performed on an outpatient basis, that is, there is no need for hospitalization. Because CVS is a relatively new procedure, it is still available only in selected locations and at specific medical centers. If a woman needs to travel to a center that performs CVS, an ultrasound is often requested from the referring obstetrician to estimate the best date for performing CVS by assessing the age and development of the fetus. An ultrasound should always be performed immediately before the CVS procedure in order to identify the location of the fetus and placenta and to make sure that there are no uterine abnormalities. If there are uterine fibroids present, they can block access to the chorion, and amniocentesis or a transabdominal CVS procedure may then be necessary. In a transabdominal CVS a needle is inserted through the abdomen into the center of the chorion to remove villi for sampling. This is similar to what is done in amniocentesis, except that in amniocentesis fluid is withdrawn from within the amniotic cavity.

SOURCE:
Hillard, Paula Adams. "The Earliest Prenatal Test." *Parents' Magazine* 64 (July 1989): 151, 152.

PROBLEMS WITH CHORIONIC VILLUS SAMPLING

A technique that experts had predicted would revolutionize prenatal diagnosis has faltered in recent studies, leading some doctors to turn back to an older, established procedure, amniocentesis.

Last month, a large randomized European trial showed that patients who used the new technique, chorionic villus sampling, experienced almost 5 percent more fetal and neonatal deaths than women who chose amniocentesis. Weeks before, British researchers reported an unusually high number of limb deformities in the children of a small group of women who had opted for the new technique.

The differences are not huge but raise concern, scientists say. Studies have also suggested that the new technique more often yields ambiguous diagnoses, so that some women have to undergo subsequent amniocentesis to clarify their babies' health.

"People should be more reserved about the technique than a few years ago," said Dr. John Hamerton, head of the department of human genetics at the University of Manitoba. "It has been subjected to a very, very critical set of trials, and they have come up with a higher risk and lower accuracy than amniocentesis. It is also more time consuming and costly. It has a number of strikes against it."

In the abstract, sampling is an attractive option since test results are returned in the third month of pregnancy, while an all-clear from amniocentesis is not available until the fifth month, by which time termination of a pregnancy can be medically complicated and more emotionally traumatic.

Dr. Tom Mead, an epidemiologist with the British Medical Research Council who directed the European trial, said that the relatively poor showing of sampling should not signal a death knell for the technique, but should help women decide which form of prenatal diagnosis to pursue. . .

Sampling is a technically difficult procedure in which the obstetrician guides a small tube through the cervix or abdominal wall into the uterus to suction cells from the hair-like projections, or chorionic villi, that form the fetus's contribution to the placenta. Some of the cells are examined immediately for chromosomal abnormalities, and others are placed in culture dishes for use in other tests. In amniocentesis the doctor simply withdraws a sample of uterine fluid, containing stray fetal cells, via a needle inserted through the abdomen.

Scientists are unsure exactly why either test causes fetal problems, although the cause is probably related to disruption of the fetus and womb by the introduction of medical instruments.

SOURCE:
Rosenthal, Elisabeth. "Technique for Early Prenatal Test Comes Under Question in Studies." *The New York Times* (July 10, 1991): B6.

CORDOCENTESIS, FETAL TISSUE SAMPLING, AND CELL SORTING

Cordocentesis

Cordocentesis, also called Percutaneous Umbilical Blood Sampling (PUBS) and fetal-blood sampling, is a four-year-old procedure that tests the fetus for genetic abnormalities, RH-factor incompatibility, and infections such as German measles, herpes and toxoplasmosis. Under ultrasound guidance, a needle is inserted through the mother's abdomen and a sample of the fetus's red blood cells is taken from the umbilical cord. The procedure can be done after the 17th week of pregnancy up until birth.

"Cordocentesis is most often used to check for chromosome abnormalities, either because the results of an amniocentesis are inconclusive or because it's late in the pregnancy and you want to get results fast," explains Usha Chitkara, MD, associate professor of obstetrics and gynecology at Mount Sinai Medical Center in New York. Unlike amniocentesis, cordocentesis produces results within a week. It is considered by some researchers to be more accurate than either amniocentesis or CVS.

Unlike some of the other testing methods, cordocentesis sometimes can offer hope when the test brings bad news. It cannot change the genetic makeup of a fetus found to have a chromosome abnormality, but if RH-factor incompatibility is detected, an anemic fetus can be saved by a blood transfusion.

The risk of miscarriage with cordocentesis is slightly more than that of amniocentesis, usually between 1 and 1.5 percent. But it's not easy to find an experienced center: at the moment, only about 25 medical centers in the country are doing the procedure.

The cost of cordocentesis is about $800 to $1,000, plus about $300 to $500 for chromosome analysis. It generally is covered by insurance.

Fetal-Tissue Sampling

This experimental technique is used to test for extremely rare and generally fatal hereditary skin disorders. Using ultrasound guidance, the surgeon inserts a needle into the amniotic sac and takes a tiny sample of fetal skin. The skin fragments also may be used to do genetic tests, but because of the invasiveness of the technique, it is never used for this purpose alone.

Researchers claim that a tissue sample taken from the back or buttocks doesn't leave a noticeable scar. However, the procedure is so rarely performed that there really isn't enough evidence to assess its risks, accuracy or long-term effects.

A few research groups are using a similar technique to take samples of fetal liver that can be tested for rare enzyme disorders.

Cell Sorting

It has been known for quite a while that a few of the fetus's cells "leak" into the mother's bloodstream after the 8th to 10th week of pregnancy. Recently a Harvard medical team isolated fetal blood cells in blood taken from a small number of pregnant women. The hope is that once extracted, the cells can be used to perform the same sort of genetic testing now done by amniocentesis and CVS—but without the risks inherent in these invasive procedures.

However, cell sorting is still a long way from reality, according to Robert Anderson, MD, co-director of the prenatal detection program at the University of California at San Francisco. Not only is it difficult to separate fetal cells from blood, but the techniques that are used to extract them often alter the cells so that they can't be reproduced—a necessity for genetic testing. What's more, it is nearly impossible to distinguish the cells of the growing fetus from those that are left over from previous pregnancies. Nonetheless, the possibility of a risk-free genetic test makes the procedure well worth pursuing.

SOURCE:

Kaplan, Janice. "Prenatal Testing: The Newest Options." *Working Woman* 15 (January 1990): 134–135.

ENDING A PREGNANCY

Unfortunately, prenatal testing technology has out-distanced medicine's ability to treat the problems the tests uncover. When trouble does turn up, couples are often emotionally devastated and unprepared to face a terrible choice—whether to bring to an end a wanted pregnancy or continue it and risk physical and mental agony for their child.

Some patients who know they're carrying a baby with Down's syndrome or other genetic anomalies that will result in mild retardation or developmental problems do continue the pregnancy. And through lots of love and, later, special help, they nurture these especially loving children.

But when prenatal testing detects a devastating genetic problem many couples choose to end the pregnancy. It's uncertain exactly what impact the U.S. Supreme Court's ruling on abortion will have for people who learn their fetus has a genetic disease. What's clear, however, is that there are very few support services available for couples who exercise the option to end a pregnancy.

Some resources are beginning to emerge, but they operate quietly, so as not to catch the attention of anti-abortionists. In the absence of specialized help, many parents seek private counseling or attend general pregnancy-loss support groups.

But unlike couples who lose pregnancies through miscarriage, those who end a wanted pregnancy may feel especially isolated and vulnerable. They are often reluctant to tell friends and family exactly what happened. "It's a very private decision," says one woman.

SOURCE:

Krance, Magda. "When Prenatal Tests Bring Bad News: Few Support Services Help Couples Cope." *American Health* 8 (July-August 1989): 11–12.

GENETIC COUNSELING

More than 95 percent of the high-risk women using prenatal diagnosis receive reassuring news—that their unborn babies do not have the disorders for which they are tested. If an abnormality is detected, the genetic counselor will share whatever information is available on the treatment of a child with the problem. In some cases, an abnormality can be treated while the baby is still in the womb.

When genetic counseling is received, counselors or referring physicians do not prescribe a particular course of action. Their role is to provide the family with a complete and accurate view of the situation—the nature of any birth defects in the family, the risk of recurrence and what a recurrence would mean in practical terms for any concerned.

Beyond the risk figures and the medical explanations, genetic counseling helps families understand the diagnoses and weigh the risks in terms of their personal values. Identical odds figures take on very different meanings to different couples, depending on the severity of the defect and on their personal beliefs and experiences. How much couples or individuals choose to learn, and what they do with that information, remains their decision.

When a birth defect is diagnosed, genetic counselors provide emotional support and understanding during a very difficult time. If there are decisions to be made—about the care of a child, about having more children, about the ability of the family to cope with ongoing problems—the parents can make more informed choices with the facts in hand.

SOURCE:

Ince, Susan. *Genetic Counseling.* March of Dimes Birth Defects Foundation. December 1987. p. 20.

RESOURCES

ORGANIZATION

March of Dimes Birth Defects Foundation. 1275 Mamaroneck Avenue, White Plains, NY 10605.

BOOKS

Rothman, Barbara Katz. *The Tentative Pregnancy: Prenatal Diagnosis and the Future of Motherhood.* New York: Penguin, 1989.

Schwiebert, Pat, and Paul Kirk. *Still to Be Born: A Guide for Bereaved Parents Who Are Making Decisions about Their Future.* Portland, OR: Perinatal Loss, 1990.

RELATED ARTICLES

Bishop, Jerry E., and Michael Waldholz. "Misfortune Telling." *American Health* (September 1990): 64–71.

Emmett-Arthur, Arielle. "Genetic Counseling." *Parents' Magazine* 64 (May 1989): 126–131.

Ferguson, J. E., and others. "Transcervical Chorionic Villus Sampling and Amniocentesis: A Comparison of Reliability, Culture Findings, and Fetal Outcome." *American Journal of Obstetrics and Gynecology* 163, no. 3 (September 1990): 926–931.

Kazilimani, Esther. "The Precautions of Prenatal Testing." *Priorities* (Winter 1990): 21–23.

Mennuti, Michael T. "Prenatal Diagnosis—Advances Bring New Challenges." *The New England Journal of Medicine* 320, no. 10 (March 9, 1989): 661–663.

Rhoads, George G., and others. "The Safety and Efficacy of Chorionic Villus Sampling for Early Prenatal Diagnosis of Cytogenetic Abnormalities." *The New England Journal of Medicine* 320, no. 10 (March 9, 1989): 609–617.

PROSTATE CANCER

(*See also:* PROSTATE ENLARGEMENT)

OVERVIEW

Prostate cancer most often arises from deep within the prostate gland not in the benign prostatic hypertrophy cells so common in older men. Over 95 percent of prostate cancers are adenocarcinomas. When viewed under a microscope, the cells in adenocarcinomas grow in patterns that have a gland-like appearance. The remaining prostate cancers are atypical adenocarcinomas, sarcomas, peripheral ductal carcinomas, adenoid cystic carcinomas, endometrioid tumors, carcinosarcomas, and malignant lymphomas.

Cancer of the prostate is one of the most common forms of cancer among American males. In the United States, approximately 1 man in 11 will develop prostate cancer during his lifetime. Found primarily in men over the age of 50, prostate cancer becomes increasingly common with each decade of life. About 80 percent of cases are diagnosed in men over 65.

The age-adjusted incidence of prostate cancer increased consistently from 45.3 to 76.4 per 100,000 from 1950 to 1985. During that period, the overall increase was 67 percent, or about a 1.8 percent increase each year. It is estimated that 99,000 new cases of prostate cancer were diagnosed in the United States in 1988. The increase in incidence is believed to be largely (but not exclusively) due to improved detection of the disease.

The true prevalence of prostate cancer (the total number of cases at a particular time) may be higher than available statistics indicate, especially in men over the age of 70. Autopsy examinations of elderly men who die from other causes often reveal previously undiagnosed cancer of the prostate. In addition, unsuspected prostate cancer is often diagnosed during microscopic examination of prostate tissue removed during surgery for other diseases of the prostate. It is not clear what the natural rate of progression would be for these early cancers, but epidemiologic studies have shown that men who have prostate cancer incidentally discovered during examination for other reasons have survival patterns similar to those of age-matched members of the general population.

Although the incidence of new cases of prostate cancer has increased steadily over the past 35 years, the mortality rate has increased only slightly. Prostate cancer was responsible for about 28,000 deaths during 1988. The 5-year survival rate for all stages of prostate cancer has improved from 43 percent in 1950 to 73 percent in 1980, due to better understanding of the epidemiology of this disease, more effective screening and detection techniques, and improved treatment.

Black men in the United States have the highest incidence rate of prostate cancer in the world. Although reliable data on black Africans are not readily available, their prostate cancer rates appear to be much lower than those for American blacks. The reasons for this apparent difference are not known. However, it appears that socioeconomic and lifestyle factors, rather than an inherent racial predisposition, explain the difference. Limited access to health care and detection of prostate cancer only after it has produced symptoms and is in an advanced stage contribute to the poor survival from prostate cancer among American black men.

SOURCE:

National Cancer Institute. *Cancer of the Prostate. Research Report.* 1990. pp. 3–4.

SIGNS AND SYMPTOMS

Often, there are no symptoms in the earliest stages of prostate cancer. When symptoms do occur, they may include some of the following problems:

- Need to urinate frequently, especially at night
- Difficulty starting urination or holding back urine
- Inability to urinate
- Weak or interrupted flow of urine
- Painful or burning urination
- Blood in the urine
- Painful ejaculation
- Continuing pain in the lower back, hips, or upper thighs

These symptoms may be caused by prostate cancer, by benign prostate conditions, or by other problems. It is important to have any of these symptoms checked by a doctor to find out what the problem is.

Benign conditions of the prostate include infections, prostate stones, and enlargement of the prostate (known as *benign prostatic hypertrophy*, or BPH). More than half of all men in the United States over the age of 50 suffer from BPH, which occurs when the prostate swells and pushes against the urethra and the bladder, blocking the flow of urine.

SOURCE:
National Cancer Institute. *What You Need to Know about Prostate Cancer.* NIH Pub. no. 86-1576, January 1988. pp. 3-4.

DETECTION AND DIAGNOSIS

Traditionally, the early detection of prostate cancer in asymptomatic men has depended on digital rectal examination, but recently, two techniques capable of detecting prostate cancer in men with a normal digital rectal examination have become available: measurement of prostate-specific antigen and transrectal ultrasonography. The prospect of using these techniques in widespread screening or early detection programs has generated considerable controversy. Both the efficacy of these techniques and the necessity for early detection of this slowly growing cancer have been seriously questioned. Because of the remarkably high prevalence of cancer in the prostate found at autopsy of men who die of other causes, the slow progression rate of the tumor, and the advanced age of men at diagnosis, patients with prostate cancer are often said to be more likely to die with rather than of their disease. On the other hand, once prostate cancer is diagnosed—whether by digital rectal examination, pathologic review of the tissue from transurethral resection, or the appearance of symptoms—treatment has generally been unsuccessful except in the cancer's very early stages. With 28,500 men dying of the disease in the United States this year, the need for earlier detection seems evident.

SOURCE:
Scardino, P. T. "Early Detection of Prostate Cancer." *Urologic Clinics of North America* 16, no. 4 (November 1989): 635.

STAGING

Several staging systems have been used for prostate cancer. The widely used American Urologic System divides prostate cancer into stages A, B, C, and D.

Stage A: Microscopic clusters of cancer cells are found in tissue samples removed during surgical treatment for benign disease; stage A disease cannot be detected by the physician during rectal examination.

A1: The tumor cells are well differentiated and are found only in one area of the gland.

A2: The tumor cells are poorly differentiated or occur in many areas of the gland.

Stage B: Cancer is confined within the capsule of the prostate; it can be felt by the physician during rectal examination.

B1: A single tumor is found in one lobe of the prostate.

B2: The cancer is more extensive, involving one or both lobes.

Stage C: The cancer extends outside the prostatic capsule to nearby tissues or organs.

Stage D: The cancer has spread to regional lymph nodes or beyond the pelvis to the bone or other organs.

D1: Only regional lymph nodes are involved.

D2: The cancer has spread to the bone, distant lymph nodes, or other distant organs.

Another important part of pre-treatment evaluation is determining the grade, or degree of differentiation, of the cancer cells. Grading is an effort to predict the aggressiveness of a tumor based on the microscopic appearance of the cancer cells. Well-differentiated cancer cells resemble their normal counterparts, while poorly differentiated cancer cells are disorganized and abnormal looking. Since poorly differentiated cells tend to spread more rapidly than well-differentiated ones, this characteristic helps the physician make recommendations about treatment.

SOURCE:
National Cancer Institute. *Cancer of the Prostate: Research Report.* NIH Pub. No. 89-528. February 1989. p. 10.

PROGNOSIS

In patients with stage A1 disease, 8% will develop distant metastases, and 2% will die of the disease within 5 to 10 years. . . .

Thirty percent of patients with clinical stage A2 tumors develop distant metastases, and 20% die within 5 to 10 years. Thus, definitive treatment is needed in most patients with stage A2.

Of those with stage B2 disease, 80% will develop distant metastases within 5 to 10 years. These patients also require definitive treatment.

More than 50% of stage C patients develop distant metastases less than 5 years after diagnosis, and 75% die within 10 years.

Most patients (85%) with stage D1 disease develop distant metastases within 5 years, and the majority die of prostate cancer within 3 years of developing distant metastases. Half of stage D2 patients die of prostate cancer within 3 years of diagnosis, 80% die within 5 years, and 90% within 10 years. Patients with bony metastases respond well to palliative radiation therapy, and to hormonal therapy to relieve pain.

Patients with tumors that have relapsed after hormonal therapy have a 90% mortality rate from prostate cancer within a 2-year period. Most die, however, within the first year after relapse.

In summary, prostate cancer continues to be a major health care problem facing our elderly male population. Improved diagnostic and treatment modalities are needed, but for now successful treatment can only be achieved through early detection, accurate staging, and judicious selection of agents.

SOURCE:
Gross, J. S. "Current Management Modalities for Prostate Cancer." *Geriatrics* 45, no. 4 (April 1990): 67–68.

PROSTATE CANCER AND IMPOTENCE

Impotence remains a common side effect of all forms of prostate cancer therapy. In the past, surgery caused impotence virtually every time, but newer surgical techniques are designed to spare the nerves involved in gaining an erection. With these nerve-sparing techniques, the incidence of impotence has fallen to between 25% and 60%.

Radiation therapy leaves men impotent 40% to 50% of the time. Hormone therapy carries a high incidence of impotence, and orchiectomy [removal of both testes] almost always causes it. Some drugs now being used seem to have less effect on sexual function. Physicians experienced in the use of radioactive pellets often have achieved low rates of impotence, and that's another reason some centers still offer the procedure.

Prostate cancer patients need considerable support and understanding from family members and physicians. Patients not only have to come to grips with the cancer and its treatment, but they also have to deal with the possible loss of sexual potency—and that can be very difficult for many men.

For patients who do experience impotence, help is available from a variety of sources. With counseling and use of penile prostheses and other devices, many impotent men can remain sexually active.

SOURCE:
"Prostate Cancer: Early Detection Saves Lives." *The University of Texas Lifetime Health Letter* 2, no. 5 (May 1990): 6.

RESOURCES

ORGANIZATIONS
American Cancer Society. National Office, 4 East 35th Street, New York, NY 10001.

National Cancer Institute. Cancer Information Service, Building 31, 9000 Rockville Pike, MD 20892.

PAMPHLETS
American Cancer Society:

Facts on Prostate Cancer. 2654-LE.

For Men Only: Prostate Cancer. 2632-LE.

National Cancer Institute:

What You Need to Know About Prostate Cancer. NIH Pub. No. 88–1576. 1988. 25 pp.

BOOK
Rous, S. N. *The Prostate Book: Sound Advice on Symptoms and Treatment.* New York: Norton, 1988.

RELATED ARTICLES
Balducci, L., M. Parker and others. "Review: Systemic Management of Prostate Cancer." *American Journal of the Medical Sciences* 299, no. 3 (March 1990): 185–192.

Guthrie, Jr., T. H., and P. Watson. "Prostate Cancer." *American Family Physician* 36, no. 4 (October 1987): 217–224.

Hardeman, S. W., R. W. Wake, and others. "Two New Techniques for Evaluating Prostate Cancer: The Role of Prostate-Specific Antigen and Transrectal Ultrasound." *Postgraduate Medicine* 86, no. 2 (August 1989): 197–208.

Lee, F., P. J. Littrup, and others. "Prostate Cancer: Comparison of Transrectal US and Digital Rectal Examination for Screening." *Radiology* 168 (August 1988): 389–394.

"The Management of Clinically Localized Prostate Cancer." National Institutes of Health Consensus Development Conference, June 15–17, 1987." *Journal of Urology* 138 (December 1987): 1369–1375.

PROSTATE ENLARGEMENT

(*See also:* PROSTATE CANCER)

OVERVIEW

It is common for the prostate gland to become enlarged as a man ages. Doctors call the condition benign prostatic hyperplasia (BPH), or benign prostatic hypertrophy.

As a male matures, the prostate goes through two main periods of growth. The first occurs early in puberty, when the prostate doubles in size. At around age 25, the gland begins to grow again. It is this second growth phase that often results, years later, in BPH.

Though the prostate continues to grow during most of a man's life, the enlargement doesn't usually cause problems until late in life. BPH rarely causes symptoms before age 40, but more than half of men in their sixties and as many as 90 percent in their seventies and eighties have some symptoms of BPH.

As the prostate enlarges, the surrounding capsule stops it from expanding, causing the gland to press against the urethra like a clamp on a garden hose. The bladder wall becomes thicker and irritable. The bladder begins to contract even when it contains small amounts of urine, causing more frequent urination. As the bladder weakens, it loses the ability to empty itself, and urine remains behind. This narrowing of the urethra and partial emptying of the bladder cause many of the problems associated with BPH.

Many people feel uncomfortable talking about the prostate, since the gland plays a role in both sex and urination. However, prostate enlargement is as common a part of aging as gray hair. As life expectancy rises, so does the occurrence of BPH. In the United States alone, 350,000 operations take place each year for BPH.

It is not clear whether certain groups face a greater risk of getting BPH. Studies done over the years have suggested that BPH occurs more often among married men than single men and is more common in the United States and Europe than in any other parts of the world. However, these findings have been debated, and no definite information on risk factors exists.

The cause of BPH is not well understood. For centuries, it has been known that BPH occurs mainly in older men and that it doesn't develop in males whose testes were removed before puberty. For this reason, some researchers believe that factors related to aging and the testes may spur the development of BPH.

Throughout their lives, men produce both testosterone, an important male hormone, and small amounts of estrogen, a female hormone. As men age, the amount of active testosterone in the blood decreases, leaving a higher proportion of estrogen. Studies done with animals have suggested that BPH may occur because the higher amount of estrogen within the gland increases the activity of substances that promote cell growth.

Another theory focuses on dihydrotestosterone (DHT), a substance derived from testosterone in the prostate, which may help control its growth. Most animals lose their ability to produce DHT as they age. However, some research has indicated that even with a drop in the blood's testosterone level, older men continue to produce and accumulate high levels of DHT in the prostate. This accumulation of DHT may encourage the growth of cells. Scientists have also noted that men who do not produce DHT do not develop BPH.

Some researchers suggest that BPH may develop as a result of "instructions" given to cells early in life. According to this theory, BPH occurs because cells in one section of the gland follow these instructions and "reawaken" later in life. These "reawakened" cells then deliver signals to other cells in the gland, instructing them to grow or making them more sensitive to hormones that influence growth.

Many symptoms of BPH stem from obstruction of the urethra and gradual loss of bladder function, which results in incomplete emptying of the bladder. The symptoms of BPH vary, but the most common ones involve changes or problems with urination, such as:

- a hesitant, interrupted, weak stream
- urgency and leaking or dribbling
- more frequent urination, especially at night

The size of the prostate does not always determine how severe the obstruction or the symptoms will be. Some men with greatly enlarged glands have little obstruction and few symptoms while others, whose glands are less enlarged, have more blockage and greater problems.

Sometimes a man may not know he has any obstruction until he suddenly finds himself unable to urinate at all. This condition, called acute urinary retention, may be triggered by taking over-the-counter cold or allergy medicines. Such medicines contain a decongestant drug, known as a sympathomimetic, which may, as a side effect, prevent the bladder opening from relaxing and allowing urine to empty. When partial obstruction is present, urinary retention also can be brought on by alcohol, cold temperatures, or a long period of immobility.

It is important to tell your doctor about urinary problems such as those described above. In 8 out of 10 cases, these symptoms suggest BPH, but they can also signal other, more serious conditions that require prompt treatment. These conditions can be ruled out only by a doctor's exam.

Severe BPH can also cause serious problems over time. Urine retention and strain on the bladder can lead to urinary tract infections, bladder or kidney damage, bladder stones, and incontinence. If the bladder is permanently damaged, treatment for BPH may be ineffective. When BPH is found in its earlier stages, there is a lower risk of developing such complications.

SOURCE:
National Institute of Diabetes & Digestive & Kidney Diseases. *Prostate Enlargement: Benign Prostatic Hyperplasia*. NIH Pub. No. 91-3012. September 1991. pp. 2-4.

SURGICAL TREATMENT

Men who have BPH with symptoms usually need some kind of treatment at some time. However, a number of recent studies have questioned the need for early treatment when the gland is just mildly enlarged. These studies report that early treatment may not be needed because the symptoms of BPH clear up without treatment in as many as one-third of all mild cases. Instead of immediate treatment, they suggest regular checkups to watch for early problems. If the condition begins to pose a danger to the patient's health or causes a major inconvenience to him, treatment is usually recommended.

Since BPH may cause urinary tract infections, a doctor will usually clear up any infection with antibiotics before treating the BPH itself. Although the need for treatment is not usually urgent, doctors generally advise going ahead with treatment once the problems become bothersome or present a health risk. The following section describes the types of treatment that are most commonly used for BPH.

Most doctors recommend removal of the enlarged part of the prostate as the best long-range solution for patients with BPH. With surgery for BPH, only the enlarged tissue that is pressing against the urethra is removed; the rest of the inside tissue and the outside capsule are left intact. Surgery usually relieves the obstruction and incomplete emptying caused by BPH. The following section describes the types of surgery that are used.

Transurethral Surgery. In this type of surgery, no external incision is needed. After giving anesthesia, the surgeon reaches the prostate by inserting an instrument through the urethra.

A procedure called TURP (Transurethral Resection of the Prostate) is used for 90 percent of all prostate surgeries done for BPH. With TURP, an instrument called a resectoscope is inserted through the penis. The resectoscope, which is about 12 inches long and ½ inch in diameter, contains a light, valves for controlling irrigating fluid, and an electrical loop that cuts tissue and seals blood vessels.

During the 90-minute operation, the surgeon uses the resectoscope's wire loop to remove the obstructing tissue one piece at a time. The pieces of tissue are carried by the fluid into the bladder and then flushed out at the end of the operation.

Although this procedure is delicate and requires a skilled surgeon, most doctors suggest using TURP whenever possible. Transurethral procedures are less traumatic than open forms of surgery and require a shorter recovery period.

Another surgical procedure is called transurethral incision of the prostate. Instead of removing tissue, as with TURP, this procedure widens the urethra by making a few small cuts in the bladder neck, where the urethra joins the bladder. Although some people believe that this procedure gives the same relief as TURP with less risk of side effects, its advantages and long-term side effects have not been clearly established.

Open Surgery. In the few cases when a transurethral procedure cannot be used, open surgery, which requires an external incision, may be used. Open surgery is often done when the gland is greatly enlarged, when there are complicating factors, or when the bladder has been damaged and needs to be repaired. The location of the enlargement within the gland and the patient's general health help the surgeon decide which of the three open procedures to use.

With all the open procedures, anesthesia is administered and an incision is made. Once the surgeon reaches the prostate capsule, he scoops out the enlarged tissue from inside the gland.

Laser Surgery. Some researchers are exploring the use of lasers to vaporize obstructing prostate tissue. Early studies suggest that this method may be as effective as conventional surgery.

SOURCE:
National Institute of Diabetes & Digestive & Kidney Diseases. *Prostate Enlargement: Benign Prostatic Hyperplasia.* NIH Pub. No. 90-3012. April 1990. pp. 5-7.

SAFETY OF TURP (TRANSURETHRAL RESECTION OF THE PROSTATE)

Although the situation began to change in the last few years, surgery has long been the only treatment for BPH. Several versions of the radical prostatectomy, involving an abdominal incision (open procedures), eventually gave way to a less-drastic procedure known as transurethral resection of the prostate (TURP). No surgical incision is necessary for a TURP, which involves the threading of a thin hollow flexible tube (catheter) through the penis via the urethra. A tiny electrified wire loop is passed through the catheter and, with the help of a fiberoptic device for viewing, the surgeon scrapes away excess prostatic tissue.

TURP was believed to be a low-risk procedure that is as effective as the open procedures and associated with lower rates of death and complications. Permanent impotence and urinary incontinence can occur after TURP, but at a far lower rate—10% and 3%, respectively—than that of the open prostatectomies. Over the last decade, however, studies began reporting TURP results that shattered the cherished beliefs of many urologists.

Among the first were studies suggesting that TURP causes the spread of cancer. The incidence of disseminated prostatic cancer was higher among those whose cancer was diagnosed accidentally while undergoing the procedure for BPH than among those whose prostatic cancer had been diagnosed via needle biopsy.

Four studies published since 1980 found similar results. Among them was a 1983 National Cancer Institute (NCI) survey of 700 prostatic cancer patients. At the time, chief investigator for the NCI study, Gerald E. Hanks, M.D., told the *Medical Tribune* (18 January 1983) that his findings generated "a lot of hate mail" from angry urologists. Co-investigator Henry M. Keys, M.D. speculated "that the mechanical scraping out of cancerous prostatic tissue may physically force malignant cells into vascular or lymphatic spaces and accelerate their tendency to spread."

The next thing to be disproved was TURP's low death rate (1%). This statistic came from researchers who followed men for only 30 days postoperatively. But three studies with longer followups showed that most of the deaths occur in the first three months after the men were discharged from the hospital. Altogether, the studies showed a 4-9% mortality rate in the 3-12 months following surgery. Death rates were substantially higher for some hospitals, particularly those with relatively few patients. Anticipating an argument from urologic surgeons that men given TURP are generally in poorer health than those given the open procedure, the investigators stated that the higher death rate was seen among low-risk as well as high-risk men. These findings came from an inspection of insurance claims data, which also showed that men given TURP had higher rates of reoperation and certain complications, such as urethral stricture.

By 1985, 95% of the prostatectomies performed in men covered by Medicare were TURP. Over 340,000 TURPS are now performed annually in the U.S.—up from 298,000 in 1980. "A dramatic change had occurred in surgical practice without any systematic assessment of whether TURP was more effective than open operations," wrote Noralou P. Roos, Ph.D. and a multi-national team of colleagues. They were explaining the impetus for their assessment of the medical records of over 50,000 men treated for BPH with either TURP or the open prostatectomy. Because so few open procedures are done in the U.S., the investigators relied on records from three other countries—Canada, Britain, and Denmark (*The New England Journal of Medicine*, 27 April 1989).

Their findings shocked the medical community and illustrated the need for better evaluation of surgical procedures. TURP was shown to be less effective in overcoming urinary obstruction than the open operation. Furthermore, the men treated with TURP were more likely to die of a variety of causes at one and eight years after surgery. It is unusual for a study involving a surgical treatment to follow up on people for eight years and, for unknown reasons, this one found the men given TURP had a higher mortality rate from heart attacks. Ironically, many surgeons pressure men into accepting prostatectomy at the onset of symptoms suggesting that the condition can only get worse and that they would live longer if the operation is not postponed until an older age.

SOURCE:
"Background: A Decade of Disillusionment Over the Safety and Efficacy of TURP." *HealthFacts* (April 1991): 4.

ALTERNATIVES TO SURGERY

Several alternatives to surgery for an enlarged prostate have been developed in recent years:

Alpha blockers. The urethra, a tube that carries urine away from the bladder, passes through the prostate on its way to the penis. An enlarged prostate narrows the urethra. It also causes muscle spasm in the lining of the urethra and in the adjoining prostate tissue. Those changes limit the flow of urine. Alpha-receptor blockers, ordinarily prescribed for hypertension, relax the prostatic-urethral muscle. In some men with an enlarged prostate, that eases the constriction enough to improve urine flow.

One of the first alpha blockers to be used for prostate trouble was phenoxybenzamine (Dibenzyline). But in some men it causes blood pressure to fall, sometimes leading to dizziness and fainting. An estimated 10 percent of patients experience decreased sexual drive; about 1 percent report impotence.

More recently, researchers have turned to two other alpha blockers, prazosin (Minipress) and terazosin (Hytrin). Those can be used to help relieve urinary symptoms in some men, with less frequent side effects.

How those two drugs will perform over the long term remains to be seen. Meanwhile, Consumers Union's medical consultants believe that they may be useful for patients who don't yet need surgery or who cannot have surgery because of other health problems. The drugs can also be used to relieve symptoms in men who are awaiting surgery.

Hormone inhibitors. Testosterone, the major male sex hormone, is converted to dihydrotestosterone (DHT) by an enzyme within the prostate. DHT causes progressive enlargement of the prostate. Certain drugs (such as Lupron, used to treat prostate cancer) can decrease testosterone production, thus limiting the amount of DHT. But lowered testosterone levels lead to impotence and loss of sexual drive.

A new experimental drug, Proscar, interferes with the conversion of testosterone to DHT. Early trials suggest that Proscar shrinks the prostate and improves urinary flow without such major side effects as impaired sexual activity. However, the drug may not be available for several years.

Balloon divulsion. Still considered an experimental procedure, balloon divulsion of the prostate has been used to improve urinary function in at least two thousand patients. This relatively simple procedure is similar to angioplasty, in which clogged coronary arteries are opened by an expanding balloon.

In balloon divulsion, a soft wire is used to push a balloon through the penis up into the constricted portion of the urethra. The balloon is filled with liquid for about 10 minutes, emptied, and removed. That pushes the surrounding tissue away from the urethra and splits the prostate, thus lessening the obstruction.

So far, there have been no reports that balloon divulsion impairs a man's potency or ability to ejaculate. However, there are recent reports of renewed symptoms after 10 to 18 months, especially among older patients.

For patients with severe symptoms, surgery may be the best choice. If the urethra is blocked completely, surgery becomes mandatory. The surgery, known as prostatectomy, involves partial removal of the new tissue growth, thus loosening the prostate's squeeze on the urethra.

SOURCE:

"Relieving Prostate Problems: An Enlarged Prostate Can Make Urination Difficult. Here's What Can Be Done about It." *Consumer Reports Health Letter* 2, no. 9 (September 1990): 66-67.

RESOURCES

ORGANIZATIONS

National Center for Treatment and Research of Prostate Diseases, Medical College of Wisconsin. Froedtert Memorial Lutheran Hospital, 9200 West Wisconsin Ave., Milwaukee, WI 53226.

National Kidney and Urologic Diseases Information Clearinghouse. Box NKUDIC, Bethesda, MD 20892.

Prostate Cancer Education Council. JAF Box 888, New York, NY 10016.

PAMPHLET

Norwich Eaton Pharmaceuticals, Inc.:

So You're Going to Have a Prostatectomy. July 1987. 12 pp.

BOOK

Rous, Stephen N. *The Prostate Book: Sound Advice in Symptoms and Treatment.* Fairfield, OH: Consumer Reports Books, 1989.

RELATED ARTICLES

"Balloon Dilation of the Prostate." *Medical Letter on Drugs & Therapeutics* 32 (June 29, 1990): 64.

Barry, Michael. "Prostate Surgery: Risk, Benefit, Uncertainty." *Harvard Medical School Health Letter* (June 1989): 5-7.

"Benign Prostatic Hypertrophy: The Most Common Cause of Prostate Enlargement." *Mayo Clinic Health Letter* 6, no. 7 (July 1988): 1-2.

"Do Balloons Cure Enlarged Prostates? Or Do They Really Do Nothing at All?" *Men's Health Newsletter* 7, no. 9 (September 1991): 1-2.

Lepor, Herbert. "Nonsurgical Approaches to BPH: Prostatectomy is the Accepted Therapy for Symptomatic Benign Prostatic Hyperplasia and Bladder Obstruction, but New Studies Focus on Drugs, Hormone Therapy, and Balloon Dilatation. Are They Reasonable Options?" *Patient Care* (December 15, 1989): 46-56.

O'Brien, Walter M. "Benign Prostatic Hypertrophy." *American Family Physician* 44, no. 1 (July 1991): 162-166.

Orandi, Ahmad. "Transurethral Resection Versus Transurethral Incision of the Prostate." *Urologic Clinics of North America* 17, no. 3 (August 1990): 601-612.

PSORIASIS

OVERVIEW

Psoriasis is a chronic skin disorder of unknown cause. It is not contagious but it is more likely to occur in individuals whose family members have it. In the United States two percent of the people have psoriasis (three to four million persons) with both sexes and all age groups involved. Each year the initial episode of psoriasis occurs in an estimated 150,000 patients.

Psoriasis derived its name from the Greek work meaning "itch." It results from an overproduction of skin cells leading to thickening of the skin and scaling. Silvery plaques occur most frequently on the scalp, elbows, knees and lower back.

There are variations in the severity of the disease. In some instances it is so mild that the persons never know they have it. In rare cases individuals have such severe psoriasis it defies therapy and causes frustration and an unending list of treatments. At its worst the disease can cover an entire body with redness and scales. Fortunately, this is uncommon. Nonetheless some of these extremely involved patients may respond to treatment with control of signs and symptoms and occasionally complete clearing of the skin.

The cause of psoriasis is unknown. Scientists speculate that a biochemical malfunction triggers the excessive skin cell production. In a person with psoriasis a skin cell matures in 3 to 4 days instead of the normal 28 to 30 days. People often experience their first attack or subsequent flare-up if their skin is injured, such as by being cut, scratched, rubbed or severely sunburned. Such a flare-up usually will occur 10 to 14 days after the skin is irritated.

Psoriasis can also be triggered by some infections, such as a strep throat and by certain drugs including lithium and propranolol.

Various diets have not been successful in curbing recurrences or improving existing psoriasis. People who live in cold weather climates usually have flare-ups in the winter when their skin dries out due to reduced humidity. Furthermore they are unable to benefit from the moderate exposure to sunlight which usually helps control psoriasis.

Psoriasis occurs in a variety of forms that differ in their intensity, duration, location, shape and pattern of scales.

The most common form starts out with red lesions that look like pimples. Gradually they enlarge and silvery scales form. While the top scales flake off easily and frequently, those below the surface stick together so that when they are removed, bleeding occurs. The small red lesions grow, sometimes merging to cover large areas. They may be shaped like a small doughnut with a clear center, coin or rough oyster shell.

Elbows, knees, genitals, arms, legs, scalp and nails are most commonly involved. The lesions will frequently appear on both sides of the body in the same areas.

Psoriasis affects the nails by pitting the surface, separating the nail from the nail bed and thickening or crumbling the nail plate. Psoriasis of the nail is difficult to treat.

Another form of psoriasis is inverse psoriasis which occurs in the armpit, under the breast, in skin folds, around the groin, in the cleft between the buttocks and around the genitals.

Guttate psoriasis begins primarily in children and young adults. Many small, red, drop-like, scaly spots appear all over the trunk, limbs and scalp. This variety of psoriasis is often preceded by a sore throat caused by group A streptococcal bacteria. It often clears up spontaneously after a few weeks.

About five percent of psoriasis patients have arthritis. Some of them have specific rheumatic diseases unrelated to the psoriasis but others have joint deformities as part of the psoriasis. This rheumatism may have characteristic distribution and x-ray findings. The arthritis of psoriasis sometimes improves when the skin manifestations of the disease improve. Anti-inflammatory medications may be helpful.

Dermatologists diagnose psoriasis by examining the skin and noting specific characteristics of the lesions. Occasionally they may need to biopsy the lesion and examine the skin under a microscope to confirm the diagnosis. There are no blood tests or other laboratory tests available for establishing the diagnosis.

The dermatologist will design an individualized treatment plan that takes into account a person's overall medical condition, age, lifestyle, severity and duration of psoriasis and expectations of treatment. Various treatments, combinations of treatments and visits to the dermatologist may be necessary before the psoriasis comes under control.

The goal in treatment of psoriasis is to relieve discomfort and slow down rapid skin cell division. Treatment varies according to the extent of the disease. Bland moisturizing creams and lotions prevent water in the skin from evaporating, improving the patient's appearance and controlling the itching often produced by dry skin.

Prescription medications containing cortisone, salicylic acid, tar or anthralin may be recommended alone or in combination with natural sunlight or ultraviolet light. Sunlight exposure helps about 95 percent of people who tan easily but must be used cautiously by people who get sunburned. Any injury to the skin may aggravate psoriasis including rubbing, scratching, vigorous brushing or combing of the hair and overmedication.

The most severe forms of psoriasis may require oral medications with or without combined ultraviolet light treatments. Depending upon circumstances, this may be achieved in the dermatologist's office, psoriasis day care center or hospital. . . .

PUVA [a combination of oral psoralen and ultraviolet light, type A] is used in patients who have failed to respond to the previously described regimens or who have more than 30 percent of their body covered. It is effective in 85 to 90 percent of the patients. Patients are given a drug called psoralen prior to being exposed to an accurately measured amount of UV-A ultraviolet light in a light box. PUVA is administered by physicians because the patient's skin must be carefully monitored. About 25 treatments are given over a two to three month span before clearing occurs. Then the patient usually requires "maintenance therapy" of around thirty treatments a year. Relapses can occur.

Because psoralen drug remains in the lens of the eye, a PUVA patent must wear a special eye gear after taking the drug and for several hours after the light treatment to prevent eye damage.

Chronic photochemotherapy increases a person's risk of skin aging, cancer and freckling. Relative contraindications for this treatment modality are young patients below the age of 18, pregnancy, previous exposure to arsenic or ionizing radiation, skin cancer or severe eye disease.

Methotrexate, [an] oral anticancer drug, can produce dramatic results, yet its use is not considered unless all other treatments have failed because it can produce serious side effects, notably liver disease. Before a patient starts a methotrexate regimen, a liver biopsy should be performed. Following that procedure, periodic studies for liver and kidney function, liver biopsies and chest x-rays are required. For the first two months of therapy, a patient should have weekly blood tests. Short term side effects include nausea, upset stomach, light headedness and feeling of "unwellness." Psoriasis tends to recur when treatment is stopped.

SOURCE:
American Academy of Dermatology. *Psoriasis.* 1987.

TREATMENT

While there is yet no cure for psoriasis, many therapies are effective in controlling symptoms and in some cases bringing about long-term remissions. Because manifestations of the disease are highly variable, treatment must be individualized. Severity—the degree of erythema and sealing, plaque thickness, and percentage of body area involved—is a useful guide to therapy. . . .

The treatments used for severe psoriasis have enough significant side effects that severe disease is best left to the expert to treat. Some of the first options for treating very widespread or severe disease include UVB light therapy, and PUVA therapy. Both forms of phototherapy can be very effective in controlling the disease, but can cause burns, eye damage, and, in the case of PUVA therapy, skin cancer in some high risk patients. Because of the dangerous side effects of most therapies for severe psoriasis, treatment is best left to physicians with special knowledge of the modalities involved.

SOURCE:
Abel, E. and others. "Insights into Psoriasis Management." *Patient Care* 23 (November 30, 1989): 104.

FUTURE TREATMENT OPTIONS

Vitamin D_3

An active form of vitamin D—1, 25-dihydroxyvitamin D_3—has demonstrated exciting potential. Used topical-ly or orally, it appears to stop skin cells from growing wildly and makes them mature normally.

Michael F. Holick, Ph.D., M.D., director of the vitamin D laboratory at Boston City Hospital, who has been studying the vitamin derivative, says 90 percent of his patients showed a marked decrease in scales and a clearing up of inflammation within two to four weeks when they applied a topical form of D_3 once a day. Sixty-five percent of the patients who took it orally once a day showed similar improvement in two to three months. Unlike current medications, active D_3 seems to have fewer side effects. None of the problems associated with the vitamin have turned up in the studies so far. However, psoriasis returns when the treatment is stopped.

This medication may be used as early as next year in Europe, says Dr. Holick, and he's hopeful that it will be approved for use in the United States within the next three. Standard vitamin D supplements are not effective, he adds, and can cause toxicity if taken in high doses.

Fish oil

This has shown some promise as an adjunct to current treatments (used alone, its effects are minimal). In a 12-week study at the Skin Research Foundation of California in Santa Monica, 24 psoriasis patients who were being treated with Acitretin were given six one-gram capsules of fish oil as a daily supplement. All showed more improvement in their condition than a control group that was taking Acitretin alone. Also, the fish oil seems to counter one of the adverse effects of the drug by lowering the levels of certain fats in the blood that the medication tends to raise.

Nicholas J. Lowe, M.D., director of the foundation, says other studies have shown fish oil enhances the effects of light therapy. The omega-3 acids found in the oil are known to reduce the levels of other acids in the body that cause inflammation, including that associated with psoriasis.

Until more research is done, it wouldn't hurt to simply eat more fish high in omega-3s, such as herring, mackerel, and salmon, says Dr. Lowe. It may help keep your skin scales to a minimum.

Acitretin

Like etretinate, this vitamin A derivative can clear severe psoriasis symptoms when taken orally once a day. But, even better, it is eliminated a lot more quickly from the body; so the side effects, such as high blood cholesterol and bone spurs, may be more manageable and reversible. It may also be safer to use in fertile women than etretinate (provided that they avoid pregnancy while taking it and for two months after taking it). It's now awaiting approval by the Food and Drug Administration.

SOURCE:

Nicholson, Leslie. "Get Tough on Psoriasis." *Prevention* 43, no. 2 (February 1991): 119-120. Reprinted by permission of *Prevention*.

MANAGEMENT OF PSORIASIS

Acute psoriatic flare-ups and the more severe cases warrant hospitalization, but with increasingly effective outpatient treatments, many people are able to avoid hospitalization altogether.

A daily home routine usually consists of a bath, using oil-rich Aveeno powder, followed by shampooing with a tar preparation (such as Polytar). To enhance absorption of the bath oil and hydration of the skin, a 20-minute bath is recommended instead of a shower. Immediately after bathing, the skin is blotted dry and the prescribed emollients—and sometimes, topical steroids—are applied. The emollients and steroids are reapplied two or three more times during the day to keep the skin from drying out.

With acute flares, patients may need to bathe and shampoo twice daily. Stronger drugs, as well as more frequent and more aggressive treatments (crude coal tar, anthralin cream, or ultraviolet light therapy, for example), are needed to achieve remission of the disease. Patients are admitted to the hospital when the side effects of the disease itself or side effects of the treatments warrant closer, more frequent monitoring.

SOURCE:

Dunn, M. L., E. B. Cockerline, and others. "Treatment Options for Psoriasis." *American Journal of Nursing* (August 1988): 1082–1083.

TREATMENT IN THE DEAD SEA

One of the most unusual approaches to coping with psoriasis is the increasingly popular trek to the Dead Sea to soak up the area's beneficial sunlight. Located below sea level, the Dead Sea offers an environment in which people can take in large quantities of ultraviolet A—which helps relieve psoriasis—without taking in too much ultraviolet B, the primary culprit in sunburn. Most of the ultraviolet B radiation is filtered out in this area because at 1,290 feet below sea level, the rays must travel a great distance through the earth's atmosphere.

Some people believe that bathing in the salty Dead Sea water also helps their condition, but that hasn't been proved, Dr. [Madeleine] Duvic [associate professor of dermatology at The University of Texas Medical School at Houston] notes. She says Dead Sea trekkers may reap psychological benefits from being able to visit with other people afflicted with psoriasis. Dead Sea light therapy typically produces disease remissions of about eight months—comparable to the results obtained in hospital- or clinic-based treatment programs.

SOURCE:
"Psoriasis: Expanding Treatment Options Offer Relief." *The University of Texas Lifetime Health Letter* 2, no. 11 (November 1990): 3, 7.

RESOURCES

ORGANIZATIONS

American Academy of Dermatology. 1567 Maple Avenue, Evanston, IL 60204.

National Psoriasis Foundation. P.O. Box 9009, Portland, OR 97207.

PAMPHLETS

California Medical Association:

"Psoriasis." *HealthTips* index 163 (October 1989): 2 pp.

National Psoriasis Foundation:

Psoriasis: How It Makes You Feel. 1987. 11 pp.

Treatment of Psoriasis: An Update. 1987. 21 pp.

RELATED ARTICLES

Able, E., and others. "Insights into Psoriasis Management." *Patient Care* 23 (November 1989): 102–115.

Bos, J. D., and others. "Use of Cyclosporine in Psoriasis." *The Lancet* 2, no. 8678–8679 (December 23, 1989): 1500–1502.

Hale, E. "Brushing off Dandruff and Other Flaky Afflictions." *FDA Consumer* (May 1988): 28–31.

Kramer, Louise. "Psoriasis Treatments that Work." *Good Housekeeping* 212 (May 1991): 211.

Morimoto, S., and K. Yoshikawa. "Psoriasis and Vitamin D_3." *Archives of Dermatology* 125 (February 1989): 231–234.

"Psoriasis Strategies." *Solutions for Better Health* 9 (July/August 1990): 26–28.

Stern, R. S. "Risk Assessment of PUVA and Cyclosporine: Lessons from the Past, Challenges for the Future." *Archives of Dermatology* 125 (April 1989): 545–547.

QUACKERY

OVERVIEW

Individuals suffering from chronic pain, chronic illness, terminal conditions, or those with an interest in unconventional remedies are susceptible to the philosophies of alternative medical practitioners and promotional health claims. Older individuals are especially prone to victimization by fraudulent concerns since it robs them of both their limited income and, often, their already fragile health. Such people often seek therapies which derive from sources other than scientific medicine. These sources include oriental medicine, homeopathy, nutritional approaches to terminal disease and holistic views of health. Individuals often ask for information or clarification regarding the areas of: 1) alternative therapies, 2) unproven methods, and 3) health fraud.

The freedom of therapeutic choice in the United States makes for a strong constituency of pro-alternative groups. Diseases still exist for which there are no cures so individuals often look for answers in unproven realms, relying on non-medical concerns such as health food stores which promote "natural" products in lieu of conventional therapies. Alternative practitioners and fraudulent purveyors find a ready audience for their philosophies and products from people who have become disillusioned with conventional medicine. Additionally, health fraud activist Stephen Barrett, MD, warns that outside the medical environment there is the larger area of books that promote questionable health ideas, talk shows that abound with guests who deliver false information and ads for health products sold by mail that are almost always misleading.

For the purpose of this discussion, alternative therapy is defined as an alternative to generally recognized surgical, radiological, pharmaceutical, or nutritional therapies. Alternatives include acupuncture, homeopathy, and macrobiotic diets. To one degree or another alternatives can also be referred to as unproven. Nutritional cancer remedies, chelation therapy, and hair analysis for allergies are viewed as unproven by the conventional medical community. Entire philosophies of practice which differ from those of scientific medicine are the foundation for some alternatives, while other philosophies are autonomous theories often promoted by a single practitioner.

Victor Herbert, MD, a health fraud activist, contends that the term unproven is a euphemism for questionable. The definition of a questionable method is that it has not successfully answered the two basic consumer protection questions of safety and effectiveness, or, has not been responsibly, objectively, reproducibly, and reliably demonstrated in humans under the auspices of a federal or academic scientific trial and been reported in the peer-reviewed or refereed medical journals. The individual should know a) if the therapy has proven to be more effective than conventional treatment; b) if it is more effective than doing nothing and letting nature take its course; or c) if it has a reasonable and objective potential for benefit which exceeds its potential for harm.

Health fraud occurs when claims for alternative therapies and unproven methods cause more harm than good, solicit money for bogus devices and remedies or remove patients from viable conventional therapies. Barrett broadly defines fraud as anything associated with false claims in the field of health. An important consideration when differentiating between fraud and an alternative therapy or unproven method is in the promotion of the product or therapy. Any promotion which promises cures without scientific evidence has the potential of being fraudulent.

The Food and Drug Administration (FDA) recognizes three categories of health fraud: economic, indirect, and direct. Economic health fraud presents no health hazard, but consumers lose money. Indirect health fraud prolongs the time before patients go for proper therapy. Direct health fraud does actual harm to a patient's health. About 90 percent of health fraud is economic, says Robert Veiga, MD, director of the medicine staff in the FDA Office of Health Affairs. Regulatory agencies like the FDA and organized medical groups like the American Medical Association and the American Cancer Society have limited funds and lack legal abilities to combat health fraud in an aggressive manner. They choose to concentrate on public education to help people differentiate between genuine and bogus claims regarding health care. This differentiation is one of the most difficult for the public to comprehend, since legitimate researchers work with investigational therapeutics and sophisticated promoters' advertising often includes a grain of truth in their pseudoscientific explanations.

SOURCE:

Sullivan-Fowler, Micaela, Terry Austin, and Arthur W. Hafner. *Alternative Therapies, Unproven Methods, and Health Fraud: A Selected Annotated Bibliography*. Pub. No. OP-137. Chicago: American Medical Association, 1988. pp. 1-2.

TOP TEN HEALTH FRAUDS

Health fraud is indeed big business in this country. *Medical World News* estimates that Americans spend about $27 billion a year on quack products or treatments. And FDA estimates that 38 million Americans have used a fraudulent health product within the past year. These products are not without risk. According to an agency survey, 1 out of 10 people who try quack remedies is harmed by side effects.

Here is FDA's list of the top 10 health frauds. Bear in mind, though, health fraud is by no means limited to these alone.

1. **Fraudulent Arthritis Products.** Arthritis affects some 40 million Americans, 95 percent of whom "are likely to engage in some form of self-treatment even after they have seen a physician," says the National Council Against Health Fraud's president, William Jarvis. Copper bracelets, Chinese herbal remedies, large doses of vitamins, snake or bee venom just don't work. Because the symptoms of arthritis go into remission periodically, individuals who try these unproven remedies may associate the remedy with the remission.

2. **Spurious Cancer Clinics.** These clinics, many of them in Mexico, promise miracle cures. Treatments use unproven and ineffective substances such as Laetrile (derived from apricot kernels) and vitamins and minerals. People who go to these clinics often abandon legitimate cancer treatments. This is particularly tragic in the case of young children because some of their cancers (such as leukemia or Hodgkin's disease) are highly curable through legitimate treatment.

3. **Bogus AIDS Cures.** Victims of incurable diseases are especially vulnerable to the promises of charlatans. AIDS is a prime example. Underground or "guerrilla clinics" offering homemade treatments have sprung up in the United States, the Caribbean, and Europe.

"When you hear the words, 'Here's the latest cure for AIDS, all you have to do is hand over the money,' beware," says Gary Lambert, vice chairman of AIDS Action, Baltimore. There is no cure for AIDS yet—proposed treatments such as massive doses of antibiotics, typhus vaccine, or herbal tea made from the bark of Brazilian trees are all unproven. Lambert recommends that people with questions about AIDS remedies check with AIDS clinical trial units located in leading hospitals throughout the country. Or call the National Institute of Allergy and Infectious Disease's hot line at 1-800-TRIALS-A. This hot line provides information on NIH-funded studies at hospitals throughout the country.

4. **Instant Weight-Loss Schemes.** With an estimated 25 percent of the American population overweight, quacks selling weight-loss gimmicks have a sizable market for their wares. Unfortunately, there is no quick way to lose weight. According to National Council Against Health Fraud's Jarvis, fraudulent weight-loss schemes are usually heralded by full-page newspaper ads promising rapid, dramatic and easy weight loss or by single news column ads that look like news stories except that the word "advertisement" is written across the top. Radio and TV ads typically list 800 telephone numbers to facilitate credit card charges and private parcel deliveries. This allows promoters to circumvent the postal service's laws against mail fraud, Jarvis says.

Some of the latest gimmicks in instant weight-loss plans have included skin patches, herbal capsules, grapefruit diet pills, and Chinese magic weight-loss earrings.

5. **Fraudulent Sexual Aids.** Products promoted to enhance libido and sexual pleasure are not new. FDA officials recently cracked down on an entrepreneur selling Chinese "Crocodile Penis Pills" purportedly prepared according to a 2,000-year-old formula for rejuvenating male sexual prowess.

FDA says no nonprescription drug ingredients have been proven safe or effective as aphrodisiacs and has acted to ban these products. Over-the-counter products that claim to increase the size of a man's penis or cure impotence or frigidity don't work. Serious health risks are associated with the use of such purported aphrodisiacs as cantharides ("Spanish fly"), a chemical derived from the dried bodies of beetles. Other ingredients of similar OTC products include strychnine (a poison), mandrake and yohimbine (poisonous plants), licorice, zinc, and the herbs anise and fennel.

Although male sex hormones, available by prescription, do influence libido and sexual performance, they have potentially serious side effects and should only be used under a physician's supervision. The agency advises that people with sexual problems should not attempt to medicate themselves but rather should seek treatment by a medical professional.

6. **Quack Baldness Remedies and Other Appearance Modifiers.** Entrepreneurs make millions of dollars trying to convince consumers to buy their versions of the fountain of youth, whether it be a remedy to grow hair or prevent its loss, a cream that removes wrinkles, or a device to "develop" the bust. Only one prescription product has been approved for growing hair on balding men: Rogaine (minoxidil). And this approval is only for a specific type of baldness. FDA has acted to ban the sale of any nonprescription hair cream, lotion, or other external product claiming to grow hair or prevent baldness. None of these products has been shown to work.

Clinical studies suggest that one product, Retin-A, may be effective in lessening certain kinds of wrinkles, and some physicians prescribe it for this purpose. This is legitimate because it is approved for treating acne and doctors may thus prescribe it for other uses. However, consumers should be aware that FDA has not evaluated safety and effectiveness data for the drug's use as a wrinkle remover.

So-called breast developers have also been used by millions of women who want larger breasts. But, as the experts point out, these devices do not increase breast size.

7. **False Nutritional Schemes.** Many Americans whose diets are not nutritionally balanced may be persuaded that some "perfect" food or product will make up for all their nutritional shortcomings. Various food products—such as bee pollen, over-the-counter herbal remedies, and wheat germ capsules—are promoted as sure-fire cures for various diseases. Though usually not harmful, neither have these products been proven beneficial.

8. **Chelation Therapy.** Promoters of this therapy claim that an injection or tablet of the amino acid EDTA, taken with vitamins and minerals, cleans out arteries by breaking down arterial plaque (deposits of cholesterol and other lipid materials). Such treatment is supposed to prevent circulatory disease, angina (chest pain), heart attacks, and strokes and is advertised as an "alternative" to heart bypass surgery. Both FDA and the American Heart Association say there is no scientific evidence that chelation therapy works. Nevertheless, patients spend as much as $3,000 to $5,000 for chelation treatments. Not only are they paying for an ineffective treatment, they are also buying a dangerous drug. EDTA can cause kidney failure, bone marrow depression, and convulsions.

9. **Unproven Use of Muscle Stimulators.** Muscle stimulators are a legitimate medical device approved for certain conditions—to relax muscle spasms, increase blood circulation, prevent blood clots, and rehabilitate muscle function after a stroke. But within the past few years health spas and figure salons have promoted new uses. They claim that muscle stimulators can remove wrinkles, perform face lifts, reduce breast size, and remove cellulite. Some even claim these handy little devices can reduce one's beer belly without the aid of sit-ups! FDA considers promotion of muscle stimulators used for these conditions to be fraudulent.

10. **Candidiasis Hypersensitivity.** *Candida* (also known as monilia) is a fungus found naturally in small amounts in the warm moist areas of the body such as the mouth, intestinal tract, and vagina. When the body's resistance is weakened, the fungus can multiply and infect the skin or mucous membranes. More serious infection occurs in individuals whose resistance has been weakened by other illnesses.

However, some promoters assert that approximately 30 percent of Americans suffer from "candidiasis hypersensitivity," which they say triggers everything from fatigue to constipation, diarrhea, depression and anxiety, impotence, infertility, and menstrual problems. To correct the problem, promoters recommend antifungal drugs and vitamin and mineral supplements.

The American Academy of Allergy and Immunology says the existence of such a syndrome has not been proven and the numerous symptoms credited to "candidiasis hypersensitivity" could be due to any number of illnesses.

SOURCE:

"Top 10 Health Frauds." *FDA Consumer* 23 (October 1989): 28–31.

CONSUMER SELF-PROTECTION

Today's quacks aren't as easy to spot as characters selling snake oil in old Westerns. Now they wear suits or lab coats and speak in scientific jargon. Some even carry medical degrees. How can you tell the difference between reliable advice and a quack promotion? Here are six warning signs to watch for:

1. Do they push vitamins?

Reputable health professionals don't recommend vitamins for a wide variety of problems. But many practitioners, including bogus nutritionists and some chiropractors, do. Sometimes they also sell vitamins, and in mega-doses at inflated prices.

Steer clear of physicians who give vitamin B12 shots for fatigue and other vague complaints. Periodic injections of B12 are appropriate only for people with documented B12 deficiency and other disorders that result in inadequate intestinal absorption of the vitamin.

In high enough doses, certain vitamins (including A, B6, C, D, and E) can cause disturbing or harmful side effects. Only individuals at risk of developing vitamin deficiencies—usually children under 2 and people with certain illnesses—stand to benefit from vitamin supplements, and then only as directed by a physician who doesn't sell them.

2. Do they give phony nutrition tests?

Practitioners looking to sell dietary supplements may promise to determine your nutritional status with any of a number of gimmicks, including amino acid analysis, cytotoxic testing, hair analysis, herbal crystallization analysis, and live-cell analysis. As screening tests for nutritional problems, they're all worthless.

Some entrepreneurs have devised questionnaires that ask about symptoms that could be due to a vitamin deficiency. But those symptoms often occur in many other conditions as well. Thus, even if a vitamin deficiency does exist, such questionnaires don't permit accurate diagnosis or responsible treatment. That requires a physical examination and specific laboratory tests.

Your physician, a registered dietitian, or a reputable nutritionist with at least a master's degree in nutrition from an accredited institution can help analyze your typical diet and recommend dietary changes.

3. Do they display fishy diplomas and certificates?

In recent years, many unaccredited correspondence schools have been issuing "degrees" in health-related areas, especially nutrition. Some require nothing more than a fee; others, just limited study. No such unaccredited school offers reliable instruction in health care. You can check a school's status by contacting your state education department, the U.S. Department of Education, or the Council on Postsecondary Accreditation.

4. Do they sell health by mail?

Most mail-order health schemes exploit the fear of being physically unattractive. Their promoters are usually "hit-and-run" artists who make a quick profit before the U.S. Postal Service intervenes. Common scams include anti-aging products, baldness remedies, blemish removers, breast developers, and miracle weight-loss plans. Ads for these products typically offer a money-back guarantee that's no more legitimate than the product.

5. Do they tout endorsements?

Companies marketing vitamins and other nutritional supplements sometimes claim that physicians or medical scientists have endorsed their products. Some of these companies establish so-called "scientific advisory boards." Such companies often make false and illegal claims for their products.

In 1986, for example, a company called United Sciences of America began marketing food supplements supposed to help prevent cancer and coronary heart disease. These products, the company claimed, had been designed and endorsed by a scientific advisory board of 16 professionals. Of the seven most prominent "board members," six—including two Nobel prize winners—had neither developed nor endorsed the company's products.

6. Do they stress the immune system?

In recent years, AIDS—acquired immune deficiency syndrome—has focused widespread public attention on the immune system and generated all sorts of immunoquackery. Some promoters, including many who had previously claimed to cure cancer, now promise to cure AIDS. Other hucksters appeal to the public by offering to boost immunity to disease in general. Since severe nutritional deficiencies can lower immunity, the quacks claim that various vitamin concoctions provide extra nutrients that will strengthen the immune system. But getting more than enough vitamins and other nutrients is no better than getting just enough of them. And most people get enough.

SOURCE:

"How to Duck the Quacks: Modern Health Hustlers Aren't Always Easy to Spot." *Consumer Reports Health Letter* 2 (July 1990): 56.

RESOURCES

ORGANIZATIONS

American Medical Association. 525 North Dearborn St., Chicago, IL 60610.

Arthritis Foundation. 1314 Spring St. NW, Atlanta, GA 30309.

Food and Drug Administration. 5600 Fishers Lane, Rockville, MD 20857.

National Council Against Health Care Fraud, Inc. Box 1276, Loma Linda, CA 90712.

PAMPHLETS

American Council on Science and Health:

Quackery and the Elderly. Special report. n.d. 10 pp.

Arthritis Foundation:

Unproven Remedies. 1987.

U.S. Food and Drug Administration:

Quackery: The Billion Dollar Miracle Business. November 1990. 5 pp.

BOOK

Barrett, Stephen. *Health Schemes, Scams, and Frauds*. Fairfield, OH: Consumer Reports Books, 1991. 256 pp.

RELATED ARTICLES

Barnhill, William. "Pulling the Plug on Quacks: Health Hucksters Can Cheat You Out of More Than Just Money." *AARP Bulletin* 32, no. 7 (July/August 1991): 2, 7.

Barrett, Stephen. "Common Misconceptions about Quackery." *Priorities* (Spring 1991): 34-36.

Barrett, Stephen. "Quack, Quack: 30 Ways to Duck Medicine's Con Artists." *American Health* (March 1991): 59-63.

Jarvis, William T. and Stephen Barrett. "How Quackery Sells." *Nutrition Forum* 8, no. 2 (March/April 1991): 9-13.

REYE SYNDROME

OVERVIEW

Reye Syndrome (aka Reye's Syndrome) is a poorly understood disease afflicting approximately one out of every million children annually. Reye Syndrome was first discovered in 1963 by an Australian pathologist, Dr. R. Douglas Reye (pronounced rye). Because it is a newly-recognized illness, the medical community is still in the process of identifying its origins and the factors contributing to its development. Until its cause is determined, parents need to be especially alert to the signs of Reye Syndrome.

Reye Syndrome strikes children between one and young adulthood, three to seven days after the start of a viral illness. Influenza (the "flu," characterized by fever, muscle aches, headache and cough) and chicken pox are the most common precursors of Reye Syndrome, but other viruses can sometimes trigger it. Usually the syndrome develops quite suddenly. The child vomits repeatedly and may exhibit unusual behavior, such as lethargy, irrationality, irritability or aggression. In some cases, a normally agreeable child becomes combative or may even hallucinate. The illness can progress rapidly to convulsions, coma, brain damage and death.

The syndrome causes an acute change in the cells of the brain and liver. These changes lead to swelling of the brain, imbalance of blood chemicals and malfunction of the liver. The liver loses its ability to filter the blood, eliminate poisons from the body, and maintain glycogen. The latter causes patients to have extremely low blood sugar, and may be one of the reasons they lapse into a coma. When any of these symptoms are present, it is important that the child be seen immediately by a physician to receive the appropriate care.

Treatment of Reye Syndrome attempts to control the swelling of the brain and correct the chemical imbalance resulting from a malfunctioning liver. Sometimes liver problems can be corrected to help prevent the accumulation of toxins in the body, and medications may be given to reduce the brain swelling so the possibility of brain damage and other complications is decreased. In essence, the main therapy for this disease is supportive care. Severe cases require surgery to relieve the pressure on the brain. For any of these procedures the patient must be monitored closely, and a respirator is often used.

The specific cause of the disease is not yet known. It is thought that it may be triggered by any number of factors, including medications, environmental toxins, or a genetic predisposition. In fact, some inherited diseases where a single enzyme is not available for an important chemical process seem similar to Reye Syndrome, but doctors are now able to distinguish between them. Studies have shown that Reye Syndrome is associated with the use of aspirin. Researchers have found a higher incidence of Reye Syndrome among children using aspirin to relieve symptoms of influenza and chicken pox than among those receiving other drugs to reduce their fevers. One should refrain from using aspirin to reduce fevers in children and adolescents. Generally, when treatment of a fever and associated symptoms is necessary, an aspirin substitute (acetaminophen) may be used.

Remember, Reye Syndrome occurs most frequently after widespread outbreaks of influenza and chicken pox. Check the ingredients of the medication you administer. Many common over-the-counter and prescription drugs, including some popular cough and cold remedies, contain aspirin. If your child develops any of the symptoms mentioned above, especially after having influenza or chicken pox, contact your physician immediately. Many children can recover fully if the disease is diagnosed and treated in time.

SOURCE:
California Medical Association. "Reye Syndrome." *HealthTips* (May 1989): 1-2.

REYE SYNDROME AND ASPIRIN

The warning on nonprescription aspirin packages cautioning against use of the drug in children and teenagers with flu or chicken pox symptoms will be strengthened as a result of findings of a Public Health Service study. In addition, the products must prominently display a statement to alert consumers to the new warning. FDA published these requirements in the June 9, 1988, *Federal Register.*

The new warning reads: "WARNING: Children and teenagers should not use this medicine for chicken pox or flu symptoms before a doctor is consulted about Reye syndrome, a rare but serious illness reported to be associated with aspirin." The current statement, required since June 1986, does not include the last phrase directly linking the disease with aspirin use.

The number of cases of Reye syndrome has declined significantly since 1980 when the link between aspirin use and the disease was first reported and publicized, and use of the drug in children has declined as well. (See "As Use of Kids' Aspirin Drops, So Do Cases of Reye Syndrome" in the October 1987 *FDA Consumer.*) The disease, although rare (101 cases were reported in 1986), is fatal in about one of four people afflicted. The symptoms—extreme fatigue, belligerence, and excessive vomiting—may arise just as a child or teenager seems to be recovering from flu or chicken pox.

The study, published in the April 10, 1987, *Journal of the American Medical Association*, verified results of a pilot study showing a significant association between Reye syndrome and the use of aspirin in children and teenagers with flu or chicken pox.

The revised warning will be a permanent requirement on all aspirin products marketed after Dec. 9, 1988.

SOURCE:
"New Reye Syndrome Warning." *FDA Consumer* 22, no. 7 (September 1988): 104.

* * *

Further evidence on the link between Reye syndrome and aspirin was reported in a study published in the May 5 [1989] *Journal of the American Medical Association.* The study was designed to answer lingering questions about potential bias in earlier studies that suggested a link between aspirin use during viral illness in children and adolescents and the subsequent onset of Reye syndrome.

The researchers found that youngsters with Reye were 35 times more likely to have used aspirin than those in the control group.

The good news about Reye syndrome is that cases have steadily declined since 1980, according to the Federal Centers for Disease Control—36 in 1987 and 20 in 1988. These are the lowest numbers since surveillance was begun in 1976. The decline is attributed to increased publicity about the association between aspirin and the syndrome.

SOURCE:
"Reye Syndrome Cases." *FDA Consumer* 23, no. 8 (October 1989): 105.

ACETAMINOPHEN AS AN ASPIRIN SUBSTITUTE

In terms of drug use, aspirin and acetaminophen are the two most widely used nonprescription analgesic/antipyretic [fever reducing] medications in the United States. For most purposes, these drugs are of equal efficacy in reducing fever and alleviating minor pain. Except in specific instances in which the superior anti-inflammatory effect of aspirin is indicated, the choice between aspirin or acetaminophen as an antipyretic or simple analgesic need not be based on efficacy. This information, in concert with the Reye syndrome association and a reassessment of the need to treat uncomplicated fever in otherwise healthy children, may suggest to physicians, parents, and pharmacists that antipyretics, in general, and aspirin, in particular, are not necessary for treating many febrile childhood illnesses.

Furthermore, acetaminophen may be a safer drug to use in treating children. Acetaminophen has fewer side effects than aspirin, is metabolized by nonsaturable kinetics and, therefore, does not tend to accumulate with repeated doses as does aspirin, and may be less toxic in overdose in young children. Also, acetaminophen is available in a liquid form and is both safer and easier to administer to young children.

SOURCE:
Arrowsmith, J. B., D. L. Kennedy, and others. "National Patterns of Aspirin Use and Reye Syndrome Reporting, United States, 1980 to 1985." *Pediatrics* 79, no. 6 (June 1987): 861.

RESOURCES

ORGANIZATION
National Reye's Syndrome Foundation. 426 North Lewis, Bryan, OH 43506.

RELATED ARTICLES
Hurwitz, E. S. "The Changing Epidemiology of Reye's Syndrome in the United States: Further Evidence for a Public Health Success." *JAMA* 260, no. 21 (December 2, 1988): 3178-3180.

Hurwitz, E. S., M. J. Barrett, and others. "Public Health Service Study of Reye's Syndrome and Medications: Report of the Main Study." *JAMA* 257, no. 14 (April 10, 1987): 1905–1911.

"Kids, Flu and Aspirin Don't Mix." *FDA Consumer* 22, no. 9 (November 1988): 11.

Meythaler, J. M., and R. R. Varma. "Reye's Syndrome in Adults." *Archives of Internal Medicine* 147 (January 1987): 61–64.

Pinsky, P. F., E. S. Hurwitz, and others. "Reye's Syndrome and Aspirin: Evidence for a Dose-Response Effect." *JAMA* 260, no. 5 (August 5, 1988): 657–661.

Stehlin, D. "As Use of Kids' Aspirin Drops, So Do Cases of Reye Syndrome." *FDA Consumer* 21, no. 8 (October 1987): 20–21.

SCHIZOPHRENIA

OVERVIEW

Schizophrenia is a term used to describe a complex, extremely puzzling condition—the most chronic and disabling of the major mental illnesses. Schizophrenia may be one disorder, or it may be many disorders, with different causes. Because of the disorder's complexity, few generalizations hold true for all people who are diagnosed as schizophrenic.

With the sudden onset of severe psychotic symptoms, the individual is said to be experiencing acute schizophrenia. "Psychotic" means out of touch with reality, or unable to separate real from unreal experiences. Some people have only one such psychotic episode; others have many episodes during a lifetime but lead relatively normal lives during the interim periods. The individual with chronic (continuous or recurring) schizophrenia often does not fully recover normal functioning and typically requires long-term treatment, generally including medication, to control the symptoms. Some chronic schizophrenic patients may never be able to function without assistance of one sort or another.

Approximately 1 percent of the population develop schizophrenia during their lives. This disorder affects men and women with equal frequency, and the information in this booklet is equally applicable to both. The first psychotic symptoms of schizophrenia are often seen in the teens or twenties in men and in the twenties or early thirties in women. Less obvious symptoms, such as social isolation or withdrawal or unusual speech, thinking, or behavior may precede and/or follow the psychotic symptoms.

Sometimes people have psychotic symptoms due to undetected medical disorders. For this reason, a medical history should be taken and a physical examination and laboratory tests should be done during hospitalization to rule out other causes of the symptoms before concluding that a person has schizophrenia.

UNUSUAL REALITIES: Just as "normal" individuals view the world from their own perspectives, schizophrenic people, too, have their own perceptions of reality. Their view of the world, however, is often strikingly different from the usual reality seen and shared by those around them.

Living in a world that can appear distorted, changeable, and lacking the reliable landmarks we all use to anchor ourselves to reality, a person with schizophrenia may feel anxious and confused. This person may seem distant, detached, or preoccupied, and may even sit as rigidly as a stone, not moving for hours and not uttering a sound. Or he or she may move about constantly, always occupied, wide awake, vigilant, and alert. A schizophrenic person may exhibit very different kinds of behavior at different times.

HALLUCINATIONS: The world of a schizophrenic individual may be filled with hallucinations; a person actually may sense things that in reality do not exist, such as hearing voices telling the person to do certain things, seeing people or objects that are not really there, or feeling invisible fingers touching his or her body. These hallucinations may be quite frightening. Hearing voices that other people don't hear is the most common type of hallucination in schizophrenia. Such voices may describe the patient's activities, carry on a conversation, warn of impending dangers, or tell the person what to do.

DELUSIONS: Delusions are false personal beliefs that are not subject to reason or contradictory evidence and are not part of the person's culture. They are common symptoms of schizophrenia and can involve themes of persecution or grandeur, for example. Sometimes delusions in schizophrenia are quite bizarre—for instance, believing that a neighbor is controlling the schizophrenic individual's behavior with magnetic waves, or that people on television are directing special messages specifically at him or her, or are broadcasting the individual's thoughts aloud to other people. Delusions of persecution, which are common in paranoid schizophrenia, are false and irrational beliefs that a person is being cheated, harassed, poisoned, or conspired against. The patient may believe that he or she, or a member of the family or other group, is the focus of this imagined persecution.

DISORDERED THINKING: Often the schizophrenic person's thinking is affected by the disorder. The person may endure many hours of not being able to "think straight." Thoughts may come and go so rapidly that it is not possible to "catch them." The person may not be able to concentrate on one thought for very long and may be easily distracted, unable to focus attention.

The person with schizophrenia may not be able to sort out what is relevant and what is not relevant to a situation. The person may be unable to connect thoughts into logical sequences, as thoughts may become disorganized and fragmented. Jumping from topic to topic in a way that is totally confusing to others may result.

This lack of logical continuity of thought, termed "thought disorder," can make conversation very difficult and contribute to social isolation. If people cannot make sense of what an individual is saying, they are likely to become uncomfortable and tend to leave that person alone.

EMOTIONAL EXPRESSION: People with schizophrenia sometimes exhibit what is called "inappropriate affect." This means showing emotion that is inconsistent with the person's speech or thoughts. For example, a schizophrenic person may say that he or she is being persecuted by demons and then laugh. This should not be confused with the behavior of normal individuals when, for instance, they giggle nervously after a minor accident.

Often people with schizophrenia show "blunted" or "flat" affect. This refers to a severe reduction in emotional expressiveness. A schizophrenic person may not show the signs of normal emotion, perhaps using a monotonous tone of voice and diminished facial expression.

Some people with symptoms of schizophrenia also exhibit prolonged extremes of elation or depression, and it is important to determine whether such a patient is schizophrenic, or actually has a bipolar (manic-depressive) disorder or major depressive disorder. Persons who cannot be clearly categorized are sometimes diagnosed as having a schizoaffective disorder.

SOURCE:
National Institute of Mental Health. *Schizophrenia: Questions and Answers*. DHHS Pub. No. (ADM) 86-1457. 1986. pp. 1-4.

PARANOID SCHIZOPHRENIA

Paranoia is a term used by mental health specialists to describe suspiciousness (or mistrust) that is either highly exaggerated or not warranted at all. The word is often used in everyday conversation, often in anger, often incorrectly. Simple suspiciousness is not paranoia—not if it is based on past experience or expectations learned from the experience of others.

Paranoia can be mild and the affected person may function fairly well in society, or it can be so severe that the individual is incapacitated. Because many psychiatric disorders are accompanied by some paranoid features, diagnosis is sometimes difficult. Paranoias can be classified into three main categories—paranoid personality disorder, delusional (paranoid) disorder, and paranoid schizophrenia. . . .

Paranoid thinking and behavior are hallmarks of the form of schizophrenia called "paranoid schizophrenia." Individuals with paranoid schizophrenia commonly have extremely bizarre delusions or hallucinations, almost always on a specific theme. Sometimes they hear voices that others cannot hear or believe that their thoughts are being controlled or broadcast aloud. Also, their performance at home and on the job deteriorates, often with a much diminished degree of emotional expressiveness.

In contrast, people with relatively milder paranoid disorders may have such symptoms as delusions of persecution or delusional jealousy, but not the prominent hallucinations or impossible, bizarre delusions of paranoid schizophrenia. Those with milder paranoid disorders are customarily able to work, and their emotional expression and behavior are appropriate to their delusional belief. Apart from their delusions, their thinking remains clear and orderly. On the other hand, those with paranoid schizophrenia are often intellectually disorganized and confused.

SOURCE:
National Institute of Mental Health. *Useful Information on Paranoia*. 1989. pp. 1-10.

CAUSES OF SCHIZOPHRENIA

Schizophrenia afflicts more than 2.5 million Americans and costs society up to $20 billion each year. Yet the hallucinations, delusions and apathy that are typical of the disease have so far eluded scientific explanation. Last week, a piece of the puzzle was firmly glued into place. A report by National Institute of Mental Health researchers yielded the clearest evidence to date that schizophrenia is a brain disorder, not a purely psychological condition, as was once argued.

The scientists used a sophisticated scanning device to examine the brain structure of 15 pairs of identical twins, one schizophrenic, the other normal, and discovered subtle anatomical differences. In the mentally ill twins, the fluid filled brain cavities called ventricles were found to be enlarged, indicating the tissue had either shrunk or developed abnormally. Similarly, brain regions involved in memory, emotion, decision making and other higher-order abilities were smaller in the afflicted twins.

Schizophrenia runs in families, and experts believe it likely that genetic vulnerability plays a role. Since the twins in the study are genetically identical, however, something other than heredity clearly is at work as well. Researchers are investigating a long list of possible culprits, some of them striking before birth, some after. Among the suspects are viral infections, oxygen deprivation and traumatic events that alter the development of neural tissue. The symptoms of the disease usually appear in adolescence or early adulthood and may be triggered by stress.

SOURCE:
"What Twins Tell Us about Schizophrenia." *U.S. News & World Report* 108 (April 2, 1990): 13–14.

TREATMENT

Antipsychotic medications (also called neuroleptics) have been available since the mid-1950's. They have greatly improved the outlook for individual patients. These medications reduce the psychotic symptoms of schizophrenia and usually allow the patient to function more effectively appropriately. Antipsychotic drugs are the best treatment now available, but they do not "cure" schizophrenia or ensure that there will be no further psychotic episodes. The choice and dosage of medication can be made only by a qualified physician who is well trained in the medical treatment of mental disorders. The dosage of medication is individualized for each patient, since patients may vary a great deal in the amount of drug needed to reduce symptoms without producing troublesome side effects.

Antipsychotic drugs are very effective in treating certain schizophrenic symptoms (for example, hallucinations and delusions). A large majority of schizophrenic patients show substantial improvement. Some patients, however, are not helped very much by such medications and a few do not seem to need them. It is difficult to predict which patients will fall into these two groups and to distinguish them from the large majority of patients who do benefit from treatment with antipsychotic drugs. . . .

Antipsychotic drugs, like virtually all medications, have unwanted effects along with their beneficial effects. During the early phases of drug treatment, patients may be troubled by side effects such as drowsiness, restlessness, muscle spasms, tremor, dry mouth, or blurring of vision. Most of these can be corrected by lowering the dosage or can be controlled by other medications. Different patients have different treatment responses and side effects to various antipsychotic drugs. A patient may do better with one drug than another.

The long-term side effects of antipsychotic drugs may pose a considerably more serious problem. Tardive dyskinesia (TD) is a disorder characterized by involuntary movements most often affecting the mouth, lips, and tongue, and sometimes the trunk or other parts of the body. It generally occurs in about 15 to 20 percent of patients who have been receiving antipsychotic drugs for many years, but TD can occur in patients who have been treated with these drugs for shorter periods of time. In most cases, the symptoms of TD are mild, and the patient may be unaware of the movements.

The risk-benefit issue in any kind of treatment for schizophrenia is an extremely important consideration. In this context, the risk of TD—as frightening as it is—must be carefully weighed against the risk of repeated breakdowns that can terribly disrupt patients' efforts to reestablish themselves at school, at work, at home, and in the community. For patients who develop TD, the use of medications must be reevaluated. Recent research suggests, however, that TD, once considered irreversible, often improves even when patients continue to receive antipsychotic medications.

SOURCE:
National Institute of Mental Health. *Schizophrenia: Questions and Answers.* DHHS Pub. No. (ADM) 86-1457. 1986. pp. 1-4.

USE OF CLOZAPINE (CLOZARIL) FOR TREATMENT

The FDA's recent approval of clozapine has attracted interest and curiosity on the part of many consumers and family members. The drug was approved for the treatment of patients with severe and persistent schizophrenia, who either have not adequately responded to, or cannot tolerate, standard antipsychotic drugs. Sandoz Pharmaceuticals manufactures and markets clozapine under the product name Clozaril.

Clozapine has unique benefits and unique risks. The benefits make it the first major innovation in antipsychotic drugs since the introduction of neuroleptics, nearly thirty years ago. The system designed to manage the risks associated with clozapine use make it an innovation in treatment modalities.

Often patients respond in as little time as a week. Some may require a much longer period, and many of those who do, show the greatest improvements. About six months is a good trial period. Once a patient responds, he/she may continue to improve for up to a year.

The benefits of clozapine are its superior effectiveness and its unique side effects profile. It treats the positive symptoms of schizophrenia such as hallucinations, delusions, blunted affect, and hostility better than any other drugs. It is also the first drug which effectively treats the negative symptoms—apathy, withdrawal, blunted emotional response, and anxiety. It accomplishes this with 30 to 60 percent of the pateints who were previously considered refractory, that is, patients who were unresponsive to standard antipsychotic drugs.

Clozapine has virtually no incidence of the muscle spasms, cramps, and posturing movements common to neuroleptic drugs and minimal incidence of the less serious neurological side effects such as restlessness, muscle rigidity, and tremor. Nor has there ever been a case of tardive dyskinesia associated with clozapine.

SOURCE:
National Alliance for the Mentally Ill. *Clozapine.* 1990. pp. 2–3.

AFFORDABILITY OF CLOZAPINE (CLOZARIL)

The patients who need the drug [clozapine] the most face a huge barrier: treatment costs nearly $9,000 a year. The drug is a patented product, available in the U.S. under the brand name Clozaril only from New Jersey–based Sandoz Pharmaceuticals, a subsidiary of Sandoz International of Basel, Switzerland. The company's explanation for the steep price is that clozapine occasionally causes fatal side effects, so patients must be required to have regular blood tests to make sure they are tolerating the drug. The expense of the tests pushes clozapine beyond the reach of the majority of schizophrenics, many of whom are poor and underinsured, and Medicaid programs in most states have not been willing to cover the cost. As a result, only 5,500 Americans have begun therapy. . . .

Several state attorneys general are investigating Sandoz for possible antitrust violations, while a handful of advocacy groups have launched lawsuits to force Medicaid to pick up the clozapine tab. But to patients with schizophrenia, these legal and legislative maneuverings mean little. All that matters to them is an impossible price tag standing between their current mental anguish and a productive life.

SOURCE:
Purvis, Andrew. "Way Out of Reach: A Schizophrenia Drug Is Too Costly for Those Who Need It the Most." *Time* (October 1, 1990): 79.

RESOURCES

ORGANIZATIONS

American Psychiatric Association. 1400 K St. NW, Washington, DC 20005.

National Alliance for the Mentally Ill. 1901 North Ft. Myer Drive, Suite 500, Arlington, VA 22209-1604.

National Depressive and Manic Depressive Association. P.O. Box 753, Northbrook, IL 60062.

National Institute of Mental Health. Public Information Branch, 5600 Fishers Lane, Rockville, MD 20857.

National Mental Health Association. 1021 Prince St., Alexandria, VA 22314.

PAMPHLET

National Alliance for the Mentally Ill:

Schizophrenia. 1990.

BOOK

Torrey, E. Fuller. *Surviving Schizophrenia: A Family Manual.* Revised Edition. New York: Harper & Row, 1987. 460 pp.

RELATED ARTICLES

Der, Geoffrey, Sunjai Gupta, and Robin M. Murray. "Epidemiology: Is Schizophrenia Disappearing?" *The Lancet* 335 (March 3, 1990): 513–516.

"Diagnosis of Schizophrenia." *The Lancet* 335, no. 8703 (June 16, 1990): 1432–1433.

Folkenberg, Judy. "New Schizophrenia Drug: Balancing Hope with Safety." *FDA Consumer* (June 1990): 17–19.

Gunby, Phil. "'Decade of the Brain' Holds Promise for Answers to Schizophrenia." *JAMA* 264 (November 21, 1990): 2483.

Johnson, Dale L. "Schizophrenia as a Brain Disease: Implications for Psychologists and Families." *American Psychologist* (March 1989): 553–555.

Martin, Ronald L. "Outpatient Management of Schizophrenia." *American Family Physician* 43 (March 1991): 921–933.

Mesulam, M. Marsel. "Schizophrenia and the Brain." *The New England Journal of Medicine* 322, no. 12 (March 22, 1990): 842–845.

SEXUALLY TRANSMITTED DISEASES

(*See also:* CHLAMYDIA; GONORRHEA; HERPES SIMPLEX VIRUS INFECTION; PELVIC INFLAMMATORY DISEASE; SYPHILIS)

OVERVIEW

Sexually transmitted diseases (STD's) also called venereal diseases, are among the most common infectious diseases in the United States today. At least 20 STD's have now been identified, and they affect more than 10 million men and women in this country each year. . . .

What are some of these basic facts? It is important to understand at least five key points about all STD's in this country today:

1. STD's affect men and women of all backgrounds and economic levels. They are, however, most prevalent among teenagers and young adults. Nearly one-third of all cases [involves] teenagers.

2. The incidence of STD's is rising, in part because in the last few decades, young people have become sexually active earlier; sexually active people today are more likely to have more than one sex partner or to change partners frequently. Anyone who has sexual relations is potentially at risk for developing STD's.

3. Many STD's initially cause no symptoms. When symptoms develop, they may be confused with those of other diseases not transmitted through sexual contact. However, even when an STD causes no symptoms, a person who is infected may be able to pass the disease on to a sex partner. That is why many doctors recommend periodic testing for people who have more than one sex partner.

4. Health problems caused by STD's tend to be more severe and more frequent for women than for men.

- Some STD's can cause pelvic inflammatory disease (PID), a major cause of both infertility and ectopic (tubal) pregnancy. The latter can be fatal to a pregnant woman.
- STD infections in women may also be associated with cervical cancer. One STD, genital warts, is caused by a virus associated with cervical and other cancers; the relationship between other STD's and cervical cancer is not yet known.
- STD's can be passed from a mother to her baby before or during birth; some of these congenital infections can be cured easily, but others may cause permanent disability or even death of the infant.

5. When diagnosed and treated early, almost all STD's can be treated effectively. Some organisms, such as certain forms of gonococci, have become resistant to the drugs used to treat them and now require higher doses or newer types of antibiotics. The most serious STD for which no effective treatment or cure now exists is acquired immunodeficiency syndrome (AIDS), a fatal viral infection of the immune system.

SOURCE:
National Institute of Allergy and Infectious Diseases. *An Introduction to Sexually Transmitted Diseases*. NIH Pub. No. 87-909A. August 1987. pp. 1–2.

MAJOR TYPES

DISEASES THAT MAY BE TRANSMITTED SEXUALLY AND THE ORGANISMS RESPONSIBLE

Disease *(Organism[s])*

- Acquired Immunodeficiency Syndrome [AIDS] *(Human immunodeficiency virus)*
- Bacterial vaginosis *(Gardnerella vaginalis; Bacteroides; Mycoplasma hominis)*
- Chancroid *(Haemophilus ducreyi)*

- Chlamydial infections *(Chlamydia trachomatis)*
- Cytomegalovirus infections (Cytomegalovirus)
- Enteric infections

  Hepatitis A (Hepatitis A virus)

  Amebiasis *(Entamoeba histolytica* [protozoan])

  Giardiasis *(Giardia lamblia* [protozoan])

  Shigellosis *(Shigellae* [bacteria])
- Genital herpes (Herpes simplex virus)
- Genital mycoplasma infections *(Mycoplasma hominis; Ureaplasma urealyticum)*
- Genital [venereal] warts (Human papillomavirus)
- Gonorrhea *(Neisseria gonorrhoeae)*
- Granuloma inguinale [Donovanosis] *(Calymmatobacterium granulomatis)*
- Group B streptoccal infections (Group B-hemolytic streptococcus)
- Molluscum contagiosum (Molluscum contagiosum virus)
- Pubic lice *(Phthirus pubis)*
- Scabies *(Sarcoptes scabiei)*
- Syphilis *(Treponema pallidum)*
- Trichomoniasis *(Trichomonas vaginalis)*

SOURCE:
National Institute of Allergy and Infectious Diseases. *Miscellaneous STD's*. NIH Pub. No. 87-909H. August 1987. p. 8.

HUMAN PAPILLOMAVIRUS

Human papillomavirus (HPV) is a virus that causes genital warts. It is one of the most common STDs in the United States. In women, it is marked by small, white bumps on the outside of the genital area or inside the vagina, rectum, or urethra (the short tube leading from the bladder to the outside of the body.) In men, lesions may occur around the anus or in or around the opening of the penis, but they may not be readily visible.

Although some warts may go away on their own, treatment is usually needed to get rid of the warts. Some types of genital warts can turn into cancer. Even after the warts have cleared up, there may still be a risk of cancer. Women who have had HPV may need to get pelvic exams and Pap tests more often than those who have never had this disease. Rarely, HPV infection can be passed on to the fetus during pregnancy or at birth.

SOURCE:
American College of Obstetricians and Gynecologists. *How to Prevent Sexually Tramsmitted Diseases*. July 1991.

PREVENTION: SAFE SEX

Each year, the number of people in the United States who contract a sexually transmitted disease (STD) increases (this includes those—both heterosexual and homosexual—with the AIDS virus).

Some may be offended by open discussions of "safe sex," but it is important that you understand what behaviors put you and your family and friends at risk of contracting disease. All of us must take responsibility for protecting ourselves and our partners. Simply addressing these issues does not imply approval of the sexual practices discussed.

Most STDs are treatable, but AIDS has no cure and death is virtually certain. Therefore, education about this disease is especially vital. Although AIDS can be spread through shared use of contaminated needles among drug abusers or, rarely, through blood transfusion, it usually is transmitted by sexual contact. The virus is present in semen and vaginal secretions and enters a person's body through the small tears in the vaginal or rectal tissues that can develop during sexual activity. AIDS is not considered to be a highly contagious disease; transmission of the virus occurs only after very intimate contact with infected blood or semen.

On the other hand, STDs such as chlamydiosis, gonorrhea, herpes, venereal warts, and syphilis are highly contagious, and many of them can be spread through even brief sexual contact. However, none of these infections is spread through casual contact such as handshaking, talking, sitting on toilet seats, or living in the same house with an infected person. The microorganisms that cause STDs, including AIDS, all die quickly once they are outside of the body.

The only sure way of preventing STDs and AIDS is through sexual abstinence or a relationship with only one uninfected person (straight or gay). If you have several partners, either heterosexual or homosexual, you place yourself at high risk of contracting disease. And at present, no vaccine is available to prevent any of the STDs.

While condoms do not eliminate the risk, correct use of a condom and avoidance of certain sexual practices can decrease the risk of contracting AIDS as well as other STDs.

The condom, also known as a prophylactic, rubber, or safe, is a thin sheath, usually made of latex rubber that covers the erect penis. When used correctly, a latex condom is effective both for preventing pregnancy and for decreasing the chance of contracting most STDs including AIDS. Condoms can be purchased over the counter at any drugstore and are available in various thicknesses, colors, and shapes. They may be lubricated or unlubricated, have a plain end or a reservoir end, and have a smooth (the most common), ribbed, or corrugated texture. They can cost as little as three for a dollar, but usually the cost ranges from 50 cents to a dollar each. Condoms sometimes are made of animal membrane; however, some experts believe that the pores in such natural "skin" condoms may allow the virus to pass through. To be effective, the condom must be undamaged, must be applied to the erect penis before any genital contact, and must remain intact and snugly in place until completion of the sexual activity.

About a third of the condoms now sold in the United States are bought by women. They can be kept in a pocket or purse until needed, and they provide protection against STDs. The condom can be placed on the erect penis of a woman's male partner as a part of the initial foreplay; a man who objects to a condom may be less opposed to wearing one if his partner puts it on for him. Most forms of female-directed contraception (i.e., the pill, the diaphragm) do not provide protection against STDs, although studies indicate that use of the spermicide nonoxynol 9, as with the vaginal sponge, does decrease the frequency of gonorrhea and chlamydiosis. Using spermicide in conjunction with a diaphragm also may help kill bacteria.

Different sexual practices carry different degrees of risk of contracting the AIDS virus. Receptive (passive) anal intercourse is the riskiest because this may damage the anal and rectal membranes and allow the AIDS virus to enter the bloodstream. The passive partner is at much higher risk of contracting the AIDS virus than is the active partner, although gonorrhea and syphilis can be transmitted from the passive partner's rectum. Most studies have focused on male homosexuals, but heterosexual anal sex probably carries the same risks.

Heterosexual vaginal intercourse, particularly with multiple partners, also carries a risk of contracting AIDS. The virus is believed to be transmitted more easily from the man to the woman than vice versa. This type of sex is how most other STDs are transmitted.

Oral/genital sex is a possible, but probably uncommon, means of transmission of the AIDS virus. However, inserting the penis in the mouth (fellatio) with ejaculation and swallowing of semen is the most common cause of throat gonorrhea; oral contact with the clitoris and vaginal opening (cunnilingus) is a frequent method of transmission of the herpes virus.

Herpes is probably the only disease that can be contracted by light (dry) kissing, but deep (French) kissing may transmit other STDs. Activities that involve only skin-to-skin contact such as hugging, massage, and mutual masturbation, with little or no exposure to body fluids, do not spread disease.

SOURCE:
Larson, David E. (ed.). *Mayo Clinic Family Health Book*. New York: William Morrow, 1990. pp. 878–879.

RESOURCES

ORGANIZATIONS

American Foundation for the Prevention of Venereal Disease. 799 Broadway, Suite 638, New York, NY 10003.

American Social Health Association. 260 Sheridan Avenue, Suite 307, Palo Alto, CA 94306.

National Institute of Allergy and Infectious Diseases. Office of Communications, National Institutes of Health, Bethesda MD 20892.

PAMPHLETS

American College of Obstetricians and Gynecologists:

Sexually Transmitted Diseases. 1984. 14 pp.

American Foundation for the Prevention of Venereal Disease:

Sexually Transmitted Diseases (STD): Prevention for Everyone. 1987. 26 pp.

California Medical Association:

"Cervical Cancer May Be Linked to Sexual Activity." *HealthTips* 371 (May 1988).

"Chlamydia." *HealthTips* WH-12. 1985.

"Genital Herpes and Pregnancy." *HealthTips* WH-20. 1985.

"Herpes." *HealthTips* 357 (May 1987).

"Screening for Gonorrhea." *HealthTips* 311 (May 1987).

March of Dimes—Birth Defects Foundation:

Sexually Transmitted Diseases. 1986.

National Institute of Allergy and Infectious Diseases:

Chlamydial Infections. NIH Pub. No. 87-909B.

Genital Herpes. NIH Pub. No. 87-909C.

Genital Warts. NIH Pub. No. 87-909D.

Gonorrhea. NIH Pub. No. 87-909E.

Pelvic Inflammatory Disease. NIH Pub. No. 87-909F.

Syphilis. NIH Pub. No. 87-909G.

RELATED ARTICLES

"CDC Releases Updated Guidelines for STD Treatment." *American Family Physician* 40 (December 1989): 199–202.

Fletcher, James L., and Ralph C. Gordon. "Perinatal Transmission of Bacterial Sexually Transmitted Diseases. Part I. Syphilis and Gonorrhea." *The Journal of Family Practice* 30, no. 4 (1990): 448–456.

MacDonald, Noni E., and others. "High-Risk STD/HIV Behavior among College Students." *JAMA* 263, no. 33 (June 20, 1989): 3155–3159.

McElhouse, Priscilla. "The 'Other' STDs: As Dangerous As Ever." *RN* 51 (June 1988): 52–59.

"STDs Near Epidemic Levels, Experts Agree." *American World News* 32 (June 2, 1989): 3–4.

"Treatment of Sexually Transmitted Diseases." *The Medical Letter on Drugs and Therapeutics* 32 (January 26, 1990): 5–10.

SINUSITIS

OVERVIEW

Sinusitis is the most common chronic illness in the country, affecting an estimated 14 percent of Americans. Many sufferers don't even realize they have the condition, dismissing their symptoms as a lingering cold. Yet, if left untreated, sinusitis—an inflammation of the sinuses—can lead to such serious diseases as asthma, bronchitis and an inflammation of the brain. Here's how to tell if you have sinusitis—and what to do about it if you do.

The sinuses are holes in the skull between the facial bones. There are four large sinuses: two inside the cheekbones (the maxillary sinuses), and two above the eyes (the frontal sinuses). There are also smaller sinuses (the ethmoidal and sphenoidal sinuses) located between the larger ones. The sinuses are lined with membranes that secrete antibody-containing mucus, which protects the respiratory passages from the onslaught of irritants in the air we breathe. (The nose and sinuses also provide the resonance in our voice—the reason Barbra Streisand won't have her nose fixed.) Sinusitis is an inflammation of the membranes lining the sinuses that may or may not be accompanied by a bacterial infection.

There are many causes of sinusitis. Allergies to dust, pollen and pet dander; indoor air pollutants such as cigarette smoke, rug shampoo, and formaldehyde (frequently used in the manufacture of carpeting, particle board and plywood); and outdoor air pollutants all can induce inflammation. Excessive dryness in homes and offices from dry-air heating and air-conditioning systems can also inflame the sinuses. A cold causes sinusitis as well.

Once the sinuses are inflamed for any reason, they are more vulnerable to bacterial infection. If the nasal congestion from a cold gets worse instead of clearing up after three to five days, it may be because the sinus membranes, inflamed and weakened by the cold virus, have been attacked by a bacterial infection. Once infected by bacteria, the sinus membranes are more sensitive to allergens and irritants and become even more inflamed. Thus, the vicious circle of chronic sinusitis is set in motion. Over time, too, the sinus membranes of those with chronic sinusitis become cracked, scarred and swollen, making them more susceptible to repeat problems. With early treatment, though, this chain of events can be stopped and sinusitis sufferers can recover fully. Often, they have become so accustomed to their symptoms that they are surprised by how much better they feel after proper care.

Untreated sinusitis can cause serious complications. It can lead to bronchitis if an infection spreads from the sinuses to the bronchial tubes. The infection can be transmitted through mucus that drips from the sinuses and nose to the throat (postnasal drip) and then into the lungs, or when it enters the bloodstream via blood vessels in the sinus membranes. Asthma can develop in the same way, or when irritation in the nasal membranes causes a reflexive spasm in the bronchial tubes. Sinusitis can also cause meningitis (inflammation of the tissue surrounding the brain and spinal cord) and osteomyelitis (bone disease), although such occurrences are rare. Meningitis results if a sinus infection breaks through the sinus membranes into the tissues of the brain; osteomyelitis develops if the sinus infection spreads into the facial bones in the sinus area.

SOURCE:

Podell, Richard N., and Beth Weinhouse. "The Cold That Won't Go Away—Sinusitis." *Redbook* 176 (February 1991): 92–93.

DIAGNOSIS

The diagnosis of sinusitis is not always straightforward. Good empiric regimens exist, but you have to maintain vigilance to avoid a smoldering chronic process or potentially serious complications. Why is the clinical diagnosis of sinusitis often not straightforward?

Since adults average two or three colds yearly, of which one-half percent are complicated by sinus infection, sinusitis is one of the most common clinical problems. The clinical diagnosis is not always obvious, however, and most patients who seek medical attention for what they think is sinusitis or "Sinus headache" actually have tension headache, upper respiratory tract viral infection, allergic rhinitis, or other conditions. Although true sinus disease is often self-limited, accurate diagnosis and treatment are important for providing symptomatic relief and preventing progression to chronic sinusitis with irreversible mucosal damage or the development of serious complications.

The classic presentation of acute sinusitis includes fever, nasal obstruction and voice nasality, nasal discharge that often is purulent, and facial pain or headache that is sometimes aggravated by bending over. Swelling of the nasal turbinates may cause anosmia [loss of sense of smell]. When pain is present, its site may suggest which sinus is affected. Maxillary sinusitis, the most common type, manifests as cheek or dental pain. Forehead pain indicates frontal sinusitis. Pain at the bridge of the nose or behind the eye suggests ethmoid sinusitis. Pain is often referred to the top of the head with sphenoidal involvement.

The classic presentation, however, may occur in only a minority of patients. Fever does not occur in 50–75% of patients, and pain may not be present. In fact, clinical and historical features do not allow you to reliably distinguish acute bacterial sinusitis from persistent viral rhinitis.

Because of the uncommon but potentially serious complications of inadequately treated sinusitis, suspect the diagnosis in any patient with an upper respiratory tract infection that is unusually prolonged—more than 7–10 days. Sinusitis is especially likely if the cold symptoms are unusually severe or accompanied by high fever, purulent nasal discharge, or periorbital edema. Some clinicians find that cough related to irritation from postnasal secretions is a relatively common finding, although it is not often described in the literature except in children.

Predisposing factors in the history may help confirm the diagnosis or indicate underlying conditions that require therapy. The two most common predisposing factors are recent upper respiratory tract viral infection and allergic disease.

Allergy provides the basis for sinus infection in about 25% of cases because of intranasal swelling and blockage of the sinus ostium. Since the roots of the upper molars are adjacent to the floor of the maxillary sinus, dental infection is also a common source of acute sinusitis, accounting for up to 10% of cases. Dental extraction sometimes causes an oroantral [mouth-sinus] fistula that may lead to contamination of the sinus space and infection.

SOURCE:

Gantz, Nelson M., and others. "Questions and Answers on Sinusitis." *Patient Care 22* (August 15, 1988): 53–55.

SINUSITIS IN CHILDREN

Historically, the inattention to sinus disease in children stemmed largely from the fact that the paranasal sinuses—the cavities that surround the nose—are not fully formed at birth. Although the ethmoid and maxillary sinuses begin to develop before birth, the sphenoid and frontal sinuses develop later. The sphenoid sinuses are not even visible on X-rays until about the age of 9.

Doctors did not expect the sinuses to cause problems before they were fully developed. But it is now known that children as young as 2, and perhaps even younger, can develop infected sinuses. If not treated properly, the problem can persist for months and recur at the slightest provocation, such as whenever the child catches a cold or develops a runny nose from an allergic reaction.

Children with chronically infected sinuses often suffer physically, academically and socially. Bad breath is a hallmark of sinusitis. Recurrent ear infections are a common complication. More rare, but also far more serious, are such complications as infections of the bone, the orbit of the eye and even the brain.

To avoid such consequences, parents and physicians must be alert to the signs of sinus problems in children, which often differ from those in adults. Sinus infections should also be treated promptly and adequately. In most cases, this means several weeks on antibiotics, even though the child may seem fine after just a few days. . . .

When a child develops a cold that lingers, think sinus infection. Symptoms of an acute infection in children include persistent nasal discharge (thin or thick, clear or colored), post-nasal drip and a cough that gets worse when the child lies down or sleeps. Fever is sometimes present, as is swelling around the eyes. A headache is rare in young children.

Older children with infected sinuses display a pattern of symptoms more like adults. They often experience nasal congestion and discharge, or a cough that gets worse at night. Their speech may sound nasal, and their sense of smell may be impaired. They may also have a sore throat, headache, facial pain, bad breath and an unpleasant taste in the mouth. When the maxillary sinuses are infected, the upper teeth often ache.

When such symptoms persist, perhaps in a more subtle form, for a month or longer, the condition is considered chronic. In young children, chronic sinusitis is often associated with fluid or infections in the middle ear, stomach pain, nausea and sometimes vomiting, loss of appetite, irritability, fatigue and malaise.

SOURCE:

Brody, Jane E. "New Appreciation of Sinus Infections in Children and What Steps Should Be Taken." *The New York Times* (December 28, 1989): 20.

TREATMENT

If a bacterial infection is present, standard antibiotics such as amoxicillin, erythromycin or sulfa drugs are usually prescribed for about ten days. Patients should also be counseled about avoiding sinusitis triggers such as cigarette smoke, dry air, dust, mold, pet dander or pollen. Your doctor may also prescribe one or more of the following remedies, which can be useful in reducing inflammation in the sinuses and nose and speeding recovery:

Decongestants. These are highly effective in treating sinusitis. They temporarily relieve symptoms and also help the healing process by draining the nose and sinuses. Decongestants like pseudoephedrine, phenylpherine and phenylpropanolamine constrict the blood vessels and shrink the sinus and nasal membranes, reducing stuffiness in the sinuses and nasal passageways. Decongestants on their own do not cause drowsiness—but those sold in combination with antihistamines might.

Over-the-counter nasal sprays. These products, which include Afrin and Dristan, are decongestants in spray form. They are effective when used for a few days, but can be addicting when used for longer periods of time. After using decongestant sprays for about three days, people usually experience a rebound effect: When they stop using the spray, they become even more congested, and need more spray to get relief. People with chronic allergies or sinus problems should limit their use of decongestant sprays to five treatments a week.

Prescription inhalers. Several types of prescription nasal inhalers can help reduce sinus inflammation. (These are not decongestants, and are not habit-forming.) Though they don't fight bacteria directly, prescription inhalers help heal sinus membranes after the bacteria have been eliminated. These drugs include Beconase, Nasalide and Vancenase—all cortisone derivatives—and Nasalcrom, a non-cortisone drug. When used as directed by a physician, they can be taken safely for months.

Expectorants. Medicines such as guaifenesin thin the mucus so it drains more easily.

Antihistamines. These medications help relieve nasal itchiness and inflammation by blocking the action of histamine, one of the body's natural inflammatory chemicals. However, they do not help mucus drain and so are less useful than decongestants for treating sinusitis. Over-the-counter antihistamines include chlorpheniramine and diphenhydramine. These drugs can cause drowsiness, so should never be used while driving or operating machinery. Newer prescription antihistamines such as Hismanol, Seldane and Tavist are less sedating.

Humidifiers and salt-water sprays. Dry-air heating systems in winter and air-conditioning in summer cause sinus membranes to dry out, crack and become vulnerable to irritants, inflammation and infection. Keeping a humidifier running in your home and office or using an over-the-counter salt-water spray (which is inhaled through the nose) five or six times a day can provide dramatic relief. . . .

Recurring sinusitis accompanied by a bacterial infection usually requires one of the new, stronger—and more expensive—antibiotics, such as Augmentin, Ceclor or Ceftin. These drugs may be given in larger doses, for a longer period of time (up to four weeks) than would be required for a brief bout of sinusitis. Your doctor may also recommend that you continue using a prescription nasal inhaler for several months to keep the inflammation down and prevent a recurrence.

SOURCE:

Podell, Richard N., and Beth Weinhouse. "The Cold That Won't Go Away—Sinusitis." *Redbook* 176 (February 1991): 93-94.

RESOURCES

PAMPHLET

California Medical Association. "Sinus Infection." *HealthTips* index 144 (February 1989): 1-2.

RELATED ARTICLES

"Chronic Sinusitis in Children." *American Family Physician* 41 (April 1990): 1234.

Edmeads, J. "The Worst Headache Ever: 1. Ominous Causes." *Postgraduate Medicine* 86, no. 1 (July 1989): 93-96, 103-104.

Goldenhersh, Margaret J., and Gary S. Rachelefsky. "Helping the Child with Sinusitis." *Patient Care* 24 (April 15, 1989): 76-80, 82, 87, 91, 94, 97.

Herrera, A. "Sinusitis: Its Association with Asthma." *Postgraduate Medicine* 87, no. 5 (April 1990): 153-156, 161, 164.

Slavin, Raymond G. "Sinusitis in Adults." *Journal of Allergy and Clinical Immunology* 81, no. 5, part 2 (May 1988): 1028-1032.

SKIN CANCER

OVERVIEW

The two most common kinds of skin cancer are basal cell carcinoma and squamous cell carcinoma. (Carcinoma is cancer that begins in the cells that cover or line an organ.) Basal cell carcinoma accounts for more than 90 percent of all skin cancers in the United States. It is a slow-growing cancer that seldom spreads to other parts of the body. Squamous cell carcinoma also rarely spreads, but it does so more often than basal cell carcinoma. However, it is important that skin cancers are found and treated early because they can invade and destroy nearby tissue. Basal cell carcinoma and squamous cell carcinoma are sometimes called nonmelanoma skin cancer. Another type of cancer that occurs in the skin is melanoma, which begins in the melanocytes. . . .

Skin cancer is the most common type of cancer in the United States. According to present estimates, 40 to 50 percent of Americans who live to age 65 will have skin cancer at least once.

Several risk factors increase the chance of getting skin cancer. Ultraviolet (UV) radiation from the sun is the main cause of skin cancer. Artificial sources of UV radiation, such as sunlamps and tanning booths, can also cause skin cancer. Although anyone can get skin cancer, the risk is greatest for people who have fair skin that freckles easily—often those with red or blond hair and blue or light-colored eyes.

The risk of developing skin cancer is also affected by where a person lives. People who live in areas that get high levels of UV radiation from the sun are more likely to get skin cancer. In the United States, for example, skin cancer is more common in Texas than it is in Minnesota, where the sun is not as strong. Worldwide, the highest rates of skin cancer are found in South Africa and Australia, areas that receive high amounts of UV radiation.

In addition, skin cancer is related to lifetime exposure to UV radiation. Most skin cancers appear after age 50, but the sun's damaging effects begin at an early age. Therefore, protection should start in childhood to prevent skin cancer later in life. . . .

The most common warning sign of skin cancer is a change on the skin, especially a new growth or a sore that doesn't heal. Skin cancer has many different appearances. For example, it may start as a small, smooth, shiny, pale, or waxy lump. Or, the cancer can appear as a firm red lump. Sometimes, the lump bleeds or develops a crust. Skin cancer can also start as a flat, red spot that is rough, dry, or scaly. Pain is NOT a sign of skin cancer. . . .

Both basal and squamous cell cancers are found mainly on areas of the skin that are exposed to the sun—the head, face, neck, hands, and arms. However, skin cancer can occur anywhere.

Another condition that can affect the skin is actinic keratosis, which appears as rough, red or brown, scaly patches on the skin. Because actinic keratosis sometimes develops into squamous cell cancer, it is known as a precancerous condition. Like skin cancer, it usually appears on sun-exposed areas but can be found elsewhere.

Changes in the skin are not sure signs of cancer; however, it is important to see a doctor if any symptom lasts longer than 2 weeks.

SOURCE:
National Cancer Institute. *What You Need to Know about Skin Cancer*. NIH Pub. No. 89-1564. August 1988. pp. 3-7.

MELANOMA

This most virulent of all skin cancers developed on the skin of 27,300 Americans in 1988. And in that year 5,800 melanoma victims died. It is important to note that the death rate is at last declining, because patients are seeking help earlier. Melanoma, like its less aggressive cousins, basal cell and squamous cell carcinomas, is almost always curable in its early stages.

Melanoma has its beginnings in melanocytes, the skin cells which produce the dark protective pigment called melanin. It is melanin which is responsible for suntanned skin, acting as a partial protection against the sun. Melanoma cells usually continue to produce melanin, which accounts for the cancers appearing in mixed shades of tan, brown and black. Melanoma has a tendency to spread, making it essential to treat.

Melanoma may suddenly appear without warning but it may also begin in or near a mole or other dark spot in the skin. For that reason it is important that we know the location and appearance of the moles on our bodies so any change will be noticed.

Excessive exposure to the sun, as with the other skin cancers, is accepted as a cause of melanoma, especially among light-skinned people. Heredity may play a part, and also atypical moles, which may run in families, can serve as markers, identifying the person as being at higher risk for developing melanoma there or elsewhere in the skin.

Dark brown or black skin is not a guarantee against melanoma. Black people can develop this cancer, especially on the palm of the hands, soles of the feet, under nails, or in the mouth.

SOURCE:
American Academy of Dermatology. *Melanoma/Skin Cancer: You Can Recognize the Signs*. TPAM 14 1/90. 1989. pp. 1-2.

TREATMENT

Treatment for skin cancer may involve surgery, radiation therapy, or cryosurgery. Sometimes, a combination of these methods is used. The doctor considers a number of factors to determine the best treatment for skin cancer, such as the location of the cancer, its size, and whether or not the cancer has spread beyond the skin. The doctor's main objective is to destroy the cancer completely while causing as little scarring as possible.

Surgery: Most skin cancers can be removed quickly and easily by surgery. Sometimes, the cancer is completely removed at the time of biopsy, and no further treatment is needed.

To remove small skin cancers, doctors commonly use a special type of surgery called curettage. After a local anesthetic numbs the area, the cancer is scooped out with a curette, an instrument with a sharp, spoon-shaped end. Then, the area is generally treated by electrodesiccation. An electric current from a special machine is used to control bleeding and kill any cancer cells remaining around the edge of the wound.

Mohs' technique is a special type of surgery used for skin cancer. It is especially helpful for treating skin cancer in cases where the shape and depth of the tumor are hard to determine. In addition, this method is used to treat skin cancers that have recurred. The cancer is shaved off one thin layer of skin at a time until the entire tumor is removed. This method should be used only by doctors who are specially trained in this type of surgery.

Sometimes, when a large cancer is removed, a skin graft may be needed. For this procedure, the doctor takes a piece of skin from another part of the body to replace the skin that was removed. Surgery to remove skin cancers, with or without skin grafts, may cause scars.

Cryosurgery: Extreme cold may be used to treat precancerous skin conditions, such as actinic keratosis, as well as skin cancers. In cryosurgery, liquid nitrogen is applied to the growth to freeze and kill the abnormal cells. After the area thaws, the dead tissue falls off. More than one freezing may be needed to remove the growth completely. Cryosurgery does not require anesthesia, but patients may have pain after treatment. A white scar may form in the treated area.

Radiation Therapy: Skin cancer responds well to radiation therapy (also called x-ray therapy, radiotherapy, or irradiation), which uses high-energy rays to kill cancer cells. This treatment is used for cancers that occur in areas that are hard to treat with surgery. For example, radiation therapy might be used to treat skin cancers of the eyelid, the tip of the nose, and the ear. Several treatments may be needed to remove all of the cancer cells. During radiation therapy, patients may notice skin reactions, such as rashes or redness, in the area being treated. Changes in skin color and/or texture may develop, becoming more noticeable many years later.

Topical Chemotherapy: Topical chemotherapy is the use of anticancer drugs in a cream or lotion applied to the skin surface. Actinic keratosis can be treated effectively with the anticancer drug fluorouracil (also called 5-FU). The 5-FU cream or lotion is applied daily for several weeks. Intense inflammation is common during treatment, but scars usually do not occur.

SOURCE:
National Cancer Institute. *What You Need to Know about Skin Cancer*. NIH Pub. No. 89-1564. August 1988. pp. 9-11.

MOLES

Melanoma can begin in an existing mole or as a new, mole-like growth. If detected early, it can be effectively treated and cured. The first warning signs of melanoma should be promptly brought to the attention of a physician:

- **Large size.** If there is an increase (gradual or sudden) in the size of a mole, it may be melanoma. Melanomas generally are at least 5 millimeters (mm) across (about ¼ inch).

- **Multiple colors.** Melanomas tend to have a variety of colors—red, white, blue, and sometimes black or dark brown—within a single mole.
- **Irregular border.** Melanomas often have uneven or notched borders.
- **Abnormal surface.** A mole may be a melanoma if it is scaly, flaky, oozing, bleeding, or has an open sore that does not heal.
- **Unusual texture.** If a mole feels hard or lumpy, it may be a melanoma.
- **Abnormal skin around a mole.** If pigment, or color, from a mole has spread to surrounding skin or if nearby skin is red or swollen or has lost its pigmentation (becomes white or gray), a melanoma may be present.
- **Unusual sensation.** A mole may be a melanoma if it itches or is painful and tender.
- **Change in appearance of the skin.** Melanomas may develop as new pigmented spots in a skin area that had been normal.

While experienced physicians, especially dermatologists, can often identify a melanoma on sight, a biopsy is the only sure way to make a diagnosis. The biopsy—surgical removal of the mole—can usually be done using a local anesthesia in a doctor's office. Suspicious-looking areas should never be burned off. By examining the tissue under a microscope, a pathologist can determine whether the growth is benign (a mole) or cancerous (a basal or squamous cell carcinoma or melanoma).

SOURCE:
National Cancer Institute. *Melanoma.* Research Report. 1988.

PREVENTION

What measures can be taken to diminish the risk of UVR [ultraviolet radiation] exposure? There is considerable information that can serve as a basis for developing a policy of "low-risk" behavior.

- First, susceptibility to UVR damage can be reduced through use of proper clothing made of tightly woven fabrics with long sleeves, long pants, wide brimmed hats, etc.
- Second, a significant reduction in certain types of UVR damage can be achieved through the proper use of physical and chemical sunscreening products. Maximum photoprotection is afforded by chemical sunscreen with SPF [sun protection factor] ratings of 15 or higher. Although most sunscreens on the market today are appropriate for UVB protection, combination sunscreens that are effective against UVB and at least part of the UVA spectrum are preferable. Waterproof sunscreens should be selected by swimmers and those who perspire sufficiently to wash off nonwaterproof products. Daily use is recommended during appropriate times throughout the year. Sunscreens should be applied before exposure, with frequent reapplications thereafter.
- Third, one must strive to enhance behavior that limits sun exposure. Data exist to suggest that 50 percent of an individual's total lifetime UVR exposure occurs by 18 years of age. Therefore, parental education with subsequent direction of the behavior of children is important during childhood. Modified schedules for outdoor activities at school, camp, daycare centers, or the beach should be considered whenever possible so as to minimize UVR exposure. Time of day and time of year have a major impact on the extent of UVR exposure. For example, on a sunny day in June between 10:00 A.M. and 3:00 P.M., fully 60 percent of the daily UVB radiation reaching the Earth's surface arrives during this period. If exposure during this time could be minimized, a significant reduction in the number of NMSC's [non-melanoma skin cancers] would almost certainly occur. Adults and children should limit their exposure during this peak period of UVR.
- Fourth, one must be aware of photosensitizing medications and chemicals because it is known that these can exacerbate the effects of UVR exposure.
- Fifth, the adverse effects of intentional UVR exposure must be considered. All evidence indicates that UVR-induced suntanning, whether from natural or artificial sources, is harmful to the skin.

SOURCE:
"National Institutes of Health Consensus Development Conference Statement." *Sunlight, Ultraviolet Radiation, and the Skin* 7, no. 8 (May 8–10, 1989): 6–7.

RESOURCES

ORGANIZATIONS

American Academy of Dermatology. P.O. Box 1661, Evanston, IL 60204.

American Cancer Society. Tower Place, 3340 Peachtree Road, NE, Atlanta, GA 30026.

American Society of Plastic and Reconstructive Surgeons. Suite 1900, 233 North Michigan Avenue, Chicago, IL 60601.

National Cancer Institute. Cancer Information Service, NIH Building 31, 9000 Rockville Pike, Bethesda, MD 20205.

Skin Cancer Foundation. 545 Fifth Avenue, New York, NY 10016.

PAMPHLETS

American Cancer Society:

Facts on Skin Cancer. 1988. 12 pp.

American Council on Science and Health:

Malignant Melanoma of the Skin: An Increasingly Common Cancer. 1986. 21 pp.

National Cancer Institute:

What You Need To Know about Melanoma. NIH Pub. No. 87-1563. 1987. 14 pp.

RELATED ARTICLES

Crutcher, William A., and Cohen, Philip J. "Dysplastic Nevi and Malignant Melanoma." *American Family Physician* 42 (August 1990): 372–385.

Goldberg, Leonard H., and Howard A. Rubin. "Management of Basal Cell Carcinoma: Which Option is Best?" *Postgraduate Medicine* 85, no. 1 (January 1989): 58–63.

Jacoby, Gail Tenikat. "The Diagnosis and Treatment of Skin Cancer." *Healthline* (October 1990): 4–6.

"Melanoma Re-Alert: Sun Protection Update: No Tan Is a Good Tan." *Health News* (June 1990): 14–15.

Morton, Donald L. "Current Management of Malignant Melanomas (editorial)." *Annals of Surgery* 212, no. 2 (August 1990): 123–124.

"Skin Cancer: Protection After 50." *Johns Hopkins Medical Letter: Health After 50* (June 1991): 4–5.

SLEEP DISORDERS

(*See also:* SNORING)

OVERVIEW

The clinical description and laboratory monitoring of sleep disorders led to their classification by the organization that represents the majority of sleep disorders specialists in the United States—the Association of Sleep Disorders Centers—into four basic categories: (1) disorders of initiating and maintaining sleep (the insomnias); (2) disorders of excessive somnolence, such as obstructive sleep apnea, narcolepsy, and sleep deprivation; (3) disorders of the sleep-wake schedule, such as jet lag and shift work; and (4) dysfunctions associated with sleep, sleep stages, or partial arousals, such as night terrors and enuresis. This classification has been used in clinical practice and research settings for the past 10 years and is the one with which most clinicians are familiar. In an effort to take into account clinical and research experience during this interim period, the American Sleep Disorders Association has developd a revised nosology. This classification groups sleep disorders into dyssomnias, parasomnias, medical or psychiatric sleep disorders, and a category called proposed sleep disorders, composed of less well-documented disorders.

SOURCE:

Richardson, Jarrett, W. "Mayo Sleep Disorders Update." (Symposium on Sleep Disorders.) *Mayo Clinic Proceedings* 65, no. 6 (June 1990): 857–860.

INSOMNIA

Insomnia is the most common sleep problem. Like other common conditions, it results from many causes and varies widely in severity and duration from patient to patient. The recent widow, the ruminative worrier, the sleepless patient with chronic obstructive pulmonary disease, the melancholic depressive person, and the executive with jet lag all share the condition of insomnia, but the cause of their problem and their therapeutic needs differ. . . .

Epidemiology of Insomnia

Every year about 20 to 40 percent of adults have difficulty sleeping, and about 17 percent consider the problem serious. Insomnia is more prevalent in women, and its prevalence increases with age and socioeconomic class. It is more prevalent in patients with medical disorders and particularly in those with psychiatric or substance-abuse disorders. Nevertheless, despite the common caricature of the person with insomnia as a neurotic hypochondriac, 85 percent of the patients with "serious insomnia" in one study neither sought professional help nor used sleeping pills. . . .

Evaluation and Classification of Insomnia

Insomnia is a subjective problem of insufficient or nonrestorative sleep despite an adequate opportunity to sleep. Since it has many causes, the clinician should search for underlying situational stressors and psychiatric, medical, or pharmacologic causes, and treat it accordingly. The duration of insomnia is probably the most important guide to evaluation and treatment. Transient insomnia (no more than a few nights) and short-term insomnia (less than about three weeks) usually occur in people with no history of sleep abnormalities. Long-term insomnia (more than three weeks) may be associated with a variety of conditions.

Transient and Short-Term Insomnia

Acute stress and environmental disturbances—among them examinations, the loss of a loved one, hospitalization, recovery after surgery, and pain—are probably the most common causes of transient and short-term insomnia. Pharmacologically induced insomnia can be caused by the use of stimulants, such as coffee and nicotine, or alcohol, and by drug side effects, such as akathisia. Rebound or withdrawal insomnia may follow the abrupt discontinuation of some hypnotic agents, especially benzodiazepines with a short half-life. In addition, some but not all studies have reported increased time awake in the early morning or increased daytime anxiety during treatment with benzodiazepine hypnotic drugs with short half-lives.

SOURCE:
Gillin, J. Christian, and Byerly, William F. "The Diagnosis and Management of Insomnia." *The New England Journal of Medicine* 322, no. 4 (January 25, 1990): 239.

DRUGS AND ALCOHOL AS SLEEP AIDS

Alcohol: Commonly self prescribed as a sleep aid, alcohol is of limited benefit. It can be relaxing and produce sleepiness early in the evening, but tolerance and withdrawal occur very rapidly. By the wee hours, sleep is likely to be disrupted. Tolerance, abuse, and dependence are common.

Antihistamines: Over-the-counter sleeping pills (Sominex, Sleep-eze, Nytol, Unisom, and others) are probably the most commonly used sleeping preparations apart from alcohol. They are not consistently effective. Residual difficulty with coordination, memory, and so forth can persist into the daytime. Antihistamines can provoke or worsen an episode of asthma, urinary retention, or glaucoma.

Benzodiazepines: These are relatives of diazepam (Valium), marketed as sleep aids. Three common ones are trade-named Dalmane, Halcion, and Restoril. They appear to reinforce the effect of a naturally occuring inhibitor of neural activity. These drugs have little effect on breathing or on the function of the heart. When the blood level is at its peak, coordination is poor, reaction time is slowed, thinking is disorganized, and memory is impaired. Hangover effects are variable, depending in part on how long the drug remains in the body. Nightmares may be more common; rebound insomnia can occur. Physical dependency can develop after prolonged use, and withdrawal is unpleasant. Lethal overdose is unusual, even with very large amounts. Alcohol exaggerates the effects and makes lethal overdose more likely. Benzodiazepines have relatively few interactions with other drugs.

Barbiturates: Formerly the standard sleeping pills, these were sold under such brand names as Seconal and Nembutal. The barbituates can depress the functioning of all electrically active tissue, including heart muscle. Although they reduce brain function broadly, barbiturates have little influence on pain perception. Tolerance and abuse are relatively common; physical dependence can develop. Lethal overdose is still fairly frequent. Combination with alcohol is particularly hazardous. Barbiturates may interfere with the action or metabolism of other drugs.

Chloral hydrate: Chloral hydrate and triclofos are similar to barbiturates in the way they act—including their tendency to leave pain perception unaffected. They are irritating to the skin, mucous membranes, and stomach but have few severe side effects at the doses used for sleep. Tolerance, dependency, and abuse occur. Nevertheless, some physicians feel that these are the least harmful sleeping medications, especially for older people.

Miscellaneous: Ethchlorvynol (Placidyl) is likely to produce neurologic side effects when it is taken and has important incompatibilities with other drugs. Overdose can be quite difficult to treat. Glutethimide (Doriden) and its chemical cousin methyprylon (Noludar) can produce addiction; withdrawal can be severe; and treatment of large overdoses is often difficult. These three drugs have little to recommend them.

SOURCE:
Gillin, J. Christian. "Sleeping Pills." *Harvard Medical School Health Letter* 15 (May 1990): 7.

NARCOLEPSY

Narcolepsy is a sleep disorder. The principal symptoms are excessive daytime sleepiness (EDS), cataplexy (loss of muscle tone), hallucinations, sleep paralysis, and disrupted nighttime sleep. Doctors also diagnose narcolepsy by measuring how quickly the patient falls asleep, and how often rapid eye movements are present at or near the onset of sleep. Excessive daytime sleepiness occurs every day, regardless of the amount of sleep obtained at night. EDS is usually experienced as a heightened sensitivity (sometimes an almost irresistible susceptibility) to becoming sleepy or falling asleep, especially in sleep-inducing situations. Patients describe the problem as sleepiness, tiredness, lack of energy, exhaustion, or a combination of these feelings, either continuously or at various times throughout the day. Sometimes sleepiness occurs so suddenly and with such overwhelming power that it is referred to as a "sleep attack." Some patients have several attacks each day. When the attack occurs during the day, sleep usually lasts for less than 30 minutes, but sometimes the patient stays asleep for several hours. Cataplexy is an abrupt loss of voluntary muscle tone, usually triggered by emotional arousal. Attacks can range in severity from a brief sensation of weakness to total physical collapse lasting several minutes. Hallucinations are intense, vivid, sometimes accompanied by frightening auditory, visual, and tactile sensations, and occur just on awakening or falling asleep. Occasionally they are extremely difficult to distingush from reality. Sleep paralysis is a momentary inability to move when waking up or falling asleep. This condition can be terrifying, especially if it occurs with a frightening hallucination. Scientists do not know what causes narcolepsy, but they think it may be due to a biochemical defect of the central nervous system. The disorder is often concentrated in families, and narcolepsy or a predisposition to it may be an inherited condition. . . .

A clear understanding of recent developments in sleep disorders medicine is essential. Any physician in general practice can easily acquire this knowledge and provide narcoleptic patients with proper medical care. Although there is no known cure for narcolepsy, several drugs help to control the symptoms. Stimulants are usually prescribed to treat EDS and sleep attacks, and certain antidepressants help control the cataplexy, sleep paralysis, and hallucinations. Narcolepsy symptoms vary from person to person, as does response to medications; also both symptoms and response are likely to change gradually over time. The proper choice of medication and dosage requires careful attention to the patient's needs and responses, and close cooperation between patient and physician.

SOURCE:
National Institute of Neurological Disorders and Stroke. *Narcolepsy*. September 1989. pp. 1, 3.

SLEEP APNEA

The word "apnea" means the absence of breathing. During sleep, our breathing changes with the stage/depth of sleep. Some individuals stop breathing for brief intervals, as often as several times per hour. This can be normal. However, when these episodes of apnea become more frequent and last longer, they can cause the body's oxygen level to decrease, which can disrupt sleep. The patient may not fully awaken, but is aroused from the deep restful stages of sleep, and thus feels tired the next day.

There are two main types of sleep apnea. The most common type is called obstructive sleep apnea, during which breathing is blocked by a temporary obstruction of the main airway, usually in the back of the throat. This often occurs because the tongue and throat muscles relax, causing the main airway to close. The muscles of the chest and diaphragm continue to make breathing efforts, but the obstruction prevents any airflow. After a short interval lasting seconds to minutes, the oxygen level drops, causing breathing efforts to become more vigorous, which eventually opens the obstruction and allows airflow to resume. This often occurs with a loud snort and jerking of the body, causing the patient to arouse from deep sleep. After a few breaths, the oxygen level returns to normal, the patient falls back to sleep, the muscles of the main airway relax, and the obstruction occurs again. This cycle is then repeated over and over during certain stages of sleep.

Most people with obstructive sleep apnea are snorers, suggesting that their main airway is already partly obstructed during sleep, but not all snorers have obstructive sleep apnea. The problem is suspected when the patient is noted to stop snoring briefly during sleep, then resumes snoring with a loud snort and/or jerking of the arms, legs, or whole body.

A less common form of sleep apnea is central sleep apnea, so named because the central control of breathing is abnormal. This control center lies in the brain, and its function can be disrupted by a variety of factors. There is no obstruction to airflow. The patient with sleep apnea stops breathing because the brain suddenly fails to signal the muscles of the chest and diaphragm to keep breathing. These patients do not resume breathing with a snort and body jerk, but merely start and stop breathing at various intervals. Although the mechanism is different than obstructive sleep apnea, sleep is still disturbed by the periodic decreases in oxygen, and the patients suffer from the same daytime symptoms. Some patients may suffer from a combination of the two causes of apnea, a disorder which is called mixed-sleep apnea.

Sleep apnea should be suspected in individuals who are noted to have excessive daytime sleepiness and other symptoms described above, especially if they are known to snore and have a restless sleep. Commonly, these patients have been loud snorers for many years, more often are male, and note that the daytime sleepiness has become a progressive problem over many months. This might first be noted by their falling asleep when not being actively stimulated, such as when watching TV, attending a lecture/movie/theatre, or reading. As the daytime sleepiness progresses, this individual may have trouble staying awake while driving a car, may fall asleep at important meetings or at unusual times, such as during eating or in the middle of a conversation. Less commonly, they may be bothered by bedwetting or impotence. The sleep problems are often aggravated by alcohol or sedative medications. They are also more readily noticed by the patient's family and friends, especially the bed partner.

SOURCE:
American Lung Association. *Sleep Apnea*. July 1989. pp. 1–2, 4.

HELP FOR SLEEP DISORDERS

If your sleep is continually disrupted and you lack initiative and energy during the day, you should seek professional help. In most cases of sleep disorder, it's best to see your own physician first, in order to sort out the general nature and severity of a sleep problem. The physician may conduct a thorough physical examination, ask you questions about your sleep habits and emotional state, and can often determine whether the sleep difficulty is related to treatable causes. However, if necessary, a referral to a mental health specialist or facility, a sleep clinic, or a sleep disorders center may be made.

The same basic service is provided by both sleep clinics and sleep disorders centers. Generally, sleep clinics are set up as part of hospitals. Sleep disorders centers may be associated with hospitals, medical centers, universities, or psychiatric or neurological institutes. Most clinics or centers primarily treat patients on referral from general practitioners and internists. However, it is possible to obtain information on specific sleep problems directly from a clinic or center or to make an appointment for a consultation.

Specialized sleep facilities usually have on their staffs experts called somnologists with training in a variety of medical and scientific fields. A sleep disorders team will often include a physician, a psychologist, a psychiatrist, and a surgeon.

Patients are typically seen as outpatients. They are interviewed thoroughly, given a battery of psychological tests and, if indicated, have their sleep patterns recorded in the laboratory for one night (sometimes two or three consecutive nights) to determine the cause of the sleep disturbance.

Fees vary, depending on the clinic or center. An entire analysis can range from a few hundred to about a thousand dollars. Insurance companies or Medicare may cover some of the cost. (This can be determined by consulting the center or your insurance company.)

SOURCE:

National Institute of Mental Health. *Useful Information On . . . Sleep Disorders*. DHHS Pub. No. (ADM) 87-1541. 1987. pp. 32-33.

RESOURCES

ORGANIZATIONS

American Narcolepsy Association. P.O. Box 1187, San Carlos, CA 94070.

American Sleep Disorders Association. 604 2nd St. SW, Rochester, MN 55902.

Association of Professional Sleep Societies. 604 2nd St. SW, Rochester, MN 55902.

Narcolepsy Network. 155 Van Brackle Rd., Aberdeen, NJ 07747.

National Institute of Mental Health. 5600 Fishers Lane, Rockville, MD 20857.

BOOKS

Hales, Dianne. *How to Sleep Like a Baby, Wake Up Refreshed, and Get More Out of Life*. New York: Ballantine, 1987.

Regestein, Quentin, and David Ritchie. *Sleep: Problems and Solutions*. Fairfield, OH: Consumer Reports Books, 1990.

Coleman, Richard M. *Wide Awake at 3:00 AM: By Choice or by Chance?* New York: W. H. Freeman, 1986.

RELATED ARTICLES

Berman, Theodore M., G. Nino-Murcia, and others. "Sleep Disorders: Take Them Seriously." *Patient Care* (June 15, 1990): 85-88, 90, 93, 96, 99-100, 103-106, 108, 111-112.

Dement, William C. "Daytime Sleepiness—Barrier to Good Health." *Executive Health Report* 26, no. 12 (September 1990): 1, 4-6.

Gillin, J. Christian, and William F. Byerley. "The Diagnosis and Management of Insomnia." *The New England Journal of Medicine* 322, no. 4 (January 25, 1990): 239-248.

"NIH Consensus Conference Studies Elderly Sleep." *Public Health Reports* 105 (November-December 1990): 641.

Richardson, Jarrett W., Paul A Fredrickson, and others. "Narcolepsy Update." *Mayo Clinic Proceedings* 65 (July 1990): 991-998.

"Sleep: Simple to High-Tech Help." *The Johns Hopkins Medical Letter* (September 1990): 4-5.

SMOKING

(*See also:* LUNG CANCER)

OVERVIEW

Cigarette smoking remains the chief preventable cause of illness and death in the United States in 1990. Smoking is responsible for approximately 390,000 deaths per year, 1 of every 6 deaths in the United States. Cigarettes cause about 30% of all cancer deaths, 30% of all cardiovascular deaths, and 80% of all deaths from chronic obstructive disease. Cigarette smoking is the cause of more than 80% of all lung cancer deaths, now the leading cause of cancer deaths in both men and women. The impact of smoking in the United States today is the equivalent of two jumbo jets crashing every day with no survivors among the 1,000 passengers.

Since the release of the first Surgeon General's Report on the Health Consequences of Cigarette Smoking, smoking prevalence among adults has decreased markedly, declining from 40% in 1965 to 29% by 1987. Although this represents significant progress in controlling the epidemic of tobacco use in the United States, 49 million adult Americans continue to smoke. Also, the decrease in smoking has not been equal across all segments of society. The rate of decline in smoking has lagged among blacks, women, the less educated, and young people. These groups must be targeted for smoking prevention efforts.

If current trends continue, by the year 2000, 22% of all adults will smoke; women will be smoking at a greater rate than men (23% vs. 20%, respectively), blacks will be smoking at a greater rate than whites (25% vs. 22%, respectively), and people who don't graduate from high school will be smoking at six times the rate of college graduates (31% vs. 5%, respectively).

Environmental tobacco smoking has been established as a cause of disease, including lung cancer, among nonsmokers exposed to other people's smoke. Environmental tobacco smoke also affects children by causing and increase in the rate of respiratory infections and slower rates of lung development.

More than 85% of smokers who quit do so on their own, without the aid of a smoking cessation program or product. Most smokers (80%) quit "cold turkey." Health concerns, followed by social concerns, are the factors most often cited by successful quitters as reasons that they choose to quit smoking. . . .

Nicotine is an addictive drug, and withdrawal from it is similar to cocaine, heroin, and alcohol. For smokers with addictive characteristics of their smoking, pharmacologic aids to stop smoking may be necessary. Nicotine polacrilix gum is currently the only pharmacologic aid to cessation licensed for use in the United States. Results of research trials using nicotine replacement gum in general clinical practice have been variable. The gum, however, appears to be helpful in controlling withdrawal symptoms for selected patients. Detailed instructions on the appropriate use of nicotine gum are necessary. Patients must be instructed to start using the gum when they quit rather than while cutting down, to use enough of the gum (up to 30 pieces per day), and to chew the gum intermittently and, in the meanwhile, parking it between the cheek and teeth so that the nicotine can be absorbed across the buccal mucosa. Other pharmacologic aids for smoking cessation, such as the nicotine patch, nicotine aerosol, nasal nicotine solution, and clonidine in oral and patch forms, are currently under investigation.

SOURCE:

Fiore, Michael C., and others. "Cigarette Smoking: The Clinician's Role in Cessation, Prevention, and Public Health." *DM: Disease-a-Month* (April 1990): 187–188, 188–189.

TEENAGERS AND TOBACCO USE

Teenagers frequently view developing cancer or any other chronic or fatal health problems as remote and unimportant possibilities. Many believe that smoking just a few cigarettes won't hurt because they can stop whenever they want. Few realize just how addictive the nicotine in cigarettes is—and how difficult it is to quit smoking. Cigarette ads have a strong impact on people between the ages of 12–18 years. Advertisements which insinuate that smoking is "in," "fashionable" and "sexy" are targeted at teenagers. Teens should realize that it is all part of a ploy to get them addicted to the nicotine, and that health and attractiveness are increased by not smoking.

Tobacco companies are now trying to promote chewing tobacco and snuff among the youth. These are not safe alternatives to cigarettes. They too lead to nicotine addiction, and they can cause mouth and throat cancer, gum disease, bad breath, tooth loss and stained teeth.

Here are some of the ways in which parents and teachers can help teenagers avoid smoking:

- Illustrate the social, non-health related consequences of smoking. These include bad breath, yellow teeth, smelly clothes and effects on friendships.
- Help teenagers recognize how easy it is to get hooked on cigarettes. Help them recognize that cigarette smoking is a powerful addiction and that addiction to any substance—drugs, alcohol or cigarettes—reduces their ability to make personal choices and control their own lives. Make sure they realize that the earlier one starts to smoke, the harder it is to quit and that many current smokers have tried to quit and find it very difficult.
- Teach teenagers to be aware of how cigarette advertising uses misleading images to manipulate them into making decisions that are dangerous to their health. Teenagers can learn to resist these media messages by developing counterarguments to them.
- Stress the harmful effects of smoking and its antisocial image in pre-teen years (age 6–10), when children are most receptive to behavior training.
- Help teenagers understand how cigarette smoking damages health. Personalize the facts by discussing how cigarettes harm teenagers in particular. Point out that the effects of cigarette smoking are immediate and are apparent in reduced physical endurance and poor athletic performance.
- Encourage peer involvement to discourage smoking. Encourage teens to educate others about the serious health risks and expense of smoking. Provide teenagers with the information they need to defend their decision not to smoke, so they can resist pressure from peers who smoke. Make sure they are aware that more and more teenagers are beginning to frown on smoking as being phony. Remind them that the norm for their age-group is not to smoke; they are in the majority if they refuse cigarettes.
- Educate parents and teachers to set an example by not smoking, and certainly not in front of the children.

SOURCE:
California Medical Association. "Teenagers and Tobacco Use." *HealthTips* index 445 (April 1990): 1–2.

SMOKING CESSATION METHODS

All smoking cessation methods have at least one thing in common—a flexible notion of what it takes to become a successful quitter. As one expert in the pharmacology of nicotine stated: "There are 56 million smokers and 56 million different individual problems." Each person has a unique perception about what it's like to quit, but in order to be successful there are several overriding considerations:

- Motivation, desire and commitment. The smoker who chooses to quit must have strong personal reasons to do so. Most cite concern about health as the main reason for quitting. Smokers who attempt to quit only because family members or best friends want them to are usually doomed to failure. Successful quitters make a firm personal commitment to stop. Along these lines, the Seventh-day Adventists' Five-day Plan centers around the key words "I choose not to smoke." The American Lung Association's self-help stop smoking manual urges participants to fill out and sign a special stop smoking contract as a form of commitment. The American Cancer Society's FreshStart guide stresses that "this time is going to be unique in that this time you are not going to smoke." Hypnotherapists and acupuncturists will not accept clients who do not have a strong personal desire to stop. Tom Wicker, syndicated columnist for *The New York Times* and former smoker, summed it up best when he wrote: "If you want to stop smoking, you can; if you merely think you ought to, you're kidding yourself."
- Timing. Kicking the habit tends to throw a smoker's life off track for a while. After all, smoking is quite a habit to break for a person who has, for example, been lighting up 20 times a day, 365 days a year, for 20 years. Trying to break the habit in the middle of an important business or family crisis is not going to pave the way to success. Smoking cessation takes lots of energy and planning. In order to succeed, the time must be right.
- Choice of method. No particular smoking cessation method is right for everyone. Surveys show that 90 to 95 percent of all smokers prefer to quit on their own or by using printed instructions, guides, or videos. The others need informal group support or counseling. But those who show the highest success rates not only reflect the highest levels of determination, but are also committed to personal change and are well aware of the reasons why they want to quit. Studies

show that these people are open to trying any one of a variety of cessation programs rather than being prejudiced toward a particular method. It is essential that the smoker plan ahead and choose the method that most closely conforms to his or her personal needs.

SOURCE:
American Council on Science and Health. *Searching for a Way Out: Smoking Cessation Techniques*. March 1985. pp. 3–4.

EFFECTIVENESS OF NICOTINE GUM IN SMOKING CESSATION

Nicotine gum is an effective aid to smoking cessation when used with a behavioral program in smoking cessation clinics or, in some instances, with a behavioral program in general medical practices. In fact, the Food and Drug Administration-approved use for the gum specifically states that the gum is to be used only with a behavioral program (Nicorette package insert, Merrell Dow Pharmaceuticals, Cincinnati, 1984). However, 99.5% of those given the gum are not in such a program but rather receive gum during a brief visit with their physician. This is because few smokers seen in general practice are willing to attend behavioral programs (2% in one study).

It is unclear whether nicotine gum is effective when used with brief interventions. . . .

Three hundred fifteen smokers who attended a family practice clinic and wished to quit smoking were assigned in a random, double-blind manner to receive either nicotine (2 mg) or placebo gum. Smokers initially received brief advice from a physician and nurse, a slide presentation and written materials (29 to 35 minutes), and a single follow-up visit (12 to 20 minutes) one week after cessation. After corrections for marital status and income, 10% of those who received nicotine gum and 7% of those who received placebo gum reported continuous abstinence for 11 months and passed observer and biochemical verification (this difference was not statistically significant). We conclude that, when used in a nonselected group of smokers along with a brief intervention in a general medical practice, the pharmacologic effects of nicotine gum to increase cessation are either small or nonexistent. . . .

We have hypothesized that the therapeutic effects of nicotine are limited to when the gum is given to dependent smokers along with intensive therapy.

SOURCE:
Hughes, John R., and others. "Nicotine vs. Placebo Gum in General Medical Practice." *JAMA* 261, no. 9 (March 3, 1989): 1300-1305. Copyright 1989, American Medical Association.

RELAPSE

Nine out of 10 smokers surveyed say they would like to kick the habit. Sometimes they are defeated by the pain of withdrawal—difficulty concentrating, cravings, irritability, anxiety, anger, headaches, nervous energy, drowsiness, coughing, and constipation. But such symptoms are short-lived and can be minimized. Exercising and drinking lots of water, for instance, help to flush nicotine from the system. The discomfort usually peaks within 24 to 72 hours of quitting, although for some people it lingers and for others fleeting pangs of withdrawal recur up to six weeks into abstinence. Every quitter does not experience every withdrawal symptom. Some experience no symptoms at all.

Abstinent smokers go into relapse at about the same rate as cocaine and heroin addicts. Eighty to 95 percent of those who make a serious effort to quit will start smoking again, usually within the first year. Unfortunately, many people regard recidivism as a sign of failure and give up hope of ever being nicotine-free. People who have quit and subsequently resumed use should take heart. Relapse is not a decree of weakness, but a measure of the addictiveness of the drug. Just one cigarette provides enough nicotine to readdict. Relapse should be viewed as a learning experience. It teaches individuals more about their patterns of use. Many people have made several efforts to give up tobacco before they were able to quit forever.

SOURCE:
Yoder, Barbara. *The Recovery Resource Book*. New York: Simon and Schuster. p. 129.

RESOURCES

ORGANIZATIONS

American Cancer Society. 4 East 35th St., New York, NY 10001.

American Lung Association. 1740 Broadway, New York, NY 10019.

Emphysema Anonymous. 7976 Seminole Blvd., Suite 6, Seminole, FL 33542.

Nic-Anon. 511 Sir Francis Drake Blvd., Glenbrae, CA 94904.

Office on Smoking and Health. Public Information Branch, Park Building, 5600 Fishers Lane, Rockville, MD 20857.

PAMPHLETS

California Medical Association:

"Teenagers and Tobacco Use." *HealthTips* 445 (April 1990): 3 pp.

National Cancer Institute:

Cleaning the Air: How to Quit Smoking . . . and Quit for Keeps. NIH Pub. No. 89–1647. April 1988. 24 pp.

BOOKS

E., Jeanne. *The Twelve Steps for Tobacco Users*. Center City, MN: Hazelden, 1984.

Rogers, Jacqueline. *You Can Stop Smoking*. New York: Pocket Books, 1987.

RELATED ARTICLES

Fiore, Michael C., and others. "Methods Used to Quit Smoking in the United States: Do Cessation Programs Help?" *JAMA* 263, no. 20 (May 23/30, 1990): 2760-2765.

Fisher, Edwin B., Jr., and others. "Smoking and Smoking Cessation." *American Review of Respiratory Disease* 142 (1990): 702-720.

McGill, Henry C., Jr. "The Cardiovascular Pathology of Smoking." *American Heart Journal* 115, no. 1, part 2 (January 1988): 250-257.

Wolf, Philip A., and others. "Cigarette Smoking as a Risk Factor for Stroke." *JAMA* 259, no. 7 (February 19, 1988): 1025-1029.

SNORING

(*See also:* SLEEP DISORDERS)

OVERVIEW

Everyone knows snoring is involuntary, but when your spouse's snoring wakes you at 3 A.M., it's difficult not to feel resentful. Chronic snoring can drive a sleep-deprived person crazy. The problem may contribute to relationship tensions and force the spouse into a separate bedroom. Sometimes not even that helps. Snoring has been recorded as loud as 80 decibels, the volume of an electric alarm clock buzzer, which might wake someone in an adjacent room. Fortunately, snoring can be cured. Some cases require professional treatment, but most respond to selfcare.

Snoring is quite common, and it increases with age. Researchers estimate that about 20% of men and 5% of women are regular snorers at age 35. But by 60, almost two-thirds of men and 40% of women have the problem.

Snoring occurs when an obstruction in the back of the throat restricts airflow during inhalation. Colds and flu cause general swelling of throat tissues (with possible tonsil enlargement), which is why many people snore for a few nights when they have upper respiratory infections. Allergies, tonsillitis, swollen glands or adenoids, and various infections may also inflame the tissues in the back of the throat enough to cause what one anonymous wit called "sleeping out loud."

Chronic snoring typically results from a loss of tone in the muscles which line the throat and support such structures as the soft palate (the rear part of the roof of the mouth) and the uvula (the "punching bag" flap of tissue which hangs from the soft palate into the throat). The loss of muscle tone is often aggravated by obesity, which compresses the throat muscles with extra tissue, or by drugs taken in the evening, which cause the throat muscles to relax, for example: alcohol, tranquilizers, and/or sedatives. Some people with allergies find their snoring is linked to use of antihistamines. Other snorers have unusually fleshy soft palates, unusually long uvulae, or nasal obstructions such as polyps or a deviated septum. A small proportion of loud sleepers have cysts or tumors on their tonsils or adenoids. Finally, receding chins sometimes alter the positioning of the tongue enough to narrow the airway and trigger noisy nocturnal inhalation.

Most snoring is associated with sleeping on one's back. Irritated spouses roused from slumber typically give the snorer a swift kick, hoping to encourage rolling over, which often changes the position of things in the back of the throat enough to open the airway and restore relative silence. But there's no need for the non-snoring spouse to be awakened. To encourage side sleeping, authorities recommend sewing a tennis ball into a pocket on the snorer's pajama back.

Elevating the snorer's head often alleviates occasional snoring due to colds or flu. Use extra pillows or place bricks under the bedposts at the head. Elevation may also help chronic snorers by keeping the tongue from dropping back against the palate. Over-the-counter decongestants might also help, for example Sudafed (psuedoephedrine) or the herbal medicine, ephedra (ephedrine, available in bulk and in commercial herbal preparations such as Breathe Easy from Traditional Medicinals). Unfortunately, decongestants often cause insomnia, but the stimulant effect, if tolerable, helps maintain muscle tone in the throat.

In addition to sleep position, seasonal snoring due to allergies may be relieved by installing air conditioning or an air filter, and by eliminating feather pillows and comforters, pulling up bedroom rugs, and banishing all pets from the bedroom.

SOURCE:
Simons, Anne. "Snore No More." *Medical SelfCare* (November-December 1989): 49–50.

DIAGNOSIS

Examination of a habitual snorer should start with a thorough look at the passages of the nose and throat. "If I see a lot of extra tissue in the throat, maybe with the tonsils and adenoids still in place, I say, 'I'll bet you snore,'" says the University of Oklahoma's Dr. Bill Moran, spokesman for the American Academy of Otolaryngology. This often looses a torrent of confession about the unhappy side effects of snoring. Explosive snoring, which half awakens the sufferer 30 to 300 times a night, leaving him dragged out the next day, requires medical attention.

Obnoxious snoring may be due to large tonsils or adenoids or blockage of the nose. Flabby muscles of the tongue and throat also encourage apnea-like snoring. Or an elongated palate that narrows the opening from the nose into the throat may team up with the uvula, the fleshy appendage you see when you open wide. With the uvula acting as a flutter valve during relaxed sleep, the result can be a high volume of sound.

Specialized diagnostic sleep centers are equipped to pinpoint the causes of all kinds of sleep problems, including apnea. Diagnosis should include a physical exam, general screening and a report on your sleep problem, says Dr. Wallace Mendelson, director of sleep-wake study programs, State University of New York at Stony Brook. If you go to such a center, expect to stay overnight and be hooked to electronic sensors that record brain waves and eye movements during sleep. Fees for a full apnea workup run from $900 to $2,000.

A center meeting standards of the American Sleep Disorders Association has on its staff an accredited clinical polysomnographer, who is a licensed medical doctor or a PhD with training and skills in diagnosing sleep disorders. For a list of accredited facilities, write to the association at 604 Second St., S.W., Rochester, Minn. 55902.

SOURCE:
Schaeffer, Charles, Kathryn Brown Ramsperger, and Suzan Richmond. "Facts on Snoring: A to ZZZ." *Changing Times* 43 (February 1989): 94.

SNORING CAUSED BY SLEEP APNEA

While simple snoring is unlikely to be more than a domestic problem, albeit a pesky one, the presence of certain additional symptoms suggest that a patient's snoring is not the stuff of cartoons, but a clue to the presence of obstructive sleep apnea syndrome. Besides the embarrassing moments of loud snoring and daytime hypersomnia, sleep apnea also has social and clinical implications, including job inefficiency, increased risk of motor vehicle accidents, and, in severe cases, nocturnal cardiac arrhythmias and cardiorespiratory failure.

According to Thomas Roth, PhD, division head, sleep disorders medicine, Henry Ford Hospital, Detroit, signs and symptoms of sleep apnea syndrome include snoring, headache, excessive sleepiness during the day, falling asleep at inappropriate times in inappropriate places, fragmented sleep patterns, frequent nocturnal awakening, and hypertension. The syndrome may, however, be marked by only a few of these symptoms: The person may be observed sleeping in a chair or while at the dinner table, for instance.

Sleep apnea most commonly affects obese men who are 30–60 years old, but may also affect women and children. According to Meir Kryger, MD, professor of medicine, University of Manitoba, St. Boniface General Hospital Research Center, Winnipeg, Canada, risk factors for sleep apnea include obesity, maxillofacial abnormalities, enlarged tonsils, male gender, cigarette smoking, and certain endocrinologic problems such as acromegaly.

Sleep apnea is classified etiologically as obstructive, central, or mixed, and snoring may occur in any of these types. Obstructive sleep apnea, or pickwickian syndrome, is caused by partial obstruction of the airway. The fricative sounds emitted by individuals with this sort of apnea and the relative lack of frequency and consistency of the noise suggest it is produced by high velocity airflow through a very small orifice created by positioning the tongue on the soft palate. (In contrast, innocuous snoring appears to result from oscillations of the soft palate that produce sound by causing abrupt fluctuations in supraglottic pressure.) Apnea ensues when the small opening is completely closed by collapse of the lateral oropharyngeal walls. When the individual wakes in response to the resultant asphyxia, the airway is reestablished; loud gasping and snoring accompany the first breaths, but sleeping is soon resumed.

An episode of obstruction may last 10–60 seconds or longer. This cycle may repeat itself every few minutes. The patient is not usually aware of the sleep-wake cycle, but the cumulative effect is the loss of slow-wave and rapid-eye-movement sleep, the factors believed to be responsible for the restorative power of sleep. As the apnea worsens, apneic episodes last much longer and are more frequent, and they result in marked reduction in arterial oxygen saturation. . . .

Treatment of obstructive sleep apnea syndrome is multifaceted. The first intervention is advice—the advice you would give anyone who wanted to control snoring:

- Lose weight (if appropriate)
- Sleep on the stomach or on a side, not on the back
- Avoid alcohol at least 3–4 hours before retiring
- Avoid pharmacologic sleep aids

- Get enough hours of sleep each night.

Additional first-line medical treatment, according to Drs. Kryger and Roth, includes use of a nasal continuous positive air pressure (CPAP) device, which supplies pressure to the upper airway and prevents the airway from collapsing while the patient is asleep. The pressure appropriate for a given patient must be determined in a sleep laboratory.

SOURCE:

"Is My Snoring Really Sleep Apnea?" *Patient Care* 23 (February 28, 1989): 107–108.

RESOURCES

ORGANIZATIONS

American Academy of Otolaryngology—Head and Neck Surgery. 1101 Vermont Ave. NW, Suite 302, Washington, DC 20005.

American Sleep Disorders Association. 604 Second St. NW, Rochester, MN 55902.

PAMPHLET

American Academy of Otolaryngology—Head and Neck Surgery:

Snoring—Not Funny, Not Hopeless.

RELATED ARTICLES

Donahue, Peggy Jo. "9 Bed-Tested Snore Stoppers." *Prevention* 41 (March 1989): 60–64.

Lipman, Derek S. "Snore No More!" *Prevention* (November 1990): 38–46.

Rees, John. "Snoring: Tackle Obesity, Smoking, and Alcohol Consumption First." *British Medical Journal* 302 (April 13, 1991): 860–861.

"Snoring: And How to Tame It." *Mayo Clinic Health Letter* (May 1991): 5.

SPORTS INJURIES

OVERVIEW

Athletes, and others who do vigorous exercise, regularly run a high risk of injuring muscles, ligaments, bones or joints. Such injuries are most common at the beginning of an athletic season and among people who begin to exercise after long periods of relative inactivity.

If you are injured during a game, you may be eager to return to the game as quickly as possible, but treatments that allow you to do this may have long-term dangers. If the injury is a cut or bruise that does not involve serious damage to muscles or ligaments, it is reasonable for your coach or trainer to relieve pain with an ice-pack or an anesthetic spray, but if there is a possibility of muscle or ligament damage, painkillers may make it possible for you to damage the tissue further without realizing it. When the extent of your injury is uncertain, or when you become unconscious, even for only a few seconds, you should take no further part in the day's play.

Remember, professional teams often employ physicians to look after their athletes, but most people do not have such an advantage. Do not return to a game after any injury until you feel certain you are all right. If you are not sure, consult a physician.

Many injuries require no treatment other than rest, and possibly physical therapy to increase the circulation of blood to damaged tissues and strengthen the affected muscles. But some injuries require surgery. If you have recurring injury, you may have to consider giving up your sport or exercise. If an injury to a ligament or bone recurs there is a strong possibility of permanent damage, and a price of not stopping the activity may be early development of degenerative joint disease or some other joint problem. Before you reach a decision, get an accurate diagnosis of the extent of the damage. This may involve X-rays, arthroscopy, or perhaps an exploratory operation.

Common injuries requiring medical attention:

March fracture: This fracture may develop in one or more of the foot bones (metatarsals) as a result of prolonged or repeated periods of excessive stress. It most commonly occurs in walkers and runners, and produces pain in the ball of the foot that worsens on exertion. Treatment consists of strapping the foot with adhesive plaster and resting it for a few weeks.

Shin splints: This condition is also known as anterior compartment syndrome and the main symptom is pain in the front of the lower leg. It occurs as a result of repeated straining of the muscles between the shin bones. The muscles become swollen and press on the blood vessels supplying them. Shin splints may also result from a stress fracture or from inflammation of the membranes covering the shin bones. In most cases, the symptoms disappear after a week or two of rest. But if pain is severe and recurrent, surgery may be necessary.

Knee injuries: Strains on the knee may stretch or rupture the ligaments around the joint, or may damage the internal ligaments or the two semicircular pads of cartilage that act as padding between the surfaces of the joint. If you have damaged your knee, you will probably need an X-ray or arthroscopy to diagnose the extent of the damage. Minor surgical repairs are often carried out during arthroscopy.

Hand injuries: Injury to the bones or tendons of the hands commonly occurs in boxing, rock climbing, handball and basketball. If you have damaged your hand, you should seek medical attention as soon as possible. If you need to have damaged tendons repaired surgically, treatment is more successful if repair is carried out soon after the injury.

Head injuries: It is possible to be knocked unconscious in most sports. If you lose consciousness even briefly after a head injury you should see a physician as soon as possible and refrain from vigorous activity for at least 24 hours.

SOURCE:

Kunz, Jeffrey R. M., and Finkel, Asher J. (eds.). "Sports Injuries." In *The American Medical Association Family Medical Guide*. Revised and updated. New York: Random House, 1987. p. 547.

FIRST AID FOR INJURIES

When should you see a doctor?

It depends both on the type of injury and, especially, on how serious it is. A severe acute injury (one that occurs suddenly) may indeed require medical attention. Call a doctor if any of the following symptoms persist: stabbing or radiating pain, numbness or tingling, significant swelling, or inability to move the injured body part.

Overuse injuries such as tennis elbow or runner's knee, which are due to the cumulative wear and tear of a repetitive movement, probably won't require a doctor's care. In fact, self-treatment is generally just what the doctor recommends. However, if pain persists for more than 10 days in spite of self-care measures, or if it is severe or is growing worse, consult a doctor.

What's the first thing you should do to treat an injury?

Apply ice. This is the most effective, safest, and cheapest form of treatment. With acute injuries such as torn ligaments, muscle strains, and bruises, start icing as soon possible. Even if you're on your way to the doctor, starting to ice the injury right away will help speed recovery. Not only does ice relieve pain, but it also slows blood flow, thereby reducing internal bleeding and swelling. This in turn helps limit tissue damage and hastens the healing process.

How should you apply ice? How often?

Although commercial ice packs are available, plain ice is fine: simply put ice cubes or crushed ice in a heavy plastic bag or hotwater bottle, or wrap the ice in a towel.

Apply the ice to the injured area for 10 to 20 minutes, then re-apply it every two waking hours for the next 48 hours. Be sure not to go over the 20-minute limit; longer than that may damage the skin and nerves.

If you start to feel mild discomfort when exercising and think it may be the first sign of an overuse injury, such as tendinitis, you may well be able to finish your activity—a set of tennis, for example. But apply ice to the tender areas right after you finish, and re-apply it several times a day for the next 48 hours.

If swelling occurs, which is likely with acute injuries, use ice in conjunction with three other measures that are often referred to as RICE:

Rest the injured body part;

apply **I**ce;

apply **C**ompression;

Elevate the injured extremity above heart level.

Resting not only reduces pain, but also helps prevent aggravating the injury. To apply compression, wrap a towel or an Ace-type elastic bandage around the injury (not so tightly that you cut off circulation). You can often combine ice and compression by holding the ice pack in place with a bandage.

When should you apply heat to an injury?

Traditionally people started applying heat to an injury soon after icing it. But heat actually stimulates blood flow and so increases inflammation. Most sports physicians and trainers now recommend that you stick with ice for at least the first 48 hours after an injury, and only then, after swelling has subsided, try heat. At that point, heat may speed up healing, help relieve pain, relax muscles, and reduce joint stiffness.

You can apply either dry heat (using a heating pad or lamp) or moist heat (a hot bath, whirlpool, hot-water bottle, heat pack, or damp towel wrapped around a waterproof heating pad). There's much debate about whether dry or moist heat is best, and for what type of injury, so check with your doctor about which is appropriate for you. If you have a heart condition, for instance, he may tell you to avoid using a hot bath or whirlpool. He will probably also advise against these if you have a fever or infection, or if the injury is bleeding. Also call your doctor if pain or inflammation gets worse after heating an injury.

The key word is "warm," not "hot." Use heating pads on low or medium settings, and keep the water in baths between 98 [degrees] and 105 [degrees] F. (The water should feel comfortable when you dip your wrist in.) Apply the heat for 20 to 30 minutes, two or three times a day. You can also use it for 5 to 10 minutes before exercising in order to reduce stiffness.

Should you take pain relievers? Will special anti-inflammatory drugs help?

Taking aspirin or ibuprofen (such as Motrin or Advil) can indeed help ease the pain and reduce inflammation of minor sprains, strains, and tendinitis. However, the other major over-the-counter pain reliever, acetaminophen (such as Tylenol), is less helpful since it has no anti-inflammatory effect.

There are more potent prescription medications, widely recommended by athletic trainers, which can eliminate pain and swelling very quickly in many cases. But these drugs—including cortisone, the strongest of all anti-inflammatory medications—can produce serious side effects. Another potential problem: they can let you ignore the pain, which is a warning sign, and allow you to exercise vigorously, perhaps resulting in permanent damage to the injured tissue. Hence such drugs should be used only under medical supervision and only for brief periods of time.

SOURCE:
"Relief: Exercise Injuries." *The University of California, Berkeley Wellness Letter* 6 (May 1990): 4–5. Excerpted from *The University of California, Berkeley Wellness Letter,* Copyright Health Letter Associates, 1990.

PREVENTION OF SPORTS INJURIES

If just the thought of pain makes you feel uncomfortable, think about this: pulled muscles are one of the most preventable of all sports injuries. Experts estimate that 80 percent of all pulled muscles are preventable! The fact that this very common injury is not being prevented tells us a lot about what kind of shape we're really in.

Here are some of factors that lead to pulled muscles.

- Inadequate conditioning—Too many people try to make up for a week of inactivity by going wild on the weekends. Thus, weekend athletes are weakened athletes who enter activity with a softening middle-aged body and a 19-year-old's enthusiasm.

You may want to sit down for this, but the reality is that the human body starts to deteriorate after about the age of sixteen. At this point we start getting stiffer, our tissues do not have the same elasticity they did in our youth, and it takes us longer to get "warmed up" for activity.

True, we are staying active longer, but for safety's sake we must realize that our body changes with age: agility, flexibility, and speed diminish; stamina and endurance decrease considerably; power and strength require more attention to simply maintain the status quo; and the "morning after" becomes a time to regret the activity of the day before.

- Insufficient warm-up—For a few people, their warm-up consists of little more than walking outside to run or getting dressed at the spa. Others simply use a poor warm-up routine. For example, the cornerstone of high school P.E. [physical education] is calisthenics. If they are part of your fitness plan, realize that they don't stretch your tight muscles, don't strengthen your weak ones, and they don't even use your muscles in the same manner you will use them in almost any given athletic endeavor. Finally, a few other people have the right idea, just not enough follow through. These people know a few simple stretches—which may or may not have any relationship to the activity they are about to enjoy—and assume that two quick minutes is "better than nothing."
- Coldness—When stretching was first popularized as a protector against injury, many individuals and teams reported an increase in muscle injuries. Runners, especially, claimed to see more injuries as a result of stretching. That's because when a muscle is very tight, either because it's cold or simply inflexible, force is more likely to tear that muscle than it is to stretch it. The key? Do a gentle warm-up until you feel yourself break into a sweat. Either try something as simple as running in place or simply enjoy a low key, comfortable few minutes of the activity you're about to undertake. Either way, as body temperature rises, muscles become more elastic and less susceptible to injury. So, warming up means exactly that. Then you can stop and stretch safely before proceeding to your chosen activity.
- Fatigue—There are two physiologic factors involved in nearly all pulled muscles: inflexibility and strength. When you are fatigued, your strength diminishes. A fatigued muscle also loses its ability to relax; thus, it remains rigid and has an increased risk of injury. So, while the stress of your chosen activity remains essentially the same, your strength over time diminishes. Once the scales tip and the stress of your activity is greater than your strength, look out: you're an accident waiting to happen.
- Muscle imbalance—I know runners whose mileage will take your breath away, but they can't lift and carry a few boxes without getting winded. They're so focused on their chosen activity that they are physical wrecks from the waist up. That's one kind of muscle imbalance and it could get them in real trouble if they decide to play a game of tennis, for example, where their weakened muscles are at major risk of injury.

However, athletes can also be simultaneously weak and strong in adjoining muscle groups. For example, runners often have strong hamstring muscles (back, lower leg), but weak quadriceps (thigh) muscles. Muscles work in pairs and the balance between quads and hams should be about 60:40. If the quads are too weak to balance the hams effectively, a strong contraction of the hams can tear the hamstring muscle. It's like picking up an object and expecting it to be very heavy, only to discover it's quite light. When you pick it up there is uncontrolled momentum of force and, in an unbalanced pair of muscles, that can cause injury.

- Prior muscle injury or scarring—If prior injury leads to muscle imbalance, we've just seen that this can be hazardous to muscular health. The perfect example is someone who has had a knee injury. Unless they have specificially rehabilitated their quadriceps muscles, former knee patients generally find they are weak in the thighs.

Likewise, a torn muscle has lost strength and is especially vulnerable to further injury. Doctors complain that too often patients do not follow their rehabilitation program and they see the patients a few weeks later after they've reinjured themselves. Sometimes you must cease activity to recover, but you lose strength at 5 percent per week and you lose endurance (your ability to sustain an activity over a period of time) in 54 hours. Even a week to ten days off will place you at tremendous risk of injury (or reinjury) if you attempt to simply pick up where you left off. A step-wise, gradual return to activity is one key to injury prevention.

Finally, injured muscle fibers do not regenerate, but heal with inelastic scar tissue. Thus, once injured, flexibility is even more important; your healthy muscles need to be in peak shape to protect their weakened comrade.

If you want to avoid a pulled muscle, your best defense is a proper warm-up and adequate stretching.

SOURCE:

McGuire, Rick. "Sports Injuries Are Preventable." *Total Health* 12 (February 1990): 18–22.

THE OVERUSE SYNDROME

Tennis elbow, Achilles tendonitis, shin splints. These are common manifestations of overuse syndrome caused by inflammation of tendons, ligaments, and other connective tissue from repetitive, frequent or prolonged exercise. Unlike sudden, traumatic muscle injuries or strains, overuse syndrome is a phenomenon brought about when the demand placed on a joint or muscle exceeds the strength or flexibility of that muscle.

One common manifestation of overuse syndrome is tendonitis, or tenderness and inflammation of a tendon from prolonged, unaccustomed exercise. Inflammation usually occurs in one of five areas: the shoulder (rotator cuff), elbow, shin, knee, or ankle. Anyone who repeatedly throws an object or swings his or her arm—swimmers, baseball players and tennis players—may be a candidate for overuse of the shoulder muscle groups. Inflammation of the knee, ankle, and shin is common in runners.

Overuse syndrome is primarily a function of changes in your regular exercise program or sports activity. Typical changes that can put excessive strain on muscles and joints include the following:

- Changing running style (flat foot to toes) or duration of your run
- Changing surfaces of tennis courts (clay to concrete)
- Changing types of shoes (flexible soles to rigid soles, or vice versa)

Generally, you can differentiate overuse syndrome from normal aches and pains of exercise by the timing and intensity of the discomfort. If you feel pain in the same tendon each time you exercise for more than one or two weeks, or if the pain worsens, you may have developed overuse syndrome.

If diagnosed early, overuse syndrome can be reduced or eliminated. But the best medicine is prevention, generally accomplished by four methods:

- Increase exercise intensity and duration gradually.
- When beginning a new weight-bearing exercise, such as tennis, aerobic dancing, or running, engage in the activity only every other day. This precaution is especially important during the first eight weeks of your new activity.
- Be aware of early symptoms. The initial symptom is tenderness in joints or muscle tendons which worsens with repeated activity and is reproducible (occurs in the same anatomical location, and develops about the same time, from workout to workout).
- Develop a routine of stretching prior to, and following, exercise. Pay particular attention to becoming more flexible in muscle groups that you use in the conditioning phase of your exercise program.

SOURCE:

LaForge, Ralph. "Preventing Overuse Syndrome." *Executive Health Report* 26, no. 8 (May 1990): 6.

RESOURCES

ORGANIZATIONS

American Academy of Pediatrics. 141 Northwest Point Boulevard, Elk Grove Village, IL 60009.

American College of Sports Medicine. P.O. Box 1440, Indianapolis, IN 46204.

American Orthopaedic Society for Sports Medicine. 70 W. Hubbard, Suite 202, Chicago, IL 60610.

BOOKS

Griffith, H. Winter. *Complete Guide to Sports Injuries: How to Treat Fractures, Bruises, Sprains, Strains Dislocations, Head Injuries*. Tucson, AZ: The Body Press, 1986. 528 pp.

Morris, Alfred F. *Sports Medicine Handbook: A Guide to the Prevention and Treatment of Athletic Injuries*. Dubuque, IA: Wm. C. Brown, 1985. 400 pp.

RELATED ARTICLES

Karkowsky, Nancy. "Exercise with Care—Fitness Is Not Risk-Free." *FDA Consumer* (May 1989): 25–26.

Pavlov, Helene. "Athletic Injuries." *Radiologic Clinics of North America* 28, no. 2 (March 1990): 435–443.

Thornton, James S. "Playing in Pain: When Should an Athlete Stop?" *The Physician and Sportsmedicine* (September 1990): 138–142.

"Weekend Warrior: The Stress and Strains of Overuse Syndrome." *Mayo Clinic Nutrition Letter* (March 1990): 2–3.

STRESS

OVERVIEW

Without stress, life would be dull and unexciting. Stress adds flavor, challenge, and opportunity to life.

Too much stress, however, can seriously affect your physical and mental well-being. A major challenge in this stress-filled world of today is to make the stress in your life work for you instead of against you.

Stress is with us all the time. It comes from mental or emotional activity and physical activity. It is unique and personal to each of us. So personal, in fact, that what may be relaxing to one person may be stressful to another. For example, if you're a busy executive who likes to keep busy all the time, "taking it easy" at the beach on a beautiful day may feel extremely frustrating, nonproductive, and upsetting. You may be emotionally distressed from "doing nothing." Too much emotional stress can cause physical illness such as high blood pressure, ulcers, or even heart disease; physical stress from work or exercise is not likely to cause such ailments. The truth is that physical exercise can help you to relax and to handle your mental or emotional stress.

Hans Selye, M.D., a recognized expert in the field, has defined stress as a "non-specific response of the body to a demand." The important issue is learning how our bodies respond to these demands. When stress becomes prolonged or particularly frustrating, it can become harmful—causing distress or "bad stress." Recognizing the early signs of distress and then doing something about them can make an important difference in the quality of your life, and may actually influence your survival.

To use stress in a positive way and prevent it from becoming distress, you should become aware of your own reactions to stressful events. The body responds to stress by going through three stages: (1) alarm, (2) resistance, and (3) exhaustion.

Let's take the example of a typical commuter in rush-hour traffic. If a car suddenly pulls out in front of him, his initial alarm reaction may include fear of an accident, anger at the driver who committed the action, and general frustration. His body may respond in the alarm stage by releasing hormones into the bloodstream which cause his face to flush, perspiration to form, his stomach to have a sinking feeling, and his arms and legs to tighten. The next stage is resistance, in which the body repairs damage caused by the stress. If the stress of driving continues with repeated close calls or traffic jams, however, his body will not have time to make repairs. He may become so conditioned to expect potential problems when he drives that he tightens up at the beginning of each commuting day. Eventually, he may even develop one of the diseases of stress, such as migraine headaches, high blood pressure, backaches, or insomnia. While it is impossible to live completely free of stress and distress, it is possible to prevent some distress as well as to minimize its impact when it can't be avoided.

When stress does occur, it is important to recognize and deal with it. Here are some suggestions for ways to handle stress. As you begin to understand more about how stress affects you as an individual, you will come up with your own ideas of helping to ease the tensions.

- Try physical activity. When you are nervous, angry, or upset, release the pressure through exercise or physical activity. Running, walking, playing tennis, or working in your garden are just some of the activities you might try. Physical exercise will relieve that "up tight" feeling, relax you, and turn the frowns into smiles. Remember, your body and your mind work together.

- Share your stress. It helps to talk to someone about your concerns and worries. Perhaps a friend, family member, teacher, or counselor can help you see your problem in a different light. If you feel your problem is serious, you might seek professional help from a psychologist, psychiatrist, or social worker. Knowing when to ask for help may avoid more serious problems later.
- Know your limits. If a problem is beyond your control and can't be changed at the moment, don't fight the situation. Learn to accept what is—for now—until such time when you can change it.
- Take care of yourself. You are special. Get enough rest and eat well. If you are irritable and tense from lack of sleep or if you are not eating correctly, you will have less ability to deal with stressful situations. If stress repeatedly keeps you from sleeping, you should ask your doctor for help.
- Make time for fun. Schedule time for both work and recreation. Play can be just as important to your wellbeing as work; you need a break from your daily routine to just relax and have fun.
- Be a participant. One way to keep from getting bored, sad, and lonely is to go where it's all happening. Sitting alone can make you feel frustrated. Instead of feeling sorry for yourself, get involved and become a participant. Offer your services in neighborhood or volunteer organizations. Help yourself by helping other people. Get involved in the world and the people around you, and you'll find they will be attracted to you. You're on your way to making new friends and enjoying new activities.
- Check off your tasks. Trying to take care of everything at once can seem overwhelming, and, as a result, you may not accomplish anything. Instead, make a list of what tasks you have to do, then do one at a time, checking them off as they're completed. Give priority to the most important ones and do those first.
- Must you always be right? Do other people upset you—particularly when they don't do things your way? Try cooperation instead of confrontation; it's better than fighting and always being "right." A little give and take on both sides will reduce the strain and make you both feel more comfortable.
- It's OK to cry. A good cry can be a healthy way to bring relief to your anxiety, and it might even prevent a headache or other physical consequence. Take some deep breaths; they also release tension.
- Create a quiet scene. You can't always run away, but you can "dream the impossible dream." A quiet country scene painted mentally, or on canvas, can take you out of the turmoil of a stressful situation. Change the scene by reading a good book or playing beautiful music to create a sense of peace and tranquility.
- Avoid self-medication. Although you can use drugs to relieve stress temporarily, drugs do not remove the conditions that caused the stress in the first place. Drugs, in fact, may be habit-forming and create more stress than they take away. They should be taken only on the advice of your doctor.

The best strategy for avoiding stress is to learn how to relax. Unfortunately, many people try to relax at the same pace that they lead the rest of their lives. For a while, tune out your worries about time, productivity, and "doing right." You will find satisfaction in just being, without striving. Find activities that give you pleasure and that are good for your mental and physical wellbeing. Forget about always winning. Focus on relaxation, enjoyment, and health. Be good to yourself.

SOURCE:
National Institute of Mental Health. *Plain Talk about Handling Stress.* DHHS Pub. No. (ADM) 85-502. 1985. pp. 1-2.

THE STRESS-DISEASE CONNECTION

Because the stress response couples physiological to emotional responses, it seems probable that stress can translate frustration into physical illness. But the precise mechanisms by which this occurs are not known. In some situations, as with tension headaches or upset stomachs, the connections appear fairly clear. On the other hand, both headaches and belly aches can occur with no emotional provocation whatever. The chain of causation is even less clear when it comes to more chronic and serious conditions such as heart disease, hypertension, and cancer.

Heart disease

If animals are subjected to repeated or prolonged stress (unavoidable electric shocks or separation from mates), they develop heart disease. How this observation bears upon the human experience is not all that clear. In the 1950s, two cardiologists popularized the concept of a "Type A" personality—the person who is competitive, time-conscious, and never able to feel approval except from the latest achievement. This personality has been widely accepted as a predictor of coronary heart disease—but not without dissent. Various personality scales are used to assess the presence of Type A traits. They seem to work for some investigators but not for others. It may also be the case that there really are two types of "fast-paced" or "hard-driven" people. Studies of management hierarchies suggest that those who rise to the top and experience real success in their lives may suffer little or not at all from their personality type. At a lower level in management, where frustration may be greater, risk of heart attack may be higher. Some authorities have suggested that the pressure of working in a situation where one has little sense of control may be more "stressful" than the sense of high-risk, high-rolling autonomy. Currently, it appears exceedingly difficult to look at a particular person and say for sure whether his personality type or behavior is contributing to heart disease.

High blood pressure

It's not clear whether emotional factors make an important contribution to chronic high blood pressure. The medical term "hypertension" is partly responsible for the widespread popular belief that tension and high blood pressure are linked, but the word doesn't imply anything about this relationship. On the other hand, behavioral scientists have shown quite clearly that meditation techniques (popularized as the "relaxation response" by Dr. Herbert Benson) can help to lower moderately elevated levels of blood pressure. These techniques, which can sometimes be self-taught but may work even better after a few sessions with an expert, are a valuable component of the approach to lowering blood pressure without medication.

Cancer

For some years, reports that destructive emotions contribute to the progress of cancer, or even cause it, have been in circulation. One popular version of this theory holds that such emotions weaken the immune surveillance mechanisms that normally hold cancer in check. A logical extension of this theory is the claim that developing more healthy emotions can help retard the progress of cancer.

These theories deserve further study, but they must be regarded as tenuous at best. Anyone, with or without cancer, can benefit from increased emotional health. That would be reason enough to offer emotional support and help to cancer patients. But the flip side of the coin—suggesting that cancer patients have somehow brought on their disease through inadequate emotional responses—is unjustified by any valid evidence, and it smacks of "blaming the victim."

Other diseases

The list of diseases that have been linked to stress is almost endless. It includes asthma, allergies, rheumatoid arthritis, ulcers, ulcerative colitis, and migraine headaches, among many others. There's an important distinction that needs to be made. Any of these chronic illnesses can be made harder to bear by a stress-laden situation, or by an emotionally inadequate response on the part of the patient. On the other hand, it is no longer possible to credit older theories that specific emotional experiences or reactions actually cause these various diseases. On the whole, it seems most likely that stress plays a nonspecific role in disease, by throwing off the body's natural ability to heal itself.

SOURCE:
Bennett, William I., Stephen E. Goldfinger, and G. Timothy Johnson. *Your Good Health: How to Stay Well, and What to Do When You're Not.* Cambridge, MA: Harvard University Press, 1987. 317–319.

BURNOUT

By definition, professionals take pride in their work; they are intelligent, conscientious, eager to learn, and want to continue growing. That is all to the good, or course. At the same time, however, these very same characteristics can sometimes lead to problems. It is just such people who, carrying their career standards to extremes, are most susceptible to burnout.

Burnout can be defined as mental, physical, and emotional exhaustion. It is the kind of "DIS-ease" that does not strike quickly—it builds up over a period of time, usually without the victim being aware of it. Then, once it takes over, it can be very difficult to deal with.

There are three stages in the development of burnout. The first is what psychologists refer to as the "Gung-Ho" stage. The potential victims regard their careers as all-important, and they are confident that an all-out effort will ensure their success. They are super conscientious and super eager; they push themselves too hard, and set unrealistic standards that are difficult to meet.

At some point, however, they realize that the appreciation and rewards they had anticipated are not coming their way, and this is a serious blow. They reach the second, "Guilt," stage of burnout. They blame themselves for their disappointment, feel that, somehow, they have done all the wrong things. To compensate, they push themselves even harder, growing more and more tired in the process.

Stage three is characterized by chronic fatigue and disillusionment . . . a "nobody out there will ever appreciate what I do" attitude. Should these negative feelings continue, complete burnout takes over.

There is really no need to ever reach such a point, though. No matter how career oriented you are, you can be alert to the warning signs of approaching burnout and take steps to deal with them.

What are these signs? Certainly, everyone feels tired, depressed, and disillusioned from time to time—that is only natural. But when these feelings persist, when you find yourself always living by the clock, crowding fun and friends out of your schedule because of the career demands you are placing on yourself, burnout could be down the road. It is time, then, to pause and take stock, assess your position, and reorganize your priorities.

Develop new interests

It may be a cliche, but variety is the spice of life. If you focus entirely on your job, the ups and downs of the daily routine will assume undue importance. Furthermore, no job can satisfy all your needs. You need a balanced life, with time for work, leisure, friends—and, equally important, time for yourself.

Work on your self image

Career-oriented people sometimes tend to be too hard on themselves. They blame themselves for failures, big and small; they agonize when they do not get the recognition they feel should be coming their way. Just hanging in there becomes an exercise in futility.

Do not waste time and energy in this way. Instead, concentrate on the good things—the things you enjoy doing, the gains you have made, the small triumphs. Make it a point to tune into yourself in positive fashion. You will feel better about yourself—and your job.

Forget "perfection"

Sure, if you want to get ahead, it is important to have high standards, but do not make yours so high that they are unrealistically out of reach. That is self-destructing. So is feeling that you must attain your career goals by a rigidly set timetable. Allow room for the inevitable changes and obstacles, time to relax and regroup.

Keep the present in perspective

Maybe you are not getting ahead as fast as you want to; maybe there are some aspects of your present situation that are not to your liking. But take the long view. Just how far have you come—and just how far can you reasonably expect to go? The promotion that went to someone else, the recognition that your should have gotten for a certain accomplishment—and, the co-worker who does not acknowledge your capabilities—all these are simply passing events. New opportunities, new people, new situations, are always in the works.

Take care of yourself

People who want to succeed need healthy bodies and keen minds—a certain amount of rest, the right kind of food, moderate exercise, time to relax with people you enjoy are all in order. When you find yourself pushing too hard, slow down. What does not get done today can always wait until tomorrow.

Many people who are susceptible to burnout let their lives be controlled by others. They are sure that if they knock themselves out, do the best possible job, success will come their way. All they have to do is sit back and wait for someone else to make the moves and decisions.

SOURCE:
Ash, Stephen. "Burnout: Causes and Cures." *Manage* 41 (March 1990): 2–3.

THE RELAXATION RESPONSE

In one study at the London School of Hygiene and Tropical Medicine, doctors tracked health records of 192 men and women ages 35 to 64. At the start of the study, each volunteer had two or more of these risk factors: high blood pressure, high cholesterol and a smoking habit of ten or more cigarettes a day.

Then some of the group took eight one-hour group lessons. They studied relaxation, meditation, managing stress and breathing exercises. Within eight weeks, doctors discovered that their blood pressures were significantly lower than those of others who were not taught to relax and breathe.

Four years later, those who had learned to meditate and breathe correctly still showed lower blood-pressure readings. Compared with those who hadn't received the eight hours of instruction, they were less likely to be in treatment for hypertension. They also were less apt to show symptoms of heart disease, or to have died of a heart attack.

Herbert Benson, M.D., associate professor of medicine at Harvard Medical School, says there are scores of other studies about the health benefits of what he calls "the relaxation response." He has studied it since the late 1960s, and his book *The Relaxation Response* became a bestseller.

You don't have to be a mystic to bring on the response, Benson says. You just focus your attention on a repeated word, sound, prayer phrase or breathing pattern. Then you disregard everyday thoughts when they come to mind. If you're distracted, you turn your mind gently back to the repetition.

During the relaxation response, Benson says, oxygen consumption decreases. Heart rate drops and breathing slows. It's the opposite of the "fight or flight" response that jump-starts us to flee or face danger or psychological stress tests. Even when the response is not being elicited, studies show a healthy drop in blood pressure—averaging ten points systolic and ten points diastolic, Benson says. "We're not talking about a drop during the relaxation response," he said. "The goal is to see healthy change during non-meditative periods."

Blood pressure declines because the relaxation response raises a kind of protective dike against stress hormones. Benson says several studies have shown that meditators become less responsive to a "fight or flight" hormone called norepinephrine. So after someone has been regularly eliciting the relaxation response, it takes more of the hormone to hike blood pressure.

SOURCE:
Williams, Gurney, III. "Don't Let Stress Number Your Days." *Longevity* (October 1990): 58–59.

RESOURCES

BOOKS

Benson, Herbert, and William Proctor. *Beyond the Relaxation Response*. New York: Berkley, 1987.

Epstein, Gerald. *Healing Visualizations*. New York: Bantam, 1989.

Gillespie, Peggy Roggenbuck, and Lynn Bechtel. *Less Stress in 30 Days: An Integrated Program for Relaxation*. New York: Plums Books/NAL, 1986. 157 pp.

Girdano, Daniel, and George Everly. *Controlling Stress and Tension: A Holistic Approach*. Englewood Cliffs, NJ: Prentice-Hall, 1986. 228 pp.

Kabat-Zinn, Jan. *Full Catastrophe Living: Using the Wisdom of Your Body and Mind to Face Stress, Pain, and Illness*. New York: Delacorte, 1990.

RELATED ARTICLES

"How to Fend Off Stress." *Good Housekeeping* (February 1991): 106, 130.

Shimer, Porter, and Sharon Ferguson. "Unwind and Destress (Part 1)." *Prevention* 42 (July 1990): 75–92.

Shimer, Porter, and Sharon Ferguson. "Unwind and Destress (Part 2)." *Prevention* 42 (August 1990): 99–117.

"Stress Can Make You Sick, But Can Managing Stress Make You Well?" *Consumer Reports Health Letter* 2 (January 1990): 1–3.

Wilkinson, Greg. "Stress: Another Chimera." *British Medical Journal* 302 (January 26, 1991): 191–192.

STROKE

OVERVIEW

Stroke is the third largest cause of death in America, after diseases of the heart and cancer. Although elderly people account for the vast majority of stroke deaths, stroke ranks third as a cause of death among middle-aged people.

Despite these statistics, there's good news. The age-adjusted death rate for stroke has been steadily declining in the U.S., dropping from 88 per 100,000 population in 1950 to 34 in 1984. The rate declined about one percent a year until 1972; after that it started dropping about five percent a year. Improvements in medical care for stroke patients and the control of high blood pressure have contributed to the decline.

A stroke is a form of cardiovascular disease. It affects the arteries or veins of the central nervous system and stops the flow of blood bringing oxygen and nutrients to the brain. A stroke occurs when one of these blood vessels either bursts or becomes clogged with a blood clot. Because of this rupture or blockage, part of the brain doesn't receive the flow of blood it needs. As a result, it starts to die.

SOURCE:
American Heart Association. *Facts about Stroke.* 1989. p. 1.

* * *

There are two main kinds of stroke. In one, a thrombotic stroke, a blood clot plugs an artery and cuts off blood circulation to parts of the brain; without a supply of oxygen, the brain cells die within minutes. The second kind, a hemorrhagic stroke, involves the rupture of a blood vessel. Blood then pours in to the brain—or the space between the brain and the skull—and brain cells die from the loss of oxygen and the sharply increased pressure within.

Roughly two-thirds of all strokes are caused by clots, which usually form in arteries that have been narrowed by a build-up of atherosclerotic plaque. A cerebral thrombosis (from the Greek *thrombus*, or clot) occurs when a clot forms within the brain itself. Such strokes usually occur at night or early in the morning, when the blood pressure is low and the blood platelets, which are responsible for clotting, are stickiest. Ten percent of such strokes are preceded by a "TIA"—a transient ischemic attack, or "mini-stroke."

A cerebral embolism (from the Greek *embolus*, or plug) is caused by a clot formed elsewhere in the body, usually the heart, that travels to the brain. (These emboli are often formed during atrial fibrillation, a disorder in which the upper chambers of the heart "quiver" rather than beat, so that blood is not entirely pumped out, but tends to pool and clot.)

A subarachnoid hemorrhage is caused by the rupture of a blood vessel on the surface of the brain so that blood fills the space between the brain and the skull. Such hemorrhages account for about 7% of all strokes. A cerebral hemorrhage is caused by the rupture of a blood vessel within the brain itself. These account for about 10% of all strokes.

SOURCE:
"Stroke: Are You at Risk?" *The Johns Hopkins Medical Letter* (April 1991): 4.

WARNING SIGNALS

The warning signals of stroke are:

- Sudden weakness or numbness of the face, arm and leg on one side of the body.

- Loss of speech, or trouble talking or understanding speech.
- Dimness or loss of vision, particularly in only one eye.
- Unexplained dizziness, unsteadiness or sudden falls.

About 10 percent of strokes are preceded by "temporary strokes" (transient ischemic attacks or TIAs). These can occur days, weeks or even months before a major stroke. TIAs result when a blood clot temporarily clogs an artery and part of the brain doesn't get the supply of blood it needs. The symptoms occur rapidly and last a relatively short period of time, usually from a few minutes to several hours. The usual symptoms are like those of a full-fledged stroke, except that the symptoms of a TIA are temporary, lasting 24 hours or less. TIAs are extremely important warning signs for stroke and shouldn't be ignored. In fact, people who've had TIAs are 9.5 times more likely to have a stroke than people of the same age and sex who haven't had a TIA.

Whenever the warning signs of stroke occur, it's important to get immediate medical attention. Don't ignore these signals! A doctor must determine whether a stroke has occurred, or a TIA, or just another medical problem with similar symptoms (seizure, fainting, migraine, or a general medical or cardiac condition). Prompt medical or surgical attention to these symptoms could prevent a fatal or disabling stroke from occurring.

SOURCE:
American Heart Association. *Facts about Stroke*. 1989. pp. 2–3.

RISK FACTORS

The best way to prevent a stroke is to reduce the factors that can cause a stroke in the first place.

Some factors that increase the risk of stroke are genetically determined, others are simply a function of natural processes, but still others result from a person's lifestyle. The factors resulting from heredity or natural processes can't be changed, but those that are environmental can be modified with a doctor's help.

Five risk factors for stroke can't be changed. These are:

- Age
- Sex
- Race
- Diabetes mellitus
- A prior stroke

The older a person gets, the greater the risk of stroke. Men are also more likely to have a stroke; blacks have a greater risk of stroke than whites. People with diabetes or who have had a prior stroke are also more likely to suffer stroke.

It is possible that precise control of diabetes may reduce the risk of stroke in diabetic patients. A national study is currently underway to find out if close control of diabetes prevents complications leading to stroke.

The major risk factors for stroke that can be decreased by treatment are:

- High blood pressure
- Heart disease
- TIAs

When these factors are present, treatment must be started and maintained. This is especially true in cases of high blood pressure, which is the most dominant factor. High-risk patients also must learn to recognize the signs of TIA and tell their physicians about them if they occur. A surprising number of people ignore the symptoms of TIA to their peril.

Besides the risk factors mentioned, there are other factors that increase the risk of stroke and can be controlled by changes in lifestyle. These include:

- Elevated blood cholesterol and lipids
- Cigarette smoking
- Excessive alcohol intake
- Obesity

These are secondary risk factors because they indirectly affect the risk of stroke by increasing the risk of heart disease (which is a primary risk factor for stroke).

Accordingly, people with a high risk of stroke may be advised by their doctors to lose weight or lower their blood cholesterol levels, exercise in moderation and quit smoking.

SOURCE:
American Heart Association. *Facts about Stroke*. 1989. pp. 3–5.

PREVENTION

Although there is no fail-safe way to prevent strokes, three basic approaches can help.

(1) The primary one is to modify risk factors, of which high blood pressure is the most important. Long-term control of hypertension reduces the chance of developing all types of strokes, and this is the single most effective form of prevention that we have. Reducing risk factors that promote atherosclerosis, notably cigarette smoking and high blood cholesterol, also helps decrease the risk of strokes, particularly those of the thrombotic type. A group of people at particularly high risk of stroke are women who have migraine headaches, take contraceptive pills, and smoke; for this group, quitting cigarettes can markedly reduce the risk.

Reduction of risk factors should be begun before there is any evidence that a stroke is impending. Other forms of prevention are used only after some evidence is found that trouble is brewing.

(2) Since blood clots play a major role in producing strokes, people who develop TIAs [transient ischemic

attacks] are often given treatment to suppress the clotting mechanism. Anticoagulant medication should, in theory, help to prevent both embolic and thrombotic strokes.

Two different types of anticoagulant drug (sometimes, inaccurately, called "blood thinners") have been tried.

Warfarin (Coumadin) interferes with the production of certain proteins necessary for coagulation of blood. The question about warfarin is whether it raises the risk of bleeding to a level that outweighs its ability to reduce the frequency of strokes. This question is currently being investigated.

Aspirin and some other related drugs prevent platelets from sticking to each other. Platelets are cell fragments that trigger clot formation; without the latticework they provide, the process of clotting is retarded. Large clinical trials have suggested that antiplatelet agents prevent strokes in people with TIAs, but these trials have not been conclusive because the studies have grouped patients with strokes or TIAs resulting from different pathological processes.

Currently, it is common clinical practice to use aspirin or a related drug for TIAs. If symptoms or other indications suggest that the real source of trouble is embolism from a clot in the heart, or if narrowing (also called stenosis) is found in one of the major arteries carrying blood to the brain, more complete anticoagulation with warfarin is considered.

(3) Finally, if a major artery is narrowed or has a damaged surface causing clots to form, then mechanically enlarging the interior space (lumen) of the artery or removing artherosclerotic plaque from the wall would be expected to improve blood flow and reduce risk. To this end, a procedure known as endarterectomy (Greek for "taking out the inner lining of an artery") has been developed.

The brain receives its blood supply through two pairs of large arteries entering the skull from the neck. The carotid arteries are located near the surface of the neck on either side of the windpipe, where the carotid pulse can usually be felt if fingertips are laid gently just under the angle fo the jaw. The vertebral arteries travel alongside the vertebral column and enter the skull, whereupon they join to form a single basilar artery. Inside the skull, the carotid and basilar arteries branch to supply the brain with many smaller vessels. Only the carotid arteries are accessible for treatment with endarterectomy.

Of the three preventive approaches, treating risk factors, and hypertension in particular, is the one supported by a general consensus; lowering high blood rpessure is clearly beneficial, and will probably protect the largest number of people. Even mild hypertension raises the risk of stroke, though it has relatively few other consequences.

Use of the anticoagulant drugs is more problematic. Although people with TIAs appear to get some protection, there is no clear support for the notion that taking aspirin every day will prevent strokes in symptom-free people.

The third and most invasive approach, endarterectomy, is controversial.

SOURCE:
"How Can We Prevent Strokes?" *Harvard Medical School Health Letter* 14, no. 10 (August 1989): 2–3.

TREATMENT

Once you have made the diagnosis of cerebral infarction, management becomes multifaceted. You will have to direct your efforts in three broad areas: general care, medical therapy, and surgical treatment.

General measures are aimed at preventing the common complications and lowering the associated morbidity and mortality.

Immediate hospitalization. The most effective intervention in stroke treatment may be limited to the first few hours. Therapeutic trials are currently concentrating on treatment during this brief window. Thus, a sudden onset of focal neurologic deficit, even if it improves, should prompt immediate evaluation in the hospital. A delay in medical attention prevents early treatment and deprives stroke victims of potential benefits.

The unpredictable course of stroke (progression or recurrence) and the associated complications require specialized personnel who can carry out early detection and intervention. This care is best accomplished in a stroke unit, if possible, or on a neurology ward that has a specialized nursing staff. . . .

Most of the currently available medications are used to prevent stroke progression or recurrence. In a few instances of stroke in evolution, they may reverse the effects. . . .

Although the use of heparin is controversial in completed stroke, it is widely used for stroke in evolution and is also indicated for recent transient ischemic attacks, small strokes, and cardioembolic stroke. Of patients with cardiogenic brain embolism, 14% will have a second event within the following 2 weeks; early anticoagulation reduces this risk by one third. Among patients with large completed infarcts, anticoagulation is sometimes delayed 48 hours in order to lower the possibility of hemorrhagic transformations; however, this must be balanced with the risk for recurrent stroke, which is highest in that same period.

Anticoagulation is empirically used for patients with partial stroke in the vertebrobasilar system because there is a substantial risk for progression. . . .

The benefits of aspirin or ticlopidine in the acute stage of stroke are unknown. Several studies have demonstrated their benefits in preventing stroke or its recurrence.

SOURCE:
Fayad, Pierre B., and Lawrence M. Brass. "Stroke: How To Treat Patients with Acute Ischemic Infarction." *Consultant* 31 (January 1991): 39–43.

REHABILITATION

Successful rehabilitation depends on the extent of brain damage, the patient's attitude, the skill of the rehabilitation team, and the cooperation of family and friends. Most stroke patients can benefit from rehabilitation, and today the outlook for stroke patients is more hopeful than ever before. Because of advances in treatment and rehabilitation, many patients are being restored to a useful life.

Stroke affects different people in different ways, depending on the type of stroke and the area of the brain affected. Brain damage from a stroke can affect the senses, speech and the ability to understand speech, behavioral patterns, thought patterns and memory. Paralysis on one side of the body can also result.

Whenever the blood supply is cut off from part of the body, the body tries to restore circulation itself. Small neighboring blood vessels get large and assume the work of damaged ones to compensate. In this way, the part of the body affected by the stroke may eventually improve or even return to normal through natural means.

Not all patients recover spontaneously, though. They need rehabilitation to learn new skills. Often old skills have been lost, so new ones are needed. Then, too, it's important to maintain and improve a patient's physical condition whenever possible.

One of the first rules of successful rehabilitation is that it must begin as soon after a stroke as possible. In the initial visit a doctor may advise proper bed positioning and recommend exercises that, in some cases, can be started the same day the stroke occurred.

Besides the primary goal of rehabilitation (helping patients develop new motor skills), nurses and other hospital personnel work to prevent secondary complications from arising. These include stiff joints, bedsores and pneumonia. They can result when a person is confined to bed for a long time.

But doctors and hospital workers aren't the only people who play a role in rehabilitation. The role of the patient's family is important, too. Family members need to understand what the stroke patient is going through and how disability can affect the patient. The situation will be easier to handle if they know what to expect, and how to handle problems that will arise once the patient leaves the hospital. A patient's will to recover and desire to be independent play a big part in recovery; the family can help by providing a warm, supportive and encouraging atmosphere.

For a stroke patient, the goal of rehabilitation is to be as independent and productive as possible, given the limitations resulting from the stroke.

SOURCE:
American Heart Association. *Facts about Stroke.* 1989. pp. 6–7.

RESOURCES

ORGANIZATIONS

American Heart Association. 7320 Greenville Ave., Dallas, TX 75231.

American Physical Therapy Association. 1156 15th St. NW, Washington, DC 20005.

American Rehabilitation Foundation. Kenny Rehabilitation Institute, 2727 Chicago Ave., Minneapolis, MN 55407.

PAMPHLET

American Heart Association:

Strokes: A Guide for the Family. 1987.

BOOKS

Conn, Foley, and H. F. Pizer. *The Stroke Fact Book: Everything You Want and Need To Know about Stroke—From Prevention to Rehabilitation.* Golden Valley, MN: Courage Stroke Network, 1988.

Frye-Pierson, J., and J. F. Toole. *Stroke: A Guide for Patient and Family.* Washington, DC: American Physical Therapy Association, 1989.

Hewer, Richard Langton, and Derick T. Wade. *Stroke: A Practical Guide towards Recovery.* Englewood Cliffs, NJ: Prentice-Hall, 1980.

Lavin, John. *Stroke: From Crisis to Victory.* New York: Franklin Watts, 1985.

RELATED ARTICLES

Adams, Harold P., Jr., Louis R. Caplan, and Eric J. Russell. "Early Care in Acute Stroke." *Patient Care* (October 15, 1990): 121–140.

Feinburg, Willam. "Antithrombotic Therapy in Stroke and Transient Ischemic Attacks." *American Family Physician* 40, no. 5 (suppl.) (November 1989): 53S–59S.

Gorelick, Philip B. "Treatment of Ischemic Stroke: Lessons from Clinical Trials." *Postgraduate Medicine* 86, no. 8 (December 1989): 107–118.

Grotta, James C. "Post-Stroke Management Concerns and Outcomes." *Geriatrics* 43, no. 7 (July 1988): 40–48.

"Is It a Stroke?" *Consumer Reports Health Letter* (June 1990): 45.

Reding, Michael J., and Fletcher H. McDowell. "Focused Stroke Rehabilitation Programs Improve Outcome." *Archives of Neurology* 46 (June 1989): 700–703.

SUDDEN INFANT DEATH SYNDROME (SIDS)

OVERVIEW

One of the most devastating tragedies that can befall young parents is the sudden death of their infant. Although such a death can occur from natural or accidental causes, more than half of such deaths are unexpected and unexplained—called sudden infant death syndrome (SIDS). SIDS is the leading cause of death in infants between the ages of 1 and 12 months in the United States and has an incidence of 1-2/1000 live births or 5,000 to 6,000 deaths per year. The peak age for SIDS is 2-4 months and it most often occurs during sleep. Although there are more cases during the winter months, SIDS can occur any time of year. Certain groups of infants are at a somewhat higher risk—including premature infants, siblings of SIDS victims (especially where there are two or more SIDS victims in a family) and infants born to substance-abusing mothers—but there are currently no diagnostic tests to identify individual infants at risk.

There is often little or no warning for the shocked parents—less than 10 percent of SIDS victims have had a history of apparent life threatening events (ALTEs). ALTEs are characterized by some combination of apnea (cessation of breathing), color change (usually pale or blue/grey), choking or gagging, and are understandably frightening to the observer, who may fear that the infant has died. Previous terms to describe these incidents—"aborted crib death" or "near death"—wrongly implied a close association between ALTEs and SIDS. In fact, most infants with an ALTE do not subsequently have SIDS. A number of supposed "causes" for SIDS have also been disproven, including DPT immunization, milk allergies and an enlarged thymus gland. There are also potential environmental hazards that can be life-threatening to babies, and even result in accidental death. Having too much space between the mattress and bedframe in a crib can result in the baby getting trapped and suffocating, for example, but these environmental hazards are not to be confused with SIDS.

Many pre- and full-term infants who have had ALTEs have been managed with home apnea/cardiac monitoring. If abnormally low heart rates or abnormally long apneas occur, an audio alarm is triggered, alerting parents to the potentially life-threatening situation. Since screening tests to determine the risks for apnea or SIDS in asymptomatic infants are not currently available, the use of home apnea/heart rate monitoring is usually recommended only for infants who have apnea or a low heart rate. Less than 10 percent of SIDS cases had apnea problems beforehand, so monitoring is not necessarily a good preventative measure for SIDS.

Home apnea monitoring is also controversial for those infants who have a somewhat increased epidemiological risk of SIDS, because the vast majority of alarms are due to recording problems and the fact that the machine is designed to be over-sensitive. Occasional shallow or deep breathing—natural in infants—can set off the alarm and panic parents. When real alarms occur, simple stimulation may awaken the infant, or often the problem resolves itself on its own. When home monitoring is recommended, physicians, parents, health care providers, monitor vendors, and community resources such as parent support groups are all necessary to make it effective. Parents and other care providers must learn how to use the monitor, infant cardiopulmonary resuscitation, and safe stimulation techniques. Monitoring can be very helpful in the management of apnea, but it is no guarantee that SIDS can be averted: SIDS has still occurred in infants during monitoring.

Infants who die suddenly and unexpectedly, but have an identifiable cause of death, are not SIDS victims. Many of these deaths may share characteristics of SIDS (they may not be anticipated or prevented) but a cause can be determined from case history and autopsy evaluation. A complete postmortem examination and case review is required in many states, including California, to make a diagnosis of SIDS. The attending physician is responsible for providing the initial diagnosis and within 24 to 72 hours, the autopsy diagnosis. In some cases, further evaluation of microscopic or culture results at autopsy may provide a cause of death. A follow-up conference as soon as possible is important to finalize the information for the parents. . . .

SIDS is tragedy for all concerned. It is generally agreed among researchers that some infants may be predisposed to SIDS due to conditions which may overwhelm brain and vital organ functions under certain stressful circumstance. It is hoped that future research on infant developmental physiology will provide answers about the cause and prevention of SIDS. Public awareness of this leading cause of infant death is important to garner national attention for continued research support.

SOURCE:
California Medical Association. "Sudden Infant Death Syndrome." *HealthTips* index 305. November 1990. pp. 1–2.

DIAGNOSIS

As infant mortality diminished in the first half of this century more attention was given to those babies dying unexpectedly and with less florid disease. The skills required to study such deaths had not, however, been developed, and the result was that diagnoses ranged from "pneumonitis" to "suffocation." The latter label led to parents being interrogated by the police and to social stigma. In 1969 a group in Seattle, believing that all of these were natural deaths, recommended that they should be registered as the sudden infant death syndrome. This approach was rapidly copied throughout the world.

The diagnosis was seductive for five reasons. First of all, it enabled doctors to tell parents that their child had died of natural causes and that no one could have prevented it. It excused all concerned from any defect in care, diagnosis, and treatment. Pathologists welcomed the diagnosis; the less they found, the more certain they could be. Because the syndrome was of unknown origin health authorities had no basis for prevention. And finally, this diagnosis facilitated the development of parent support groups and the raising of money for research. Those concerned in research and support became media sensitive, and all concerned looked for the day when a genius would find "the cause."

This, then, is the setting in which armchair theories surface monthly. Yet, as the diagnosis is open, parents relate every new theory to themselves. If it concerns some obscure reflex, brain enzyme, or organism they are content, but any theory that reflects on the care of their child makes them feel threatened. They react, and they are supported by doctors who have developed an interest in their welfare. . . .

Questions are now beginning to be asked, including: Is there such an entity as the sudden infant death syndrome or is it a convenient diagnostic dustbin? If, as has been alleged, 5–10% of sudden infant deaths are infanticide is the label the sudden infant death syndrome facilitating infanticide? The justification for retaining the sudden infant death syndrome is the supposed benefit to parents, but who is benefiting—the doctors or the parents? The "no cause; no guilt" approach has never been subjected to any controlled trial; nor is there any evidence that a parent of a victim of cot [crib] death has greater need for help than one given a diagnosis of meningitis or of "cause unknown." To abolish the sudden infant death syndrome as a registerable cause of death would simply put the clock back to 1960. Among research workers there is much vested interest against change. Lip service is paid to possible multiple causes, but each acts as if his or her own theory is universal.

SOURCE:
Emery, John L. "Is Sudden Infant Death Syndrome a Diagnosis? Or Is It Just a Diagnostic Dustbin?" *British Medical Journal* 299, no. 6710 (November 18, 1989): 1240.

CAUSES

The explanation for sudden infant death syndrome, a mysterious malady that kills 8,000 American babies each year, seems to lie in the developing brain, scientists are concluding.

The research emphasis is shifting to the brain, they say, because 20 years of painstaking study into other organ systems, including the heart and lungs, have failed to explain why seemingly healthy infants die in their sleep. Moreover, recent insights into brain chemistry and advanced imaging techniques are making the new brain studies possible.

While scientists say they are still far from knowing the underlying cause of sudden infant death, most experts now believe that SIDS babies have a subtle brain abnormality.

Some researchers believe the abnormality could lie in the brain stem, which controls breathing and heart rates. Others believe the problem may lie in brain areas controlling sleep patterns or learning processes. Still others are looking at centers that control specific functions, like tongue muscles or regulation of body heat.

The new work is being mounted as scientists discard a popular theory linking crib death to apnea, a breathing disorder. Although thousands of babies have been fitted with monitoring devices that sound an alarm when their breathing becomes irregular during sleep, the incidence of crib death has not fallen, SIDS experts say.

"SIDS researchers are in shock from the loss of their favorite pet theory," said Dr. Bruce Beckwith, a professor of pathology and pediatrics at the University of

Colorado. "The situation is verging on the chaotic. We've had lots of ideas but few hard facts."

SOURCE:
Blakeslee, Sandra. "Crib Death: Suspicion Turns to the Brain." *The New York Times* (February 14, 1989): 17.

* * *

New evidence from a pair of pediatricians at the Washington University School of Medicine in St. Louis suggests that a subtle form of suffocation may be the true culprit in one-quarter to one-half of all suspected SIDS cases. Their conclusion, published in last week's *New England Journal of Medicine,* reflects a growing suspicion among doctors that the position in which these babies slept, face down, may have played a major role in their death.

With the help of the Consumer Product Safety Commission, Dr. James Kemp and Dr. Bradley Thach obtained information about 25 infants who died face down. All of the babies had been sleeping on soft cushions, filled with polystyrene beads, intended for infants. The two colleagues began their investigation with a simple test. Each held one of the suspect pillows to his own face and tried to breathe through it. "If you breathe into it for a minute or two, you're OK," says Kemp, an expert in the physiology of infant airways. "But after that you really feel out of breath and uncomfortable."

Even though the cushion had not prevented them from breathing, the air they exhaled had become trapped in the beads. So when they inhaled, they drew in stale air that was low in oxygen. "You end up breathing back in what you've just breathed out," Thach explains. "All the oxygen gets used up." Adults have enough lung power to suck in sufficient oxygen through the pillow, but Kemp and Thach determined that babies could not. By testing rabbits that had the same lung size as infants, the pediatricians proved that rebreathing into the bead-filled cushions was fatal for babies. The two investigators also determined that any movement by the children to free themselves only buried their faces deeper into the pillows.

SOURCE:
Gorman, Christine. "Beware of the Pillow: Researchers Uncover a New Culprit in the Mystery of Sudden Infant Death Syndrome." *Time* (July 8, 1991): 48.

PREVENTION

Nearly all affected parents wonder if there might have been something they could have done to prevent their baby's death. The answer is that there still is no way to determine which baby will die of SIDS. Presently, there is no certain way anyone can prevent the death.

SIDS occurs in all social, economic, ethnic and racial groups in the United States. There are, however, certain groups of babies who are at slightly increased risk. For example, statistics indicate that there is a higher incidence of SIDS among premature and low birth weight infants as well as among twins and triplets. SIDS is also more frequent among babies born to teenagers, mothers who smoke heavily or abuse drugs and those who have not received good prenatal care. Other groups at increased risk are babies of American Indians, black and poor families. Although the previously mentioned groups have more of a chance of having a baby die of SIDS, most victims of SIDS have few or none of the risk factors mentioned.

SIDS is not predictable or preventable at this time. However, there are actions that parents may take to decrease the risk, not only for SIDS but also for other infant problem. Health professionals should encourage mothers to take good care of themselves during pregnancy and to obtain good prenatal care to decrease their risk.

SOURCE:
National SIDS Foundation. *Facts about SIDS.* July 1989. p. 3.

* * *

In 1986, several branches of the National Institutes of Health held a Consensus Development Conference on Infantile Apnea and Home Monitoring. A major conclusion was that home monitoring of normal infants is inappropriate, even if an infant had apnea associated with prematurity. Monitoring should be considered only for children who have had unexplained, apparently life-threatening events requiring resuscitation or vigorous stimulation, preterm infants who continue to have severe apnea at the time they would otherwise be ready for hospital discharge, and infants with certain other specific diseases or conditions such as central hypoventilation. Evidence does not justify monitoring infants who are siblings of victims of SIDS, have had an apparently life-threatening event requiring resuscitation or vigorous stimulation, or were tracheostomized or born to cocaine- or opiate-abusing mothers.

SOURCE:
Herbst, John J., Dorothy Kelly, and others. "New Findings Shed Light on SIDS." *Patient Care* 22 (May 15, 1988): 61.

RESOURCES

ORGANIZATIONS

American Sudden Infant Death Syndrome Institute. 275 Carpenter Drive, Atlanta, GA 30328.

National Sudden Infant Death Foundation. 8200 Professional Pl., Suite 104, Landover, MD 20785.

PAMPHLET

Public Health Service, Sudden Infant Death Syndrome Program:

Fact Sheet: What is SIDS? n.d. 2 pp.

BOOKS

DeFrain, John, Jacques Taylor, and Linda Ernst. *Coping with Sudden Infant Death.* Lexington, MA: Lexington Books, 1982. 115 pp.

Golding, Jean, Sylvia Limerick, and Aiden MacFarlane. *Sudden Infant Death: Patterns, Puzzles, and Problems*. Seattle: University of Washington Press, 1985. 264 pp.

RELATED ARTICLES

Cotton, Paul. "Sudden Infant Death Syndrome: Another Hypothesis Offered but Doubts Remain." *JAMA* 263 (June 6, 1990): 2865–2866.

Kemp, James S., and Bradley T. Thach. "Sudden Death in Infants Sleeping on Polystyrene-filled cushions." *The New England Journal of Medicine* 324, no. 26 (June 27, 1991): 1858–1864.

Martinez, Fernando D. "Sudden Infant Death Syndrome and Small Airway Occlusion: Facts and a Hypotheses." *Pediatrics* 87 (February 1991): 190–198.

Meadow, Roy. "Suffocation, Recurrent Apnea, and Sudden Infant Death." *The Journal of Pediatrics* 117, no. 3 (September 1990): 351–357.

"Sudden Infant Death Syndrome Despite the Use of Home Monitors." *American Family Physician* 39 (April 1989): 329.

SYPHILIS

(*See also:* CHLAMYDIA; GONORRHEA; PELVIC INFLAMMATORY DISEASE; SEXUALLY TRANSMITTED DISEASES)

OVERVIEW

Syphilis, which swept through Europe in a devastating epidemic during the late 15th century, is now readily treated with antibiotics. However, in many areas of the United States syphilis is on the rise. In 1986, about 70,000 cases were reported to the U.S. Public Health Service. This sexually transmitted disease (STD), which in its late stages can cause mental disorders, blindness, and death, is caused by a corkscrew-shaped bacterium called *Treponema pallidum*.

The infection is acquired by direct contact with the sores of someone who has an active infection. Although the bacterium is usually transmitted through the mucous membranes of the genital area, the mouth, or the anus, it also can pass through broken skin on other parts of the body. A pregnant woman with syphilis can transmit the disease to her unborn child, who may be born with serious mental and physical problems. The syphilis bacterium is very fragile, however, and the infection is rarely, if ever, spread by contact with objects such as toilet seats or towels.

Because the early symptoms of syphilis can be very mild, many people do not seek treatment when they first become infected. However, untreated infected people can infect others during the first two stages of the disease, which can last for up to 2 years.

SOURCE:
National Institute of Allergy and Infectious Diseases. *Syphilis.* NIH Pub. No. 87-909G. August 1987. p. 1.

* * *

Syphilis, which is known as the great imitator because it mimics so many other diseases, is making its strongest comeback in 40 years in the United States. And it is fooling a generation of doctors who have rarely, if ever, seen a case.

Many doctors are scurrying to textbooks and flocking to lectures to learn about the unusual ways the bacterial infection can damage organs at any age, from newborns to the elderly.

Specialists from pediatricians to pathologists have mistaken the sores of syphilis for cancers, abscesses, hemorrhoids, hernias and other conditions. Pediatricians have mistaken the sniffles that can result at birth from congenital syphilis for the flu. Other doctors also have mistaken different forms of syphilis for dizziness from Meniere's disease and multiple sclerosis. . . .

New cases of syphilis are at the highest level since 1949.

Dr. Willard Cates Jr., an expert at the Federal Centers for Disease Control in Atlanta, said the centers expect about 50,000 cases to be reported in 1990, as against 41,942 in 1949. The reporting of syphilis is the most reliable of all the sexually transmitted diseases.

The surging number of cases reflects social and economic factors like changing sexual habits; drug abuse, particularly trading sex for crack; rising rates of pregnancy among teenagers who do not use contraceptives to protect against infection, and declining support for public health services, which has limited tracing some cases.

Some epidemics occur because a microbe develops resistance to antibiotics, but the spirochete that causes syphilis still is killed by penicillin, the drug that has been used to treat it since World War II. . . .

The surge is primarily among black and Hispanic heterosexual men and women in cities. A primary factor is the trading of sex for drugs. Women who give birth to babies with syphilis are more likely to have used crack while pregnant and less likely to have received prenatal care.

Health officials are also deeply concerned about the links between syphilis and AIDS. The open sores of syphilis are believed to make it easier for the AIDS virus to enter the body.

SOURCE:
Altman, Lawrence K. "Syphilis Fools a New Generation." *The New York Times* (November 13, 1990): B7.

SYMPTOMS

The first symptom of primary syphilis is a usually painless open sore called a chancre ("shan-ker"). The chancre can appear within 10 days to 3 months (usually 2 to 6 weeks) after exposure. Because the chancre is ordinarily painless and sometimes occurs inside the body, it may go unnoticed. It is usually found on the part of the body exposed to the bacteria, such as the penis, the vulva, or the vagina. A chancre also can develop on the cervix, tongue, lips, or fingertips. The chancre disappears within a few weeks, but the disease continues. If not treated during the primary stage, the disease may progress through three other stages.

Secondary syphilis is marked by a skin rash that appears anywhere from 2 to 12 weeks after the chancre disappears. The rash may cover the whole body or appear only in a few areas, such as the palms of the hands or soles of the feet. Because active bacteria are present in these sores, any physical contact—sexual or nonsexual—with the broken skin of an infected person may spread the infection at this stage. The rash may be accompanied by flu-like symptoms such as mild fever, fatigue, headache, sore throat, as well as patchy hair loss, swollen lymph glands throughout the body, and other problems. The rash usually heals within several weeks or months, and the other symptoms subside as well. The signs of secondary syphilis occasionally come and go over the next 1 to 2 years. Like the symptoms of the primary stage, those of secondary syphilis can be very mild and go unnoticed.

If untreated, syphilis then lapses into a latent stage during which the patient is no longer contagious. Many people who are not treated will suffer no further consequences of the disease. However, from 15 to 40 percent of those infected go on to develop the complications of late, or tertiary, syphilis, in which the bacteria damage the heart, eyes, brain, nervous system, bones, joints, or almost any other part of the body. This stage can last for years, or even for decades. Late syphilis, the final stage, can lead to mental illness, blindness, heart disease, and death.

SOURCE:
National Institute of Allergy and Infectious Diseases. *Syphilis*. NIH Pub. No. 87-909G. August 1987. pp. 1–2.

DIAGNOSIS AND TREATMENT

Syphilis has sometimes been called "the great imitator" because its early symptoms are similar to those of many other diseases. People who have more than one sex partner should consult a doctor about any suspicious rash or sore in the genital area. Those who have been treated for another STD such as gonorrhea should be tested to be sure they have not acquired syphilis.

There are three ways to diagnose syphilis: a doctor's recognition of its symptoms, microscopic identification of syphilis bacteria, and blood tests.

To diagnose syphilis by identifying the bacteria, the doctor takes a small amount of tissue from a chancre and has it examined under a special "darkfield" microscope. Blood tests also provide evidence of infection, although they may give false negative results (not show signs of infection despite its presence) for up to 6 weeks after the infection occurred. Interpretation of blood tests for syphilis can be difficult, and repeated examinations are sometimes necessary to confirm the diagnosis. In some patients with syphilis (especially in the latent or late stages), a lumbar puncture (spinal tap) must be done to check for infection of the nervous system.

The most common of the screening tests are the VDRL (Venereal Disease Research Laboratory) test and the rapid plasma reagin (RPR) test. These tests can result in false-positive results in people with autoimmune disorders or certain viral infections and may be insensitive in primary, latent, and tertiary syphilis.

More accurate blood tests specifically detect the patient's immune response to the syphilis bacterium. These tests include the fluorescent treponemal antibody-absorption (FTA-ABS) test that can accurately detect 70 to 90 percent of cases. Another specific test is the *T. pallidum* hemagglutination assay (TPHA). Because these tests detect syphilis antibodies (proteins made by a person's immune system to fight infection), they are not useful for diagnosing a new case of syphilis in patients who have had the disease previously, because once antibodies are formed against the syphilis bacteria, the antibodies remain in the body.

Syphilis is treated with penicillin, administered by injection. Other antibiotics can be used for patients allergic to penicillin. A person usually can no longer transmit syphilis 24 hours after beginning therapy. A small percentage of patients do not respond to the usual doses of penicillin. Therefore, it is important that patients have periodic repeat blood tests to make sure that the infectious agent has been completely destroyed and there is no further evidence of the disease. In all stages of syphilis, proper treatment will cure the disease, but in late syphilis, damage already done to body organs cannot be reversed.

SOURCE:
National Institute of Allergy and Infectious Diseases. *Syphilis*. NIH Pub. No. 87-909G. August 1987. pp. 2–3.

RESOURCES

ORGANIZATIONS

American Federation for the Prevention of Venereal Disease. 799 Broadway, Suite 638, New York, NY 10003.

American Social Health Association. P.O. Box 13827, Research Triangle Park, NC 27709.

RELATED ARTICLES

"Gonorrhea and Syphilis Pose Renewed Threats." *Patient Care* 22 (April 30, 1988): 23–24.

Nettina, Sandra L. "Syphilis: A New Look at an Old Killer." *American Journal of Nursing* 90 (April 1990): 68–70.

"Screening for Sexually Transmitted Diseases: Syphilis." *American Family Physician* 42 (September 1990): 691–693.

"Syphilis: An Old Ailment is on the Rise Again." *Mayo Clinic Health Letter* (December 1990): 4–5.

THYROID DISORDERS

OVERVIEW

The thyroid gland is a butterfly-shaped organ located in the front of the neck, just over the windpipe. It produces iodine-containing hormones which regulate the rate at which body cells use energy and produce heat. The growth and development of all the body's tissues are dependent on the thyroid gland's proper functioning.

If the thyroid gland is either overactive or underactive, it can create health problems. Measuring the blood levels of hormones secreted by the thyroid gland, and the pituitary gland which controls it, is the most common test for detecting thyroid gland disorders.

The person with too little secretion of thyroid hormone—called hypothyroidism—has general symptoms of slowing down—of coldness, sluggishness, dry skin and scanty hair growth. In more serious cases, there is a characteristic thickening of the skin, a condition called myxedema. Sometimes a child is born without a thyroid gland. Recognizing and treating this defect early is extremely important to prevent serious problems with both physical and mental development.

Fortunately, deficient production of thyroid hormone in either a child or an adult can be simply and effectively treated by replacing the normal amounts of this chemical the body requires.

At the opposite extreme, the person with an overactive thyroid gland—called hyperthyroidism—may have an increase in body metabolism, which results in weight loss in spite of an increased appetite, excessive warmth and sweating, noticeably trembling hands, pounding of the heart and, in some cases, bulging eyes. Along with these symptoms, the thyroid gland may swell. This swelling is called a goiter.

Medication is effective in slowing down an overactive thyroid. Because improvement may be only temporary, the physician may decide on more permanent measures, such as eradicating it with radioactive iodine or, less often, surgical removal of the overactive thyroid tissue.

Goiter—enlargement of the thyroid gland—is common, but does not necessarily mean that anything is wrong with the production of thyroid hormones. Sometimes the gland enlarges because of an inflammation, which can be either acute and painful or chronic and painless. Some persons have a goiter because of a hereditary defect. Some women may develop a goiter temporarily during pregnancy because there is an increased need for the hormone then and the gland enlarges to meet this additional need.

Goiter used to be rather common among persons who lived in parts of the country which were iodine deficient. This particular type of goiter has almost disappeared in this country through the widespread use of iodized salt and the addition of iodine to animal food and fertilizer.

The thyroid gland, like all other tissues in the body, may be affected by tumor growth. If a goiter is caused by a malignant tumor, it is removed surgically. Sometimes an extremely large goiter, although benign, may be removed because it is a source of discomfort or because it is inconvenient or embarrassing.

SOURCE:
California Medical Association. "The Thyroid Gland." *HealthTips* index 108 (August 1990): 1–2.

HYPOTHYROIDISM AND HYPERTHYROIDISM

An underactive thyroid gland causes hypothyroidism (the opposite of hyperthyroidism). Its name comes from the Greek hypo for under and thyreos for shield-shaped.

The group of symptoms and findings that develop after several years of untreated hypothyroidism is termed myxedema.

The thyroid hormone has such significant effects on growth and development that deficiencies can lead to various health problems. In extreme cases, deficiency states can lead to mental retardation in infants and young children and to a slowing of mental processes, an in ability to maintain normal body temperatures, and even heart failure in adults.

In hypothyroidism, the body's normal functioning rate, its basal metabolic rate, is slowed. The shortage of thyroid hormone causes the body to slow down, leaving the patient feeling mentally and physically sluggish.

In some cases, failure of the pituitary gland to produce a hormone called thyroid-stimulating hormone (TSH) causes hypothyroidism. More often, the thyroid gland gradually is destroyed by an abnormal antibody. In other cases, the cause of the hypothyroidism is unknown. In still others, the treatment for hyperthyroidism may produce hypothyroidism by working too well. In these cases the thyroid hormone status is reversed (from an excess of the hormone to a deficiency); this condition may be temporary or permanent. In some rare instances, infants are born without thyroid glands.

Hashimoto's disease (lymphocytic thyroiditis) may also be a cause of hypothyroidism.

Although it is not a common ailment, hypothyroidism is not unusual. It can occur in anyone of either sex or any age. However, middle-aged women are most commonly affected, and it is most likely to remain undiagnosed in elderly persons. . . .

Hyperthyroidism (also known as overactive thyroid disease) occurs when the thyroid gland produces excessive amounts of thyroid hormone. Its name is derived from the Greek hyper, which means over, and thyreos, for shield-shaped, describing the appearance of the thyroid gland.

The two forms of hyperthyroidism are Graves' disease (also known as toxic diffuse goiter) and hyperfunctioning nodular goiter (sometimes called Plummer's disease, named for an early physician at the Mayo Clinic). Both forms involve the excessive manufacture of the thyroid hormone thyroxine.

Graves' Disease

The functions of the thyroid gland ordinarily are controlled by a hormone secreted by the pituitary gland. In Graves' disease, the thyroid gland is stimulated excessively by an abnormal antibody, and the normal thyroid-stimulating hormone (TSH) from the pituitary cannot be detected in the blood. The production of thyroid hormones is abnormally high. The amount of thyroxine in the blood also is high.

Hyperthyroidism involves an increase in the body's normal energy expenditure (that it, its basal metabolic rate). One manifestation of this change is an increased appetite because the body will demand more fuel for its added activity. The body generates excessive heat, so that patients with hyperthyroidism feel warm when others may be cool or comfortable. They may have a tremor of the hands with warm, sweaty palms. The heart pounds forcibly at a rapid rate. Occasionally the heart develops a rapid irregularity (atrial fibrillation). They also may have difficulty sleeping.

If you have hyperthyroidism, your thyroid gland will be enlarged, but often so slightly that it isn't noticeable. The abnormal antibody that stimulates the thyroid also has effects on the eyes and may cause protrusion, widening of the lids, excessive tearing and redness, and sometimes double vision.

SOURCE:

Larson, David E. (ed.). Mayo Clinic Family Health Book. New York: William Morrow, 1990. pp. 727, 730.

THYROID FUNCTION TESTS

Until recently, doctors lacked a sensitive test of "thyroid function"—a way to gauge if the gland was over- or underactive and by how much. But now a sophisticated new test can diagnose thyroid problems that have gone unrecognized in the past. And it allows doctors to gauge the optimum dose of replacement thyroid hormone that best suits each patient's needs.

The old thyroid function test measures blood levels of the main thyroid hormone, thyroxine. But a wide range of thyroxine levels can be considered "normal." A "low-normal" reading may be O.K. for one person's metabolism but too skimpy for another's. Using a highly sensitive technique, the new test measures a different hormone, thyroid stimulating hormone, or TSH.

TSH comes from the pituitary gland and does what its name suggests: stimulates the thyroid to release its hormone. The pituitary sends out TSH in response to the amount of thyroid hormone it senses in the blood. A high TSH level tells you the thyroid isn't making enough hormone.

Normal TSH levels vary less than normal levels of thyroid hormone, making TSH values easier to interpret. A low thyroxine reading, for example, suggests—but doesn't prove—that you have hyperthyroidism. Using the new TSH test, your doctor may not need to do other blood tests; a high TSH level confirms that hypothyroidism is present. And in most cases, the test can detect both hypo- and hyperthyroidism.

SOURCE:

"Do You Have a Thyroid Problem?" *Prevention* (July 1990): 53.

TREATMENT

Whatever your thyroid problem, chances are you take thyroid hormone to treat it. In hypothyroidism, thyroid hormone restores metabolism to normal. And most people diagnosed with hyperthyroidism ultimately take thyroid hormone, too. . . .

Today's thyroid medicine of choice is levothyroxine sodium. This newer, manmade version of natural thyroid hormone costs only about 15 cents a day.

But, unfortunately, not everyone uses the synthetic type. A study published last year in the *Journal of the American Medical Association* (May 12, 1989) found that many older people still take the natural kind, obtained from the thyroid glands of slaughtered animals. But in this case, "natural" may not be as healthy as synthetic. The thyroid hormone obtained from animals is unpredictable. The kind of animals used, what they ate, the season they were slaughtered—all can cause the hormone's potency to vary from one batch to another.

By contrast, the synthetic variety is pure, standardized from batch to batch and identical in chemical structure to human thyroid hormone. Many doctors have switched their patients from natural to synthetic thyroid, and some believe that all patients should switch. . . .

It's now known that thyroid hormone should be used only for specific disorders, such as hypothyroidism, benign goiter, thyroid nodule and cancer of the thyroid. Taking unnecessary thyroid probably isn't dangerous for most people but it's risky for some. If you're on thyroid medication but think you might not need it, don't discontinue therapy on your own. You can withdraw safely, but only under a doctor's care.

SOURCE:
"Do You Have a Thyroid Problem?" *Prevention* (July 1990): 50–52.

THYROID CANCER

Cancer of the thyroid is the most common endocrine malignancy but is an uncommon cancer, comprising only about 1 percent of invasive cancers. It is estimated that there will be about 12,400 new cases in 1991, 9,100 in women and 3,300 in men. People with these malignancies are usually treated successfully.

Although invasive thyroid cancer is uncommon, doctors often have to diagnose and treat thyroid nodules, since about 4 percent of adults develop them. Thyroid cancer commonly appears as a "cold" nodule, meaning that it does not take up radioactive iodine. About 20 percent of cold nodules are cancer.

Most cases occur between 25 and 65 years of age, and the age at diagnosis is one of the most important factors in predicting prognosis. Men under 40 and women under 50 have significantly lower rates of recurrence and better survival rates than older patients.

There are three types of thyroid cancer: well-differentiated, undifferentiated, and medullary carcinoma. Eighty percent are well-differentiated, and include papillary carcinomas and follicular carcinomas.

Papillary carcinomas are generally slow growing, with an 80 percent overall survival at 10 years. Even if tumor cells spread to regional lymph nodes or the lungs, survival may be more than 10 years. Tiny, clinically insignificant papillary carcinomas are found in 5 to 10 percent of thyroid glands examined at routine autopsies.

Follicular carcinomas occur in patients about 10 years older than those who get papillary carcinomas. Although these tumors are also usually slow growing, they behave somewhat more aggressively than papillary carcinomas.

Three percent of thyroid cancers are undifferentiated (anaplastic) carcinomas. They grow rapidly, behave aggressively and respond poorly to treatment.

Medullary carcinomas make up about 5 percent of thyroid cancers. These tumors secrete calcitonin, a tumor marker that is helpful in diagnosis and follow-up and also in screening relatives of those affected, since this tumor may occur on a familial, or inherited, basis. In the syndromes of multiple endocrine neoplasia (MEN), the cancer may be associated with tumors in other endocrine organs, such as pheochromocytoma of the adrenals, parathyroid cancer and islet cell cancer.

Other tumors that can arise in the thyroid gland include sarcomas, lymphomas, epidermoid carcinomas and teratomas. The thyroid gland can also be a site of metastasis from other cancers, especially cancers of the lung, kidney and breast, and melanoma.

SOURCE:
Dollinger, Malin. "Thyroid." In *Everyone's Guide to Cancer Therapy*. Kansas City: Andrews and McMeel, 1991. pp. 538–539.

RESOURCES

ORGANIZATIONS

American Thyroid Association. Walter Reed Army Medical Center, Washington, DC 20307.

Thyroid Foundation of America, Inc. Massachusetts General Hospital (ACC 7305), Boston, MA 02114.

BOOK

Bayliss, R. I. S. *Thyroid Disease: The Facts*. New York: Oxford University Press, 1982.

RELATED ARTICLES

Bartuska, Doris Gorka. "The Thyroid Factor." *Healthline* (June 1990): 5.

Lipman, Marvin. "Hypothyroidism: Avoidable 'Aging'." *Consumer Reports Health Letter* (October 1990): 78–79.

Salman, Karl, Jeffrey L. Miller, and others. "Selection of Thyroid Preparations." *American Family Physician* 40, no. 5 (November 1989): 215–219.

Santos, Edith T. de los, and Ernest L. Mazzaferri. "Thyrotoxicosis: Results and Risks of Current Therapy." *Postgraduate Medicine* 87, no. 5 (April 1990): 277–294.

Utiger, Robert D. "Therapy of Hypothyroidism: When Are Changes Needed?" *The New England Journal of Medicine* 323 (July 12, 1990): 126.

TOXIC SHOCK SYNDROME

(*See also:* MENSTRUATION)

OVERVIEW

Toxic shock syndrome (TSS) is a rare condition which occurs in association with infections caused by the *Staphylococcus aureus* bacterium. This organism is normally found on the skin and in the vagina and it does not produce a harmful effect. On occasion, however, it can cause skin infections and even abscess formations. In severe cases, the toxin produced by the bacteria is absorbed into the blood stream and causes TSS. The toxin appears to produce its effects by directly damaging the cell membranes in the tissues on the surface of the body.

The illness occurs most frequently in young menstruating women, but has been reported to occur in men and non-menstruating women of all ages. Although a definite explanation is not yet available, observations indicate that menstruating women who use tampons face a greater risk of becoming ill with TSS than women who do not. Ninety percent of the cases are associated with the use of tampons. Studies have shown that tampons, especially super-absorbent tampons, may produce conditions in the vagina which enable the bacteria to grow and produce the toxin. It is thought that tampons may dry, scratch or tear the lining of the vagina and that this environment speeds the body's absorption of the toxin. Other cases of TSS have developed from abscesses in association with surgical wound infections, abrasions, infected burns, shingles and a number of other conditions including leaving diaphragms or contraceptive sponges in place for several days.

An individual with TSS may experience any number of a wide variety of symptoms. Typically, the syndrome begins abruptly with a fever (frequently above 102°F), accompanied by headache, sore throat, vomiting, diarrhea, abdominal cramping and generalized aching. A rash, resembling a sunburn, may appear during the first two days of the illness and is often followed three to four days later by peeling skin, usually on the palms and soles. The patient often develops a progressive illness and is frequently in shock when presented for care. Adult respiratory distress syndrome, acute renal failure and abnormalities in literally every organ system may also be present. This syndrome can be fatal. Although TSS is rarely fatal in mild cases, the overall fatality rate is approximately five percent. Prompt diagnosis and treatment are essential.

Treatment for TSS depends on the severity of the case. If an abscess is present or a tampon in place, it should be removed. Most cases require hospitalization, and may require treatment in intensive care facilities. Shock is treated by the administration of intravenous fluids, which helps the body maintain steady blood pressure. Antibiotics are used to treat the infection.

Most patients recover within 7 to 14 days. However, recurrences are common among those women who developed the syndrome during menstruation. Since it is difficult to completely eradicate the staphylococcus organism from the vagina, up to one-third of these patients have a recurrence of the illness within six months. These recurrences have most frequently occurred during a menstrual period. For this reason, women who have had TSS are advised not to use tampons for several months following the illness. The recurrent illness is usually not as severe as the initial episode.

Women can reduce the risk of developing TSS by avoiding the use of tampons. Those who prefer to use tampons can reduce their risk by using them every other day of their period at the time of their heaviest flow, never leaving a tampon in place for longer than four hours, minimizing their use of high-absorbency tampons and never wearing a tampon during sleeping hours or for an entire day. They should use sanitary pads at night; this allows any vaginal irritation to heal, cutting down on the risk of infection. Women between the ages of 15 and 24 should be especially careful about tampon usage as they appear to be at a higher risk of contracting TSS than older women. If a woman develops a high fever and vomiting during her menstrual period, she should contact her doctor immediately.

SOURCE:
California Medical Association. "Toxic Shock Syndrome." *HealthTips* index WH-53 (December 1989/January 1990): 1–2.

TREATMENT

No treatment protocols for toxic shock syndrome are universally accepted. The need for hospitalization should be determined by the severity of the illness, tempered by the availability of follow-up care.

In all suspected cases, caution should be exercised since the illness may progress from mild to life-threatening within a matter of hours.

Treatment of an acute episode of toxic shock syndrome consists of supportive measures tailored to the patient's symptoms. The administration of a Beta-lactamase-resistant antibiotic during the acute episode has been shown to significantly reduce the risk of recurrence during subsequent menses. To date, no study has shown a clear advantage of parenteral over oral antibiotics. As in any potentially serious infection, the choice of antibiotic should be backed by sensitivity testing of cultures of the specific offending agent.

Seriously ill patients require aggressive intravenous fluid therapy, careful monitoring of cardiac and renal function, and close observation to detect any pulmonary dysfunction. Critically ill patients are best managed with the placement of an arterial line, a urethral catheter, and a pulmonary artery balloon-flotation catheter to assess cardiac function. Patients with acute blood loss secondary to coagulopathy may require fluid replacement with packed red blood cells and coagulation factors, as well as large volumes of isotonic crystalloid solutions. If fluid resuscitation alone is insufficient to restore perfusion to the vital organs, vasopressor therapy with dopamine is indicated.

At present, there is no convincing rationale for the use of glucocorticoids in patients with acute toxic shock syndrome. However, when other measures have proved inadequate, there is no reason to withhold steroids. Some investigators suggest that patients with refractory hypotension be given naloxone (Narcan) to antagonize the endorphins released during great stress. These endogenous endorphins are believed to depress cardiac function. When toxic shock stems from a localized infection, such as an abscess or cellulitis, surgery is indicated to drain the abscess or debride devitalized tissues.

SOURCE:
Bryner, Charles L., Jr. "Recurrent Toxic Shock Syndrome." *American Family Physician* 39, no. 3 (March 1989): 160.

PREVENTION—USE OF LOW ABSORBENCY TAMPONS

Prodded by a consumer watchdog group, the FDA has finally standardized tampon absorbency labeling. Beginning this month, it will be easier for a woman to choose the tampon with the lowest effective absorbency she needs—a step that will help protect her from toxic shock syndrome (TSS).

It took eight years and a lawsuit by the Ralph Nader-founded Public Citizen Health Research Group to get the FDA to act. But at last the new regulation is in effect, making each brand's "junior," "regular," "super" and "super plus" directly comparable.

Until now each manufacturer could use its own method of assigning absorbency ratings. In some cases, says the FDA, one brand's regular was actually more absorbent than another's super.

Helping women choose tampons with the least absorbency is important: TSS is thought to be caused by toxins produced by bacteria found in the presence of highly absorbent tampons.

Says Public Citizen attorney Patti Goldman: "It took too long. If they'd acted faster, lots of women could have been spared toxic shock."

The disease is not associated with sanitary napkins, and so new labeling also advises women to alternate between tampons and pads to further reduce their risk.

Last year, toxic shock struck one in 100,000 women of menstrual age—down considerably from the estimated seven to 13 cases per 100,000 in 1980 when the syndrome first surfaced. Dr. Anne Schuchat, a medical epidemiologist at the CDC, attributes the improved statistics to changes in tampon design—from high to medium absorbency—and to the fact that women are now using tampons intermittently.

SOURCE:
Newman, Jennifer. "With Tampons, Less is More: Now Consumers Know What They're Buying." *American Health* 9 (March 1990): 16–17.

RESOURCES

PAMPHLETS
Food and Drug Administration:

Toxic Shock Syndrome & Tampons. HHS Pub. No. (FDA) 90–4169. 1990. 7 pp.

Toxic Shock Syndrome Is So Rare You Might Forget It Can Happen. HHS Pub. No. (FDA) 85-4192. 1985. 7 pp.

RELATED ARTICLES

Farley, Dixie. "Preventing TSS: New Tampon Labeling Lets Women Compare Absorbencies." *FDA Consumer* (February 1990): 6–9.

Williams, Glyn R. "The Toxic Shock Syndrome: Many Cases Are Not Associated with Menstruation." *British Medical Journal* 300 (April 14, 1990): 960.

ULCERS

OVERVIEW

Ulcers are crater-like sores, generally a quarter to three-quarters of an inch in diameter but sometimes as large as an inch or two in diameter, that form in the lining of the stomach (gastric ulcers), or just below the stomach, at the beginning of the small intestine, in the duodenum (duodenal ulcers). The stomach is a great bag of muscle that crushes and mixes food with the digestive "juices," hydrochloric acid and pepsin. If the lining of the stomach or duodenum is damaged in one place or another, the acid and pepsin (thus the name, peptic ulcers) go to work on the lining as they would on food, breaking it down as though to digest it.

An ulcer is the result of an imbalance between aggressive and defensive factors. On the one hand, too much acid and pepsin can damage the stomach lining and cause ulcers; on the other hand (and more commonly), the damage comes first, from some other cause, making the stomach lining susceptible to the depredations of even an ordinary level of gastric acid.

The principal damagers of the stomach lining's defenses appear to be the bacteria *Helicobacter pylori* and nonsteroidal anti-inflammatory drugs (NSAIDs) such as aspirin, ibuprofen (Motrin, Advil, Nuprin), naproxen (Naprosyn, Anaprox), or piroxicam (Feldene). This is why older people, who often take NSAIDs—for arthritis, for example—are especially susceptible to ulcers. Just how *Helicobacter pylori* damages the stomach lining has not been completely explained; it may be that the bacteria is merely an opportunistic invader of already-damaged tissue. In any case, it has been shown in several studies that eliminating the bacteria leads to the prolonged healing of ulcers.

Smoking, drinking, and genetic makeup are also associated with ulcers. Smoking doubles your chances of getting ulcers; it will also slow the healing of ulcers and make them likely to recur. Studies on alcohol consumption and ulcers have been less conclusive, although alcoholic cirrhosis has been linked to an increased risk of ulcers, and heavy drinking has been shown to delay the healing of ulcers.

There have been studies that have linked stress and ulcers, but the difficulty of measuring stress—and, even more importantly, or gauging an individual's response to stress—have made it impossible to reach any well-supported conclusions about the connections between stress and ulcers. If there is a connection, it may be that the harried executive or parent loses crucial hours for relaxing and sleeping, replaces meals with cocktails and snacks, and counteracts hangovers with coffee and—worst of all—aspirin, thus doing the sort of harm to the stomach that encourages ulcers. Meanwhile, the roles of *Helicobacter pylori*, NSAIDs, and smoking are clear—and lead to clear strategies for treatment.

SOURCE:

"Ulcers: New Thinking on Causes and Cures." *Johns Hopkins Medical Letter: Health after 50.* (December 1990): 4.

DIAGNOSIS

If your doctor suspects ulcers, he or she will usually order what's known as an upper GI (gastrointestinal) series—an x-ray of your esophagus, stomach and duodenum. You will swallow a chalky liquid that contains barium, which makes the ulcer visible on the x-ray. The doctor may also order a gastroscopy, in which a flexible tube-shaped device with special light-conducting properties will be put down your throat to enable your doctor to see the ulcer and obtain tissue samples for microscopic examination to determine if the ulcer is cancerous. Some physicians may prefer to order a gastroscopy as the first diagnostic test instead of an x-ray.

SOURCE:

"Ulcers: New Thinking on Causes and Cures." *Johns Hopkins Medical Letter: Health after 50.* (December 1990): 5.

TREATMENT

Antacids

Still of value in ulcer treatment (mostly for duodenal ulcers), antacids neutralize the acid, relieve pain and promote mucosal healing. Antacids come in tablet or liquid form—liquids being the most effective. They are best taken one to three hours after meals and at bedtime. Their appeal is limited by rather short-lasting action. Aluminum hydroxide and magnesium hydroxide are the longest acting forms. Calcium carbonate (found in Tums and Rolaids) gives rapid relief but is apt to trigger "acid rebound"—a surge of acid after two or three hours. One big problem with antacids is failure to take the right amount: people often self-medicate without advice and stop taking the medication as soon as the pain vanishes, rather than continuing until the ulcer heals. Most antacids have some side effects—varying with the type chosen. Magnesium—containing brands commonly cause diarrhea. Aluminum compounds may cause constipation and prolonged therapy can disrupt mineral metabolism (possibly also contributing to the risks of Alzheimer's disease). Antacids rich in sodium should be avoided by people with high blood pressure and kidney or heart disease. Some antacids interfere with the action of other drugs, notably warfarin, digoxin, anticonvulsants, some antibiotics and anti-inflammatories.

Gastric acid suppressors (that reduce or arrest gastric acid secretion)

- Histamine H2-receptor blockers (acid-reducing drugs) have transformed ulcer management. Taken as tablets, H2-blockers act on the stomach's surface "receptors" and prevent release of histamine, one of the substances that stimulates hydrochloric acid secretion, inhibiting acid build-up. (Histamine is also involved in allergic reactions, but the receptors are different: ulcer drugs don't cure allergies.) The end result of H2-blocker treatment is less stomach acid which permits healing. These drugs can reduce ulcer pain within a few hours of the first dose, allowing ulcers to heal in a few weeks. The first of the H2-blockers on the market, cimetidine, introduced in the early 1970s, revolutionized ulcer treatment. Besides cimetidine (Tagamet) and ranitidine (Zantac), acid-suppressing drugs include the more recent famotidine (Pepcid) and nizatidine (Axid)—a single bedtime dose healing a duodenal ulcer in four weeks and a gastric ulcer in six to eight weeks.

Side-effects of H2-blockers, especially cimetidine, include dizziness, mental confusion and sleepiness (especially frequent in the elderly). They can also cause impotence in men and breast enlargement. The H2-blockers may also interact with other drugs (such as warfarin, theophylline and Valium).

- Proton-pump inhibitors. The recently approved and now available drug, omeprazole, is 10 times more powerful in suppressing stomach acid production than the H2-blockers, able to promote duodenal ulcer healing in two to four weeks, not necessarily as swift with gastric ulcer. This potent acid-inhibitor can suppress about 95 percent of stomach acid production. It is especially useful for treating people whose ulcers fail to respond to H2-receptor blockers or other medications and those with Zollinger-Ellison syndrome. Side effects include diarrhea, cramps, indigestion, gas (bloating) in some people.

Anti-cholinergics (inhibitors of acetylcholine)

In wide use before the arrival of the H2-receptor blockers but now mainly of historical interest, these drugs are still occasionally used in conjunction with new medications to treat stubborn ulcers and for the Zollinger-Ellison syndrome.

Gut lining protectors or barrier shields (ulcer coating, "cytoprotective" agents)

- Sucralfate (Sulcrate or Carafate)—an aluminum salt of sucrose—doesn't alter stomach acid levels, but coats the ulcer (crater), forming a barrier across which hydrochloric acid and pepsin cannot pass, permitting it to heal. Taken two to four times a day and at bedtime, sucralfate has fewer side effects than H2-blockers. However, about five percent of those on it report nausea, constipation or a metallic taste in the mouth. No clinically significant drug interactions have been reported.

Prostaglandin-like medications (a new class of synthetic prostaglandins with potent anti-ulcer properties)

- Misoprostol (Cytotec), a synthetic prostaglandin-E, is especially valuable for people such as arthritics who take ASA/aspirin or other NSAIDs that suppress natural prostaglandin production. Newly available in Canada, misoprostol decreases acid production and enhances the mucosal defences. Healing rates roughly parallel those with H2-receptor blockers, but one big advantage of the synthetic prostaglandins is their ability to combat the damaging effects of NSAIDs. (Misoprostol is highly effective in healing aspirin-induced ulcers.) Moreover, the latest studies suggest it can also protect against NSAID-induced kidney damage (a recently reported adverse effect of these anti-inflammatory drugs.) Misoprostol may be prescribed together with anti-inflammatories for arthritics. However, misoprostol's side effects—experienced by nine to 13 percent of patients—may limit its use, especially diarrhea, abdominal cramps and menstrual disturbances. Used inappropriately, it may cause uterine contractions and spontaneous abortion, so should never be prescribed to childbearing women. Other occasional adverse effects are headache, dizziness, fever and flushing. The long term effects are unknown.

Antibacterials

- Colloidal bismuth suspensions such as Pepto-Bismol (bismuth subsalicylate) might promote ulcer healing not by influencing gastric acid levels but by increasing prostaglandin secretion and suppressing *H. pylori* infections. Combination therapy with bismuth plus antibiotics may help to eradicate intestinal infections—therapy that's still experimental.

SOURCE:
"Drugs Used to Treat Peptic Ulcer Disease." *University of Toronto Faculty of Medicine Health News* 8, no. 5 (October 1990): 4.

* * *

Every year, 1 American in 1,000 develops an ulcer in the lining of the stomach. Most often appearing in people over 40 years of age, stomach ulcers can occur in people of all ages, including children. Stomach ulcers and ulcers that form in the esophagus and in the lining of the duodenum (the upper part of the small intestine) are called peptic ulcers because they need acid and the enzyme pepsin to form. Duodenal ulcers are the most common type, tend to be smaller than stomach ulcers, and heal more quickly, though much of what can be said about the cause, diagnosis, treatment, and future outlook for duodenal ulcers is also true for stomach ulcers. . . .

Stomach ulcers tend to recur, though this is less likely if the right kind of drug treatment is continued. If ulcers do return often, if they do not respond to medication, or if complications develop, surgery may become necessary. The failure of the ulcer to heal or to stay healed is one of the most important reasons for surgery. (In some cases, the failure to heal may indicate an ulcerating cancer.) Surgery has some risks and may have unpleasant aftereffects. For this reason, the doctor will help to determine whether surgery is necessary.

SOURCE:
Malagelada, Juan R. "About Stomach Ulcers." *National Digestive Diseases Information Clearinghouse Fact Sheet.* NIH Pub. No. 87-676. January 1987. pp. 1, 3.

RESOURCES

ORGANIZATION
National Digestive Diseases Information Clearinghouse. Box NDDIC, Bethesda, MD 20892.

PAMPHLETS
National Digestive Diseases Information Clearinghouse:

Bleeding in the Digestive Tract. NIH Pub. No. 89-1133. 1986.

Peptic Ulcers. (Patient Information Pamphlet).

National Institutes of Health, Office of Medical Applications of Research:

"Therapeutic Endoscopy and Bleeding Ulcers." *NIH Consensus Development Conference Statement* 7, no. 6 (March 6-8, 1989): 1–22.

BOOK
Decker, John L., and Paul N. Maton. *Understanding and Managing Ulcers.* New York: Avon, 1988.

RELATED ARTICLES

Clearfield, Harris R., and Richard A. Wright. "Update on Peptic Ulcer Disease." *Patient Care* (February 15, 1990): 28–40.

Feldman, Mark, and Michael Burton. "Histamine2-Receptor Antagonists: Standard Therapy for Acid-Peptic Diseases." (Second of Two Parts). *The New England Journal of Medicine* 323, no. 25 (December 20, 1990): 1749–1755.

Gilbert, Greg, Chao H. Chan, and Eapen Thomas. "Peptic Ulcer Disease: How to Treat It Now." *Postgraduate Medicine* 89, no. 4 (March 1991): 91–93, 96.

Lieberman, David. "Endoscopic Therapy for Bleeding from the Upper Gastrointestinal Tract." *Postgraduate Medicine* 87, no. 4 (March 1990) 75–88.

Ohning, Gordon, and Andrew Soll. "Medical Treatment of Peptic Ulcer Disease." *American Family Physician* (April 1989): 257–270.

URINARY INCONTINENCE

OVERVIEW

The National Institutes of Health estimates that at least 10 million Americans are stricken by urinary incontinence extreme enough to cost $10.3 billion annually to manage the problem. . . .

Women are far more prone to the problems than men for several reasons. For one thing, childbirth exerts a heavy toll on the bladder and the sphincter muscle that controls the urethra, the opening to the bladder. For another, men are equipped with a second sphincter muscle, inside the penis, that further thwarts an undesirable passage of urine during ejaculation. . . .

The problem for women mounts rapidly with age, as the loss of female hormones after menopause leads to a thinning and weakening of the urethral lining that is supposed to keep the bladder closed except during urination. Older men are also likelier to become incontinent as a result of prostate disease and neurological disorders like Alzheimer's. Several large epidemiological surveys have revealed that among people over 60, almost 40 percent of women and 20 percent of men are incontinent.

By far the most common kinds of incontinence are stress incontinence and urge incontinence. In stress incontinence, the bladder outlet is physically injured and allows urine to leak out when the abdomen presses down on the bladder, as happens during exercising, sneezing, and the like. Urge incontinence, so named because a person feels a desperate urge to urinate, results from the bladder spasming when it should be relaxed. Stress, urge or a combination of the two account for about 85 percent of all cases of incontinence.

For mild to moderate stress incontinence, exercises to strengthen the muscles that hold in urine can be very helpful, and there have been some improvements on Kegel exercises, the program for strengthening the pelvic muscles through rapid, repeated muscular contractions. . . .

When stress incontinence becomes severe, surgery is often the only remedy, but doctors are now trying a non-surgical approach to repairing the damaged urethra. Collagen is injected under the surface of the urethral lining, creating a mound of tissuelike material and allowing the urethra to close up again. Collagen injections can also be used to help lift a bladder that had dropped out of its proper position. The method is now in clinical trials at about six medical centers around the country. . . .

To treat both urge and stress incontinence, doctors often start patients on biofeedback or behavioral modification programs, in which people are taught to gradually lengthen the time between runs to the bathroom.

Urge incontinence is also amenable to medications that soothe the bladder spasms by blocking certain chemicals of the nervous system. One new drug, Micturin, is now in clinical trials in eight centers around the United States and seems quite promising, physicians said. Unlike other anti-spasm medications, Micturin can be taken in a single dose that lasts for 24 hours.

SOURCE:

Angier, N. "New Focus on Urinary Incontinence." *New York Times* (October 25, 1990): B7.

CONSEQUENCES OF URINARY INCONTINENCE

UI is extremely costly in both social and financial terms. Research on women reveals that UI causes depression and embarrassment, as well as limitation of routine activities, such as travel outside the home, visits with family and friends, and sexual activity. It is a major cause of institutionalization, and the widespread use of catheters to manage UI in nursing home residents increases the risk of recurrent urinary tract infection. Pervasive urine odor in nursing homes can discourage potential visitors and lower resident and staff morale.

Conservative estimates of the financial burden of UI are placed at over $10 billion. In 1983, the U.S. Surgeon General estimated that UI accounted for $8 billion in costs in nursing homes alone (Resnick). An NIH consensus Conference on UI in 1988 put the costs of UI care for those living in the community at twice that of nursing home residents (institutionalized persons constitute about 15% of those with UI). These figures represent a very large public and private expenditure, exceeding the total budget of the National Institutes of Health, the entire costs of the school lunch program for U.S. children, and dialysis for U.S. citizens with end-stage renal disease.

SOURCE:
Zones, J. S. "Urinary Incontinence Emerges as a Significant Health Issue." *Network News* (May/June 1990): 1.

TREATMENT

- Exercises often help. Many experts suggest Kegel or pelvic floor exercises as the first line of defence for stress and urge incontinence. Some will benefit, some will not. Exercises are now recommended not only for women, but also increasingly for men with moderate stress incontinence. . . .
- Bladder or behavior training using special bladder drills is another effective therapy for those with urge or stress incontinence, using breathing and relaxation to suppress the urge to urinate. People are taught to "hold on" for increasing times, and to void at regular, scheduled intervals, the interval being gradually extended over the weeks and months of training to the normal three to four hour lapse between voidings. The retraining scheme teaches people to resist urgency, and urinate by the clock rather than because of the urge. The cure rate is around 10–15 percent, with marked improvement in 75 percent of cases.
- Combined bladder training, Kegel exercises and variations on these strategies help many to overcome incontinence. They are sometimes also combined with hypnosis, biofeedback and other behavioural therapies. The training requires commitment and is generally best for younger or middle age groups.
- Medications for incontinence include muscle calmants (for urge incontinence) and estrogens for the stress type—which build up the genital tract's lining tissues. Some drugs work by dampening bladder contractions or increasing bladder capacity. But self-medicating with over-the-counter products is strongly discouraged without specific medical advice.
- Calcium channel blockers, which are widely used heart drugs, and the tricyclic antidepressant, imipramine (Desmopressin), can be useful for calming and drying out a leaky bladder but may cause undesirable urinary retention and are therefore not commonly used for incontinence.
- Bladder surgery in women with severe stress incontinence can be 90 per cent successful. The vaginal sling operation creates a hammock under the urethra to give support, and other operations can be used. More complicated surgical procedures include implantation of an artificial sphincter—a cuff which can be inflated to squeeze the urethra, impeding urine flow. Surgery is also used for overflow incontinence.
- Contigen injection using a type of collagen injected into the urethral lining is a promising new treatment for stress incontinence. Types of teflon have also been tried. The advantage of contigen injections is that they can be done as a rapid office procedure under local rather than general anesthetic. Preliminary results are encouraging. Ontario studies show a success rate of 60 per cent in men and 96 per cent in women. The procedure is already offered in certain specialist centres in Ontario (some University of Toronto hospitals) and British Columbia.
- For nocturnal enuresis (nighttime bedwetting) a small dose of Desmopressin may resolve the problem.

SOURCE:
"Treatment for Incontinence—Often Successful." *Health News* (University of Toronto) (June 1991): 8.

KEGEL EXERCISES

Dr. Arnold Kegel began researching the effectiveness of strengthening the pelvic floor muscles (those that hold the urinary and intestinal tracts and the reproductive organs in place) in the 1940s. Commonly prescribed during pregnancy to help prevent hemorrhoids and to ease labor by giving women greater control over the birth canal, Kegel exercises are an effective means of improving control over urination. These exercises reportedly increase sexual pleasure as well.

Kegel exercises are particularly helpful to those with stress or urge incontinence, because they increase ability to stop urine flow. Lying on a floor or bed, successively tighten the vaginal muscles, as if you were stopping urine flow, then the muscles of the anus, as if you were stopping a bowel movement. If you are unsure whether you are using the proper muscles, sit on a toilet and try actually stopping and starting urination as you begin to urinate. If you cannot stop urine flow, it means either that your muscles are weak, or that you are using the wrong ones. Biofeedback methods may be helpful to those who have difficulty identifying or controlling these muscles on their own.

Once you have identified these two muscle sets, tighten them in turn, pulling upward and inward. Hold these muscles tight, counting slowly to three, breathing slowly and deeply, and then relax. Do this five to ten times several times a day, increasing the number and length of contractions, and the number of sets over time. Eventually, you should be contracting the muscles for ten seconds or longer.

SOURCE:
"Kegel Exercises: Good for Women of All Ages." *Network News* (May/Jun 1990): 3.

BEDWETTING (ENURESIS)

Enuresis or bedwetting is an involuntary release of urine by night, day or both in children over age five, in the absence of any congenital (inherited) or physical abnormalities. Nighttime enuresis is usually due to a delay in the development of normal bladder control—slow maturation of the complex urine-voiding system. If there are no other symptoms or abnormalities, bedwetting is considered a common variant of normal development. (Male bedwetters outnumber girls by two to one up to age 11, after which the sexes even out.) . . .

While disruptive to a family, upsetting and uncomfortable for the child, bedwetting must be kept in perspective. For the most part, it is an "inconvenience," not a grave problem especially in younger children, more a housekeeping annoyance than a medical abnormality. Nocturnal bedwetters are not misbehaving; they do not do it on purpose. Many parents erroneously criticize, scold or punish an enuretic child. But parental disapproval only aggravates the situation and engenders shame and guilt in a child who cannot help wetting. Scolding won't cure the problem and parental pressure or criticism only worsens matters and may seriously diminish self-esteem in an incontinent child. If undertaken at all, treatment should include reassurance, perhaps gentle attempts to increase bladder holding or possibly use of an alarm system. In some cases, medication helps to dry up the urine flow for special occasions (a weekend away, a holiday or going to camp). Despite the fact that enuresis is usually beyond the child's control, many parents can't help becoming irritated by it. Some feel belittled, believing that their child's bedwetting reflects their own shortcomings as parents. A 1981 U.S. study found that 61 percent of parents with enuretic children were "very distressed" by their offspring's bedwetting, a third of them severely punishing the bedwetter. Yet punishment only makes life miserable for the child and cannot solve a transient condition that's not under conscious control.

SOURCE:
"Bedwetting: Usually Just a Transient Annoyance." *Health News* (June 1990): 11–12.

RESOURCES

ORGANIZATIONS

Continence Restored. 407 Strawberry Hill Avenue, Stamford, CT 06902.

Help for Incontinent People (HIP). P.O. Box 544, Union, SC 29379.

Simon Foundation for Continence. Box 835, Wilmette, IL 60091.

PAMPHLET

National Institutes of Health:

"Urinary Incontinence in Adults." *National Institutes of Health Consensus Development Conference Statement* 7, no. 5 (October 3–5, 1988). U.S. GPO 229-567-41181, 1989. 11 pp.

BOOKS

Burgio, K. L., and L. Pease. *Staying Dry: A Practical Guide to Bladder Control.* Johns Hopkins University Press. 1990. 176 pp.

Chalker, R., and C. Whitmore. *Overcoming Bladder Disorders.* Fairfield, OH: Consumer Reports Books, 1990. 368 pp.

RELATED ARTICLES

Farley, D. "Incontinence Comes Out of the Closet." *FDA Consumer* 21 (March 1987): 4–9.

"Incontinence: A Problem You Can Cure." *Johns Hopkins Medical Letter: Health After 50* (May 1991): 4–6.

Marks, J. L., and J. K. Light. "Male Urinary Incontinence: What do you Do?" *Postgraduate Medicine* 83, no. 7 (May 15, 1988): 121–127, 130.

Resnick, N. M. "Urinary Incontinence in the Older Person." *Harvard Medical School Health Letter*, suppl. (August 1990): 9–14.

Sloane, B., and N. Baum. "Urinary Incontinence in Women: Evaluation in the Primary-Care Office." *Postgraduate Medicine* 84, no. 5 (October 1988): 251–259, 262.

Thomas, Anita M., and Janice M. Morse. "Managing Urinary Incontinence with Self-Care Practices." *Journal of Gerontological Nursing* 17, no. 6 (June 1991): 9–14.

Turpie, I. D., and J. Skelly. "Urinary Incontinence: Current Overview of a Prevalent Problem." *Geriatrics* 44, no. 9 (September 1989): 32–38.

"Urinary Incontinence in Adults." *JAMA* 261, no. 18 (May 12, 1989): 2685–2690.

Walzer, Y. "Female Urinary Incontinence: Discerning the Exact Cause." *Postgraduate Medicine* 83, no. 7 (May 15, 1988): 78–92.

URINARY TRACT INFECTIONS

(*See also:* CYSTITIS)

OVERVIEW

Most urinary tract infections start in the lower urinary tract. Bacteria enter through the urethra and spread upward to the bladder causing cystitis, a bladder infection. Urethritis, an infection of the urethra, usually occurs at the same time.

Occasionally, bacteria that have infected the bladder travel up the ureters to the kidneys causing pyelonephritis, a kidney infection.

Urinary tract infections are usually caused by bacteria from the bowel that live on the skin near the rectum or in the vagina. These bacteria can spread and enter the urinary tract through the urethra. They then travel up the urethra causing infections in the bladder and, sometimes, in other parts of the urinary tract.

Sexual intercourse is one of the causes of urinary tract infections. Women may be prone to urinary tract infections after sexual relations because of their anatomy. In front of the vagina is the opening of the urethra. During intercourse, bacteria in the vaginal area could be massaged into the urethra by the back and forth motion of the penis. Bladder infections also tend to occur in women who change sexual partners or begin having sexual intercourse more frequently. Although it is rare, some women get an infection each time they have sex.

Waiting too long to urinate can also result in urinary tract infections. The bladder is a muscle that stretches to hold urine and contracts to expel it. If you go for hours without urinating, the bladder muscle is stretched beyond its normal capacity. Overfilling the bladder like this gradually weakens the muscle so that it can't contract with enough force to expel all of the urine it holds. Some urine remains in the bladder after urination. Any time this happens, the risk of a urinary tract infection increases.

There are certain other factors that increase your chances of having a urinary tract infection. If you are pregnant, if you had urinary tract infections as a child, if you are past menopause, or if you have diabetes, you are more likely to have an infection than other women.

Symptoms of urinary tract infections can come on suddenly. The first sign of a bladder infection is a strong urge to urinate (urgency) that cannot be delayed. As urine is released, a woman will feel a sharp pain or burning sensation (dysuria) in the urethra. Very little urine is eliminated and the urine may be tinged with blood. The need to urinate returns minutes later (frequency). Soreness may occur in the lower abdomen, in the back, or in the sides.

This cycle may repeat itself many times during the day or at night (nocturia). Most people normally urinate about six times a day, so if you are urinating more often, you may have a bladder infection.

If the bacteria enter the ureters and spread to the kidneys, symptoms such as back pain, chills, fever, nausea, and vomiting may develop in addition to the symptoms of a lower urinary tract infection.

Symptoms linked with a urinary tract infection, such as painful urination, can be caused by other problems such as infection of the vagina or vulva. Only your doctor can make the correct diagnosis. It is up to you to let your doctor know when you are aware of any of these changes.

Urinary tract infections are diagnosed on the basis of the number of bacteria and white blood cells found in a urine sample. To detect the presence of bacteria and white blood cells, a sample of your urine is examined under a microscope and also cultured in a substance that promotes the growth of bacteria. A pelvic exam may be needed as well.

SOURCE:
American College of Obstetricians and Gynecologists. *Urinary Tract Infections.* 1984. pp. 3–5.

URINARY TRACT INFECTIONS IN WOMEN

Because a woman's anatomy leaves her vulnerable to the bacteria that cause urinary-tract infections, one woman in four develops at least one infection in her lifetime, and many are plagued by recurrent infections.

Though most urinary-tract infections, commonly known as UTI's, do not pose a serious health hazard, they often lead to frequent, urgent, and painful urination.

The infections are usually caused by bacteria that commonly inhabit the skin of the anal area. Because a woman's urethra—the tube that carries urine from the bladder—is so short and close to the anal area, those bacteria can enter the bladder and cause a UTI.

Whether a urinary-tract infection takes hold in the bladder or spreads to the kidney depends mainly on the type of bacteria and on how long the infection goes untreated. There are three levels of infection:

Asymptomatic bacteriuria. Bacteria are present in the urine, but there are no symptoms. This "silent" infection can usually be detected by a routine urinalysis or urine culture.

Cystitis. This is a bladder infection, which is by far the most common type of UTI. You experience a frequent need to urinate, or a strong urge even when there's no need. The bladder wall becomes inflamed, causing pain in the lower abdomen and a burning sensation when you urinate.

Pyelonephritis. Bacteria have infected the kidney. Symptoms can include chills, fever, nausea, vomiting, and kidney pain, usually felt on either side of the small of the back. If it's left untreated, pyelonephritis can eventually lead to kidney damage.

Women who suffer from recurrent UTI's may be able to help prevent infection by taking these steps:

- Drink plenty of fluids. Ideally, that means a glass of water every two to three hours to flush out the bladder.
- Urinate frequently and completely. Don't hold your urine. The less time bacteria spend in the bladder, the less likely they are to cause infection.
- Urinate after sexual intercourse. Then drink more water to force urination several hours later as well.
- If you use a diaphragm, don't leave it in place any longer than necessary. (Oral contraceptives do not appear to increase the risk of infection.)

Many other suggestions are commonly offered to women who are prone to UTI's. Although there's little or no proof that they work, some of those tips seem sensible. Chief among them is the usual advice always to wipe from front to back after urination or a bowel movement.

Women with recurrent UTI's are also typically advised to take precautions, such as cleansing or a change of condoms, during sexual activities that might transfer bacteria from the anal area to the vaginal area.

Studies have found no difference in frequency of infection between women who use tampons and those who use menstrual pads. Whichever type you use, it makes sense to change tampons or pads often (if possible, every three to four hours) to discourage the growth of bacteria.

If mild symptoms of a urinary-tract infection begin to develop, you may be able to flush out the bacteria by drinking even more water. Some studies have suggested that the popular folk remedy, cranberry juice, is effective against mild infection. But it's likely that the effect is due to the water, not the cranberries, in the juice.

Another popular home remedy for mild infection is taking large doses of vitamin C to acidify the urine. However, that has not been found to inhibit the growth of bacteria.

SOURCE:
"What To Do about Urinary Tract Infections." *Consumer Reports Health Letter* 2 (October 1990): 73–74.

TREATMENT

Many urinary tract infections might perhaps spontaneously vanish even without treatment. But today's approach is to treat symptomatic cases with antibiotics geared to kill the causative bacteria. Most cases clear up quickly with a short course of antibiotics such as: amoxicillin, trimethoprim-sulfamethoxazole (Bactrim or Spectra), nitrofurantoin (Furadantim), and/or the newer quinolone products, such as norfloxacin (Noroxin), enoxacin and ciprofloxacin. The drugs are taken either as a single, large dose, or as a three to seven day course. Treatment is ideally continued until all symptoms are gone and a midstream urine sample becomes free of bacteria. A repeat infection requires another course of antibiotics. If an infection persists, more of the same antibiotic or a different drug may be tried as bacteria easily mutate and resistant forms may surface. If the UTI is associated with sexual activity, an antibiotic pill taken directly after intercourse may prevent cystitis.

For recurrent infections that return four, five or more times yearly, physicians may prescribe nightly, low-dose antibiotics for several months, with periodic checks to make sure that resistant strains aren't emerging (which would call for a change of drug). Sometimes people are given antibiotic tablets to keep at home, in case symptoms reappear. Should this happen they are instructed to collect a midstream sample before starting on the antibiotics so that a lab test can verify the causative agents. (NB. The urine sample shouldn't be left around as bacteria multiply fast at room temperature!)

SOURCE:
"Urinary Tract Infections Irritating but Rarely Dangerous." *Health News* (University of Toronto) 6 (December 1988): 3–4.

POSITIVE BENEFITS OF CIRCUMCISION

Routine circumcision of male newborns remains controversial. Roberts and Thompson debate the advantages and disadvantages of this procedure.

Recent studies have found that urinary tract infections are up to ten times more common in uncircumcised boys than in circumcised boys. According to Roberts, who takes the affirmative view, sequelae from urinary tract infections, such as pyelonephritis and end-stage renal disease due to renal scarring, might increase if circumcision were less widely practiced. Because of this evidence, the American Academy of Pediatrics has changed its policy. Previously, the policy stated that there are no absolute medical indications for routine circumcision. The policy now states that "circumcision may result in decreased incidence of urinary tract infection."

In the opposing view, Thompson points out that most data about the relationship between circumcision and urinary tract infections are not from prospective studies. Newborns from lower socioeconomic groups are more likely to be uncircumcised and to acquire infections, and data not corrected for these factors may be suspect. In addition, although circumcision is usually a benign procedure, it is not totally without side effects or complications. These include pain, hemorrhage, infection and surgical trauma. With the exception of pain, complications are rare. Yet it may be argued that an elective procedure with any risks should not be performed in the absence of conclusive evidence of benefit.

Although the authors disagree on whether neonatal circumcision should be routinely performed, both agree that the risks and benefits of circumcision should be discussed with all parents. (*Journal of Family Practice* 31 (August 1990): 185, 189.)

SOURCE:
"The Debate over Routine Circumcision: Tips from Other Journals." *American Family Physician* 43 (January 1991): 226.

RESOURCES

ORGANIZATIONS

American College of Obstetricians and Gynecologists. 600 Maryland Ave. SW, Suite 300 East, Washington, DC 20024.

National Institute of Arthritis, Diabetes, and Digestive and Kidney Diseases. Westwood Building, Room 657, Bethesda, MD 20205.

National Kidney Foundation. Two Park Avenue, New York, NY 10003.

PAMPHLETS

National Institute of Arthritis, Diabetes, and Digestive and Kidney Diseases:

Understanding Urinary Tract Infections. NIH Pub. No. 88-2097. 1988.

National Kidney Foundation:

Urinary Tract Infection. 1986. 6 pp.

BOOK

Chalker, Rebecca, and Kristene E. Whitmore. *Overcoming Bladder Disorders: Compassionate, Authoritative Medical and Self-Help Solutions for Incontinence, Cystitis, Interstitial Cystitis Prostate Problems, Bladder Cancer*. Fairfield, OH: Consumer Reports Books, 1990. 368 pp.

RELATED ARTICLES

"Editorials." *American Family Physician* 41, no. 3 (March 1990): 817–822, 824.

Johnson, Mary Anne G. "Urinary Tract Infections in Women." *American Family Physician* 41, no. 2 (February 1990): 565–571.

Lipsky, Benjamin. "Urinary Tract Infections in Men: Epidemiology, Pathophysiology, Diagnosis, and Treatment." *Annals of Internal Medicine* 110, no. 2 (January 15, 1989): 138–150.

Renner, John H. "Urinary Infections Common to Women." *Healthline* (May 1990): 12–13.

Wiswell, Thomas E. "Routine Neonatal Circumcision: A Reappraisal." *American Family Physician* 41, no. 3 (March 1990): 859–863.

UTERINE FIBROIDS

(*See also:* DILATION AND CURETTAGE [D&C]; HYSTERECTOMY)

OVERVIEW

Uterine fibroids, technically called leiomyomata but also called fibromyomas or myomas, are noncancerous growths on the uterus. Fibroids are thought to arise from the growth and division of a single muscle cell that develops within the muscular wall of the uterus, the myometrium. Fibroids may occur singly but are typically multiple in number. Although they start off within the wall of the uterus (intramural), they can grow toward the inside of the lining of the uterus (submucosal) or toward the surface (subserosal). If they grow away from the surface, they may develop a stalk—a pedunculated fibroid. They can range in size from small, pea-size lumps to very large masses (eight to ten inches or larger in diameter), which distort the uterus, making it large, bulky, and irregular in contour.

It is not well known what causes fibroids, although there may be some familial tendency to develop them. There does appear to be a link with the female hormone estrogen, as fibroids may increase in size during pregnancy, when estrogen levels are high, and decrease in size after menopause when estrogen levels are low. The growth of fibroids is unpredictable. They may remain relatively stable, or they may increase in size rapidly. They may be totally symptomless, or they may cause problems. The majority of women with fibroids (up to 80 percent) have no symptoms. If symptoms do occur, they may include a heavier menstrual flow or one of longer duration, increased menstrual cramping and backache, irregular or unpredictable bleeding, and lower-abdominal pressure, which is often described as an achy or heavy feeling or which may be associated with the need to urinate more frequently. Only very rarely do fibroids become cancerous (probably fewer than 0.1 percent).

SOURCE:
Hillard, Paula Adams. "What Are Uterine Fibroids?" *Parents* (March 1989): 183.

TREATMENT

When your clinician first diagnoses small leiomyomas, it is unlikely that you will need immediate surgery. Unless you have severe hemorrhage (bleeding) or unbearable pain, it will be safe for you to take time to think about your alternatives.

The first step is to be certain that leiomyomas are the cause of your symptoms or abnormalities. If you are having irregular bleeding or your uterus is enlarged, your clinician will probably recommend a D&C without delay to be certain that you don't have an unrelated malignancy, or a simple problem like uterine polyps. Similarly, prompt evaluation will be necessary if your clinician feels a mass in the area of your ovary. The mass is likely to be a leiomyoma if you have other leiomyomas on your uterus as well, but it is essential to be sure that unsuspected ovarian cancer is not present.

Once your diagnosis is confirmed, treatment options for fibroid tumors are:

- Wait; have frequent pelvic exams to detect rapid or excessive growth.
- Have myomectomy surgery to remove only the leiomyoma(s) and repair the uterus as much as possible.
- Have a hysterectomy.
- Consider drug treatment to induce temporary menopause (available in research programs).

Leiomyomas are unlikely to shrink or disappear on their own until after menopause. After menopause, no new leiomyomas are likely to develop, and those already present usually shrink in size. If symptoms have not been a problem before menopause, they rarely will be after menopause.

Before menopause, it is more likely that your leiomyomas will continue to grow and that you will gradually notice more and more symptoms. In the premenopausal years, leiomyomas usually do not improve with time; nor is there any simple medical treatment. . . .

If you would like to become pregnant in the future, you may want to consider myomectomy. Myomectomy may also be recommended if your clinician suspects that leiomyomas are causing infertility or repeated miscarriage. New laser techniques for myomectomy utilizing laser surgery are now available in some communities, and laser can be used in conjunction with traditional surgery (laparotomy) to decrease uterine bleeding as each leiomyoma is cut free from the uterine wall. Some types of fibroids can be located and removed with a hysteroscope and cautery.

In most cases, though, myomectomy surgery involves a standard 5-inch abdominal incision and postoperative recovery similar to that for abdominal hysterectomy. Your surgeon is likely to ask for your consent to possible hysterectomy when you plan myomectomy surgery. In some cases the location and size of the leiomyomas makes uterine repair technically difficult or even impossible, so hysterectomy may be necessary. Be sure to discuss this issue with your surgeon beforehand.

SOURCE:
Stewart, Felicia H., Gary K. Stewart, and others. *Understanding Your Body: Every Woman's Guide to a Lifetime of Health.* New York: Bantam. 1987.

GnRH AGONISTS (GONADOTROPIN-RELEASING HORMONE)

The one exception to the stagnant state of fibroid research involves a drug called leuprolide [Leupron]. Though the Food and Drug Administration has only approved the drug to treat prostate cancer, its ability to turn off male and female hormones has led doctors to try it for fibroids. Studies show that three months of injections of the drug, which can be given daily or in long-acting monthly doses, can cut the size of fibroids in half and decrease their blood supply.

Once the drug is stopped, however, the uterus returns to its previous state, fibroids and all. And the side effects of the drug have discouraged many doctors from prescribing it: Because it cuts off estrogen, the drug induces a temporary menopausal state, complete with such side effects as hot flashes and vaginal dryness. Also, women taking leuprolide experience an increased rate of bone loss—a problem that's disturbing, even though lost bone is quickly replenished when the drug is stopped.

Giving women small doses of estrogen and progesterone to compensate for the hormone drain can prevent reduction in bone mass, according to one small study. Still, doctors are hesitant to give the drug for more than six months because of the osteoporosis risk as well as the possibility of other, unforeseen, long-term side effects. Its main uses are to shrink large fibroids before surgery, making them easier to remove, and to help some women near menopause to avoid surgery. For them, taking the drug for short periods can sometimes provide temporary relief until menopause, when the growths shrink on their own.

These studies are not only exciting for their own sake, they may provide the field of fibroid research with a needed shot in the arm. By depriving fibroids of their natural growth fuel—estrogen—leuprolide sets up an artificial condition that may help answer some of the basic questions.

SOURCE:
Ranard, Ann. "The 'Good' Problem." *Health* (March 1990): 69.

* * *

The synthesis of the first gonadotropin-releasing hormone (GnRH) agonist in 1972 was followed by the development of a new class of drugs, the GnRH analogs, with potential widespread therapeutic applications in gynecology. Not since the development of oral contraceptives has there been so much excitement and enthusiasm among basic scientists, clinical investigators, and practitioners of reproductive medicine. It is anticipated that the GnRH agonists will have a major impact on gynecologic care in the 1990s.

Uterine leiomyomas are a common gynecologic problem that often present with symptoms related to enlarged uterine size, excessive bleeding, or both. Because these neoplasms are estrogen dependent, it follows that a GnRH agonist-induced hypogonadal state will lead to a reduction or resolution of symptoms related to excessive myoma size or bleeding. . . . Unfortunately, most women experience a relatively rapid reversal of these therapeutic effects after cessation of GnRH agonist treatment. The transient nature of these beneficial effects has limited the efficacy of GnRH agonists as a primary medical therapy for uterine leiomyomas. In addition, the profound hypoestrogenic environment induced by GnRH agonists has raised concerns regarding the safety of long-term GnRH agonist treatment. . . .

Treatment of women with uterine leiomyomas with GnRH agonists has been shown to result in a reduction in uterine and fibroid size, a decrease or abolition of menstrual flow with a resultant increase in hemoglobin concentrations, and a decrease in intraoperative blood loss in women undergoing hysterectomy or myomectomy. Long-term GnRH agonist treatment is limited by concerns about increased bone resorption and other hypoestrogenic side effects. Future research will focus on the safety and efficacy of long-term GnRH agonist hormone add-back regimens and preoperative treatment.

SOURCE:

Friedman, Andrew J., Susan M. Lobel, and others. "Efficacy and Safety Considerations in Women With Uterine Leiomyomas Treated With Gonadotropin-Releasing Hormone Agonists: The Estrogen Threshold Hypothesis." *American Journal of Obstetrics and Gynecology* (October 1990): 1114–1115, 1119.

RESOURCES

ORGANIZATION

American College of Obstetricians and Gynecologists. 600 Maryland Ave. SW, Suite 300 East, Washington, DC 20024.

RELATED ARTICLES

Dranov, Paula. "An Unkind Cut." *American Health* (September 1990): 36–41.

Podolsky, Doug. "Saved From the Knife: New Treatments Mean Many Women Can Avoid Hysterectomy." *U.S. News & World Report* (November 19, 1990): 76.

Ranard, Ann. "Fibroids—Are They Dangerous?" *Redbook* (September 1990): 28, 30.

Vollenhoven, B. J., A. S. Lawrence, and others. "Uterine Fibroids: A Clinical Review." *British Journal of Obstetrics and Gynaecology* 97 (April 1990) 285–298.

White, Evelyn C. "The Fibroid Epidemic (Uterine Tumors Affect Many Black Women) (Includes Related Information About Detection, Treatment, and Protection Against Fibroids)." *Essence Magazine* (December 1990): 22.

VACCINES

(*See also:* FLU; MEASLES)

OVERVIEW

When smallpox was wiped out in the 1970s, the achievement seemed to herald a new era of control over disease through immunization. Measles was on the decline, and officials predicted it would be eradicated altogether by 1982.

Yet measles, while down dramatically from the pre-vaccine years, is on the rebound. Health authorities cite two probable reasons: not all children are vaccinated, and a single dose of the vaccine does not provide full immunization in all cases.

Ideally, a second vaccination against measles would be given to all people born after 1956. (Virtually everyone born before 1957 has had the disease and is immune.) But public health officials say present resources—the supply of vaccine and the funding to administer it—couldn't accommodate that demand. Instead, a second dose may be offered to those adults born after 1956 who are most likely to be exposed to measles (new health care workers, teachers, and college students, for example). Routine immunization guidelines for children will add a second dose.

The resurgence of measles illustrates that certain vaccinations can be critical for adults—and not just to protect travelers from exotic diseases. In fact, you may face added danger from "childhood" diseases.

Measles, for example, can be especially harmful to adults, possibly leading to pneumonia, encephalitis, and even death. Mumps, which has also made a comeback, can cause inflammation of the sexual organs and other severe complications in adults. (In October 1987, mumps struck at least 116 people who worked on the floor of the Chicago futures exchange.)

The proportion of people who are not protected against tetanus and diphtheria increases with age. Recent surveys indicate that at least 40 percent of people over the age of 60 lack adequate protection from those two diseases. Rubella is usually mild in adults, but it can be devastating to a developing fetus, often resulting in miscarriage or birth defects.

Don't assume you were protected as a child. Even if you were, some vaccines (tetanus, diphtheria) need to be updated periodically.

Piecing together an immunization history is a challenge for many adults. If you're completely or partially unvaccinated, your physician can help you determine an appropriate course of action. The first step will be to round up your medical records. If they are incomplete or raise doubts, antibody tests can check your exposure to some diseases or their vaccines. Or your physician may simply administer certain vaccines.

For some adults, however, the known risk from a vaccine may be greater than the possible risk of infection from the disease itself. That's often the case with pregnant—or potentially pregnant—women, whose fetuses may be endangered. Vaccination is especially risky during the three months before and after becoming pregnant. Vaccines can also pose risks to people who have certain disorders or who take drugs that lower their immunity.

Before you travel, consult your local or state health department to see if your destination requires vaccinations.

SOURCE:

"Why Immunize? Those Shots Are Not Just Kid Stuff." *Consumer Reports Health Letter* (September 1989): 6–7.

DTP VACCINE

One of the best ways to prevent Diphtheria, Tetanus and Pertussis is through immunization with DTP vaccine. DTP is actually three vaccines—Diphtheria, Tetanus, and Pertussis—combined into one shot. Five DTP shots are needed for complete protection, with the first shot given at 2 months of age. Young children should be given three DTP shots in the first year of life and a fourth shot at about 15 or 18 months of age. A fifth shot, or booster, is given between the fourth and sixth birthdays to children.

DTP vaccine provides protection against tetanus in over 95 percent of those who get the recommended number of shots. The diphtheria and pertussis parts of the vaccine are not quite as effective, but still prevent the diseases in most children. They also make the diseases milder for those who do catch them.

Children 7 years of age and older should take a different vaccine called Td. Td does not contain the pertussis part of the vaccine, because pertussis is not very serious in older children. Td also has less of the diphtheria part, because reactions to diphtheria vaccine occur more often among older children, especially those who have had previous doses. Booster shots of Td vaccine should be taken every 10 years throughout life.

There is a third vaccine preparation called DT, which contains the full diphtheria and tetanus parts, but no pertussis part. DT is given to children under 7 who should not receive the pertussis vaccine. Generally, these are children who have had certain reactions, such as very high fever or convulsions, after a previous DTP shot. Report any reactions to your health care provider. He or she can then determine whether your child should continue to receive DTP or should receive DT instead.

With DTP vaccine, most children will have a slight fever and will be cranky for up to 2 days after getting the shot. Half will develop some soreness and swelling in the area where the shot was given. Occasionally, more serious side effects occur. Out of about every 330 DTP shots given, one child develops a temperature of 105°F or greater. About one child in 100 experiences continuous crying lasting 3 hours or more, and about one in 900 experiences unusual, high-pitched crying. Convulsions may occur once in about 1,750 shots. Episodes of limpness and paleness may also occur about once in 1,750 shots. Children who have previously had convulsions (from any cause) may be more likely to have another one after shots containing pertussis vaccine (DTP).

If your child has a history of convulsions or other neurologic disorders, check with your doctor before having that child vaccinated with DTP. Even though the risk of such children suffering serious reactions following a DTP shot is still very small, the risk is higher than in other children. Children whose brothers and sisters or parents have a history of convulsions are also slightly more likely to have a convulsion following a DTP shot. However, this risk is so small and the benefits of DTP so great that most children should still be immunized. Usually these convulsions are caused by fever, and not the vaccine itself. Some experts suggest that fever-reducing drugs (acetaminophen-based products such as Tylenol™), given at the time of vaccination and every 4-6 hours over the next 2 to 3 days, will reduce the likelihood of fever and therefore should also reduce the likelihood of fever-associated convulsions. Most experts believe that convulsions with fever do not cause any permanent damage to the child.

More serious reactions to DTP are very uncommon. Rarely, permanent brain damage has been reported after a child has been vaccinated with DTP. However, most experts now agree that DTP has not been proven to be a cause of brain damage. Side effects from DT or Td vaccine are not common and usually consist only of soreness and slight fever. As with any drug or vaccine, there is a very slight possibility that other serious problems, or even death, could occur. Some people have questioned whether DTP shots might cause Sudden Infant Death Syndrome (SIDS), but studies have not shown this to be the case.

SOURCE:
Public Health Service, Centers for Disease Control. *Parents Guide to Childhood Immunization*. 1991. pp. 6-8.

DTP VACCINE—SAFETY CONCERNS

By far the vaccine that has inspired the most fear is the whole-cell pertussis shot (so called because it's made of entire dead bacteria). Linked with complications ranging from fever to seizures, the vaccine is even accused of causing brain damage and death.

Other vaccines have come under scrutiny as well: Measles and mumps vaccines, given as part of the MMR shot (measles, mumps, rubella), can cause fever, rashes and swollen glands in children. (Rubella, the other part of the shot, has been suspected of sometimes causing rheumatoid arthritis when given to adults.) The oral polio vaccine can in extremely rare instances actually cause the disease.

The pertussis vaccine, however—usually given in a series beginning at two months of age—is the subject of worldwide controversy. In the mid '70s fear of adverse vaccine reactions in Great Britain drove immunization rates down to near 30% for pertussis. Several years later, as the "herd immunity" effect of group vaccination wore off, whooping cough cases began to climb. The English reported 66,000 cases in 1978—compared with an annual rate between 2,000 and 17,500 for the years 1969 through 1977. As the disease spread, more and more people opted to get shots.

Today, 75% to 80% of the English are immunized and the case load dropped to 11,700 last year. In 1976, Japan's pertussis vaccination rate dropped to about 10% but now is back up to over 80% in part because of a new, purified form of the vaccine. Sweden, however, hasn't vaccinated against pertussis since 1979, and the disease is prevalent.

Today, some scientists are saying the worst fears about the vaccine simply aren't justified.

SOURCE:
Flippin, Royce. "The Vaccine Debate: Kids at Risk?" *American Health* (July/August 1990): 50.

DTP VACCINE—EVIDENCE OF SAFETY

The article by Griffin et al. in this issue of [*JAMA*] is the third recent controlled study that has examined the risk of seizures and other acute neurological illnesses after immunization with pertussis-containing vaccines. In these three studies, which involved about 230,000 children and 713,000 immunizations, no evidence of a causal relationship between pertussis vaccine and permanent neurological illness was found. . . .

It is now the last decade of the 20th century, and it is time for the myth of pertussis vaccine encephalopathy [degeneration of brain tissue] to end. Historically, it is not surprising that physicians tended to blame pertussis immunization for severe neurological events and deaths. First of all, when pertussis immunization was undertaken, we already had vaccines and antitoxins (smallpox and rabies vaccines and tetanus antitoxin) that caused encephalitis, anaphylaxis, and immunologic neurological illness. Reactions were noted in temporal association with early attempts at pertussis immunization. The initial vaccines were not standardized, and it is likely that some of the initial reactions were the result of excess endotoxin, other vaccine ingredients, or immunization methods. However, it is clear from the studies reviewed above that the major problem has been the failure of observers to separate sequences from consequences. The two are not synonymous.

The national immunization programs in the United States have enjoyed enormous success. In particular, the universal use of pertussis vaccine has prevented death and retardation in thousands of children over the last 40 years. Unfortunately, over the last 8 years the vaccine has been under attack because of the historical medical belief that it can cause brain damage. This belief was never a major medical concern because the benefit of the vaccine was clearly much greater than even the perceived risk. Unfortunately, because of the sensationalistic media, the organization of a group of parents who attribute their children's illnesses and deaths to pertussis vaccine, and the unique destructive force of personal injury lawyers, we now have a national problem that shouldn't be. . . .

We need to end this national nonsense. To do this, we need vaccine information relating to risks and benefits that represent true scientific evidence (such as reviewed in this report) and not the wishes of special interest groups. Second, we need to revise the recommendations for vaccine contraindications so that they reflect the knowledge of 1990. Last, new vaccines are needed, not to prevent nonexistent problems such as "pertussis vaccine encephalopathy," but to decrease the many disquieting reactions, such as high fever, persistent uncontrollable crying, and hypotonic hyporesponsive state, that do occur with presently available whole-cell pertussis vaccines.

SOURCE:
Cherry, James D. "'Pertussis Vaccine Encephalopathy': It Is Time to Recognize It as the Myth that It Is." *JAMA* 263, no. 12 (March 23/30, 1990): 1679-1680.

DTP VACCINE—PRECAUTIONS

Most kids who get the pertussis vaccine have no serious side effects. But in rare instances, major complications do arise. The CDC has now developed the following checklist to help identify high-risk kids who should not get the pertussis portion of the DTP vaccine.

- Anyone over age seven.
- Children with a fever-related illness.
- Those with a history of convulsions (with or without fever).
- Children undergoing immunosuppressive therapy.
- Children with an underlying neurological disorder, such as epilepsy or infantile spasms.

Children who've had one of the following reactions to a previous DTP shot should not receive any more pertussis shots: allergic hypersensitivity; fever of 105 [degrees] or higher within 48 hours of the shot; a collapse or shock-like state within 48 hours; persistent crying for three or more hours, or unusually high-pitched crying within 48 hours; convulsions (with or without fever) within three days; impaired or reduced consciousness within a week.

The grassroots organization Dissatisfied Parents Together lists the following as high-risk factors not officially recognized by the CDC:

- Any illness, including runny nose, cough, ear infection or diarrhea, up to one month prior to a DTP shot.
- A family member who has reacted severely to DTP.
- A personal or family history of severe allergies.
- Premature delivery, low birth weight or birth complications.
- A family history of convulsions.

SOURCE:
Flippin, Royce. "The Vaccine Debate: Kids at Risk?" *American Health* (July/August 1990): 52.

MUMPS AND RUBELLA

Mumps Immunization

To be considered immune from mumps, a child must be able to provide (1) proof of physician-diagnosed mumps, (2) laboratory evidence of mumps immunity, or (3) evidence of having been vaccinated with live mumps virus vaccine at age 12 months or older. All healthy children who have never had mumps should be vaccinated on or after their first birthday. If you are not sure, it is safe to have your children vaccinated or revaccinated against mumps, even though they may be immune. The vaccine, which has been in use since 1967, also can be given to older children and adults. It is very effective, and one injection gives a child long-lasting protection.

Mumps vaccine is usually given in the combination vaccine MMR, which also protects against measles and rubella. MMR is routinely given at 15 months of age. Many children will get a second dose of mumps vaccine when they get a second MMR shot during their school years.

Laws requiring schoolchildren to be immunized against mumps now exist in 39 of the 50 states. States with weak or no school requirements have more cases of mumps.

Rubella Immunization

All healthy children should be immunized after their first birthday. The rubella vaccine, which has been in use since 1969, is highly effective and one injection produces long-lasting, probably lifelong, protection.

Rubella vaccine is available by itself or in combination vaccines that protect against measles and rubella (MR); or measles, mumps and rubella (MMR). These vaccines should be given at 15 months of age.

Experts also recommend that adolescents and adults who are not known to be immune to rubella should receive rubella vaccine (or MMR if they might also be susceptible to measles or mumps). This is especially important for women of childbearing age. Even if you have had an illness which a doctor told you was rubella, this is not proof of immunity since rubella can be easily confused with other illnesses. You should consider yourself immune to rubella only if (1) you can document that you were vaccinated against rubella on or after your first birthday, or (2) you have the results of a blood test stating that you are immune.

If there is any doubt, it is safe to get vaccinated or revaccinated against rubella, even if you are already immune.

Women should not receive rubella vaccine if they are pregnant or might become pregnant within 3 months. However, if you **are** vaccinated against rubella while you are pregnant, it is not ordinarily a reason to interrupt the pregnancy, because there is no known risk of damage to the unborn child.

All 50 states have laws requiring schoolchildren to be immunized against rubella.

SOURCE:
Centers for Disease Control. *Parents Guide to Childhood Immunization.* 1991. pp. 17-18, 20-21.

INFLUENZA AND PNEUMOCOCCAL VACCINES FOR ADULTS

Influenza

Influenza vaccination is recommended yearly. Those at greatest risk for severe complications of influenza should have priority in vaccination programs: (1) adults with chronic cardiopulmonary disease severe enough to require either regular medical follow-up or hospitalization in the last year, and (2) residents of nursing homes and other chronic care facilities. Others who would benefit from vaccination include medical personnel who have extensive contact with high-risk patients; healthy adults over age 65; and adults with chronic metabolic or renal disease, those with anemia, and those receiving immunosuppressive drugs. Vaccination is recommended also for otherwise healthy adults who provide essential community services.

Local reactions (erythema and tenderness) at the site of injection are common, but fevers, chills, and malaise (which lasts in any case only 2-3 days) are rare. Like measles, mumps, and yellow fever vaccines, influenza vaccine is prepared using embryonated chicken eggs, and persons with a history of anaphylaxis to eggs should not be vaccinated.

Pneumococcal Pneumonia

Pneumococcal vaccine contains purified polysaccharide from 23 of the most common strains of *Streptococcus pneumoniae,* which cause 90% of bacteremic episodes in the USA. Although the efficacy of pneumococcal vaccine has been questioned, it is presently recommended for patients at increased risk for developing severe pneumococcal disease, especially asplenic patients and those with sickle cell disease. It is also recommended for adults who are at increased risk of developing pneumococcal disease, including those with chronic illnesses (e.g., cardiopulmonary disease, alcoholism, cirrhosis, cerebrospinal fluid leaks), those who are immunocompromised (e.g., patients with Hodgkin's disease, lymphoma, chronic renal failure, nephrotic syndrome, and asymptomatic or symptomatic HIV infection), and those taking immunosuppressive medications. In addition, it is recommended for all individuals over 65 years of age. A single dose of vaccine usually confers lifelong immunity. Revaccination every 5-6 years should be considered only in those at highest risk of fatal pneumococcal infection (e.g., asplenic patients) and those known to have a rapid decline in antibody titers (e.g., nephrotic syndrome, transplant recipients, renal failure). Revaccination should also be considered for high-risk individuals previously immunized with the older 14-valent vaccine. Since immunocompetent patients respond best to the vaccine, it should be given before splenectomy or starting chemotherapy if that can be anticipated.

Mild reactions (erythema and tenderness) occur in up to 50% of recipients, but systemic reactions are uncommon. The incidence of adverse reactions with revaccination is unknown but is probably related to the interval between vaccinations. Early reports suggested frequent adverse reactions when revaccination occurred within 1-2 years. Subsequent reports have indicated few adverse reactions when revaccination occurs 5 or more years later.

SOURCE:

Schroeder, Steven A., and others (eds.). *Current Medical Diagnosis & Treatment 1991.* Norwalk, CT: Appleton & Lange, 1991. pp. 935-936.

RESOURCES

BOOKS

Fisher, Barbara Loe. *A Shot in the Dark*. Avery Publishing, 1991.

Guide for Adult Immunization. Philadelphia: American College of Physicians, 1990.

RELATED ARTICLES

Centers for Disease Control, Immunization Practices Advisory Committee (ACIP). "General Recommendations on Immunization." *JAMA* 262, no. 2 (July 14, 1989): 187–191.

Centers for Disease Control, Immunization Practices Advisory Committee (ACIP). "General Recommendations on Immunization." *JAMA* 262, no. 3 (July 21, 1989): 339–340.

Gillum, Jack E., and others. "Current Immunization Practices: 1. Polio, Diphtheria, Tetanus, Pertussis, Measles, Mumps, Rubella, and Influenza." *Postgraduate Medicine* 85, no. 2 (February 1, 1989): 183–198.

Griffin, Marie R., and others. "Risk of Seizures and Encephalopathy After Immunization with the Diphtheria-Tetanus-Pertussis Vaccine." *JAMA* 263, no. 12 (March 23/30, 1990): 1641–1645.

"Immunization Update: Why Are Adults Getting Childhood Diseases? What Protection Do You Need?" *Mayo Clinic Health Letter* (August 1990): 4–5.

U.S. Preventive Services Task Force. "Childhood Immunizations." *American Family Physician* 40, no. 4 (October 1989): 115–118.

VASECTOMY

DEFINITION

Vasectomy, a procedure for male sterilization involving the bilateral surgical removal of a portion of the vas deferens. Vasectomy is most commonly performed as an office procedure using local anesthesia. The procedure is also performed routinely before removal of the prostate gland to prevent inflammation of the testes and epididymides. Potency is not affected. A signed and witnessed form indicating informed consent is usually required before performance of the procedure.

SOURCE:
Mosby's Medical and Nursing Dictionary. 3d ed. St. Louis: Mosby, 1990. p. 1226.

OVERVIEW

Vasectomy is a safe and effective method of male sterilization. The procedure and necessary follow-up care can usually be performed in an office setting. Failure of the procedure may be due to incorrect identification of the vas, recanalization or the presence of an accessory vas. Vasectomy is an effective method of male sterilization that can be offered by family physicians. The procedure is safer and less expensive than female sterilization and can be performed in the office with minimal equipment.

Vasectomy is indicated for the sterilization of men who no longer wish to be fertile. The procedure must be considered permanent. Although vaso vasostomy [reconnection or reversal] can be performed, it is not always successful. Therefore, if the patient has any doubt about his future desire to father children, vasectomy should not be performed.

While most patients seeking vasectomy are married with several children, there are other legitimate reasons for men to seek sterilization. These may include the health of the patient's partner, marriage to a woman who already has children, and a careful decision by a couple who does not want to have children. While many physicians hesitate to sterilize childless individuals, thoughtful counseling and detailed informed consent will reduce medical and legal liability while permitting these patients to choose the family planning method that best suits their needs. . . .

Although a variety of vasectomy techniques are advocated, all have the same goal: permanent interruption of the vas deferens. To achieve this, the vas must first be correctly identified and divided, and at least one of the cut ends must be permanently obstructed. Many surgeons recommend that the sheath of the vas deferens between the divided ends should also be obliterated. . . .

The most difficult aspect of the procedure is locating the vas deferens. This is accomplished by compressing the tissue within the scrotal sac above the testis and feeling for the typically firm tube. Once identified, the vas can be manipulated close to the skin and away from adjacent structures.

SOURCE:
Greenberg, M. J. "Vasectomy Technique." *American Family Physician* 39, no. 8 (January 1989): 131, 132.

RISKS OF TESTICULAR CANCER

A small study of men who had vasectomies has found that an unexpectedly large number later developed testicular cancer.

The researchers urged that other scientists undertake larger studies to verify the findings and to determine the risk, if any, of the increasingly popular form of contraception. Earlier studies have shown conflicting results about a link between vasectomy and testicular cancer.

The study involved 3,079 men who had a vasectomy in one hospital in Edinburgh from 1977 to 1987. Vasectomy involves severing the tubes that transport sperm, to prevent the ejaculation of sperm during intercourse. Eight of the men developed testicular cancer; only about two cases would be expected in a group that size.

The Scottish team, headed by Dr. A. R. J. Cale at Bangour General Hospital in Edinburgh, reported their findings in the Feb. 10 issue of *The British Medical Journal.* They urged that doctors carefully check their patient's testicles for evidence of a cancer before and after the procedure.

Testicular cancer is relatively uncommon in the United States. The American Cancer Society in Atlanta says that testicular cancer will affect 5,900 men this year and cause 350 deaths.

The new report raises "an issue that is important to pursue," said Dr. Gerald P. Murphy, a urologist who is the cancer society's chief medical officer; he agreed on the need for further studies.

Doctors advise men to be alert to any change in size or shape of the testicles, regardless of whether they have had a vasectomy.

A study reported in England three years ago showed findings similar to those from Edinburgh. The earlier study suggested that the tumors had been present at the time of surgery.

Four larger studies combining data from several medical centers did not find a link between vasectomy and testicular cancer. However, the researchers said an even larger study would be needed to determine whether the link was valid.

In the new Scottish study the average interval between vasectomy and the diagnosis of testicular cancer was 1.9 years. The range was from three months to four years. The relatively short time interval, the Scottish researchers said, raises the question whether vasectomy could accelerate growth of small tumors already present in the testicles and overlooked at the time of surgery.

It is not known why vasectomy would accelerate tumor growth. Earlier studies have shown immunological changes after the procedure.

SOURCE:

Altman, L. K. "Study Raises Question of Cancer-Vasectomy Link." *The New York Times* (March 6, 1990): C3, col. 3.

VASECTOMY REVERSAL (VASOVASOSTOMY)

Vasectomy has been one of the most commonly performed operations in the United States over the past several years. Subsequently, the frequency with which vasectomy reversal has been performed has increased dramatically because many of these vasectomized men desire to regain their fertility. The most common reason for requesting a vasovasostomy is divorce followed by remarriage and the desire to have children with the new wife. Other motivating factors include the desire for more children, religious conversion, change of heart about the idea of being sterile, and, rarely, loss of a child.

The popularity of vasovasostomy in recent years can be attributed to improvements in operative techniques, instruments, optics, and, most importantly, results. Controversy continues regarding the most effective operative technique. From a review of the relevant literature on the subject, we have concluded that (1) surgeons who perform the procedure with regularity obtain better results than those who do it occasionally; (2) the use of stents is not advantageous if the anastomosis [surgical joining of two ducts] is watertight; (3) the use of optical aids probably increases the success rate; and (4) the relative merit of specific techniques such as the two-layer microscopic anastomosis cannot be evaluated definitively because of the lack of data.

SOURCE:

Yarbro, E. S., and S. S. Howards. "Vasovasostomy." *Urologic Clinics of North America* 14, no. 3 (August 1987): 515.

RESOURCES

ORGANIZATIONS

Association for Voluntary Sterilization Inc. 122 E. 42nd Street, New York, NY 10168.

Planned Parenthood Federation of America. 810 Seventh Avenue, New York, NY 10019.

BOOK

Shapiro, H. I. *The New Birth Control Book: A Complete Guide for Women and Men.* New York: Prentice-Hall, 1988. 288 pp.

RELATED ARTICLES

Alderman, P. "The Lurking Sperm: A Review of Failures in 8879 Vasectomies Performed by One Physician." *JAMA* 259, no. 21 (June 3, 1988): 3142–3144.

McCormack, M., and S. Lapointe. "Physiologic Consequences and Complications of Vasectomy." *Canadian Medical Association Journal* 138 (February 1, 1988): 223–225.

Raifer, J., and C. J. Bennett. "Vasectomy." *Urologic Clinics of North America* 15, no. 4 (November 1988): 631–634.

Shanberg, A., and others. "Laser-Assisted Vasectomy Reversal: Experience in 32 Patients." *The Journal of Urology* 143 (March 1990): 528–530.

Sidney, S. "Vasectomy and the Risk of Prostatic Cancer and Benign Prostatic Hypertrophy." *The Journal of Urology* 138, no. 4 (October 1987): 795–797.

WEIGHT CONTROL DIETS

(*See also:* EATING DISORDERS; OBESITY)

OVERVIEW

Are you looking for a way to lose weight—quickly and easily? You may be tempted to try one of the widely advertised weight-loss programs that use liquid diets, require special diet regimens, or claim to have medically-qualified staff.

But, before you pay for any weight-loss program, take note: while many diet programs may help you lose weight, there is little published evidence that most people maintain that weight loss for any significant time.

Being obese has serious health consequences and losing weight can help reduce those risks. Some experts suggest that losing even 30 percent of excess weight can significantly decrease some obesity-related consequences.

If you want to lose weight permanently, scientific evidence suggests it is important to make lifelong changes in how you eat and exercise. The Council on Scientific Affairs of the American Medical Association says that only through gradual long-term changes like these can you effectively lose weight and keep it off.

Be skeptical, then, of approaches that promise, easy, quick, or permanent weight loss. Such loss is likely to be short-term.

The Diet Programs

Dieting in the United States is a big business. A multi-billion dollar industry caters to approximately 34 million overweight American adults, millions of whom are dieting at any given time.

As most dieters know, to lose a pound of weight, you need to reduce caloric intake or increase caloric demand by 3,500 calories. To help dieters do this, many professional weight-control programs offer special dietary and exercise plans, as well as psychological support. Many such programs are independently operated through local hospitals, clinics, and physician-specialists. Two widely-advertised programs are:

Very low calorie diet (VLCD) programs. VLCD programs generally use 400 to 800 calorie-a-day liquid diet formulas as part of a 12 to 16 week supplemented fast. They are often called "semi-starvation" diets. Available only through physicians in their offices or through hospital-based programs, VLCD programs require careful medical screening and constant medical supervision.

Most VLCD programs are targeted to people who are severely obese, those about 30 percent or more above their ideal body weight. Some VLCD programs now also accept individuals who are 20 percent or more above their ideal body weight. Typical weight loss may be around 3 pounds per week for women and about 5 pounds per week for men. VLCD programs cost about $2,000 to $3,000, but some expenses may be reimbursed through health insurance.

Diet clinics/food plans. Many of these programs are 1,000 to 1,500 calorie-a-day diets, where weight loss averages one or two pounds a week. You usually follow a carefully controlled menu plan. In some cases, you may be required to purchase specially packaged meals available only from the company—and not reimbursable through health insurance. The costs for these programs vary considerably, ranging from $250 to $1,000 or more. Be wary of initial low-price offers that may not include all costs.

The Health Consequences

Being obese has serious health consequences. Complications include increased risk of heart disease, stroke, high blood pressure, diabetes, gallstones, some forms of cancer, and other illnesses.

Losing weight can help reduce these risks. In general, the more slowly you lose weight and the longer you maintain that weight loss, the safer that diet will be for you.

But dieting itself is not without risk. Studies have reported that patients on VLCD or other rapid-weight loss programs may run an increased chance of developing gallstones. Less severe consequences of dieting include: dizziness, diarrhea, constipation, fatigue, muscle cramps, bad breath, temporary hair loss, headaches, potassium deficiencies, and irregular menstrual cycles.

Because of the possible health complications associated with dieting, you may wish first to ask your physician whether a particular program is right for you. This is particularly important for those with diabetes, high blood pressure, or heart, liver, or gallbladder disease. In addition, parents may want to check with their physician before placing their children on a diet program. Pregnant women generally are advised not to go on a diet program.

Questions to Ask

If you are thinking of trying a diet program, getting answers to the following questions may be helpful.

What does the diet program require you to do?

Decide whether the diet program's requirements—such as calorie restrictions—are acceptable to your level of commitment. Find out what the diet regimen includes. Are counseling and exercise included? Must you purchase special foods or vitamins from the company sponsoring the program? Decide if a diet program that requires using only selected products will be practical or affordable in the long run.

How much does the program cost? How do you pay for it?

You can judge the costs of programs by adding up all fees and charges, including prices for initial membership and/or weekly fees, food, supplements, maintenance, and counseling. Then compare costs. Find out how payment is required. Some programs charge large upfront fees that you may not get back if you drop out. Others allow you to pay as you go. Be aware that many people who begin diet programs drop out early.

What are the health risks associated with the diet program?

The National Council Against Health Fraud cautions consumers about diet programs that do not reveal risks about the specific program, as well as about weight loss in general. Some diet programs are riskier than others, and some are better suited for certain kinds of people. For example, only those significantly overweight should consider enrolling in a VLCD program.

What kind of professional supervision is provided?

When considering a diet program, you may wish to find out how qualified the staff is to monitor your progress. Ask about the credentials of anyone represented as an "expert" in dieting. A fully-staffed program frequently includes registered dieticians, registered nurses, clinical psychologists, and exercise therapists, as well as physicians.

What kind of maintenance program is provided and at what cost?

Learning how to keep weight off—through a maintenance program—is just as important as losing weight. While many diet programs can help you lose weight, the track record for helping customers maintain weight loss is not nearly as good. Ask if the maintenance program is offered as part of the total package—or optional at additional cost. Find out what the maintenance program consists of, how long it lasts, and what you must do. Inquire whether counseling, exercise, and group meetings are included. Remember that the longer the program focuses on helping you change your eating and exercise patterns, the greater the chances of long-term success. If the diet program is not seriously committed to helping you maintain a sensible eating and exercise program—possibly for the rest of your life—you may want to look elsewhere.

SOURCE:
Federal Trade Commission. "Diet Programs." *Facts for Consumers* (September 1990).

COMPARISON OF NINE MAJOR PROGRAMS

All diet programs have the same objective—to help you lose weight—but they vary in their approach. With over-the-counter products such as Slim Fast and Ultra Slim Fast, for example, you're essentially self-prescribing. The "real food" diets, like Weight Watchers and Jenny Craig, try to help you slim down without special shakes or formulas. And the very low-calorie programs—HMR, Medifast, and Optifast—are medically supervised and usually require clients to be at least 20 percent over ideal weight to participate. Even within these major categories, however, there is considerable variation. And some people may fare better with one variety than another. Still, applying a common set of questions to all weight-loss regimens can help you evaluate which might be best for you. When we asked nine of the nation's best-selling diet plans the nine questions that follow, we came up with the answers that appear [here].

1. Is this a diet you could live with indefinitely?

2. What is the recommended rate of weight loss?

3. Does the program take individual differences into account to determine caloric needs?

4. To what extent does the plan educate the client about nutrition, behavior modification, and the importance of exercise?

5. Does the program put you in contact with professionals such as physicians, registered dietitians, and psychotherapists?

6. What percentage of clients reach goal weight and maintain their losses?

7. Does the program offer a maintenance plan once the weight is lost?

8. What is the nature of the advertisements and endorsements?

9. How much does it cost?

Diet Workshop, real food diet without special products

1. yes

2. 1½ to 2 pounds/week

3. variations within set program

4. 1 hour/week in group setting

5. no—contact is with trained "graduates" of program

6. estimated 1 in 10 reach goal by finishing program; 71% of those remain within 2 pounds of goal weight after 6 months according to one 12-year-old study

7. yes—4 weeks, but lifelong visits are encouraged and are free for those who maintain their losses

8. testimonials

9. $14 for membership, $9/week until maintenance phase is reached

Health Management Resources (HMR), a medically supervised very low calorie diet

1. no

2. 3- to 5-pound loss expected/week

3. variations within set regimen (520- to 800-calorie formulas, but physician has discretion to adjust calorie intake as he or she sees fit)

4. 1½ hours/week in group setting (generally with a registered dietitian), often accompanied by individual telephone follow-up)

5. yes—hospital-based team approach with physicians, etc.

6. 62% of clients reach goal weight by finishing program (according to clinical data collected monthly by company); about 60% of weight loss is maintained after 2 years (according to 2 company studies unpublished in a medical journal)

7. yes—weekly meetings for 18 months

8. testimonials plus extensive statistics in promotional materials based on company data

9. averages $2,775 for entire program

Jenny Craig, real food diet that requires pre-packaged meals until maintenance phase

1. no

2. 1 to 2 pounds/week

3. variations within set regimen

4. 14 1-hour video classes with discussion leader plus weekly, 20-minute one-on-one sessions with counselor

5. no—college graduates implement program

6. approximately 1 in 10 finish program; 92% of those stay within 7 pounds of goal weight—no time frame given (numbers based on spokesperson's estimate; no published data available)

7. yes—monthly meetings for 1 year to help people learn to make their own food choices, but life-long visits are encouraged

8. celebrity testimonials plus client case studies

9. $185 for membership, $60 to $70/week for food

Medifast, liquid fast dispensed from individual physician's office; program support varies greatly, depending on intensity of doctor's approach

1. no

2. 3 to 5 pounds/week

3. modification of set plan is left to physician's discretion

4. one-on-one counseling (usually weekly) and/or group program called LifeStyles (frequency decided upon by doctor, but at least once a week)

5. yes—how many depends on size and scope of physician's practice

6. of the clients who finish the program (figure not available), 65% remain within 4 pounds of goal weight after 1 year (spokesperson's estimate; no published data available)

7. yes—weekly meetings for 5 months

8. information about obesity as "disease" plus testimonials

9. averages $1,700 to $1,900 ($50/week)

Nutri/System, real food diet that requires pre-packaged foods until maintenance phase

1. no

2. 1½ to 2 pounds/week

3. variations within set regimen

4. 30-minute weekly group meetings plus 10-minute individual meetings with nutrition "specialist"

5. no—most who implement program are college graduates

6. not available

7. yes—1 year transition to self-chosen diet by eating pre-packaged Nutri/System meals 2 days/week while selecting foods independently the other 5 days

8. "dieting DJ" testimonials

9. company would not estimate

Optifast

1. no

2. up to 1 to 2% of body weight/week

3. variations within set regimen (420- and 800- calorie formulas, but physician has discretion to raise calorie intake if patient is losing weight too rapidly)

4. 1½ hours/week in group setting plus individual weekly meetings with physician for at least 21 weeks and at least 1 individual meeting with a registered dietitian)

5. yes—hospital-based team approach with physicians, etc.

6. Direct answer on goal weight not available. Average weight loss for Optifast patient is approximately 20% of starting weight (according to company data unpublished in medical journal); approximately 60% of patients complete 6-month program (according to company spokesperson); on average, between 50% and 67% of weight lost is maintained for 1 year (data on 1,429 patients published in the *International Journal of Obesity*)

7. yes—7 weekly meetings, 26 additional biweekly meetings

8. discuss medical team approach and describe other components of program plus some before-and-after pictures

9. $2,500 to $3,500 for 26-week program

Slim Fast/Ultra Slim Fast, an over-the-counter product

1. not without dependence on a product that averages about $500 a year

2. up to individual

3. no—self-regulated

4. no educational or support programs

5. no professional supervision of any kind

6. unknown

7. no

8. celebrity testimonials

9. $8 to $12/week

Weight Loss Clinic, real food diet that does not require special products

1. yes

2. average of 2- to 3-pound loss/week

3. variations within set regimen

4. one-on-one meetings with staff member up to 5 days/week lasting approximately 5 to 10 minutes

5. program implemented by registered nurses, licensed practical nurses, registered dietitians, individuals with a bachelor's degree in nutrition, and company-trained counselors

6. proportion of clients who finish program not available; of those who do, 76% remain within 2 pounds of goal weight after 1 year and 67% maintain weight loss after 2 years (according to 1 study unpublished in a medical journal)

7. yes—2 days/week for 6 weeks followed by at least 6 monthly meetings

8. testimonials

9. averages $60/week

Weight Watchers

1. yes

2. 1 to 2 pounds/week

3. variations within set regimen

4. 45-minute weekly group meeting plus Q&A period

5. no—trained "graduates" implement program

6. not available

7. yes—at least once a week for 6 weeks followed by free lifetime membership for those who maintain their losses

8. testimonials of "graduates"

9. $12 to $20 for membership plus $7 to $9/week until maintenance

SOURCE:
"Smart Losers' Guide to Choosing a Weight-Loss Program." *Tufts University Diet and Nutrition Letter* 8, no. 6 (August 1990): 5–6.

DANGERS OF YO-YO DIETING

Yo-yo dieting—repeated attempts at rapid weight loss with subsequent rapid weight regain—is doing a lot more harm than keeping people from losing weight. That's because each cycle of weight loss and regain puts the dieter at a greater risk of overall weight gain. And each time a rapid weight loss and regain occurs, muscle tissue is lost and body fat increases.

What causes this phase of yo-yo dieting? The overly rapid weight loss can be achieved by three major routes. First, severe caloric restriction should never be attempted without medical supervision. Behavior modification is strongly recommended.

Second, high-protein/low carbohydrate diets can cause rapid weight loss. Severely reducing carbohydrates temporarily eliminates large amounts of fluid—the quickest means of weight loss.

A third means of rapid weight loss are eating disorders such as anorexia and bulimia. Compulsive binge-purge behavior produces abrupt fluid changes similar to low carbohydrate diets.

But yo-yo dieters don't simply lose weight; they rapidly regain it (a phenomenon known as rebound). Weight regain can often occur simply by terminating a diet. This rebound phase, however, can occur simply by altering the composition of the calories you consume (the ratio of protein, fat and carbohydrates). For example, when a low-carbohydrate diet is abandoned, increasing carbohydrate intake promotes rehydration. For every gram of carbohydrate consumed, there are up to four grams of associated water that may contribute to an increase in total body weight.

There are also psychological factors which influence yo-yo dieting, particularly the feeling of being deprived. There may also be a decreased ability to stay on a diet as it becomes more difficult to maintain restrictions.

But whatever the cause, the results are disheartening and potentially dangerous. Imagine you are a yo-yo dieter. With each cycle of loss and regain, there's a net weight gain. You literally get fatter and fatter as muscle tissue is replaced by body fat.

As your percent body fat increases, it becomes increasingly difficult to lose weight because your metabolism slows down. This cycle affects more than your waistline. Each cycle puts added strain on your cardiovascular system as your heart works harder to accommodate your increased body weight. Additional pressure is put on your joints; arthritis can flare up and gastrointestinal distress increases, and changes in blood chemistry are likely.

And, sadly, the very realization that you've gained weight again can prompt you to start yet another—probably futile—diet.

How can you avoid this yo-yo syndrome? I recommend these steps:

- Monitor your food intake and get regular exercise. Diet or exercise alone is not enough.
- Learn to "balance" calories. Vary the foods you eat, never eliminating any one basic food group.
- Keep a food diary. Record all calories eaten in a week, and divide by seven to get your daily caloric intake. Reduce this intake by 500 calories a day, and you'll lose about one pound a week. This means you're losing predominantly fat.

My advice to yo-yo dieters—and to anyone who wants to avoid this syndrome—is to change your lifestyle, not simply your diet. Only a sustained change in eating habits can get pounds off and keep them off.

SOURCE:

Minear, Alisa. "Preventing Yo-Yo Dieting." *Executive Health Report* 26 (February 1990): 7.

VERY LOW-CALORIE (LIQUID) DIETS

Our national fascination with the literal ups and downs of celebrity weight watchers like Oprah Winfrey or Elizabeth Taylor is understandable. More than one in four of us checks in at 20% more than our ideal body weight (that's the standard definition of obesity); 34 million of this group, their health at stake, need to lose at least 35 pounds. Does the latest variation on crash dieting, the very-low-calorie (VLC) diet, at last offer a safe and effective solution? Crash diets go in and out of style rapidly as more than half the nation—not only the obese but many who are only moderately overweight—periodically grasp at the latest slimming panacea. Although statistics aren't available, it's estimated that fewer than 5% of these dieters actually manage to reach their ideal weight; and of those who do, more than 90% gain it back within a year.

The VLC diet, extreme though it is, has earned medical recognition as sound therapy for people whose obesity puts them at risk for such problems as diabetes, hypertension, and heart disease. On the other hand, such drastic dieting is generally regarded as overkill for people who simply want to lose a few pounds from their hips or thighs. Nor do all doctors or researchers agree that even seriously obese patients benefit from VLC-diet programs over the long term. But the new—and important—wrinkle is that VLC-diet programs are being administered by hospitals and physicians who keep close tabs on their patients' health.

No extreme diet (less than 1,200 calories a day) should in fact be undertaken without a doctor's advice. Strict monitoring is essential when calories are limited to 400 to 800 a day—in effect, a "modified fast." VLC-diet calories come from powdered dietary supplements available by prescription only. They contain 33 to 75 grams of egg- or milk-derived protein, varying amounts of carbohydrate, and RDA levels of most other nutrients. They're a far cry from the over-the-counter "liquid protein" supplements of the 1970s, withdrawn when the Centers for Disease Control reported 60 deaths attributable to their use. The protein in these early supplements was collagen-based; its inadequate amino-acid composition (plus possibly a lack of carbohydrates) led to a dangerous loss of lean muscle mass, including heart muscle. Also, these early diets didn't provide for adequate potassium intake, which may have resulted in serious disturbances of heart rhythm.

The new supplements, mixed with liquid, are taken three to five times a day at meal and snack times. Other than eight glasses or more of water a day, that's all you get. (Some programs do allow you to munch on raw vegetables to satisfy the need to chew.) Reportedly, hunger pangs are rarely a problem, possibly because low intakes of calories lead to the manufacture of substances called ketones that are thought to suppress hunger. More important, regular electrocardiograms (ECGs), blood and urine tests, and visits to the doctor are part of the package—which also includes essential regimens of exercise, nutrition education, and support groups.

Obviously none of this comes cheap: cost to the patient is about $400 to $600 a month, and VLC-diet programs usually last three months. After one to three months on a maintenance diet of 1,250 to 1,500 calories, the patient may repeat the program. Some critics have accused hospitals and clinics of promoting this costly process to bolster sagging revenues.

Studies made by researchers conduction VLC-diet programs indicate high rates of short-term success. Two- to five-pound losses per week are common, and over three months most patients lose 40 to 60 pounds. As yet there are few long-term studies to indicate how many people manage to keep the weight off permanently—and it is weight-loss maintenance that ultimately validates any weight-reduction program.

SOURCE:
"Very-Low-Calorie Diets." *The University of California, Berkeley Wellness Letter* 5 (January 1989): 4. Excerpted from *The University of California, Berkeley Wellness Letter*, Copyright Health Letter Associates, 1989.

RESOURCES

BOOK
Bennion, Lynn J., Edwin L. Bierman, and others. *Straight Talk About Weight Control: Taking the Pounds Off and Keeping Them Off.* Fairfield, OH: Consumer Reports Books, 1991.

RELATED ARTICLES
"A Comparison of Weight Loss Programs." Environmental Nutrition (December 1990): 4-5.

Donahue, Peggy Jo. "Inside America's Hottest Diet Programs: Part One—Optifast." *Prevention* 42 (January 1990): 52-57, 127-134.

Donahue, Peggy Jo. "Inside America's Hottest Diet Programs: Part Two—Nutri/System." *Prevention* 42 (February 1990): 55-59, 124-133.

Fletcher, Anne M. "Inside America's Hottest Diet Programs: Part Five." *Prevention* 42 (May 1990): 49, 102-104, 106-108, 110, 112.

Fletcher, Anne M. "Inside America's Hottest Diet Programs: Part Three—Weight Watchers." *Prevention* 42 (March 1990): 54-64.

Hughes, Rebecca. "Inside America's Hottest Diet Programs: Part Four—Diet Center." *Prevention* 42 (April 1990): 64-72.

Paulsen, Barbara K. "Position of the American Dietetic Association: Very-Low-Calorie Weight Loss Diets." *Journal of the American Dietetic Association* 90 (May 1990): 722.

YEAST INFECTIONS (VAGINITIS)

OVERVIEW

Candidiasis (also called fungus or yeast infection or moniliasis) is the most common type of vaginal infection that causes symptoms of irritation. It is often hard to get rid of, and recurrences are common.

Many women with this infection do not notice a discharge, but if it is present it is usually described as an odorless, white, "cheesy" discharge. The main symptom of this type of inflammation is intense itching, burning, and redness of the vaginal tissues.

Candidiasis is caused by a fungus, like yeast. Although it can affect any woman, candidiasis is more frequent among women who are pregnant, diabetic, or obese. These conditions can alter the body's metabolic balance and vaginal acidity and promote the growth of the fungus.

The use of antibiotics and birth control pills also make a woman more prone to get this disorder. Antibiotics stimulate the growth of the fungus and eliminate certain protective bacteria. Birth control pills produce chemical changes in the vagina similar to those of pregnancy. In both cases, the fungus has a chance to overdevelop and cause inflammation.

If the physical exam and lab tests reveal that candidiasis is present, your doctor will prescribe medication to destroy the fungus causing the problem. This may include vaginal suppositories or tablets or application of a cream or gel into the vagina. The medication may be somewhat messy—you may need to wear a sanitary napkin during treatment. Your doctor will advise you in detail about what is involved.

In most cases, candidiasis will be cured with treatment. However, the infection resists treatment in some women—especially pregnant and diabetic women—and a cure may take some time. Conditions that spur the growth of candidiasis will also have to be changed in order to get rid of the vaginal infection completely.

SOURCE:
American College of Obstetricians and Gynecologists. *Vaginitis: Causes and Treatments*. 1984. pp. 4–5.

SUSCEPTIBILITY TO YEAST INFECTIONS

Several factors increase susceptibility to yeast infections, particularly pregnancy, prolonged antibiotic use and perhaps birth control pills (still debated). During pregnancy, vaginal yeasts increase because of decreased vaginal acidity and a higher output of female hormones which raise glycogen (carbohydrate) levels, favouring candidal growth. Poor ventilation in the genital area may exacerbate or perpetuate (but not cause) yeast infections. Tight underwear or jeans may trap the infection against the vulva. Other predisposing factors include: menopausal thinning of the vaginal wall; diabetes; cuts/abrasions in the genital area; poor hygiene (soiled underwear and transfer of fecal yeasts); and douching. Dietary sugar and a defect in milk sugar (lactose) metabolism may predispose some women to yeast infections. For them, eliminating dairy products from the diet and cutting down on sugar may help to curb candidiasis. While there's no proof that diet alters susceptibility to vaginitis, abnormal carbohydrate metabolism (as in diabetes) can increase the sugar content of vaginal secretions. And since yeasts feed on sugar, conditions that raise vaginal glucose levels could promote their growth.

SOURCE:
"Vaginitis: Common and Annoying, but Curable." *Health News* (University of Toronto) 6 (April 1988): 4-8.

TREATMENT

In general, local application of antifungal therapy is effective in treating yeast vaginitis. There do, however, seem to be two distinct types of patients with this condition. The most common type of patient has isolated, infrequent vaginal yeast infections that respond readily to topical therapy. The other group of patients have frequently recurring infections that may become chronic and even intractable. Most providers of women's health care are familiar with this condition of recurrent yeast vaginitis. A large number of antifungal agents are currently available for the treatment of vulvovaginal candidiasis. There are two major classes of modern antifungal agents; the polyenes (nystatin, amphotericin) and the imidazole derivatives. The earlier imidazoles (miconazole and clotrimazole) and the newer imidazoles (butoconazole and ketoconazole) now provide the mainstay of antifungal therapy, although the polyenes may still be employed effectively. For relief of simple yeast vaginitis, numerous agents in various doses have been successfully employed with success rates that vary from 70-95%. Nystatin vaginal suppositories can be inserted twice daily for 10 days or twice daily for 7 days, followed by once daily for 7 days. This has been a widely used regimen for years. The use of topical imidazole agents has become the mainstay of therapy in recent years. In comparative clinical trials, the cure rate of the imidazoles have at least equaled and usually surpassed those of nystatin. The earlier imidazoles (miconazole and clotrimazole) have been effective agents when used as intravaginal creams or suppositories.

SOURCE:
Landers, Daniel V. "The Treatment of Vaginitis: Trichomonas, Yeast, and Bacterial Vaginosis." *Clinical Obstetrics and Gynecology* 31, no. 2 (June 1988): 475.

YEAST INFECTION—OVER-THE COUNTER DRUGS

Yeast infections struck 13.6 million women last year. Instead of going to their doctors, many of these women can now go to their drugstores to find relief. The FDA has approved the active ingredient in two of the most commonly prescribed antifungal drugs for nonprescription use. By the first of March, Monistat (miconazole nitrate) and Gyne-Lotrimin (clotrimazole) should be on drugstore shelves.

That's good news for women with recurrent yeast infections who must pay for each office visit. For those with a suspected first time infection, however, the label advises a doctor visit for confirmation. Women who are pregnant or think they may be pregnant, as well as women who have had more than four yeast infections in a year's time, are also urged to use the product under a doctor's supervision.

"It's an acknowledgment that women can take charge of their health," says Raquel Arias, M.D., assistant clinical professor of obstetrics and gynecology at the University of Southern California. "Once you've had a yeast infection, you know what the symptoms [itching, a thick, white odorless discharge, burning] are." Not all doctors are as enthusiastic. "What most women call yeast infections really aren't," says Attila Toth, M.D., associate professor of obstetrics and gynecology at New York Hospital-Cornell Medical Center. "And even if a woman makes a correct diagnosis, yeast infections can mask other more serious conditions, such as sexually transmitted diseases."

The smartest course: Use the medication only if you are familiar with yeast infection symptoms from previous attacks. If symptoms don't clear within a week, consult your doctor.

SOURCE:
"Prescription Drug for Yeast Infections Goes Over the Counter." *Glamour* 89, no. 3 (March 1991): 76.

YOGURT AS ALTERNATIVE TREATMENT

Just one cup of yogurt a day may prevent vaginal infections caused by the yeastlike fungus, *Candida albicans*. This condition—commonly known as a "yeast infection"—troubles just about every woman at some time in her life and, in an estimated 10 percent of women, is a recurring problem.

Researchers at Long Island Jewish Medical Center in New Hyde Park, New York, studied 15 women with chronic yeast infections. Each had suffered at least five such infections in a year. For six months of the project, each patient ate a cup of plain yogurt daily. During the next six months, they were asked not to eat any yogurt at all. Eileen Hilton, M.D., an infectious disease specialist and head of the study, found that the group suffered three times more yeast infections during the non-yogurt period than they did during the first half of the study.

The study indicates that only yogurt containing the bacteria *Lactobacillis acidophilus* interferes with Candida's growth. So check the label.

SOURCE:
"Yogurt Fights Yeast Infections." *Redbook* (September 1990): 32.

PREVENTION

There are some things women can do when they have vaginitis or when they want to prevent future attacks:

- Discontinue use of tampons while under treatment. Also, since underwear and pantyhose made from synthetic fibers often increase heat and moisture in the vulval area, switch to cotton underwear and pantyhose with cotton crotches if you are prone to frequent infections. For the same reason, don't wear skintight pants.

- Avoid sexual intercourse while undergoing treatment. Have your sex partner checked by the doctor if you get repeated infections.
- Practice good feminine hygiene. Wash the vulval and anal areas with mild soap and water at least once daily, and after each bowel movement, if possible. Always wipe from front to back, away from the vagina. The bowels harbor bacteria and fungi that can travel over to the vulval area.
- Don't douche unless the doctor says to. By disturbing the normal acidity of vaginal secretions, douching may create more problems than it cures.
- Make it a rule that anything that goes into the vagina—pessaries, diaphragms, and other contraceptive devices, for example—be scrupulously clean.
- Take the medication for as long as the doctor prescribes. Some women stop the medication when they feel better, but that's an invitation to recurrent infections.

SOURCE:

Food and Drug Administration. Zamula, Evelyn. *On Yeast Infections and Other Female Irritations.* DHHS Publication No. (FDA) 85-1121. (July/August 1985): 3.

RESOURCES

RELATED ARTICLES

Foxman, Betsy. "The Epidemiology of Vulvovaginal Candidiasis: Risk Factors." *American Journal of Public Health* 80, no. 3 (March 1990): 329-331.

McCue, Jack D. "Evaluation and Management of Vaginitis: An Update for Primary Care Practitioners." *Archives of Internal Medicine* 149 (March 1989): 565-568.

"Management of Vaginitis." *American Family Physician* 40 (October 1989): 288-289.

Reed, Barbara D., Werner Huck, and others. "Differentiation of *Gardnerella vaginalis, Candida albicans,* and *Trichomonas vaginalis* Infections of the Vagina. *The Journal of Family Practice* 28, no. 6 (June 1989): 673-680.

Spiegel, Carol A. "Vaginitis/Vaginosis." *Clinics in Laboratory Medicine* 9, no. 3 (September 1989): 525-533.

INDEX

A

C

E

F

I

J

K

N

O

Q

R

T

U

V

W

Y

Z